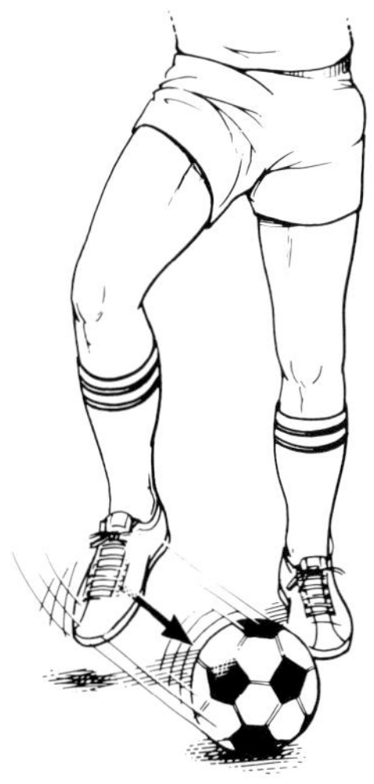

Morrie E. Kricun, Series Editor

Imaging of Sports Injuries

CLINICAL DIAGNOSTIC IMAGING SERIES

Morrie E. Kricun, Series Editor

Professor
Department of Radiology
Hospital of the University of Pennsylvania
Philadelphia, Pennsylvania

Imaging of Vertebral Trauma
by Richard H. Daffner

Imaging of the Foot and Ankle
by D.M. Forrester, Morrie E. Kricun, and Roger Kerr

Imaging of the Pelvis
Edited by Madeleine R. Fisher and Morrie E. Kricun

Imaging Strategies in Pediatric Orthopaedics
by Gerald A. Mandell, H. Theodore Harcke, and S. Jay Kumar

MRI of the Knee
by Peter L. Munk and Clyde A. Helms

Imaging of Sports Injuries
by Thomas H. Berquist

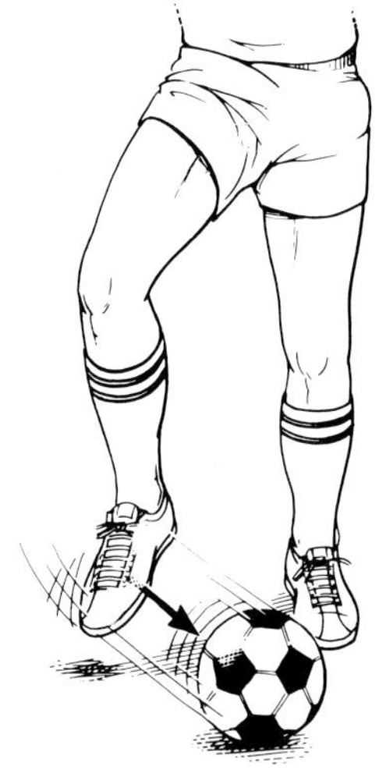

Morrie E. Kricun, Series Editor

Imaging of Sports Injuries

Thomas H. Berquist, MD, FACR
Chairman
Diagnostic Radiology
Mayo Clinic Jacksonville
Jacksonville, Florida

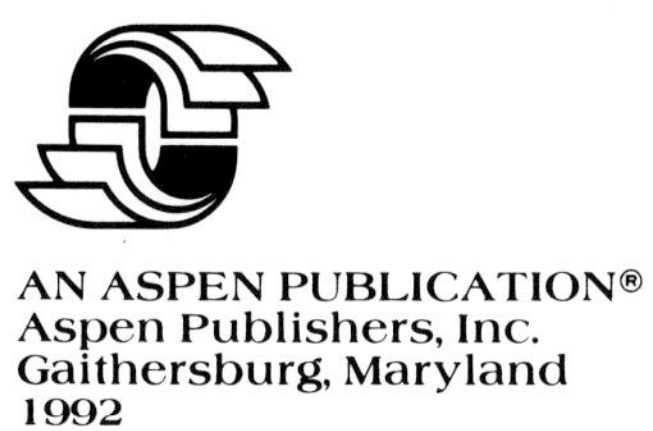

AN ASPEN PUBLICATION®
Aspen Publishers, Inc.
Gaithersburg, Maryland
1992

Library of Congress Cataloging-in-Publication Data

Berquist, Thomas H. (Thomas Henry), 1945—
Imaging of sports injuries / Thomas H. Berquist.
p. cm.—(Clinical diagnostic imaging series)
Includes bibliographical references and index.
ISBN: 0-8342-0296-4
1. Sports—Accidents and injuries—Imaging. I. Title. II. Series.
[DNLM: 1. Athletic Injuries—radiography. QT 260 B532i]
RD97.B48 1992
617.1'027—dc20
DNLM/DLC
For Library of Congress
92-7532
CIP

Editorial Services: Barbara Priest
Library of Congress Catalog Card Number: 92-7532
ISBN: 0-8342-0296-4

Printed in the United States of America

1 2 3 4 5

To my student athletes
Matthew, Andrew, and Aric

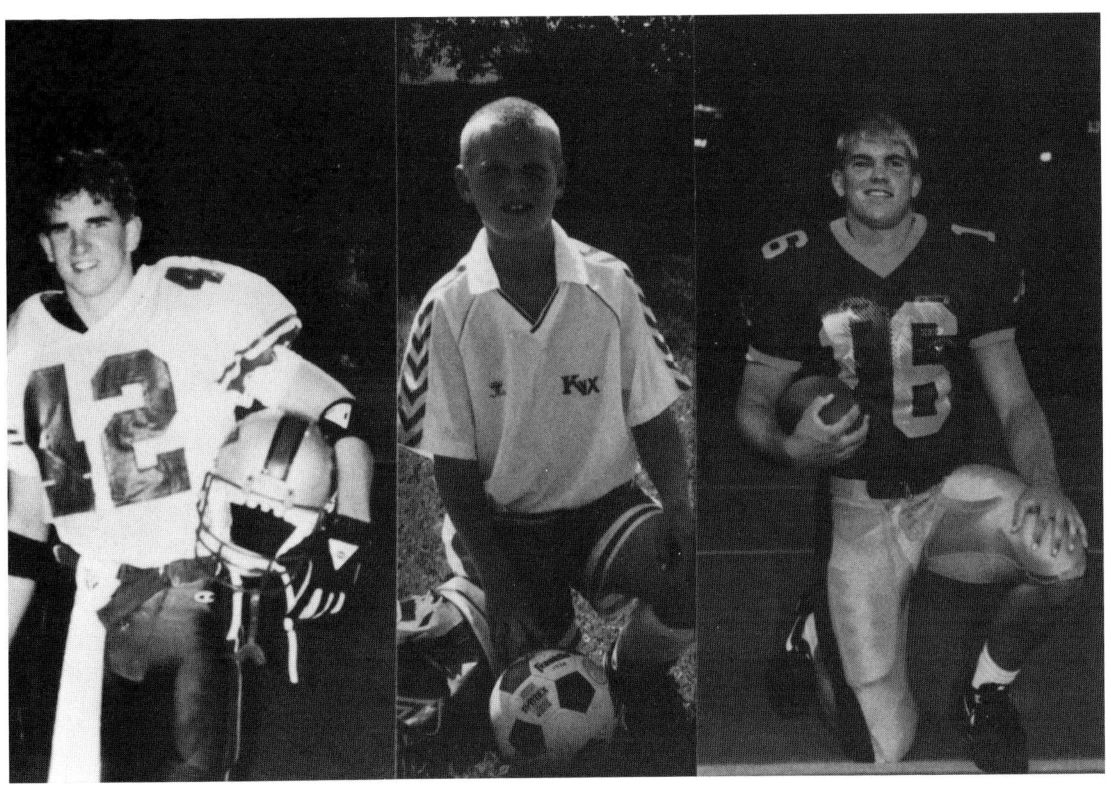

Matt Drew Aric

Table of Contents

Series Foreword xi

Preface xiii

Acknowledgments xv

Chapter 1—Epidemiology and Categories of Sports Injuries 1

General Epidemiological Considerations 1
Categories of Sports Injuries 4

Chapter 2—Diagnostic Techniques 11

Routine Radiography, Tomography, and Magnification Radiography 11
Ultrasound 15
Skeletal Scintigraphy 16
Computed Tomography 19
Magnetic Resonance Imaging 20
Angiography 22
Myelography 24
Arthrography and Tenography 25
Thermography 26

Chapter 3—The Spine 31

Introduction and Anatomy 31
Cervical Spine Trauma 37
Thoracolumbar Spine Trauma 57

Chapter 4—Pelvis and Hips **67**

Anatomy 67
Imaging of the Pelvis and Hips 71
Fractures 80
Soft Tissue and Miscellaneous Injuries 92

Chapter 5—Femur and Thigh **99**

Anatomy 99
Femoral Shaft Fractures 100
Imaging of Femoral Shaft Fractures 101
Soft Tissue Injuries 102
Imaging of Soft Tissue Injuries 104

Chapter 6—The Knee **107**

Introduction 107
Anatomy 107
Imaging of the Knee 110
Patellar Disorders 119
Fractures 127
Ligament, Meniscus, and Soft Tissue Injuries 135
Miscellaneous Injuries 146

Chapter 7—Tibia, Fibula, and Calf **155**

Anatomy 155
Fractures 157
Soft Tissue Injuries 157

Chapter 8—Foot and Ankle **167**

Introduction 167
Anatomy 167
Soft Tissue Trauma 176
Ankle Fractures 190
Talar Fractures and Dislocations 201
Calcaneal Fractures 206
Midfoot and Forefoot Injuries 209
Stress Fractures 215

Chapter 9—Shoulder and Arm **221**

Introduction 221
Anatomy 221
Imaging Techniques 226
Fractures, Dislocations, and Osseous Injuries 242
Soft Tissue Trauma 253

Chapter 10—Elbow and Forearm **265**

Introduction 265
Anatomy 265
Imaging Techniques 268

Soft Tissue Injuries 278
Fractures and Osseous Injuries 285

Chapter 11—Hand and Wrist 303

Introduction 303
Anatomy 303
Imaging Techniques 311
Fractures and Dislocations 324
Soft Tissue and Miscellaneous Injuries 348

Chapter 12—Stress Fractures 357

Introduction 357
Radiographic Evaluation 357
Summary 364

Index 367

Series Foreword

Skeletal and soft tissue injuries occurring from sports play an important part in the practice of radiology and orthopaedic surgery. Recent advances in musculoskeletal imaging and in practical magnetic resonance imaging have greatly aided physicians in the diagnosis, work-up, and follow-up of patients with musculoskeletal trauma. This is especially true with patients who have experienced soft tissue injuries.

Imaging of Sports Injuries is an outstanding book that is timely and focused. Based on Dr. Berquist's vast experience in orthopaedic radiology and magnetic resonance imaging, this state of the art book is well organized and written in a style that is enjoyable and easy to read. It is beautifully illustrated with crisp radiographs and line drawings, and it contains hundreds of pertinent current references. The format is practical, with especially helpful introductory chapters on epidemiology, terminology, and imaging techniques. The rest of the chapters deal with individual anatomic areas. Discussions of the various injuries are thorough, and include mechanisms of injuries, utilization of imaging modalities, and imaging observations.

Dr. Berquist has provided a wealth of practical and clinically useful information dealing with sports injury problems faced by clinicians daily. He is to be congratulated for producing such a fine text. I consider it a privilege to write this foreword and to have this book as a part of the *Clinical Diagnostic Imaging* series.

Morrie E. Kricun, MD
Professor
Department of Radiology
Hospital of the University of Pennsylvania
Philadelphia, Pennsylvania

Preface

Athletic injuries continue to increase in organized or varsity athletics and in the general population because of the increased interest in fitness. Skeletal injuries, with the exception of stress fractures, are usually easily diagnosed with conventional radiographic techniques. Newer modalities, specifically magnetic resonance imaging, have had a significant impact on detection, classification, and management of soft tissue injuries.

Clinicians and radiologists must be familiar with the utility of the numerous imaging techniques and invasive procedures (arthrography, tenography, and diagnostic and therapeutic injections) available for diagnosis, treatment, and follow-up evaluation of sports injuries. This text is designed to discuss thoroughly bone and soft tissue sports injuries. Clinical data, including mechanism of injury and optional imaging of specific injuries, will be discussed.

Introductory chapters serve to familiarize readers with commonly used terminology, epidemiology, and background data on imaging techniques. Specifically Chapter 2, Diagnostic Techniques, discusses basic principles, indications, and contraindications of specific radiographic techniques. Chapter 2 is primarily intended for nonradiologists, who may not be familiar with the basic principles of the numerous imaging techniques.

Chapters 3 through 11 are anatomically oriented. Basic anatomy, specific imaging techniques, and injuries are discussed for each anatomic region (skull and facial injuries are not included). Treatment of injuries is noted when appropriate, but complete discussion of treatments of all injuries is beyond the scope of this text. Finally, Chapter 12 discusses stress fractures.

This text provides a thoroughly referenced resource for radiologists, clinical residents (orthopaedic surgeons, emergency physicians, physical therapists, and the like), and practitioners in sports medicine centers who deal with diagnosis and treatment of sports injuries.

Acknowledgments

Preparation of this text required the support of numerous individuals. Many colleagues provided daily assistance on selecting the case material. I especially wish to thank my colleagues in diagnostic radiology and orthopaedic surgery.

The Department of Photography provided the quality prints of images. John Hagan from Medical Graphics was responsible for all the excellent illustrations that demonstrate mechanisms of injury and injury classifications. This text would not have been possible without his assistance.

The manuscript was prepared by my secretaries, Cindy Franke and Becky Richmond. They deserve special thanks for their diligence in preparing the lengthy bibliographies and tables and in obtaining permissions for borrowed materials.

Finally, I wish to thank my editors, Jack Bruggeman and Barbara Priest, and the production staff of Aspen Publishers.

Chapter 1

Epidemiology and Categories of Sports Injuries

Over the last several decades the interest and levels of participation in both organized sports and leisure or fitness activities have expanded dramatically. The increasing numbers of participants at both levels, along with the broad spectrum of age groups involved in athletic activities, have greatly expanded the number of sports-related injuries and their impact on medical practice. This chapter serves as an introductory review of the epidemiology of sports injuries and is intended to provide a general overview of the magnitude of this problem in today's medical practice. Table 1-1 lists the sports or athletic activities, with specific references when appropriate, that will be considered in the later anatomic chapters of this text.

GENERAL EPIDEMIOLOGICAL CONSIDERATIONS

The incidence and severity of sports-related injuries vary significantly depending upon the activity, the physical condition of the participant, and the age and sex of the individual.[2,4,9,10,15,16,20,32,33,36,40,42,45,49,52] Part of the difficulty in evaluating injuries and defining the epidemiology is the definition itself.[2,4] As noted above, there are many factors that affect this definition. Some authorities define an injury as any abnormality that requires medical treatment. Others require evidence of diminished performance or lost time by the participant before an injury is considered documented. Noyes et al[40] exclude the lumps, bumps, and bruises and suggest that, when data on injury are collected, an injury should be defined as an event that is sports related and results in keeping the participant out of practice or competition on the day after the injury or any injury requiring medical attention.

With this in mind, it is useful to consider the types of injuries that occur in males and females during childhood and

Table 1-1 Organized Team and Individual Sports or Activities

Aerobic dancing[43,47]	Ping-Pong[5]
Archery	Pocket billiards
Badminton[5]	Polo
Baseball[2]	Racquetball[5,27]
Basketball[2]	Riflery
Bowling	Rodeo
Boxing	Rugby
Canoeing	Running—jogging[23,24,34,42,46]
Crew[31]	Sailboarding[29]
Cricket	Sailing
Cross country[23,42,46]	Scuba
Cycling[19,55]	Skating[3,53,58]
Diving	Skiing—cross country[7,26,53]
Fencing	Skiing—snow[7,26,37,44,48]
Field hockey	Skiing—water
Figure skating[15]	Soccer[6,15,17]
Football[12,38,54]	Softball
Golf	Squash[5,27]
Gymnastics[28]	Swimming[7,15]
Handball[5,13,39]	Synchronized swimming
Horseback riding[7,57]	Tennis[5,11,27]
Ice hockey[15,21,22,51]	Track[15,23,35,51]
Judo	Track and field[15,23,56]
Karate	Trap and skeet
Lacrosse	Triathalon
Martial arts	Volleyball[7]
Mountain climbing[1]	Water polo
Orienteering[14]	Weight lifting[7]
Parachuting[8]	Wrestling[7]

Table 1-2 Ten Most Common Overuse Injuries

Male Children		*Female Children*		*Adult Males*		*Adult Females*	
Injury	%	*Injury*	%	*Injury*	%	*Injury*	%
Osgood-Schlatter disease	18	Nonspecific knee synovitis	16	Achilles tendinitis or bursitis	18	Achilles tendinitis or bursitis	16
Sever disease	8	Osgood-Schlatter disease	13	Jumper's knee	15	Nonspecific knee synovitis	16
Ankle overpronation, flatfoot, or both	8	Shin splint syndrome	15	Iliotibial tract friction syndrome	14	Patellar chondromalacia	9
Achilles tendinitis or bursitis	7	Ankle overpronation, flatfoot, or both	11	Meniscus lesion	12	Knee instability	9
Nonspecific knee synovitis	7	Lower back insufficiency	11	Shin splint syndrome	10	Shin splint syndrome	9
Ankle instability with synovitis	5	Ankle instability with synovitis	9	Flexor tendinitis of the foot	8	Plantar fasciitis	9
Hamstring syndrome	5	Achilles tendinitis or bursitis	7	Supraspinatus tendinitis	7	Tension neck	9
Trochanteric bursitis	5	Extensor tendinitis of the foot	7	Nonspecific knee synovitis	6	Jumper's knee	7
Shin splint syndrome	4	Sever disease	5	Knee instability	5	Osgood-Schlatter disease	7
Osteochondritis dissecans of the knee	3	Patellar chondromalacia	5	Extensor tendinitis of the foot	5	Flexor tendinitis of the foot	7

Source: Kannus P, Niitymäki S, Järvinen M, *Clinical Pediatrics* (1988;27:333–337), JB Lippincott.

adulthood while they are participating in common sports. In all these categories, injuries can be considered either acute or chronic (overuse syndromes). As expected, in children most acute injuries result in fractures of the growth plates or avulsion fractures. Long bone fractures and soft tissue injuries are less common. Kvist et al[20] reviewed 1124 sports injuries in children 6 to 15 years of age. Sixty-nine percent of these injuries occurred in boys. Of these, 21% were sports related. Boys were most commonly injured in ice hockey (36%) and football (20%), and girls were most commonly injured in skating (18%) and horseback riding (18%). One-fourth of the injuries involved the head and neck, 36% involved the upper extremities, 33% the lower extremities, and 4% the trunk. Types of acute injury included fractures (26%), sprains or strains (24%), and contusions (22%). Only 9% of injuries required hospitalization. Obviously, the region studied and the popularity of specific sports geographically have a significant impact on the incidence and types of injuries.

Overuse injuries or syndromes are as common in children as in adults. As expected, most overuse injuries involve the lower extremities in both children and adults. By definition, an overuse injury is defined as a long-standing or recurrent musculoskeletal problem that was not initiated by an acute injury.[30] Table 1-2 lists the 10 most common diagnoses for overuse syndromes in male and female children and adults.[15]

In adults, as in children, the incidence of injuries in men is significantly higher than in women. The ratio is nearly 2:1.[16] Table 1-3 lists the most common sites of injury in men and women reported by Kannus et al.[16] Locations of these injuries will of course vary depending upon the size of the epidemiologic study and the sports participated in. These data are collaborated by studies in college and high school athletics. McLain and Reynolds[32] reviewed 1283 student athletes involved in organized high school athletics. The overall injury rate was 22%. The largest injury rate occurred in football (61%). Sprains and strains accounted for 57% of all injuries (Table 1-4). Table 1-5 lists the percentage of injuries and days lost as a result of injury in 24 common varsity high school sports. As noted in Table 1-5, in most sports the number of days lost due to injury is significantly greater in girls than in boys.

Meeuwisse and Fowler[34] reviewed 712 intercollegiate athletes in 24 different sports and demonstrated an injury rate of 38% for men and 32% for women. Serious injuries were significantly more common in men. Ice hockey had the highest player injury rate, but football had the greatest absolute

Table 1-3 Ten Most Common Sites of Injury in Adults

Women		*Men*	
Injury Site	%	*Injury Site*	%
Knee	29	Knee	27
Ankle	10	Ankle	10
Lower back	9	Lower back	9
Lower leg	6	Shoulder	7
Metatarsal region	3	Achilles tendon	7
Toes	3	Lower leg	4
Calf	3	Hip	3
Achilles tendon	3	Elbow	3
Sole	2	Heel	3
Hip	2	Calf	3

Source: Kannus P, Niitymäki S, Järvinen M, *British Journal of Sports Medicine* (1987;21:37–39), British Association of Sport and Medicine.

Table 1-4 High School Athletic Injuries (280 Injuries per 1283 Students)

Type of Injury	*Percentage of Total Injuries*
Sprain	34
Strain	23
Contusion	13
Fracture	10
Tendinitis	7
Articular subluxation	3
Concussion	3
Knee injury	1
Other	6

Source: McLain LG, Reynolds S, *Pediatrics* (1989;84:446–450), American Academy of Pediatrics.

Table 1-5 Injury Severity in High School Athletics

Sport	*Percentage of Athletes With Injuries*	*Days Lost to Injury*
Football	61	7
Gymnastics		
Boys	40	10
Girls	46	19
Wrestling	40	23 (boys)
Basketball		
Boys	37	12
Girls	31	29
Volleyball	17	8
Baseball	15	22 (boys)
Cross-country		
Boys	13	4
Girls	7	27
Soccer		
Boys	13	11
Girls	17	10
Softball	13	9 (girls)
Track		
Boys	10	23
Girls	18	32
Badminton	7	5
Field hockey	6	3
Water polo		
Boys	5	5
Girls	0	0
Tennis		
Boys	0	0
Girls	3	10
Golf	0	0
Swimming		
Boys	0	0
Girls	0	0
All	22	

Source: McLain LG, Reynolds S, *Pediatrics* (1989;84:446–450), American Academy of Pediatrics.

number of injuries. As expected, the knee was the anatomic region most frequently involved.[34] In this group of athletes acute injuries were more common in men, with an acute injury rate of 62% compared to an overuse syndrome rate of 38%, women had an acute injury rate of 42% and an overuse syndrome rate of 58%. Table 1-6 summarizes the injury rates in some of the more common intercollegiate sports.[34]

In the adult and older adult population, unorganized physical activity is increasingly common. In these age groups, the most common physical activities include running and racket sports. Matheson et al[25] reviewed sports-related injuries in 685 elderly and 722 young adults. A clear relationship between a given sport and the type of injury was not identified in 104 of 685 cases in the older age group. Fitness classes and field sports were more commonly seen to be associated with injuries in the younger group, whereas racket sports, walking, and low-intensity sports were more commonly associated with injuries in the older group. Table 1-7 summarizes the activity and location of injuries in young and older adults.[25] As expected, most injuries involved the lower extremity. This was evident in both younger and older adult populations. Certain types of injuries are more common in the older population, such as metatarsalgia, plantar fasciitis, and meniscal

Table 1-6 Intercollegiate Athletic Injuries

Sport	*Number of Injuries*	*Common Anatomic Locations*			
		First		*Second*	
Football					
Men	83	Knee	24%	Shoulder	22%
Track and field					
Men	20	Thigh	15%	Shoulder	15%
Women	20	Leg	40%	Foot	25%
Rowing					
Men	11	Knee	36%	Shoulder	18%
Women	19	Knee	37%	Back	16%
Hockey					
Men	29	Knee	31%	Ribs	14%
Rugby					
Men	25	Shoulder	36%	Back	16%
Basketball					
Men	13	Knee	31%	Ankle	23%
Women	11	Leg	45%	Ankle	27%
Volleyball					
Men	7	Knee	33%	Shoulder	33%
Women	13	Knee	23%	Ankle	23%
Cross country					
Men	9	Foot	33%	Thigh	22%
Women	10	Ankle	30%	Leg	30%
Soccer					
Men	10	Knee	30%	Nonspecific	
Women	8	Leg	38%	Nonspecific	
Swimming					
Men	7	Shoulder	29%	Neck	29%
Women	5	Shoulder	60%	Nonspecific	

Source: Meeuwisse WH, Fowler PJ, *Canadian Journal of Sport Sciences* (1988;13:35–42), Canadian Association of Sport Sciences.

Table 1-7 Sports-Related Injuries in Adults

	Older (685)		Younger (722)	
Sport	Men (%)	Women (%)	Men (%)	Women (%)
Running	24.9	6.6	22.3	18.2
Racquet sports	10.7	5.1	5.5	2.8
Multiple sports*	9.8	5.4	6.9	5.0
Walking	7.7	5.4	0.8	1.4
Low-intensity sports†	4.4	2.6	1.3	0.4
Skiing	4.1	2.0	2.4	3.3
Fitness class‡	2.0	2.8	3.0	9.9
Water sports	1.2	0.7	1.5	0.9
Ice sports§	1.4	0.2	2.6	0.5
Cycling	0.9	0.3	0.7	0.7
Field sports‖	0.9	0.0	6.0	1.6
Weightlifting	0.7	0.2	1.8	0.6

Numbers in parentheses are raw values.

*Individuals in this group were participating in two or more sports at the time of injury, preventing the clear identification of a relationship between the onset of injury and any single activity.

†Low-intensity sports include curling, golf, horseback riding, sailing, bowling, table tennis, and shooting.

‡Fitness classes are aerobic dance classes.

§Ice sports include hockey and skating.

‖Field sports include football, rugby, and soccer.

Source: Matheson GO, MacIntyre JG, Taunton, JE, Clement DB, Lloyd-Smith R, *Medicine and Science in Sports and Exercise* (1989;21:379–385), Williams & Wilkins.

knee injuries. Patellofemoral pain syndrome and stress fractures or periostitis are more common in younger adults.

CATEGORIES OF SPORTS INJURIES

Most physicians clearly understand the specific types of skeletal and articular injuries. Soft tissue injuries and the terminology used for them can be confusing, however. Therefore, a review of the common types of osseous and soft tissue sports injuries is provided so that the reader will be familiar with these terms as they appear in the remainder of the text.

Fractures and Dislocations

A fracture has been defined as a complete or incomplete break in the continuity of bone, cartilage, or both.[50] There have been many common labels and eponyms that have been used to describe the various types of fractures and fracture-dislocations. Listed below are common terms for fractures and dislocations that will be used throughout the text.

Closed Fracture (Simple Fracture)

A closed or simple fracture is a fracture that results in only two fragments with intact overlying skin and soft tissues (Fig. 1-1).[50]

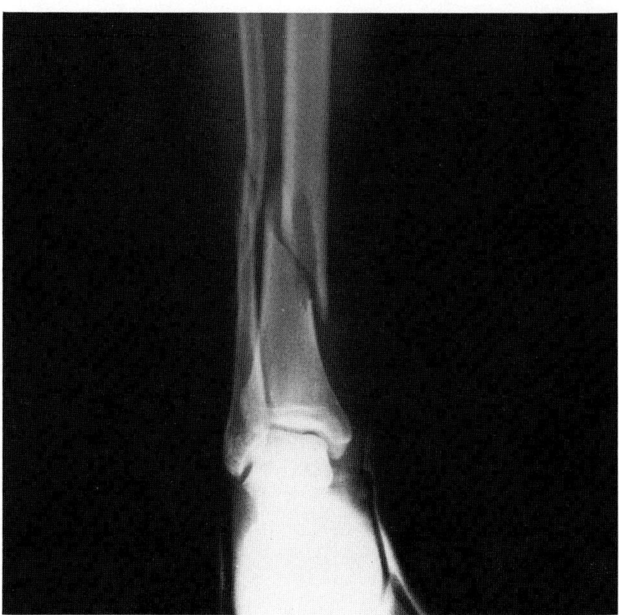

Fig. 1-1 Complete fractures of the distal tibia and fibula. There was no soft tissue loss over the fracture sites (closed fracture). The tibial fracture is a simple spiral fracture. The fibular fracture is comminuted.

Open Fracture (Compound Fracture)

An open or compound fracture occurs when there is disruption of the soft tissues, so that the fracture site communicates with the outside environment.[50]

Complete Fracture

A complete fracture is one that involves both cortices (Fig. 1-1).[5,50]

Comminuted Fracture

A comminuted fracture is typically a complete fracture resulting in more than two fragments. These are usually the result of high-velocity injury and are more frequently open or compound injuries (Fig. 1-1).[5,50]

Avulsion Fracture

Avulsion fractures result from rapid forced contraction of a muscle at its attachment or from the resistance force of a strong ligament. These injuries typically occur at bony prominences, which serve as the attachment sites of muscle tendon units and ligaments (Fig. 1-2).[5,50]

Incomplete Fracture

An incomplete fracture is one that involves only one cortex of the involved bone. Listed below are several categories of incomplete fracture that are commonly seen, particularly in children.

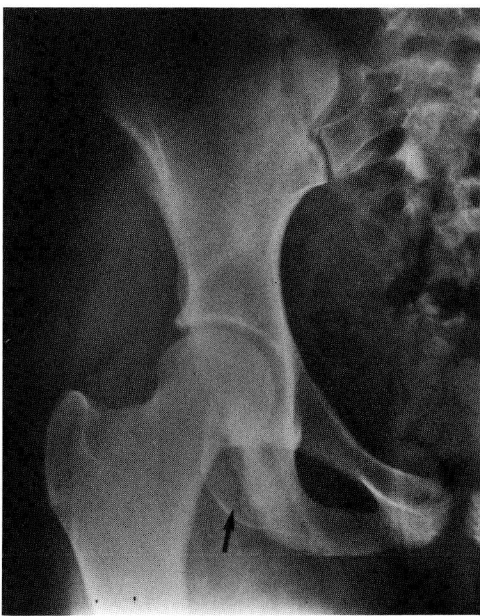

Fig. 1-2 Avulsion fracture of the ischial tuberosity (arrow) due to hamstring muscle contraction. *Source:* Reprinted from *Imaging of Orthopedic Trauma* ed 2 by TH Berquist, 1991, Raven Press, © Mayo Foundation.

1. Torus fracture: A torus fracture is an incomplete fracture that results in buckling of the cortex (Fig. 1-3).[5]
2. Greenstick fracture: A greenstick fracture occurs when there is interruption of one cortex with angling at the fracture site resembling a broken branch (Fig. 1-4).[5,50]
3. Microfracture or bowing fracture: With this fracture a bending occurs, and there may be no obvious defects in the cortex. This fracture commonly occurs in the radius and ulna in young children (Fig. 1-5).[5]

Growth Plate or Physeal Fracture

These are often subtle fractures involving the growth plate and associated metaphysis or epiphysis; they typically occur in children but certainly occur before closure of the growth plates. This group of fractures has been classified by Salter and Harris (Fig. 1-6). Type I fractures involve the growth plate but spare both epiphysis and metaphysis. Type II fractures involve the growth plate and exit through the metaphysis. In type III fractures, the fracture involves the growth plate and exits through the epiphysis. Type IV fractures involve both epiphysis and metaphysis, extending through the growth plate. Type V fractures are essentially impaction or crush injuries of the growth plate.

Stress Fracture

Stress fracture results from repeated trauma to a normal bone (Fig. 1-7).[5,50]

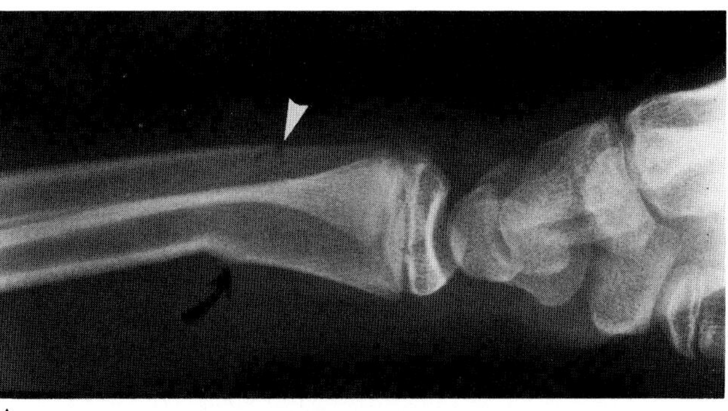

A

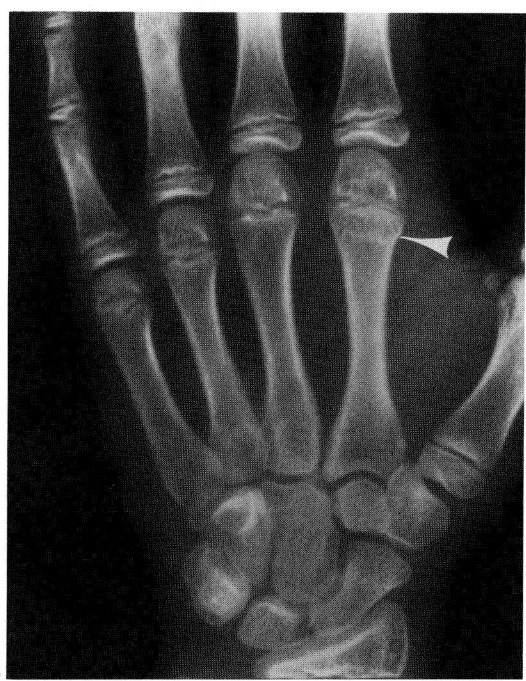

B

Fig. 1-3 Torus fractures. (**A**) Lateral view of the wrist with a torus fracture of the distal radius (curved arrow) and incomplete fracture of the distal ulna (upper arrow). *Source:* Reprinted from *Imaging of Orthopedic Trauma* ed 2 by TH Berquist, 1991, Raven Press, © Mayo Foundation. (**B**) Subtle torus fracture (arrowhead) of the second metacarpal neck.

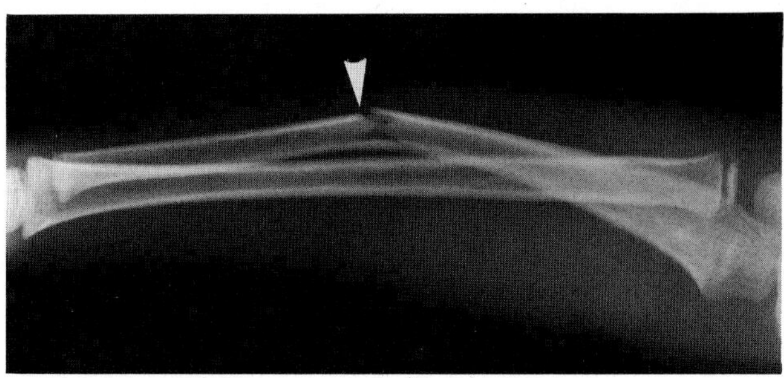

Fig. 1-4 Greenstick fracture of the midulna. *Source:* Reprinted from *Imaging of Orthopedic Trauma* ed 2 by TH Berquist, 1991, Raven Press, © Mayo Foundation.

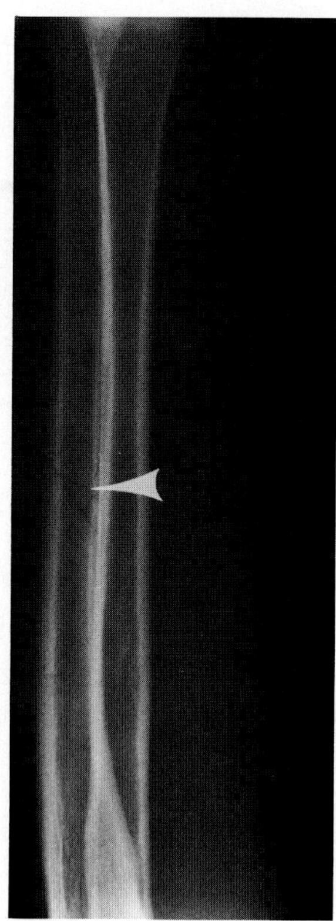

Fig. 1-5 Microfracture of the midulna (arrow).

Pathologic Fracture

A pathologic fracture is a fracture through an area of abnormal bone, such as in metabolic disease or a neoplastic process.[5,50]

Dislocation

Dislocation is an injury to an articulation or joint such that the resulting position of the two articular surfaces is completely displaced (Fig. 1-8).

Subluxation

Subluxation is an injury to an articular region or joint such that a portion of the articular surfaces still remains in contact (Fig. 1-9).[5]

Fracture-Dislocation

Fracture-dislocation is an injury that contains a fracture of the osseous structure along with dislocation of the adjacent articulation.[5,50]

Soft Tissue Injuries

Numerous terms are used to describe minor and major soft tissue injuries. General terms are described here. More specific anatomic terms are discussed in later chapters as they relate to specific regions.

Contusion

A contusion is defined as a direct blow against a soft tissue structure resulting in bruising of the skin and underlying soft tissues. This results in capillary rupture with an infiltrative type of bleeding and edema in the traumatized tissues (Fig. 1-10).[41]

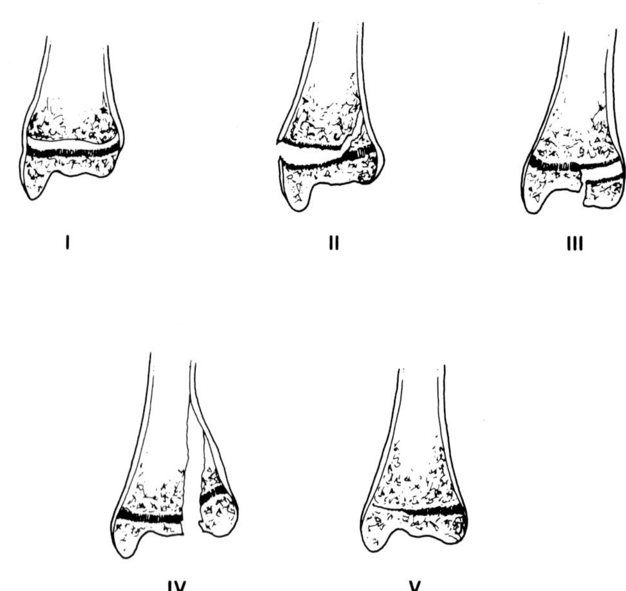

Fig. 1-6 Illustration of growth plate fracture classification by Salter and Harris. *Source:* Reprinted from *Imaging of Orthopedic Trauma* ed 2 by TH Berquist, 1991, Raven Press, © Mayo Foundation.

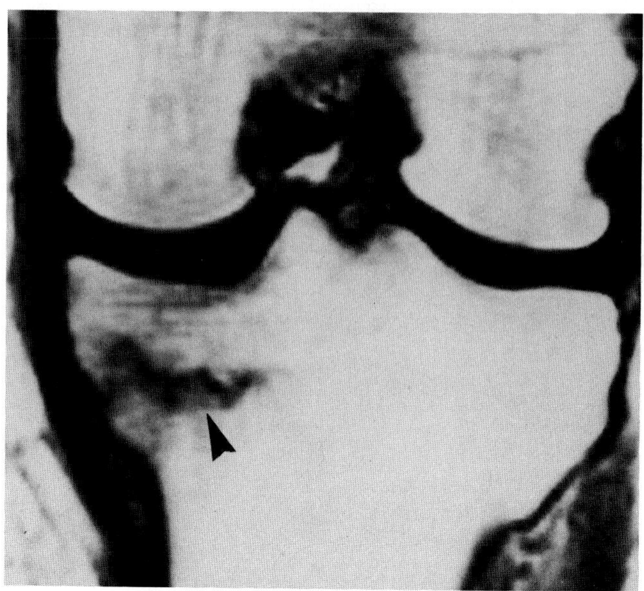

Fig. 1-7 Coronal (SE 500/20) magnetic resonance (MR) image of the knee demonstrating an upper tibial stress fracture (arrowhead). Radiographs were normal.

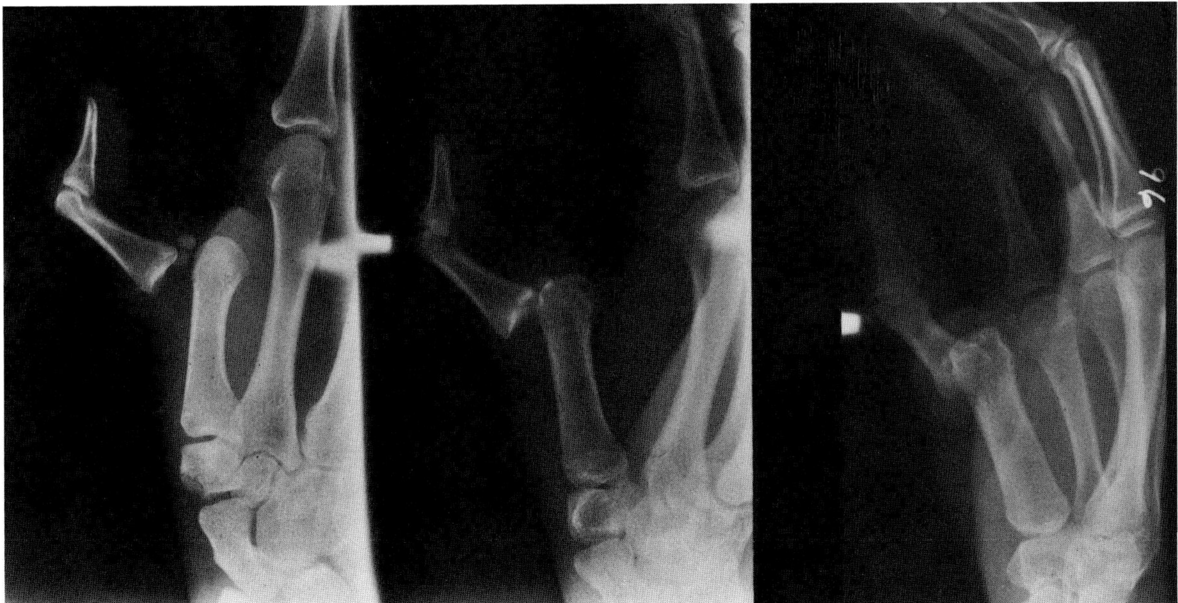

Fig. 1-8 Three views of the right thumb demonstrating a dislocation of the metacarpophalangeal joint.

Hemorrhage

Hemorrhage is defined as a poorly defined or infiltrative bleed into the soft tissues (Fig. 1-11).[5]

Hematoma

A hematoma differs from a hemorrhage in that it is a well-defined, restricted collection of blood (Fig. 1-12).[5]

Strain

Strain is injury to a muscle tendon unit and can be either acute or chronic. These injuries are typically classified as first, second, and third degree. With first-degree strains there are no appreciable disruptions of the muscle or tendon fibers, and only local inflammatory changes will be noted. There is also typically no loss of strength or decrease in motion. Second-degree strains result in partial damage to the muscle tendon

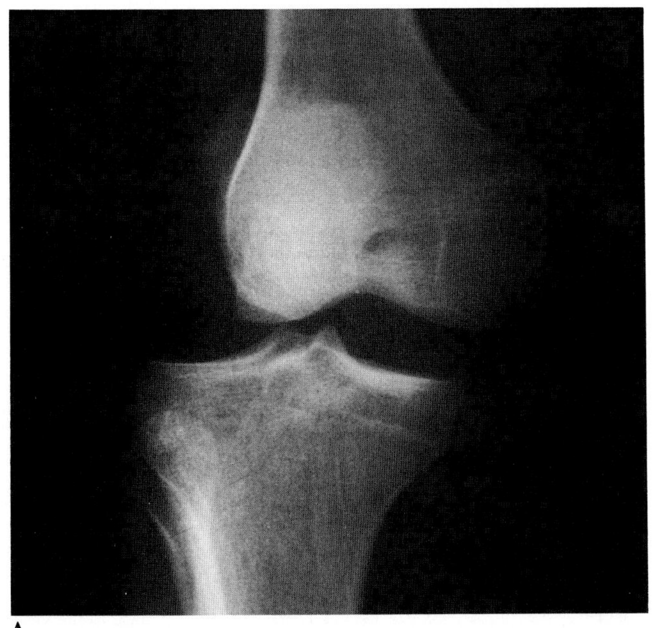

A

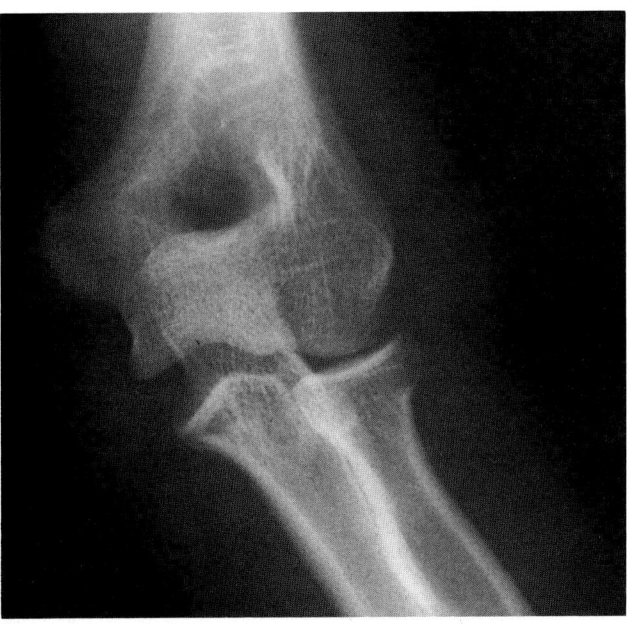

B

Fig. 1-9 Subluxations of the knee (**A**) and elbow (**B**) with various degrees of articular incongruency.

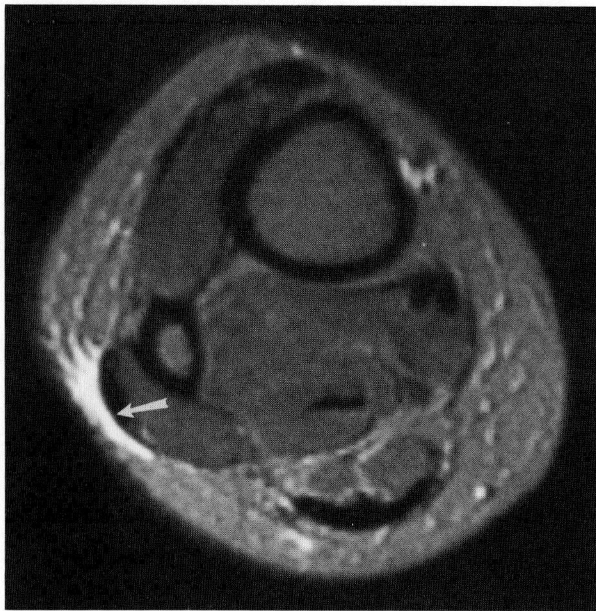

Fig. 1-10 Axial T2-weighted MR image (SE 2000/60) of the ankle demonstrating a high-signal contusion (arrow) over the peroneal tendons.

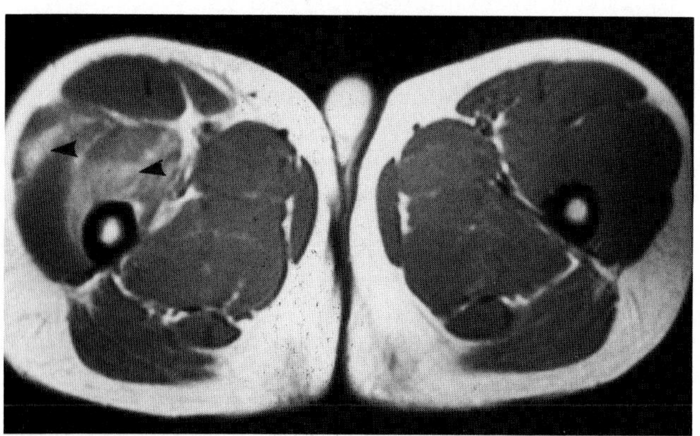

Fig. 1-11 Axial T2-weighted MR image (SE 2000/30) of the thighs demonstrating hemorrhage into the vastus lateralis and intermedius muscles (arrowheads).

unit, although less than 50% of the unit is typically involved. There is usually detectable loss of strength with this degree of injury. Third-degree strain is a complete rupture of the muscle tendon unit.

Sprain

Sprains are injuries to ligaments resulting from overstress that can cause variable degrees of ligament disruption (Fig. 1-13). First-degree sprain involves only a few fibers with little resulting hemorrhage into the ligament. A second-degree sprain, like a second-degree strain, involves 50% or less of the ligament. A third-degree sprain results in complete disruption of the ligament. A sprain-fracture is an injury that results essentially in avulsion of a piece of bone along with the ligament.[41]

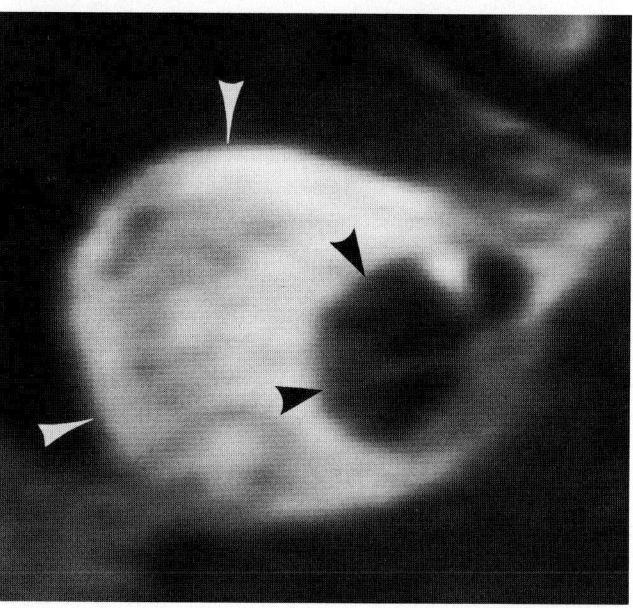

Fig. 1-12 Axial T2-weighted MR image (SE 2000/60) demonstrating a hematoma (white arrowheads) at the origin of the hamstring tendons (black arrowheads).

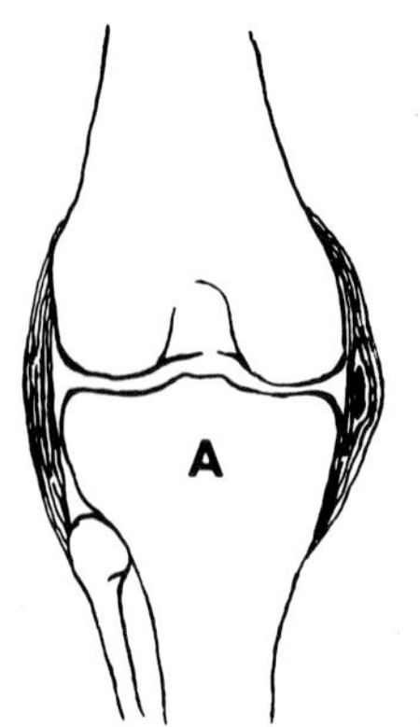

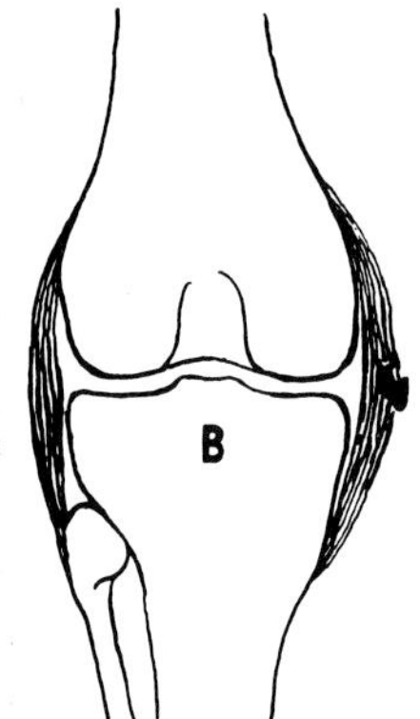

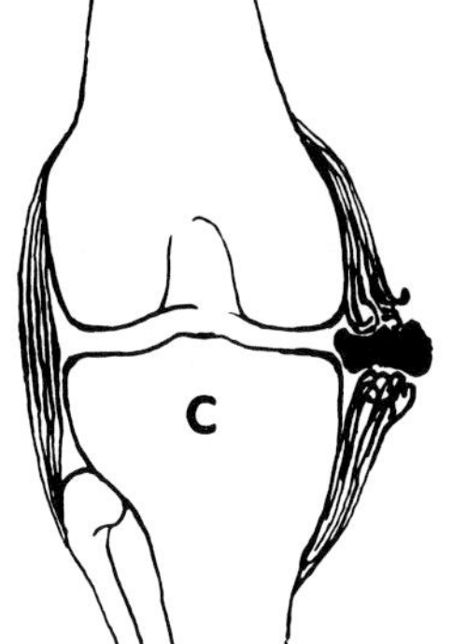

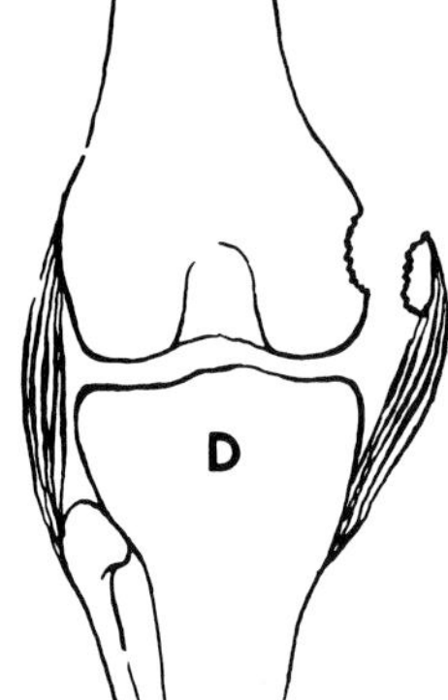

Fig. 1-13 Illustration of the degrees of ligament sprain. (**A**) First degree, (**B**) second degree, (**C**) third degree, (**D**) fracture sprain. *Source:* Reprinted from *Treatment and Injuries to Athletes* (p 64) by DH O'Donoghue with permission of WB Saunders, © 1984.

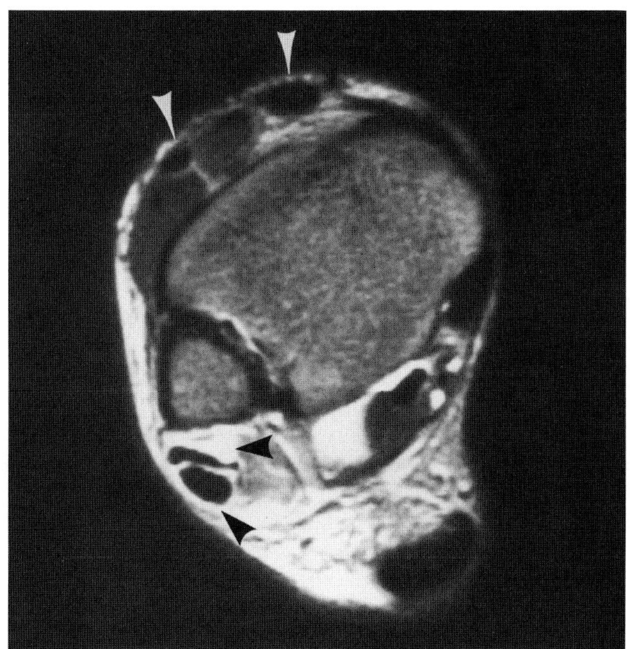

Fig. 1-14 Peroneal tenosynovitis. Axial T2-weighted MR image (SE 2000/60) demonstrating fluid (black arrowheads) around the peroneal tendons. There is no fluid around the extensor tendons anteriorly (white arrowheads).

Myositis Ossificans

This is a frequent complication of contusion and hematoma involving muscles near their origins or insertions onto bone. The term is often used to describe several conditions. The term actually implies inflammation of the muscle with subsequent ossification. More commonly, however, there is ossification of the infiltrative blood along the muscle origin on the bone. Another type of myositis ossificans occurs when there is actually linear bone formation lying within the muscle but separated from the bone by a layer of soft tissue or periosteum.[5,16,18]

Nerve Injury

Nerve injuries may result from direct blows that cause contusion of the involved area or from stretching of the nerve such as may occur with ligament disruption in widening of an articulation, resulting in stretching of the nerve on the involved side.[5,16,18]

Overuse Syndromes

As noted above, an overuse syndrome is defined as a long-standing or recurrent musculoskeletal injury. Specific terms are defined in anatomic chapters that follow. Certain basic terms are commonly used, however, and are defined here.

Tenosynovitis

This is inflammation of the synovium surrounding a tendon due to chronic overuse (Fig. 1-14).

Bursitis

Bursitis is inflammation of a bursa or numerous bursae associated with the joints. These inflammatory changes occur most frequently in the shoulder, elbow, and trochanteric region.

Osteochondritis

Osteochondritis is an articular fragmentation with or without separation. This is also commonly referred to as a transchondral fracture.

REFERENCES

1. Addiss DG, Baker SP. Mountaineering and rock-climbing injuries in US national parks. *Ann Emerg Med.* 1989;18:975–979.
2. Back FJG, Erich WBM, Kemper ABA, Verbeek ALM. Sports injuries in school age children: an epidemiologic study. *Am J Sports Med.* 1989;17: 234–240.
3. Baker BE. Current concepts in the diagnosis and treatment of musculotendinous injuries. *Med Sci Sports Exerc.* 1984;16:323–327.
4. Bernard AA, Corlett S, Thomsen E, et al. Ice skating accidents and injuries. *Injury.* 1988;19:191–192.
5. Berquist TH. *Imaging of Orthopedic Trauma.* 2nd ed. New York: Raven; 1991.
6. Chard MD, Lachmann SM. Racquet sports—patterns of injury presenting to a sports injury clinic. *Br J Sports Med.* 1987;21:150–153.
7. de Loës M, Goldie I. Incidence rate of injuries during sport activity and physical exercise in a rural Swedish municipality: incidence rates in 17 sports. *Int J Sports Med.* 1988;9:461–467.
8. Ekstrand J, Nigg BM. Surface-related injuries in soccer. *Sports Med.* 1989;8:56–62.
9. Ellitsgaard N. Parachuting injuries: a study of 110,000 sports jumps. *Br J Sports Med.* 1987;21:13–17.
10. Gibson T. Sports injuries. *Baillieres Clin Rheumatol.* 1987;3: 583–600.
11. Gregg JR, Torg E. Upper extremity injuries in adolescent tennis players. *Clin Sports Med.* 1988;7:371–385.
12. Halpern B, Thompson N, Curl WW, Andrews JR, Hunter SC, Boring JR. High school football injuries: identifying the risk factors. *Am J Sports Med.* 1987;15:S113–S117.
13. Hoeberigs HJ, van Galen WCC, Philipsen H. Pattern of injury in handball and comparison of injured versus noninjured handball players. *Int J Sports Med.* 1986;7:333–337.
14. Johansson C. Injuries in elite orienteers. *Am J Sports Med.* 1986;14: 410–415.
15. Kannus P, Niittymäki S, Järvinen M. Athletic overuse injuries in children. *Clin Pediatr.* 1988;27:333–337.
16. Kannus P, Niittymäki S, Järvinen M. Sports injuries in women: a one-year prospective follow-up study at an outpatient sports clinic. *Br J Sports Med.* 1987;21:37–39.
17. Keller CS, Noyes FR, Buncher CR. The medical aspects of soccer injury epidemiology. *Am J Sports Med.* 1987;15:S105–S112.
18. Kellett J. Acute soft tissue injuries—a review of the literature. *Med Sci Sports Exerc.* 1986;18:489–500.

19. Kiburz D, Jacobs R, Reckling F, Mason J. Bicycle accidents and injuries among adult cyclists. *Am J Sports Med.* 1986;14:416–419.

20. Kvist M, Kujala UM, Heinonen OJ, et al. Sports-related injuries in children. *Int J Sports Med.* 1989;10:81–86.

21. Lorentzon R, Wedren H, Pietilä T. Incidence, nature, and causes of ice hockey injuries. A three-year prospective study of a Swedish elite ice hockey team. *Am J Sports Med.* 1988;16:392–396.

22. Lorentzon R, Wedren H, Pietilä T, Gustavsson B. Injuries in international ice hockey. A prospective, comparative study of injury incidence and injury types in international and Swedish elite ice hockey. *Am J Sports Med.* 1988;16:389–391.

23. Marti B, Vader JP, Minder CE, Abelin T. On the epidemiology of running injuries. The 1984 Bern Grand-Prix study. *Am J Sports Med.* 1988; 16:285–294.

24. Matheson GO, Clement DB, McKenzie DC, Taunton JE, Lloyd-Smith DR, MacIntyre JG. Stress fractures in athletes. A study of 320 cases. *Am Orthop Soc Sports Med.* 1987;15:46–58.

25. Matheson GO, MacIntyre JG, Taunton JE, Clement DB, Lloyd-Smith R. Musculoskeletal injuries associated with physical activity in older adults. *Med Sci Sports Exerc.* 1989;21:379–385.

26. Matter P, Ziegler WJ, Holzach P. Skiing accidents in the past 15 years. *J Sports Sci.* 1987;5:319–326.

27. Maylack FH. Epidemiology of tennis, squash, and racquetball injuries. *Clin Sports Med.* 1988;7:233–243.

28. McAuley E, Hudash G, Shields K, et al. Injuries in women's gymnastics. The state of the art. *Am J Sports Med.* 1987;15:558–565.

29. McCormick DP, Davis AL. Injuries in sailboard enthusiasts. *Br J Sports Med.* 1988;22:95–97.

30. McKeag DB. The concept of overuse: the primary care aspects of overuse syndromes in sports medicine. *Primary Care.* 1984;1:43–59.

31. McKenzie DC. Stress fracture of the rib in an elite oarsman. *Int J Sports Med.* 1989;10:220–222.

32. McLain LG, Reynolds S. Sports injuries in a high school. *Pediatrics.* 1989;84:446–450.

33. McMaster PE. Tendon and muscle ruptures. *J Bone Joint Surg Am.* 1933;15:705–722.

34. Meeuwisse WH, Fowler PJ. Frequency and predictability of sports injuries in intercollegiate athletes. *Can J Sports Sci.* 1988;13:35–42.

35. Messier SP, Pittala KA. Etiologic factors associated with selected running injuries. *Med Sci Sports Exerc.* 1988;20:501–505.

36. Miller TW, Heck LL, Kight JL, McCarroll JR, Shelbourne KD, Van Hove ED. A clinical and radiological review of stress fractures in competitive and non-competitive athletes. *Indiana Med.* 1987;80:942–949.

37. Morrow PL, McQuillen EN, Eaton LA, Bernstein CJ. Downhill ski fatalities: the Vermont experience. *J Trauma.* 1988;28:95–100.

38. Nicholas JA, Rosenthal PP, Gleim GW. A historical perspective of injuries in professional football. *JAMA.* 1988;260:939–944.

39. Nielsen AB, Yde J. An epidemiologic and traumatologic study of injuries in handball. *Int J Sports Med.* 1988;9:341–344.

40. Noyes FR, Lindenfeld TN, Marshall MT. What determines an athletic injury? *Am J Sports Med.* 1988;16(suppl 1):365–368.

41. O'Donoghue DH. *Treatment and Injuries to Athletes.* 4th ed. Philadelphia: Saunders; 1984.

42. Paty JG Jr. Diagnosis and treatment of musculoskeletal running injuries. *Semin Arthritis Rheum.* 1988;18:48–60.

43. Pickard MA, Tullett WM, Patel AR. Sports injuries as seen at an accident and emergency department. *Scott Med J.* 1988;33:296–297.

44. Pliskin M, D'Angelo M. Atypical downhill skiing injuries. *J Trauma.* 1988;28:520–522.

45. Renstrom P. Swedish research in sports traumatology. *Clin Orthop.* 1984;191:144–158.

46. Robbins SE, Gouw GJ, Hanna AM. Running-related injury prevention through innate impact-moderating behavior. *Med Sci Sports Exerc.* 1989;21: 130–139.

47. Rothenberger LA, Chang JI, Cable TA. Prevalence and types of injuries in aerobic dancers. *Am J Sports Med.* 1988;16:403–407.

48. Sherry E, Clout L. Deaths associated with skiing in Australia: a 32-year study of cases from the Snowy Mountains. *Med J Aust.* 1988;149: 615–618.

49. Shiff HB, MacScarraigh ET, Kallmeyer JC. Myoglobinuria rhabdomyolysis and marathon running. *Q J Med.* 1978;188:463–472.

50. Shultz RJ. *The Language of Fractures.* Baltimore: Williams & Wilkins; 1972.

51. Sim FH, Simonet WT, Melton LJ, Lehn TA. Ice hockey injuries. *Am J Sports Med.* 1987;15:S86–S96.

52. Stanitski CL. Common injuries in preadolescent and adolescent athletes. *Sports Med.* 1989;7:32–41.

53. Steinbrück K. Frequency and aetiology of injury in cross-country skiing. *J Sports Sci.* 1987;5:187–196.

54. Thompson RR. A study of the type and cost of football injuries. *Minn Med.* 1986;69:656–658.

55. Tucci JJ, Barone JE. A study of urban bicycling accidents. *Am J Sports Med.* 1988;16:181–184.

56. Watson MD, DiMartino PP. Incidence of injuries in high school track and field athletes and its relation to performance ability. *Am J Sports Med.* 1987;15:251–254.

57. Whitlock MR, Whitlock J, Johnston B. Equestrian injuries: a comparison of professional and amateur injuries in Berkshire. *Br J Sports Med.* 1987;21:25–26.

58. Williamson DM, Lowdon IMR. Ice-skating injuries. *Injury.* 1986;17: 205–207.

Chapter 2

Diagnostic Techniques

There are multiple imaging techniques that are of diagnostic importance for evaluating sports injuries. Table 2-1 lists the major techniques used in musculoskeletal evaluation.

Proper application of these techniques is essential in obtaining optimal diagnostic information. This chapter provides background information and indications for each of the modalities listed in Table 2-1. This information is applied in subsequent chapters in discussing the radiographic evaluation of sports injuries.

ROUTINE RADIOGRAPHY, TOMOGRAPHY, AND MAGNIFICATION RADIOGRAPHY

Routine Radiography

Routine radiography remains the mainstay for diagnosis of skeletal injuries. This section discusses basic background material necessary for obtaining radiographic studies of consistently high quality. Specific positioning techniques are discussed in anatomic chapters that follow.

Thorough radiographic evaluation of any condition requires high-quality films. These cannot be obtained without properly functioning equipment, proper screen and film combinations, and technical consistency. Communication among the examining physician, the radiologist, and the technologist is essential to obtain the proper views and to ensure consistent patient positioning for optimal evaluation of the injury.

At the Mayo Clinic we typically use a three-phase, 12-pulse X-ray generator; Eimac AZ92 X-ray tubes with a 0.6-mm focal spot; and four-way floating tables. Radiography of the axial skeleton is performed at a 48-inch source-to-film distance (Bucky grid technique, 16:1 ratio) with Kodak X-omatic cassettes, Kodak Lanex medium screens, and Kodak TML film. Extremity radiographs are obtained with Kodak Lanex fine screens and Kodak TML film.

For the acutely traumatized patient we use a dedicated radiographic room adjacent to the emergency department. The equipment includes a Kermath Versitome table with a U-arm system capable of performing all routine radiographs as well as tomography in the lateral, oblique, anteroposterior, and transaxial directions. The room is also equipped with a modern life-support system. With such a dedicated emergency unit, one can obtain radiographs in all directions without moving the patient. The same film and screens are used in the trauma room.

Table 2-1 Diagnostic Techniques in Orthopaedic Trauma

- Routine radiography
  - Conventional tomography
    - Linear motion
    - Complex motion
  - Magnification radiography
- Ultrasound
- Skeletal scintigraphy
- Computed tomography
- Magnetic resonance imaging
- Angiography
- Myelography
- Arthrography and tenography (with or without diagnostic injections)
- Thermography

Selection of the proper recording medium (films and screens) is essential in obtaining radiographs of consistently high quality. The choice of screen and film combinations is complicated by the number of combinations available. There are approximately 40 different screens and 80 different films on the market. Various screen and film combinations can produce radiographs with a broad spectrum of sensitivity, contrast, and resolution characteristics. Generally, the optimum combination will be a compromise among the image quality desired, available equipment, and patient exposure factors.[4,16,18]

What is considered an optimal system should be determined within each institution. In theory, multiple screen and film combinations would be needed to obtain optimal results for each specific radiographic examination; this approach increases the potential for human error and inconsistency, however. Many departments select one screen and film system for all examinations or purchase different types of cassettes to assist in identification of the combinations within the department. In general, we use a 300-speed system for the axial skeleton and proximal extremities and an 80-speed system for the distal extremities.[2,3,6]

Proper choice of screen and film combinations will help maintain consistent radiographic quality. Consistency in selecting proper exposure factors, however, may be an even larger problem.

Patient size and the body part being examined specifically affect the exposure factors (peak kilovoltage and milliampseconds) required for optimal radiographs. We prefer to use a system that can be applied throughout the department and can provide uniform quality. Measuring the body part to be examined and referring to standardized charts available in each examining station result in more uniform quality. The charts remove the guesswork in deciding which exposure factors should be used.

In addition to proper exposure factors, certain basic principles of physics must be applied. The focal spot should be as small as practical to reduce geometric unsharpness or blurring. The central portion of the beam should be as perpendicular to the cassette as possible to minimize distortion of the object being radiographed. This also ensures that adjacent structures will be recorded in their true spatial relationships. The body part to be examined should be placed parallel to the film to minimize magnification, blurring, and distortion. The body part should be placed as close as possible to the cassette.[16]

Motion of either the equipment or the body part during the examination results in blurring of the image. Thus short exposure times are necessary, especially in severely injured or uncooperative patients. This will assist in reducing the lack of clarity in the image due to motion. Proper positioning as well as reduced motion can also be aided by using positioning wedges and props. This not only assists the patient in maintaining the proper position but also ensures consistency in positioning. Consistency in positioning is especially desirable with skeletal injuries because multiple follow-up studies are often performed. Slight changes in position may make observation of fracture healing and other orthopaedic problems more difficult.

The hand, wrist, foot, and ankle may be difficult to position because of overlap of osseous structures. In these situations it may be useful to obtain fluoroscopically positioned spot films. Subtle position changes can be monitored so that the structure is optimally positioned. Motion studies are also useful, and positioning for stress views is optimized with fluoroscopic control (Fig. 2-1).[4]

Proper radiation protection must be given to the patient, radiology department staff, and any assistants who may be required to aid in patient positioning. When it is necessary to hold or position patients (as in acute trauma or when children are involved), it is often best to enlist the aid of persons not normally engaged in radiographic work. For instance, parents may be best able to calm and reassure children. Assistants should wear lead gloves and aprons during the procedure.[2–4]

Multiple factors must be considered in discussing patient exposure. Proper positioning and exposure factors will prevent unnecessary retakes. Proper collimation not only decreases patient exposure but also increases image quality. Gonadal shielding should be undertaken when it will not obscure needed information. The Bureau of Radiological Health recommends shielding when the gonads lie within 5 cm of the primary beam in patients of reproductive age, assuming that the objective of the examination will not be compromised.[6]

Filtration with a minimum of 2.5 mm of aluminum equivalent is required with fluoroscopic and radiographic units capable of generating more than 70 kVp. This reduces the soft radiation that increases patient exposure but is of no diagnostic usefulness.[6] Proper choice of screen and film combination may reduce patient exposure by as much as 400%. Technical factors such as high peak kilovoltage also reduce patient exposure. Therefore, the highest practical peak kilovoltage (the amount that produces the needed subject contrast) should be used.

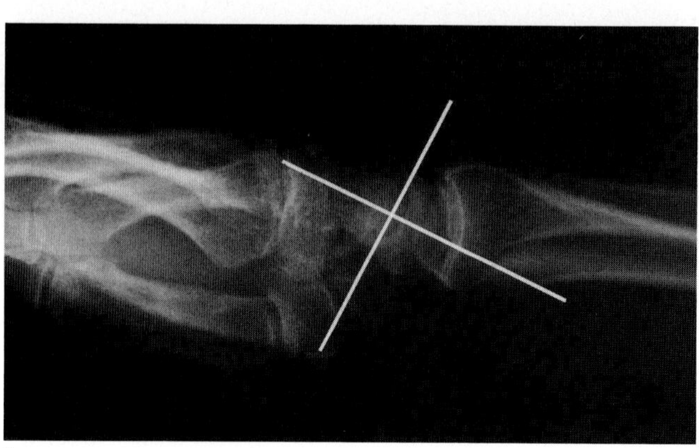

A

Fig. 2-1 Fluoroscopically positioned wrist images in a tennis player with chronic wrist pain. (**A**) In the lateral position the scapholunate angle (white lines) is increased to just over 90°.

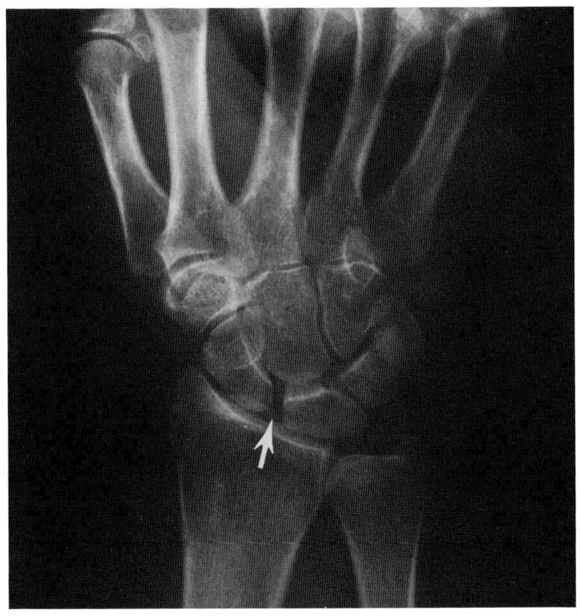
B

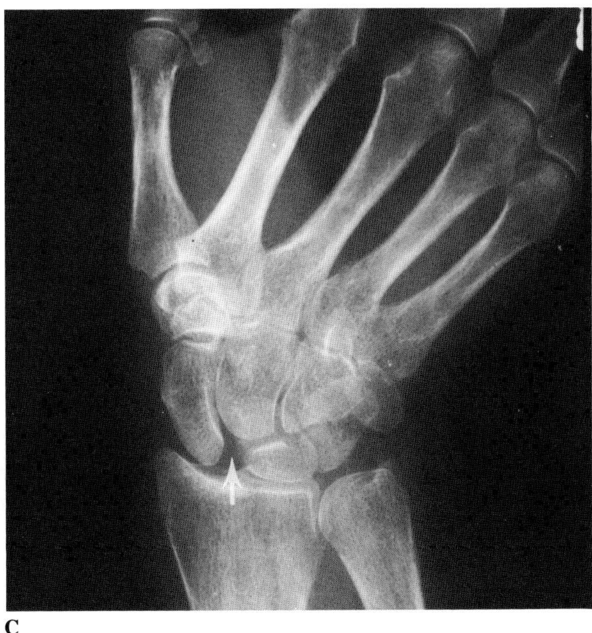
C

Fig. 2-1 contd (B) The posteroanterior clenched fist position shows widening of the scapholunate space (arrow), which increased as the wrist was moved into ulnar deviation (**C**). Diagnosis was scapholunate ligament tear.

Tomography

Conventional tomography provides a method of blurring out unwanted information the better to visualize desired structures. Laminography, planography, and stratigraphy are terms that have been applied to this technique. The technique was developed by two Dutch investigators (Ziedes des Plantes and Bartelink) in 1931.[5] During the exposure, the X-ray tube and film move in two parallel planes but in opposite directions. Speeds are maintained at a constant relationship.

Tomography is a useful addition to conventional films when more detailed information is required (Fig. 2-2).[1,4,15,17,19] Conventional tomography provides an image of any selected plane in the body while blurring structures above and below that plane.[12] Basic equipment for linear tomography includes an X-ray tube, a connecting rod that moves about a fixed fulcrum, and a cassette and film. As the film moves in one direction, the tube moves in the opposite direction. Only the plane of interest remains in sharp focus on the tomogram. Planes above and below will be blurred. Commonly used tomographic motions include simple (linear) and complex (circular, hypocycloidal, elliptical, and trispiral).

An understanding of tomography requires a basic knowledge of blurring and section thickness. Blurring refers to the effect of the tomographic system on objects outside the focal plane. It depends upon the amplitude of tube travel, the tube's orientation, and the distance of the tube from the focal plane. Section thickness refers to the plane that is in sharp focus on the film. It is inversely dependent on (but not proportional to) the amplitude of tube travel. Therefore, the greater the tomographic angle, the thinner the section.[4,7] Skeletal tomograms are typically obtained in 1- to 3-mm slices.

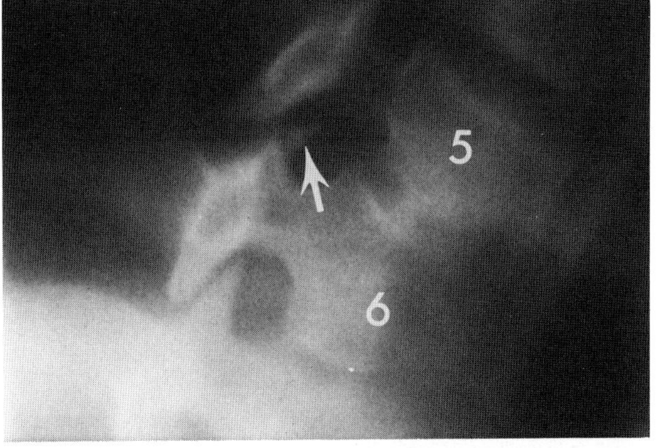

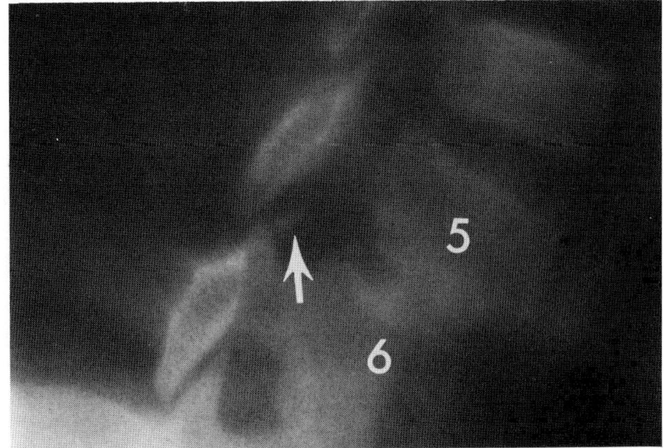

Fig. 2-2 Cervical tomography in a football player with nerve root symptoms after a rotation-compression injury. Routine films were normal. Tomograms of the lower cervical region demonstrate a chip fracture of the facet (arrows) with slight subluxation of C-5 on C-6.

For evaluating skeletal structures (which have high inherent contrast), wide-angle tomography with an arc of 30° to 50° is usually preferred. With the wide angle, maximum blurring of objects outside the focal plane occurs, and therefore phantom (unreal or unwanted) images are less likely to be produced. For standard skeletal tomography we use a CGR Stratomatic, which is capable of performing linear (longitudinal, transverse, and diagonal), circular, and trispiral motions. Linear and circular tube travel may be 20°, 30°, or 45°. In trispiral studies the angle is always 45°. 3M XUD film with Lanex regular screens (200-speed system) in special carbon fiber front cassettes are used at a 48-inch source-to-film distance. A Bucky grid with a 12:1 ratio is used. Exposure factors will vary with the body part being studied.

The type of tomographic motion used may greatly influence the radiographic findings. There are advantages to simple and complex motion studies. Increased blurring of objects occurs outside the plane in focus because of the greater distance that the tube and film move during the complex motion exposure. This results in elimination of streaking (incomplete blur) in an image of a structure when its long axis is aligned with the tube and film motion, as seen in linear tomography.[7] Complex motion has a decreased tendency to produce phantom images. The more complex the motion, the less the likelihood of phantom images. Linear tomography has the advantage of shorter exposure time, which may be useful in uncooperative patients. Linear motion may also be more useful when metal fixation devices are in place.

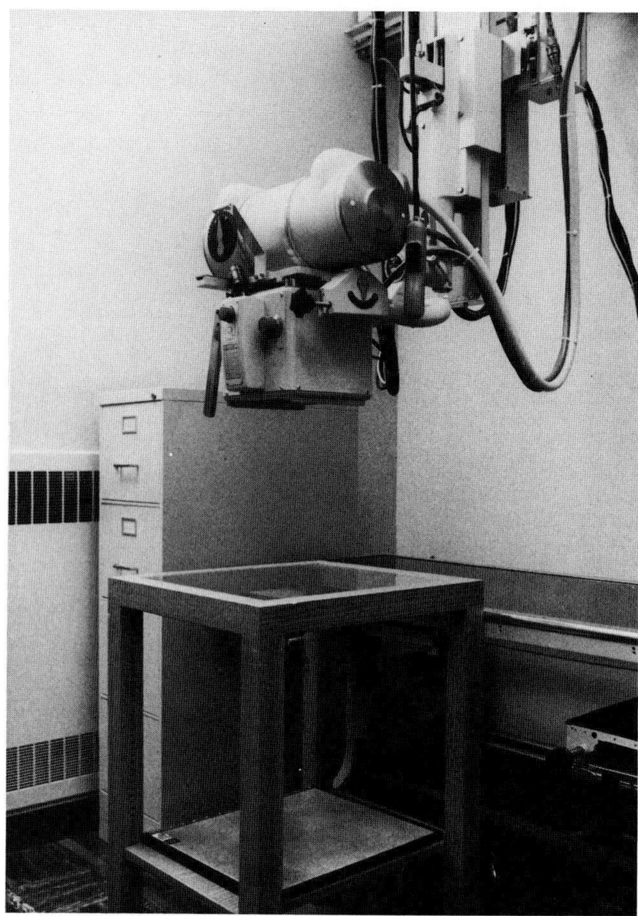

Fig. 2-3 Magnification position device with film at the lower level. The part to be examined is placed on the upper level.

Magnification Radiography

Magnification radiography was first introduced in 1940 but did not gain popularity until the last decade.[7] The technique provides accurate and detailed assessment of subtle skeletal abnormalities in articular, metabolic, infectious, neoplastic, and traumatic disorders.[4,9,10,11,13,14,21]

A thorough understanding of the equipment and principles of magnification is necessary to obtain high-quality magnification radiographs. Proper selection of the X-ray tube is the key to success. We use a Machlett DX78E tube with a 0.20-mm focal spot (as specified by the manufacturer). The actual focal spot size (grid-biased) measures 0.10 mm when a star text pattern is used in accordance with the specifications of the National Electrical Manufacturers Association.[10,20] High-speed rotation of the anode is necessary to prevent X-ray tube damage under heavy exposure conditions. A three-phase generator is also preferred.

For magnification hand films we use a 44-inch source-to-film distance, Kodak NMB single-emulsion film, Kodak single Min-r intensifying screens (used as rear screens), and exposure factors of 60 kVp, 30 mA-s, and 1.25 seconds. The body part being examined is supported on a Lucite stand 24 inches above the film. This results in a magnification factor of 2.2× to 1.0× (Fig. 2-3).

Magnification radiography is based on two geometric principles. First, the size of the image is proportional to the distance between the object and the film; second, the smaller the focal spot of the X-ray tube, the sharper the image.[8,10,20] A focal spot size of 0.30 mm or less is required for magnification radiography. Increased image size occurs as the distance between the object and film increases and as the distance between the focal spot and the object decreases, other factors remaining constant.[7,10] Geometric magnification is defined as the ratio of the source-to-film distance to the source-to-object distance for a point-source focal spot.

Radiation exposure to the skin is increased in magnification radiography because of the short source-to-skin distance. The size of the entrance field (in skull and abdominal magnification) is significantly reduced, however, thereby lowering total body exposure to nearly the equivalent dose obtained with conventional techniques. Entrance exposure to the skin for the magnified hand by means of the technique described above measures 246 mR (Webbels W. 1988. Exposure data, St. Mary's Hospital). This exposure is higher than that for the routine hand films (26 mR) but is acceptable because the magnification technique is used only in selected cases.[11,21] Also, the hand is among the least radiosensitive body parts. The overall high-quality image is the advantage of this technique. Increased effective sharpness, reduced effective noise, increased subject contrast (the air gap reduces the scattered radiation reaching the film), and improved visual effect of the enlargement contribute to high-quality radiographs. When the technique is properly performed, anatomic structures are better defined than those visualized in conventional radiographs observed with a magnifying lens.

Limitations of magnification include the following: Imaging is limited to small areas, proper positioning of the area of interest may be difficult, and high relative skin exposure and long exposure times may result in limited tube-loading capabilities.[19]

ULTRASOUND

The term *ultrasound* refers to mechanical vibrations whose frequencies are above the limit of human audible perception (about 20,000 Hz or cycles per second). Medical ultrasound imaging utilizes frequencies in the range of 2 to 10 MHz.[37,39] A central component of any ultrasound instrument is the transducer, which contains a small piezoelectric crystal. It serves as both the transmitter of sound waves into the body and the receiver of the returning echoes. When a brief alternating current is applied to the crystal, it vibrates at a characteristic frequency. By applying this vibrating transducer to the skin surface (through an acoustic coupling medium such as mineral oil or gel), the mechanical energy is transmitted into the body as a brief pulse of high-frequency sound waves. The advancing wave front interacts with tissues in various poorly understood ways and generates small reflected waves that return to the transducer. These cause the crystal to vibrate again, thereby generating an electric signal that is conducted back to the machine, where it is processed and displayed. With B-mode ultrasound imaging, the returning echoes are displayed as dots of light on a television screen, with the position of the dot on the screen corresponding to the position in the body where the echo was generated. In this way, the ultrasound image represents a cross-sectional display of the underlying anatomy. Unlike computed tomography (CT), in which the geometric constraints of the scanner itself limit the possible scanning planes, any conceivable plane or section can be obtained with modern ultrasound instruments. Such scanning flexibility can be of great value in demonstrating the continuity or discontinuity of adjacent structures.[37,39]

Real-time ultrasound scanners generate rapid, sequential B-scan images that permit high-speed continuous viewing.[22,25,29,37–39] These instruments can display dynamic events, such as a pulsating vessel, or they can be moved across the body to provide continuous viewing of the underlying anatomy. Gray-scale image processing is utilized, whereby the returning echoes (depending on their amplitude) are assigned 1 of up to 64 shades of gray for final display. The resulting images, therefore, demonstrate not only the major boundaries between soft tissue structures but also the structures' internal parenchymatous texture. This permits characterization of diffuse pathologic processes as well as detection of space-occupying lesions.

High-resolution images of superficial soft tissue structures can be obtained by using high-frequency sound waves (up to about 10 MHz).[36] It is a fundamental principle of ultrasound that the higher the frequency of the sound, the better the resolution of the images. Nevertheless, it is also fundamentally true that high-frequency sound waves are attenuated more rapidly in the soft tissues and therefore cannot penetrate deeply. The result of these counterbalancing effects is that one can obtain submillimeter resolution but only for structures located within about 5 cm of the skin surface.

Doppler ultrasound techniques reflect changes in frequency of moving structures. This technique is commonly used to evaluate blood flow. The Doppler effect is based on changes in observed frequency due to either object or observer motion. Changes in frequency indicate that motion or flow is present. When flow is toward the ultrasound source, Doppler frequency is increased. If flow or motion is in the opposite direction of the emitted wave (away from the source), the frequence decreases. Most new vascular ultrasound imagers offer both Doppler and color flow techniques. This provides more accurate assessment of vascular disease and flow abnormalities.

Perhaps the most severe limitation of diagnostic ultrasound imaging is the inability of sound waves to penetrate gas and bone. The strength of an echo generated at the boundary between any two tissues is related to differences in the acoustic impedance of the tissues (a physical property generally dependent on density). Because the acoustic impedances of bone and air are so different from those of human soft tissues, almost all sound energy is reflected off a soft tissue–bone or soft tissue–gas interface, leaving essentially no sound energy left to penetrate and thus image deeper structures. The strong echo reflected off such an interface overwhelms the transducer and is displayed as useless noise or artifact in the image.

Because this fundamental physical principle prevents ultrasound from passing from soft tissue into bone, the applications of this modality for skeletal lesions are limited.[37,39]

Initially, the most frequent musculoskeletal application of ultrasound was for distinguishing fluid from solid tissue, which is particularly useful in the characterization of the internal consistency of masses.[23] A simple fluid collection, such as an uncomplicated cyst, will be represented sonographically as an echo-free area, whereas solid tissue or the cells and debris within some fluid masses (such as abscesses) will provide interfaces for sound reflection and will therefore be echogenic. Some masses, of course, will demonstrate a complex pattern with both solid and cystic elements. In addition to characterizing a mass by the number of echoes generated within it, it is also important to assess the manner in which sound is transmitted through the mass. Fluid-containing structures cause little attenuation of the sound beam and thereby demonstrate a characteristic ultrasound finding, so-called enhanced through-transmission. This finding takes the form of stronger or brighter echoes deep to the fluid structure. Solid lesions cause greater attenuation of sound and therefore lack the finding of acoustic enhancement. By evaluating both the internal echogenicity of a mass and the ease of sound propagation through it, one can in virtually all instances characterize the basic contents of the mass as fluid, solid, or mixed. Although such a broad categorization is by no means histologically specific, such information, combined with appropriate clinical data, can often be helpful in patient management.

A common anatomic region where ultrasound has come to play a key role in diagnostic soft tissue evaluation is the popliteal fossa.[24,30,32,35] Masses or swelling in this area, whether pulsatile or not, can be difficult diagnostic problems for the clinician. Ultrasound has been successful in imaging popliteal artery aneurysms, popliteal cysts, abscesses, hematomas, and malignant tumors. In addition, patients with acute calf pain can be evaluated by ultrasound to differentiate pseudothrombophlebitis (due to ruptured popliteal cyst) from true thrombophlebitis.[38]

In recent years the musculoskeletal applications for ultrasonography have expanded significantly (Table 2-2).[26–28,31,33] Musculoskeletal injuries, such as rotator cuff tears, and other muscle, tendon, and ligament injuries are frequently investigated with ultrasound (Fig. 2-4). Complications of trauma, particularly venous thrombosis, can also be assessed with ultrasonography.[26,31,34] These applications are discussed more completely in specific anatomic chapters.

Table 2-2 Musculoskeletal Applications of Ultrasound

Soft tissue masses (cystic or solid)
Trauma
Muscle tears
Hematomas
Foreign bodies (wood, glass, metal)
Vascular disease
Joint effusions
Arthropathies

Sources: Harcke HT, Grissom LE, Furkelstein MS, *American Journal of Roentgenology* (1988;150:1253–1261), American Roentgen Ray Society; Kaplan PA, Matamoros A, Anderson JC, *American Journal of Roentgenology* (1990;155: 237–245); Sarti DA, Sample WF, *Diagnostic Ultrasound: Text and Cases*, 1980, GK Hall and Co.

SKELETAL SCINTIGRAPHY

Bone scintigraphy developed by way of a progression that began with studies of [^{32}P]orthophosphate tissue distribution conducted in the 1930s.[40] Radiopharmaceuticals currently used in bone scanning include compounds with P–O–P bonds (phosphates) and P–C–P bonds (phosphonates). The phosphonates are the current agents of choice because of their stability and soft tissue clearance rates are better than those of phosphates. The phosphate and phosphonate reagents come in sterile, pyrogen-free, lyophilized form with stannous ion as a reducing agent. Technetium-99m is reduced from the +7 to the +4 state and forms a chelate with the diphosphonate. After compounding, the material is checked for acceptability by quality control procedures, commonly by means of thin-layer or paper chromatography. The material is injected intravenously. Its localization in bone is dependent on blood flow and osteoblastic activity. The most widely accepted mechanism of localization is held to be chemisorption to the hydroxyapatite crystals of the bone mineral matrix. Approximately 50% of the mineral is cleared by the kidneys and excreted in the urine. Good hydration and an interval between administration and scanning of approximately 3 hours allow for soft tissue clearance and improved target-to-background ratios.[40,61,62]

Another important radiopharmaceutical in the case of orthopaedic patients with suspected bone infection is ^{67}Ga-labeled citrate. In the 1950s Ga isotopes were originally studied as potential bone-scanning agents. Although they do localize in bone, the available isotopes at that time were not satisfactory for imaging. Later, ^{67}Ga was shown to localize in tumors and sites of infection, which remains its major role today. The mechanism of localization of Ga in infection sites is not well understood, but it appears to be related to the binding of Ga to transferrin and lactoferrin, leukocyte labeling, and/or direct bacterial uptake.[51] The optimal time from injection to scanning is 24 to 48 hours. Because Ga is deposited in bone, care must be taken in the interpretation of Ga uptake when bone or joint infections are being sought. A sequence of ^{99m}Tc and ^{67}Ga scans may be necessary to differentiate reactive bone from inflammatory lesions.

A new agent that has proven useful in bone and joint infections is ^{111}In-labeled autologous white blood cells.[55,56,58] White blood cells migrate to sites of infection, and localization in the area of bone implies an infectious process. Images may be taken at 4 and 24 hours after the administration of the labeled white cells. Another new agent that may prove useful in bone and joint infections is ^{111}In-labeled polyclonal human immunoglobulin G.[56,58]

The Anger gamma camera is the imaging instrument used for all bone imaging. The camera allows total-body surveys with a moving table or moving detector. Selected views can also be obtained with this instrument. Radioactivity from the area of interest passes through a lead collimator and enters a sodium iodide crystal. The photon deposits its energy in the crystal. The crystal in turn gives off photons of light, which are converted to electrons by the photocathode of the photomultiplier tubes. These electrons are amplified by the photomultiplier tubes and processed, with the resulting data being placed on film or entered into a computer for further analysis.

Collimators are designated according to the resolution and energy levels at which they can be used (ie, low energy for ^{99m}Tc-labeled agents, medium energy for ^{111}In-labeled white

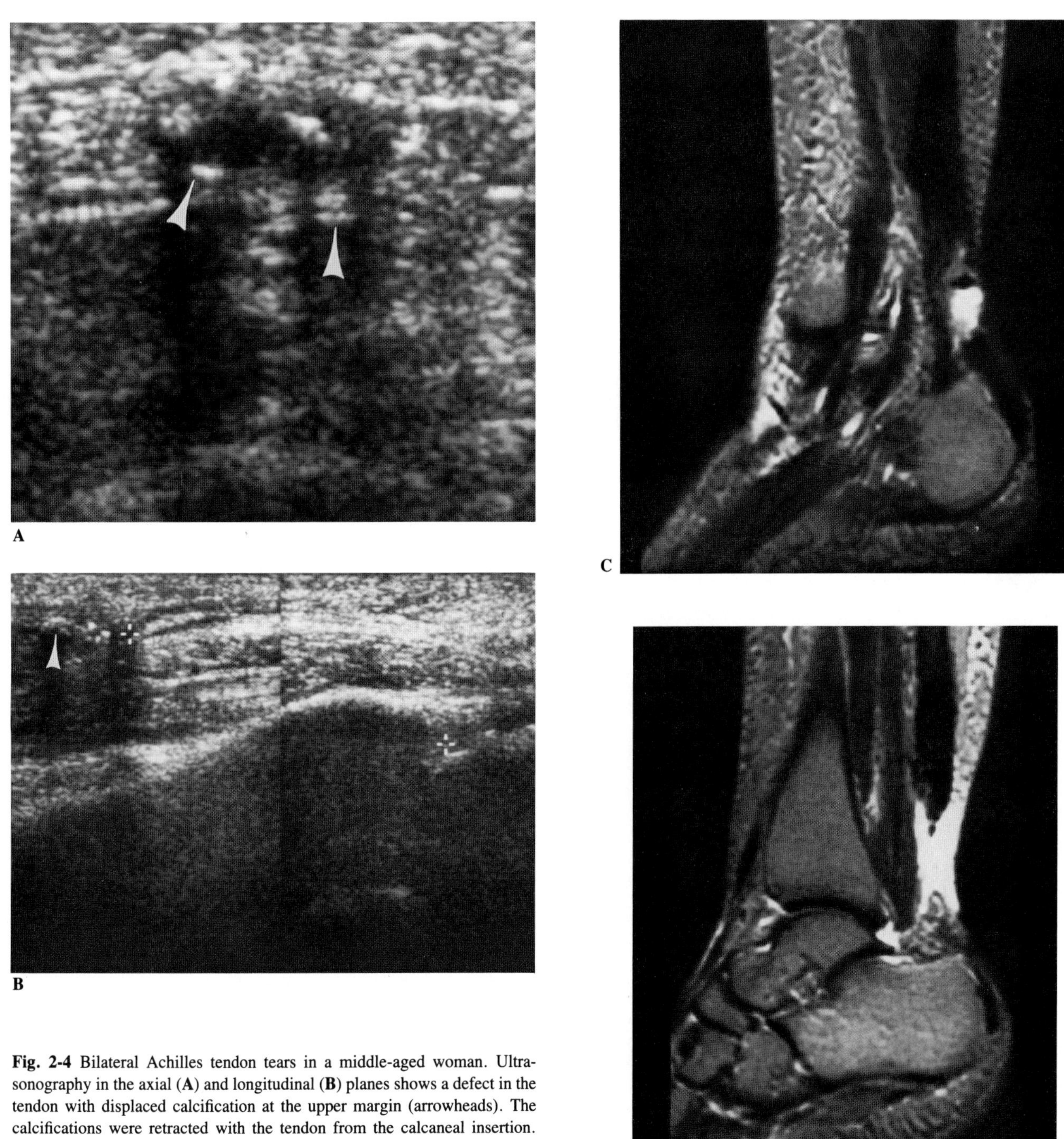

Fig. 2-4 Bilateral Achilles tendon tears in a middle-aged woman. Ultrasonography in the axial (**A**) and longitudinal (**B**) planes shows a defect in the tendon with displaced calcification at the upper margin (arrowheads). The calcifications were retracted with the tendon from the calcaneal insertion. Sagittal (SE 2000/60) magnetic resonance (MR) images (**C** and **D**) demonstrate the changes more clearly.

cells or ^{67}Ga studies, and high energy for ^{131}I-labeled agents). Collimator holes can be parallel or nonparallel; converging collimators magnify slightly. The pinhole collimator is a single hole that allows magnification of an area of interest with some geometric distortion.[40]

Although there are many indications for the use of bone scanning in clinical practice, the most common use is in oncology for detection and follow-up of metastatic bone disease, primarily from prostatic, breast, and lung cancer or primary bone tumors. The orthopaedic uses of bone scanning primarily include diagnosis of trauma and infection, determination of vascularity, compartmental evaluation of degenerative arthritis of joints, and evaluation of patients with painful prostheses. Secondary uses include evaluation of elevated serum alkaline phosphatase levels and diagnosis of patients who present with bone pain of undetermined etiology.[40,42–46,52]

Trauma

Bone scanning can provide important information in patients with known or suspected trauma.[40,41,47,52] Routine radiographs will easily demonstrate the site of fracture in most patients with a clinical history of trauma. In these uncomplicated cases bone scintigraphy will not add significant additional information. When the initial X-ray studies are normal, however, as may occur with subtle fractures of the pelvis, proximal femur, or carpal bone,[46] the bone scan may play a role in directing the course of management (Fig. 2-5). Fractures will show focal areas of increased uptake early, with 80% being visible in 24 hours and 95% in 72 hours,[40,50,54] although in elderly patients more time is often required for the onset of activity at the fracture site. Bone scanning is also helpful in patients suspected of having stress fractures (Fig. 2-6). The scan will detect stress fractures earlier than radiography, and if cessation of the stress is instituted the radiograph may never become positive.[47,60,63] A negative scan implies that the symptoms are not due to a stress fracture. Finally, in the battered child syndrome the bone scan may show the extent of the bone trauma, allowing directed radiographic confirmation. The scan may also demonstrate bone contusion not seen radiographically.

Other uses for bone scanning are currently being explored. Animal models show that sequential studies can use radionuclide imaging to evaluate fracture healing,[59] although this has not been convincingly demonstrated in humans. The question of bone viability after trauma, such as in the formal neck fracture, can also be evaluated with bone scanning.[48,49] Finally, focal areas of intense increased uptake in the spine may indicate pseudarthrosis in patients with ankylosing spondylitis or after fusion. This finding in an otherwise normal patient may indicate spondylosis.[40,52]

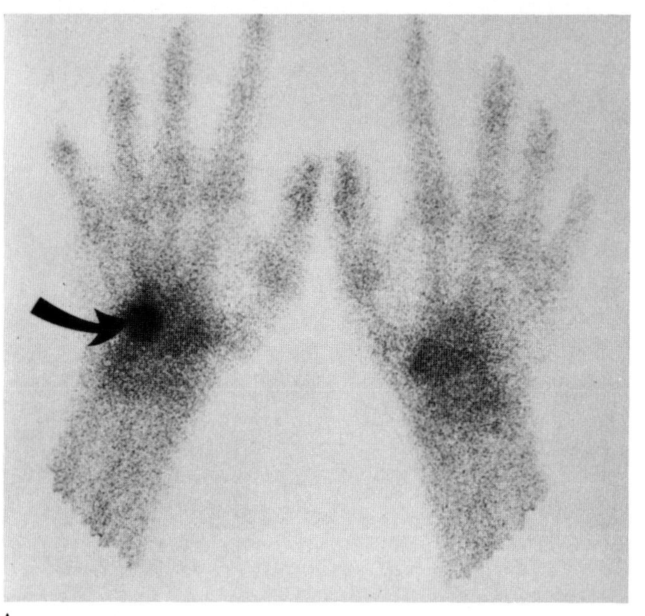

A

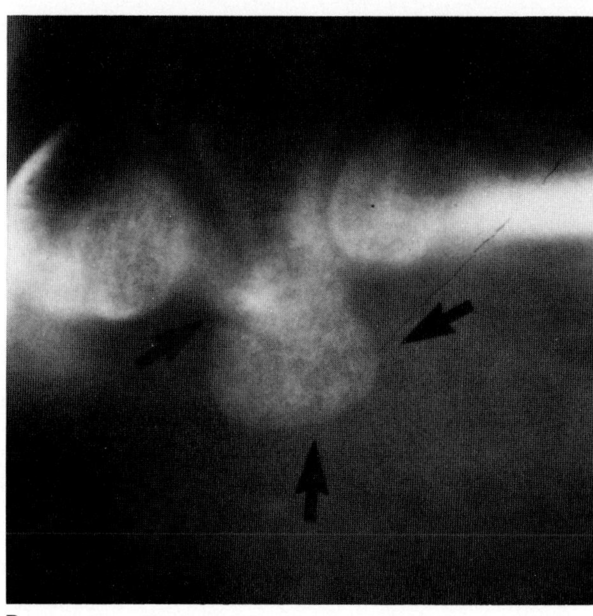

B

Fig. 2-5 Radiographic examination of a golfer with pain in the palm of her hand. Routine radiographs were normal. (**A**) Technetium-99m bone scan shows focal uptake in the ulnar aspect of the wrist (arrow). (**B**) Tomogram of this region demonstrates a subtle fracture (arrows) of the hamate hook.

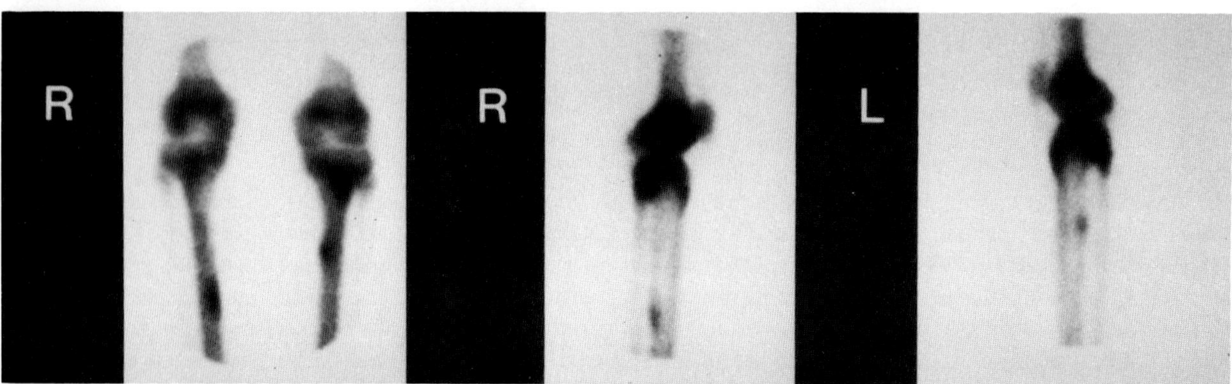

Fig. 2-6 Bone scans in a jogger with bilateral tibial pain demonstrating focal uptake in both tibias due to stress fractures.

Vascularity of Bone

The vascularity of bone can be assessed with the use of radiotracers. As mentioned above, bone scanning has a potential clinical role in evaluating femoral head vascularity after fracture. In a patient suspected of having Legg-Calvé-Perthes disease, the bone scan will demonstrate a lack of tracer before radiographic findings appear.[44,52] The results of one large series showed a sensitivity of 98%, a specificity of 95%, and an accuracy of 96%.[44] After revascularization, the bone scan may reveal increased activity in the femoral head. Elderly patients with painful knees may show intense activity in the metaphysis of the tibia or femur as a result of osteonecrosis.[53] Bone scintigraphy may also play a role in the early evaluation of bone grafts, detecting vascularity in the first postoperative week. Studies performed later may not be accurate because uptake may occur in a thin area of new cortical bone and may not demonstrate true graft viability.[40]

Infection

Bone scanning is helpful in the evaluation of patients with suspected osteomyelitis.[57] There are pitfalls in its use, however, especially in neonatal osteomyelitis, in patients with orthopaedic appliances, and in patients with recent trauma or surgery. Gallium- and indium-labeled white cells can be helpful in these instances.

Further Clinical Applications

The bone scanning agents accumulate in the arthritides. Although the pattern of localization may help differentiate between rheumatoid arthritis and the rheumatoid variants, the scan is less specific than radiographic findings, and its ability to aid in the diagnosis and follow-up of patients with arthritis is uncertain. When it is important to assess accurately the compartmental involvement in osteoarthritis of the knee, the bone scan is more sensitive than radiographs or arthrography.[40,52]

COMPUTED TOMOGRAPHY

The introduction of CT has played a major role in improving imaging of most structures in the body and has resulted in a decrease in the use of more invasive imaging modalities, such as angiography. It has a secondary role in skeletal imaging because in most areas it has not supplanted the routine radiograph. CT of the musculoskeletal system, however, can provide additional information in a number of sports injuries.[65–69,75,76,78,85,89]

CT scanners use highly collimated X-ray beams, highly efficient detectors, and computer-image reconstruction and display to produce images that have superior contrast resolution but slightly less spatial resolution than routine radiographs. CT thus provides better display of soft tissues than any plain film technique. In addition, the transverse axial orientation of the images is a useful supplement to the plain film examination of skeletal structures.[76,83,89]

All CT scanners have three components: the scanning gantry, the computer, and the display console. The scanning gantry contains the X-ray source, detection system, and couch and positioning system for the patient. The patient lies on the horizontal couch and moves through a circular opening in the vertically oriented scanning gantry, passing through the field of the X-ray source and detectors. Although many gantry systems can be tilted a few degrees from the vertical, the orientation of the system permits only transverse axial images to be obtained in most cases. Therefore, sagittal and coronal images are usually obtained by computer reformatting of the transverse axial image data rather than by direct scanning. Certain regions such as the facial bones and peripheral extremities can be positioned to obtain direct coronal or sagittal data. In a typical CT scanner the X-ray tube moves through 360° at small increments (as many as 1200 increments or more) during a single CT scan slice. The X-ray detectors (which can be fixed or rotated opposite the X-ray tube) take several hundred measurements of X-ray transmission at each increment. Each slice requires one or more seconds depending upon the scanner used. In critically injured patients or patients with respiratory difficulty, fast scanners are required. Electron beam CT scanning, in which there are no moving parts, allows scan times as short as 50 msec. The use of subsecond scan times greatly enhances CT images in this patient population. Dynamic images of the extremities can also be obtained in this manner.[67,89]

The data from the X-ray detectors are processed by a computer that uses an algorithm (a series of mathematical formulas) to manipulate the data and to reconstruct an image of the scanned object. Reconstruction time for a single image varies from 1 to 60 seconds. The computer divides the scanned area into a matrix (eg, 256 × 256 or 512 × 512) of small squares (picture elements or pixels). An X-ray attenuation coefficient is determined for each square by applying the reconstruction algorithm to the data obtained by the detectors. Each square is then assigned a CT number related to the attenuation coefficient (with the CT number of water being 0). The numbers are displayed on the final image as various shades of gray, with the highest numbers (eg, for air) being black.[89]

Because the X-ray beam in the scanner has a finite thickness (from 3 to 13 mm for most scanners), the X-ray attenuation coefficient calculated by the computer for each pixel actually represents the average coefficient of a volume of tissue rather than a plane. The pixel thus actually represents a volume element or voxel. This can introduce a significant artifact, called a partial volume effect, into the final image. This occurs when two objects that have different X-ray attenuation coefficients (eg, bone and fat) are both included in the volume scanned. Because the pixels displayed on the monitor screen are represented as the average attenuation coefficient of the contents of the voxel, the number for the voxel containing both bone and fat will be somewhere between the actual attenuation coefficients of bone and fat. This partial volume artifact can result in significant errors. For example, a fracture line in the transverse plane of the scan can be missed because it is averaged in with the bone in the rest of the voxel.

The reconstructed image is displayed on a console that allows the operator to manipulate the window width (range of CT numbers in the gray scale) and the window level (center of the gray scale) optimally to display either bone detail or soft tissues. In addition, the operator can obtain sagittal or coronal reconstructions of the scanned object by means of computer reconstruction of the transverse image data.

Many CT scanners can also produce digital radiographs of any area of the body by moving the patient through the X-ray beam with sampling at intervals from the X-ray detectors. These digital images are of lesser quality than routine radiographs but can be quite useful for localization purposes.

The X-ray dose delivered by a CT scan varies with a number of factors, some related to the CT unit (eg, transverse spatial resolution, slice thickness, and scan noise) and some related to the individual examination (eg, the number of slices obtained and the degree of overlap of the slices). In general, the dose is greater than that for a single radiograph but less than that for conventional tomograms of the same body part. CT doses may vary from less than 1 rad to more than 10 rads.[65,82]

The radiologist should review the patient's history and the indication for the examination to tailor the procedure to the patient's problem. In most cases, contiguous slices 1 cm thick are adequate, although in evaluation of small lesions or anatomically complex areas such as the spine thinner slices at overlapping intervals are required. The latter is especially important if three-dimensional reconstruction is contemplated.[72,74,85–88] Anatomic symmetry is useful in evaluating CT images of the skeletal system, and therefore care should be taken to position the patient symmetrically within the scanner. The contralateral side should be included whenever possible. The gastrointestinal tract can be opacified with oral or rectal contrast medium if a lesion in the abdomen or pelvis is suspected. Administration of intravenous contrast agents by rapid infusion or bolus technique with rapid acquisition of multiple slices may be useful in detecting subtle soft tissue lesions or in detecting the relationship of pathology to major vessels. Nonionic contrast material has supplanted ionic contrast material in patients with contrast allergy, significant cardiovascular disease, or certain other specific contraindications. In these patient groups nonionic medium provides an increased margin of safety. The radiologist should monitor the procedure and manipulate the display controls (window level and window width) to ensure optimal display of both bones and soft tissues. Images of bones should be viewed at wide window width settings and high window levels; soft tissues are best displayed at narrower window widths and lower levels.

The quality of the CT image is affected by a number of variables beyond the control of the examiner. In general, individual muscles, vessels, and nerves are optimally imaged when surrounded by fat. Thus the scan is less helpful in examining thin patients, infants, or the distal extremities.[65,73] Patient motion produces significant degradation of image quality. This can be especially troublesome in a severely injured or uncooperative patient. Metallic objects such as joint prostheses, internal fixation devices, and surgical clips produce artifacts that may obscure detail in the region of interest.[74]

CT is particularly useful in examination of the bones in areas of complex anatomy such as the pelvis, hips, sacrum, spine, shoulders, and face.[72,77,78,81,83,88] In addition, some areas that cannot be displayed easily on routine radiographs, such as the sternoclavicular joints, are optimally seen on the cross-sectional images obtained by CT.[70] Occult fractures not visible on plain films or tomograms may be detected, especially in the spine.[64,65,69,78,79,84] Some investigators have found CT to be more useful than plain film tomography in the evaluation of the vertebral column after trauma.[64] Most have found that CT adds valuable information to routine radiographs in the majority of cases, although most cases studied by CT have been selected instances rather than consecutive cases of trauma. In addition to the presence of a fracture, CT can demonstrate bone, disc, blood, or foreign bodies in the spinal canal.[72,79] Nonionic contrast medium may be introduced for better delineation of the spinal canal.[85] Plain films are still essential because CT may miss horizontal fractures (fractures parallel to the plane of the scan slice, such as odontoid fractures) owing to the partial volume effect or improper slice selection. In addition, it is difficult to detect vertebral body compression fractures, subluxations, and increased intervertebral distance on CT scans alone.[79]

CT scans of the shoulder, hip, or pelvis after trauma aid in the display of the spatial relationships of the fracture fragments before and after reduction. CT may detect intraarticular fragments that prevent reduction and require operative intervention.[69,76,78,80] Three-dimensional reconstruction is most often used to assist with surgical planning for these complex fractures.[72,86,88]

CT can accurately detect soft tissue injuries and is especially important in evaluating the abdomen after trauma.[87] Evaluation of periarticular soft tissue injuries in the extremities is also possible, however. Magnetic resonance imaging (MRI) and, in some cases, sonography may be better suited in this setting.[71,73]

MAGNETIC RESONANCE IMAGING

Resonance properties of nuclei were first reported by Block and Purcell. Early work in the field was initiated by Damadian and Lauterbur.[104] Since then, clinical interest in MRI as an imaging modality has increased rapidly. Technologic advancements have progressed significantly, resulting in improved image quality and patient throughput and in some cases improved specificity.[90–98,102,107,108]

The principles of MRI are beyond the scope of this small chapter. The reader is referred elsewhere for more detailed discussions.[92,109]

Clinical Techniques

MRI has rapidly become an accepted technique in evaluation of the musculoskeletal system, specifically soft tissue trauma but also articular and skeletal injuries.[91,92,103,110] Respiratory motion is not a significant problem in the extremities as it is in the chest and upper abdomen, so that examination of the extremities is easily accomplished with MRI. Images can be obtained in the coronal, sagittal, oblique, and transaxial planes. In addition, soft tissue contrast is superior to that in CT and other imaging techniques.

With conventional pulse sequences, normal anatomic tissues have fairly characteristic signal intensities. Fat and medullary bone have the highest signal intensity and appear nearly white on MR images. Signal intensity of articular cartilage is between that of muscle and medullary bone. It has been suggested that the different image appearance of articular meniscal cartilage is probably due to variations in the type of collagen and content of water of these structures.[101] Water content of articular cartilage is higher (75% to 80%) than that of menisci. Menisci ligaments and tendons appear black on MR images. These structures are composed of predominantly type I collagen (articular cartilage is type II) and contain less water.[101] Therefore, articular cartilage typically has a gray appearance on MR images, and the latter tend to appear dark or black. Blood vessels also appear black if flow is normal. Signal intensity in vascular structures may vary, however, depending upon the velocity of flow and other pulse sequence variables. Cortical bone is white on CT images and often causes a significant beam-hardening artifact, decreasing the ability to evaluate juxtacortical soft tissues. Cortical bone is black on MR images, and there is no artifact. This allows adjacent soft tissues to be evaluated more easily.

MR examinations must be conducted differently than conventional radiographic or CT examinations. Patient selection, patient positioning, coil selection, and pulse sequences must be carefully considered to optimize image information and patient throughput.[90,92]

Patient Selection

The MRI gantry is more confining than a conventional fluoroscopic unit or CT scanner. Patients are typically positioned in the center of the cylindric magnet during the examination. Despite this apparent drawback, problems with claustrophobia are noted in only about 2% to 5% of patients.[92] Patients with claustrophobic tendencies seem to tolerate MR examinations more easily when they are in the prone position. The prone position makes positioning of the foot and ankle more difficult, and this should be considered when evaluating patients with disorders in this region. When necessary, mild sedation with oral diazepam may be helpful in patients with some degree of claustrophobia.

The patient's clinical status must also be considered. When significant discomfort or inability to maintain necessary positions is a problem, the examination may be difficult to complete. Premedication with diazepam or meperidine may be useful in these cases. Initially there was concern that severely ill patients requiring cardiac and respiratory monitoring would be difficult if not impossible to examine because ferromagnetic anesthesia equipment cannot be moved into the magnet room or near the gantry without affecting the images. Experience shows, however, that patients can be successfully monitored with proper equipment. Typical equipment includes a blood pressure cuff with plastic connectors, chest bellows for respiratory evaluation, and an electrocardiographic (ECG) telemetry system. Respiratory rate and ECG are monitored on a Saturn monitor. Generally satisfactory monitoring can be achieved in patients without affecting image quality.[92]

Magnetic fields may affect certain metallic implants and electrical devices.[111,112] In most situations, the exact chemical structure of surgically implanted materials cannot be determined.[102] Nevertheless, early efforts to determine which implants are potentially dangerous to the patient or may affect image quality have been successful.[90,92,98,106–108] Synchronous pacemakers convert to the asynchronous mode when placed in a magnetic field. The pacemaker power pack may also torque in the magnetic field. In addition, significant image degradation may occur if the power pack is in the region being examined.[107] Numerous heart valves and other metallic materials have been studied and the artifacts generated are negligible without significant risk to the patient.[92,106]

The majority of surgical clips used at the Mayo Clinic are not ferromagnetic. A significant number of aneurysm clips (approximately 75%) are ferromagnetic, however, and torquing can be demonstrated in a magnetic environment.[106] Therefore, patients with aneurysm clips or pacemakers are currently not examined with MRI.

Manufacturers of most orthopaedic appliances (plates and screws, joint prostheses, etc) generally use high-grade stainless steel, cobalt, titanium, or multiphase alloys. These materials are usually not ferromagnetic but may contain small quantities of iron impurities. All the orthopaedic appliances at our institution have been tested for magnetic properties and heating. No heating or magnetic response has been detected.[92] External fixation devices, although bulky, may not be ferromagnetic and can be easily checked with a hand-held magnet before imaging. Early experience with metal implants at low and high field strengths (0.15 to 1.5 T) shows that artifacts are more significant at higher field strengths.[92] Evaluation of patients with casts and bulky dressings is also possible with MRI without causing significant problems with image quality.

Patient Positioning and Coil Selection

Patient positioning considerations include body part, patient size, and expected examination time. Typically the patient is examined with the most closely coupled coil possible to achieve the maximum signal-to-noise ratio and best basal resolution (Fig. 2-7).[90,92,99] Signal-to-noise ratios may increase four to six times with a limb coil compared to head or body coils.[99] The knee, leg, foot, and ankle can be examined in the circumferential extremity coil or with flat coils. Both are available with high-field magnets and should be used when they fit the clinical setting. With noncircumferential surface coils (flat or incomplete circle), the depth of view is limited. This can result in loss of uniform signal in structures farther from the coil. As a rule, the depth of view of the flat coils is approximately half the diameter or width of the coil.[99] A coil with a larger opening may be used when comparison with the opposite extremity is required. Recently, dual coils have become available for evaluation of both extremities simultaneously.

Position and course of the anatomic structures being studied must also be considered. Coronal and sagittal MR images do not necessarily have less significant partial volume effects than axial CT images. This must be kept in mind when the extent of disease processes in the coronal and sagittal planes is evaluated. When possible, image planes should be chosen to fit the structure being studied. This may require off-axis oblique planes for optimal evaluation of these anatomic regions.

Pulse Sequences and Imaging Parameters

Selection from among the different pulse sequences (inversion recovery, spin-echo, partial saturation, chemical shift, and gradient-echo techniques) and the many available echo times (TE) and repetition times (TR) at first seems cumbersome. Current experience indicates, however, that most musculoskeletal injuries can be evaluated with simple T1- and T2-weighted spin-echo sequences.[92] Short TE, TR spin-echo sequences are T1-weighted and can be performed quickly, providing excellent anatomic detail. Long TE, TR sequences are T2-weighted and are particularly useful for evaluating hemorrhage and other traumatic changes in the muscles, tendons, ligaments, and other soft tissues. More specific information regarding pulse sequences is presented in the anatomic chapters for imaging evaluation of specific traumatic conditions.

Clinical Applications

Superior soft tissue contrast, multiple image planes, and excellent spatial resolution give MRI many advantages over other techniques in evaluating soft tissue, articular, and even subtle osseous trauma (Fig. 2-8).[105] With MRI all structures can be examined; ultrasound is less versatile by comparison (Fig. 2-4). MRI is also of value in studying conditions that may be associated with trauma such as osteonecrosis and infection.[100] Specific changes seen with these conditions are described later in specific anatomic chapters.

ANGIOGRAPHY

Angiography is useful in the diagnosis and treatment of vascular injuries after blunt, penetrating, or operative trauma.[113–115,119–122,124] Vascular injuries include intimal injury, arterial transection or thrombosis, pseudoaneurysm, arteriovenous fistula, and venous thrombosis or transection.[125] Vascular trauma may be asymptomatic or may result in hemorrhage, pulse deficits, expanding masses, bruits, or signs of distal ischemia.[123] In addition, repetitive minor trauma, usually occupationally related, may result in vascular injury as serious as that produced by major trauma.[113] Ultrasound, CT, and new angiographic MRI techniques have

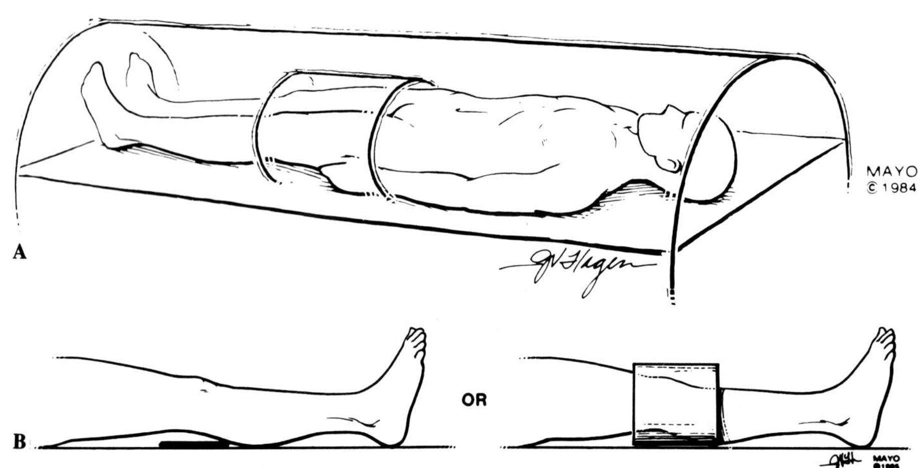

Fig. 2-7 Illustrations of patients positioned in the MR gantry with the body coil (**A**) and flat and circumferential knee coils (**B**). *Source:* Reprinted from *Magnetic Resonance Imaging of the Musculoskeletal System* by TH Berquist, 1990, Raven Press, © Mayo Foundation.

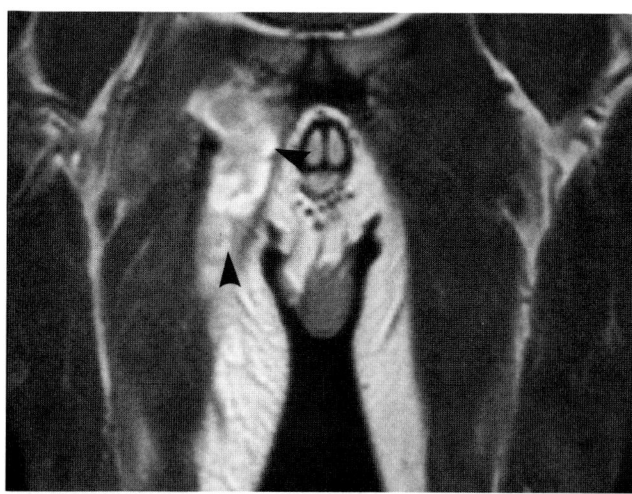

Fig. 2-8 MRI in a runner with acute groin pain. Coronal T2-weighted image (SE 2000/60) of the upper thighs shows a hematoma (arrowheads) due to an adductor muscle tear.

reduced the need for diagnostic angiography in many of the above conditions.

In addition to its use in diagnosis, angiography can be used to treat some arterial lesions by transcatheter introduction of embolic materials to produce temporary or permanent vessel occlusion. These techniques are most helpful in the patient with posttraumatic pelvic hemorrhage, the majority of which is due to arterial sources.[118] The bleeding arteries can be accurately localized and then occluded through the catheter, resulting in a high rate of successful cessation of the hemorrhage. In addition, some cases of pseudoaneurysm and arteriovenous fistula can be treated by transcatheter embolization.[120,125,126]

The angiogram should be performed on dedicated angiographic equipment if possible because this results in the highest quality films and the most flexibility in obtaining multiple views and various film series. A number of contrast media and catheter shapes are available, depending upon the type of study performed and the preference of the angiographer.

Digital subtraction angiography (DSA) can image vessels with less contrast agent than required for traditional film scans.[116] This technique links a computer with an X-ray fluoroscope and allows high-quality images of arteries to be made after intraarterial injection of contrast medium. The information from the fluoroscopic images is digitized, and the computer then subtracts an image made before injection of contrast material from images made after injection. The only difference between the two images, the contrast material in the blood vessels, is then enhanced by the computer, allowing excellent vascular images to be obtained. Initially this technique was used with intravenous injections, but because of poor image quality this has been largely abandoned. Currently DSA studies use intraarterial injections of contrast medium. The images obtained are perfectly adequate for the diagnosis of arterial occlusion in most areas of the body and in many cases will also allow detection of fine detail, such as intimal injuries. The main role of DSA in trauma patients is to decrease the amount of contrast medium used because these patients have multiple injections of contrast medium for various diagnostic tests.[116]

Technique

The angiographic examination and all other imaging examinations should be tailored to the clinical problems of the patient. The imaging evaluation should be designed in such a way that no tests that might interfere with a subsequent angiogram are performed. For example, oral or rectal contrast media should not be administered before angiography. In addition, care should be exercised in the amount of intravenous contrast material given both before and during the angiogram because large volumes of intravenous contrast material can have serious effects on renal function. One should be certain that the patient's other injuries can be stabilized long enough to allow angiography to be performed before surgical intervention is required. If not, the angiogram can be delayed. The angiographer should direct attention initially to the area of greatest clinical suspicion; survey examinations of the rest of the body should be performed afterward if the patient's condition and the amount of contrast medium used permit.

In most cases a transfemoral route by means of the Seldinger technique with selective catheterization of the affected vessel is the preferred approach for performance of the angiographic examination. In a few cases this route is not available owing to the extent of pelvic trauma or coexisting vascular disease. In these cases an axillary approach can be used. Complications of these techniques can occur at the puncture site (hemorrhage, arterial obstruction, pseudoaneurysm, or arteriovenous fistula), can result from the guide wire or catheter (vessel perforation, intimal damage, or distal embolization), or may be systemic (contrast medium reactions or cardiac and neurologic abnormalities). The incidence of complications is higher with the axillary than the transfemoral approach mainly because of an increase in the number of puncture sites and neurologic complications.[117]

Indications

Angiography can accurately identify the vast majority of trauma-induced arterial lesions. Despite years of experience with its use, however, the indications for angiography after trauma are still not well defined. In the extremities, some physicians advocate performing angiography in every case of blunt or penetrating trauma that occurs near a major vessel, whereas others favor angiography only when physical findings such as pulse deficit or bruit are present (Fig. 2-9).[123,124] Venography may be useful in a few cases to define venous injuries.

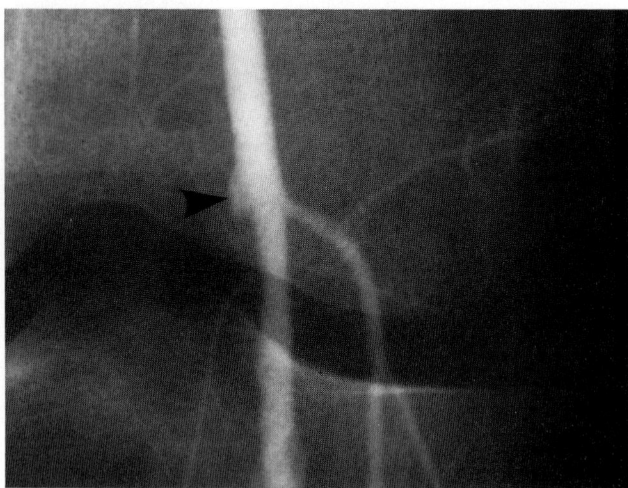

Fig. 2-9 Angiogram of the lower extremity showing an intimal injury (arrowhead) after trauma.

MYELOGRAPHY

Positive-contrast myelography has been accomplished for many years and provides useful information regarding the bony spinal canal, spinal cord, and nerve roots.[128] Until recently positive-contrast examination of the spinal canal was performed with film or fluoroscopic studies. The advent of CT of the spine has added a new imaging technique. The combination of CT and intrathecal contrast medium has provided an additional technique for evaluation of the posterior spinal structures that is complementary to conventional myelography (and occasionally more definitive).[130,132] More recently MRI has been substituted for myelography for many clinical problems.

Routine myelography is accomplished with the patient in the prone position on a radiographic table equipped for 90° tilt in either direction. Plain films should be thoroughly examined before the examination because subtle changes on these films may dictate changes in filming sequence and appropriate needle placement for the myelogram. Routinely a 20- to 22-gauge needle is introduced into the L2–3 interspace. Because of the level of the conus, puncture at a higher site is undesirable. If the needle is placed in a lower position, it may create artifacts, making it difficult to identify L-4 and L-5 pathology. This is, of course, a common location for lumbar disc disease. Spinal puncture should be made with fluoroscopic guidance to ensure an ideal midline position for the needle. This allows better positioning of the needle in the subarachnoid space for injection. After a single-wall midline puncture, cerebrospinal fluid should be collected for laboratory studies when indicated. The contrast material (typically nonionic or of low osmolality) is then injected under fluoroscopic observation to confirm its presence in the subarachnoid space. In most cases, 12 to 14 mL of contrast agent is all that is required. Fourteen to 20 mL of low-osmolality contrast medium (eg, Isovue 200) may be needed if the entire spine is being studied.

Filming for myelograms consists of a series of anteroposterior, cross-table lateral, and oblique exposures through the region of potential disease. Tilting the table under fluoroscopic control produces gravity-directed flow of the contrast material, allowing one to evaluate the site of interest.

In myelography with low-osmolality (nonionic), water-soluble contrast medium, several changes from the older iophendylate technique are employed.[127,129,131,133] The patient should be well hydrated, and any anticonvulsant therapy should be continued.

A small needle is used (20- to 22-gauge) because the contrast agent has low viscosity. A major advantage of the new nonionic and water-soluble contrast agents (eg, metrizamide) is that they need not be removed from the spinal canal after the procedure. These contrast agents are totally absorbed from the cerebrospinal fluid space and excreted through the kidneys in 24 to 48 hours. Although these agents are more directly irritating to the central nervous system than iophendylate, they are considered to have less potential to cause the late complication of arachnoiditis. Arachnoiditis has been attributed to iophendylate in certain cases. The lower risk of arachnoiditis with use of metrizamide is primarily due to the total disappearance of metrizamide through its early absorption.[134]

After myelography with a water-soluble agent the patient should be kept well hydrated, and the head should be elevated approximately 45° for several hours. This prevents the immediate ascent of a bolus of contrast medium into the intracranial region. Should this occur, the incidence of complications such as seizure is significant. With iophendylate the patient should be kept supine, well hydrated, and still with as little head movement as possible for at least 6 to 8 hours. If headaches occur after the myelogram, they should be treated supportively.

Although myelography is rarely indicated immediately after acute spinal trauma, in such cases the procedure is conducted quite differently. The needle must be positioned away from the lesion, often resulting in a lower puncture site or a C-1 puncture.[132] Only a small amount of cerebrospinal fluid should be removed in cases of potential obstruction. The fluid should be examined carefully, and if blood is present the significant risk of arachnoiditis must be recognized. In these situations, the water-soluble agents are the contrast materials of choice.[136]

Patient positioning may be a significant problem after acute injury. This may require additional equipment to stabilize the spine and to assist in controlled patient motion in directing the flow of contrast material.

In practice, myelography is most commonly used for definitive diagnosis or exclusion of herniated discs. This has changed significantly in recent years owing to the increased application of CT, with or without metrizamide, in evaluation of the spinal canal.[130,132] Other indications for conventional myelography include spondylosis or spinal stenosis, spinal tumors, congenital malformations, and arteriovenous malformations. Myelography is rarely indicated after acute spinal trauma. CT and conventional tomography will usually provide the necessary information. In selected patients myelography may be useful in defining the level of epidural obstruction after trauma or surgery and in localizing cervical nerve root avulsions.[132,135]

ARTHROGRAPHY AND TENOGRAPHY

Arthrography and tenography are extremely useful, benign procedures. Before the advent of MRI, these techniques were most frequently employed in the knee, shoulder, and hip; almost any accessible articulation may be evaluated, however (Fig. 2-10).[139] In recent years MRI has replaced knee arthrography, and MRI is also becoming an accepted technique for the shoulder.

To obtain the maximum amount of information, arthrography or tenography should be performed by an experienced radiologist with a thorough understanding of the patient's clinical situation.[137] Review of routine radiographs is essential. These films may provide clues that dictate subtle changes in film technique, which views may be required, and which contrast medium may be best suited for the procedure. Simply stated, these techniques should be tailored to the individual patient and not performed as a set procedure.

Equipment

Radiographic equipment should provide excellent detail and allow adequate work space to simplify patient positioning and needle placement. We prefer an overhead fluoroscopic tube with a small focal spot (no larger than 0.6 mm) and a 48-inch source-to-target distance. This provides better geometric positioning and resulting film quality than a conventional fluoroscopic suite with the X-ray tube under the table. The overhead tube allows better access to the patient, making the procedure less difficult to perform. This table, which is movable, can be used for all types of arthrography and interventional orthopaedic procedures.

The arthrogram set is devised so that all arthrograms and injections can be performed with the same tray. The tray includes the following items: four sterile drapes, one sterile drape with a 4-inch center hole, six absorbent 6 × 6 gauze sponges, one 5-mL syringe, two 10-mL syringes, one 30-mL syringe, one cup for contrast material, and extension tubing. A needle box is kept in the room. This contains 22- and 18-gauge spinal needles, 1½-inch 18- and 22-gauge needles, and ⅝-inch 25-gauge needles. Needle selection will vary depending on the joint to be studied and the size of the patient.

Additional items include vials of nonbacteriostatic saline solution for joint aspiration and irrigation, culture vials for aerobic and anaerobic bacterial and fungal studies, specimen tubes for synovial fluid analysis, and 1% lidocaine (Xylocaine). Betamethasone (Celestone) and 0.25% bupivacaine (Marcaine) are also stocked for diagnostic and therapeutic injections. Sterile conventional and leaded surgical gloves also should be available in the arthrographic suite. An additional necessity is an emergency tray or cart in case of contrast medium reactions or other unforeseen emergencies.

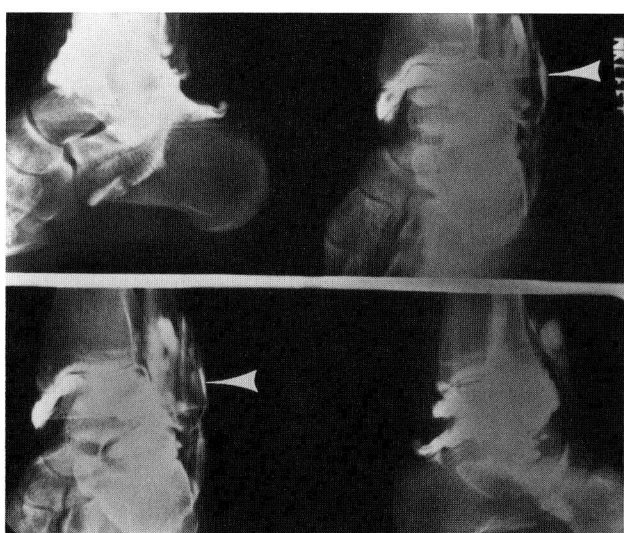

Fig. 2-10 Four views of an ankle arthrogram. There is filling of the peroneal tendon sheaths (arrowheads) due to a lateral ligament tear.

Arthrography and tenography may be performed with positive-contrast material, air, or double-contrast techniques that use both a positive-contrast medium and air or carbon dioxide. Several contrast media are available. We most commonly use Hypaque-M-60 (Winthrop). Renografin-60 and Reno M-60 (Squibb) may also be used. Iodine content (approximately 47% with Hypaque-M-60) does not differ significantly from that in other arthrographic contrast media. Sodium content with these contrast agents is less than that with other diatrizoates, however, resulting in less irritation. Extracapsular injection is particularly painful if the sodium content of the contrast medium is too high. New nonionic, low-osmolality agents are not frequently used in our practice.

Because of increased osmolality and rapid absorption, contrast medium becomes rapidly diluted in joints and tendon sheaths, resulting in loss of detail on the radiographs. This may occur in 5 to 10 minutes after the injection. If an effusion is present in the joint, the detail may deteriorate even more rapidly. This can be prevented to some degree by combining 0.3 mL of 1:1000 epinephrine with the contrast material.[138] Epinephrine may cause systemic side effects, however, and should not be used in patients with cardiac disease. Epinephrine is generally reserved for cases that require tomography or CT in addition to conventional views. Tomography requires significantly more time, and if epinephrine is not used the image quality may be decreased.

Metrizamide, which is used in myelography, is a water-soluble contrast medium that has also been investigated for arthrographic purposes. Metrizamide also remains in the joint longer and has a lower incidence of postarthrographic effusion compared to Urografin-60 and Conray-282.[142,143] New low-osmolality contrast agents may also play a role but have not been used extensively for arthrotenography because of their cost.

In the shoulder, knee, and elbow, double-contrast technique provides increased articular detail. We routinely use room air rather than carbon dioxide. Room air is less expensive and readily available, and we have not experienced any complications. Rarely, room air alone is used in patients with a significant history of allergy to contrast media.

Complications

Articular and tendon sheath injections are benign procedures with little risk of significant complications. Freiberger and Kaye[138] reported an incidence of infection of 1 per 25,000 cases. Effusions may occur after arthrography whether contrast medium or air alone is used. The effusion usually appears within 12 hours of the arthrogram and results in pain and stiffness of the involved joint.[138] Eosinophilic infiltration of the synovium has also been demonstrated[141] and may explain postarthrographic pain and swelling. Regardless of the etiology of the effusion and discomfort, they do not usually constitute a significant problem, especially when the diagnostic usefulness of the procedure is considered. This difficulty seems to be less of a problem after double-contrast studies, perhaps because of the smaller volumes of contrast medium used with this technique.[140] Also, air may remain in the joint for up to 10 days, which will result in increased crepitation in the joint.

Patients should be questioned concerning allergies to iodinated contrast media before arthrography is performed. Allergy to contrast agents must be considered but is extremely rare, patients with allergy numbering fewer than 1 per 1000 in the series reported by Freiberger and Kaye.[138] Urticaria is the usual reaction experienced, and often no treatment is required. Antihistamines may be used in more severe cases of urticaria. Most reactions to contrast medium develop within 15 to 30 minutes of the injection. When necessary, premedication with steroids can be useful.[144] MRI should be considered in patients with contrast agent allergies in most situations, however.

THERMOGRAPHY

Increase in body temperature in response to disease is a well-known process. Although not commonly used in practice at the Mayo Clinic, thermography provides a method of documenting surface temperature changes.

Infrared energy emitted by the body can be measured with special chemical and/or photoelectric methods. The radiation emitted is related to the surface area, energy emitted, and fourth power of the absolute temperature. The body's infrared energy ranges in wavelength from 3 to 75 μm (peak, 9.3 μm).[154]

Several thermographic techniques have been developed. These include contact thermography, telethermography, and computed thermography.[146,154,155] Contact thermography is performed with a flexible sheet containing cholesterol esters that is placed over the area of interest. Infrared energy changes the black cholesterol crystals to different colors depending upon the energy absorbed by the sheet. The sheet is photographed in position to document the different colors or energy levels. This allows abnormal vascular patterns and areas of increased temperature to be documented.[154,155] Telethermography uses an optical mirror system to measure infrared energy. The mirrors (thermistors) convert infrared energy into electrical energy for CRT display. Permanent images are obtained or created from the CRT.[154] Computed thermography uses multiple thermistors. The signals are converted to actual numbers. An image is not formed.[154]

Thermographic evaluation of patients requires a carefully controlled environment, including temperature, humidity, and ventilation. Patients should avoid excessive sun exposure for 2 days before the examination. Food, liquids, and medications are restricted for at least 2 hours before the examination.[154,155]

Thermography was initially used to evaluate breast cancer.[153] In recent years arthropathies, deep venous thrombosis, reflex sympathetic dystrophy, herniated discs, and sports injuries have been studied with thermography.[145–152,156–158] The degree of inflammation and blood flow to an area can be correlated with the temperature elevation. After treatment of injuries, their physiologic evolution can be evaluated using thermographic techniques.[146] Thermographic features can be correlated with physical findings, especially in patients with injuries that may not require more sophisticated imaging to follow their course.

REFERENCES

Routine Radiology, Tomography, and Magnification Radiography

1. Apple JS, Martinez S, Allen NB, Caldwell DS, Rice JR. Occult fractures of the knee: tomographic evaluation. *Radiology*. 1983;148: 383–387.

2. Ballinger PW. *Merrill's Atlas of Roentgenographic Positions and Standard Radiologic Procedures*. St Louis, MO: Mosby; 1982.

3. Bernau A, Berquist TH. *Orthopedic Positioning in Diagnostic Radiology*. Baltimore: Urban & Schwarzenberg; 1983.

4. Berquist TH. *Imaging of Orthopedic Trauma*. 2nd ed. New York: Raven; 1991.

5. Berrett A, Brunner S, Valvassori GE. *Modern Thin Section Tomography*. Springfield, IL: Thomas; 1973.

6. Bureau of Radiological Health. *Gonadal Shielding in Diagnostic Radiology*. Rockville, MD: Bureau of Radiological Health; 1975. Food and Drug Administration publication FDA 75-8024.

7. Curry TS, Dowdey JE, Murry JR. *An Introduction to the Physics of Diagnostic Radiology*. 4th ed. Philadelphia: Lea & Febiger; 1990.

8. Eastman Kodak Co. *The Fundmentals of Radiology*. 12th ed. Rochester, NY: Eastman Kodak; 1980.

9. Fletcher DE, Rowley KA. Radiographic enlargements in diagnostic radiology. *Br J Radiol*. 1951;24:598–604.

10. Genant HK, Kunio D, Mall JC, Sickles EA. Direct magnification for skeletal radiography. *Radiology*. 1977;123:47–55.

11. Gordon SL, Greer RB, Wiedner WA. Magnification roentgenographic technique in orthopedics. *Clin Orthop*. 1973;91:169–173.

12. McCullough EC, Coulam CM. Physical and dosimetric aspects of diagnostic geometrical and computer assisted tomographic procedures. *Radiol Clin North Am*. 1976;14:3–24.

13. Milne E. Magnification radiology. *Appl Radiol*. 1976:12. Editorial.

14. Nemet A, Cox WF. The improvement of definition of X-ray image magnification. *Br J Radiol.* 1956;29:335–337.

15. Norman A. The value of tomography in the diagnosis of skeletal disorders. *Radiol Clin North Am.* 1970;8:251–258.

16. Orhan HS, Showalter CK, Koustenis GH, et al. *A Sensitometric Evaluation of Film-Screen-Chemistry-Processor Systems in the State of New Jersey.* Rockville, MD: Bureau of Radiological Health; 1982.

17. Pavloy H, Torg JS, Freiberger RH. Tarsal navicular stress fractures: radiographic evaluation. *Radiology.* 1983;148:641–645.

18. Picus D, McAlister WH, Smith E, Rodewald S, Jost GR, Evens RG. Plain radiography with a rare-earth screen: comparison with calcium tungstate screen. *AJR.* 1984;143:1335–1338.

19. Resnick D, Niwayama G. *Diagnosis of Bone and Joint Disorders.* Philadelphia: Saunders; 1988.

20. Wagner LK, Cohen G, Wong W, Amtey SR. Dose efficiency and the effects of resolution and noise detail perceptibility in radiographic magnification. *Med Phys.* 1981;8:24–32.

21. Weiss A. A technique for demonstrating fine detail in the bones of the hand. *Clin Radiol.* 1972;23:185–187.

Ultrasound

22. Bluth EI, Merritt CRB, Sullivan MA. Gray scale ultrasound evaluation of the lower extremities. *JAMA.* 1982;247:3127–3129.

23. Braunstein EM, Silver TM, Martel W, Jaffe M. Ultrasonographic diagnosis of extremity masses. *Skeletal Radiol.* 1981;6:157–163.

24. Carpenter JR, Hattery RR, Hunder GG, Bryan RS, McLeod RA. Ultrasound evaluation of the popliteal space. Comparison of arthrography and physical examination. *Mayo Clin Proc.* 1976;51:498–503.

25. Cooperberg PL, Tsang I, Truelove L, Knickerbocker WJ. Grey scale ultrasound in the evaluation of rheumatoid arthritis of the knee. *Radiology.* 1978;126:759–763.

26. Dorfman GS, Froelich JA, Cronan JJ, Urbanek PJ, Herndon JH. Lower extremity venous thrombosis in patients with acute hip fractures: determination of anatomic location and time of onset with compression sonography. *AJR.* 1990;154:851–855.

27. Farin PU, Jaroma H, Harju A, Simakallio S. Sonographic evaluation. *Radiology.* 1990;176:845–849.

28. Fornage BD, Scheruberg FL, Rifkin MD. Ultrasound examination of the hand. *Radiology.* 1985;155:785–788.

29. Gompels BM, Darlington LG. Grey scale ultrasonography and arthrography in evaluation of popliteal cysts. *Clin Radiol.* 1979;30:539–545.

30. Gordon GV, Edell S. Ultrasonic evaluation of popliteal cysts. *Arch Intern Med.* 1980;140:1453–1455.

31. Harcke HT, Grissom LE, Furkelstein MS. Evaluation of the musculoskeletal system with sonography. *AJR.* 1988;150:1253–1261.

32. Hermann G, Yeh HC, Lehr-James C, et al. Diagnosis of popliteal cysts: double contrast arthrography and sonography. *AJR.* 1981;137: 369–372.

33. Holder J, Fretz CJ, Terrier F, Gerber C. Rotator cuff tears: correlation of sonographic and surgical findings. *Radiology.* 1988;169:791–794.

34. Kaplan PA, Matamoros A, Anderson JC. Sonography of the musculoskeletal system. *AJR.* 1990;155:237–245.

35. Lawson TL, Mittler S. Ultrasonic evaluation of extremity soft tissue lesions with arthrographic correlation. *J Can Assoc Radiol.* 1978;29:58–61.

36. Leopold GR. Ultrasonography of superficially located structures. *Radiol Clin North Am.* 1980;18:161–173.

37. Sarti DA, Sample WF. *Diagnostic Ultrasound, Text and Cases.* Boston: Hall & Co; 1980.

38. Swett HA, Jaffe RB, McIff EB. Popliteal cysts: presentation as thrombophlebitis. *Radiology.* 1975;115:613–615.

39. Winsberg F, Cooperberg PL. *Real Time Ultrasonography.* New York: Churchill Livingstone; 1982.

Skeletal Scintigraphy

40. Brown ML. Skeletal scintigraphy. In: Berquist TH, ed. *Imaging of Orthopedic Trauma.* 2nd ed. New York: Raven; 1991:16–19.

41. Campbell G, Warnekros W. Tarsal stress fracture in a long distance runner. *J Am Podiatry Assoc.* 1983;73:532–536.

42. Collier BD, Johnson RP, Carrera GF, et al. Chronic knee pain assessed by SPECT: comparison with other modalities. *Radiology.* 1985;157:795–802.

43. Collier BD, Kir MK, Mills BJA, et al. Bone scan: a useful test for evaluating patients with low back pain. *Skeletal Radiol.* 1990;19:267–270.

44. Danigelis JA. Pinhole imaging in Legg-Perthes disease: further observations. *Semin Nucl Med.* 1976;6:69–82.

45. Desai A, Alavi A, Dalinka M, Brighton C, Esterhai J. Role of bone scintigraphy in the evaluation and treatment of nonunited fractures: concise communication. *J Nucl Med.* 1980;21:931–934.

46. Ganel A, Engel J, Oster Z, Farine I. Bone scanning and assessment of fractures of the scaphoid. *J Hand Surg.* 1979;4:540–543.

47. Geslien JE, Thrall JH, Espinosa JL, Older RA. Early detection of stress fractures using Tc-99m polyphosphate. *Radiology.* 1976;121:683–687.

48. Greiff J. Determination of the vitality of the femoral head with Tc-99m–Sn-pyrophosphate scintigraphy. *Acta Orthop Scand.* 1980;51: 109–117.

49. Greiff J, Lanng S, Hoilund-Carlsen PF. Early detection by Tc-99m–Sn-pyrophosphate scintigraphy of femoral head necrosis following medial femoral neck fractures. *Acta Orthop Scand.* 1980;51:119.

50. Gumerman LW, Fogel SR, Goodman MA, et al. Experimental fracture healing: evaluation of radionuclide bone imaging: concise communication. *J Nucl Med.* 1978;19:1320–1323.

51. Hoffer P. Gallium: mechanisms. *J Nucl Med.* 1980;21:282–285.

52. Holder LE. Clinical radionuclide bone imaging. *Radiology.* 1990; 176:607–614.

53. Lotke PA, Ecker ML, Alavi A. Painful knees in older patients: radionuclide diagnosis of possible osteonecrosis with spontaneous resolution. *J Bone Joint Surg Am.* 1977;59:617–621.

54. Matin P. The appearance of bone scans following fractures, including immediate and long-term studies. *J Nucl Med.* 1979;20:1227–1231.

55. Merkel KD, Brown ML, Dewanjee MK, Fitzgerald RH. Comparison of indium-labeled leukocyte imaging with sequential technetium-gallium scanning in the diagnosis of low-grade musculoskeletal sepsis. *J Bone Joint Surg Am.* 1985;67:465–476.

56. Oyen WJG, Claessens RAMJ, vanHorn JR, van der Meer JWM. Scintigraphic detection of bone and joint infections with indium-111 labeled nonspecific polyclonal human immunoglobulin. *J Nucl Med.* 1990; 31:403–412.

57. Rosenthal L, Kloiber R, Damten B, Al-Majed H. Sequential use of radiophosphate and radiogallium imaging in the differential diagnosis of bone, joint, and soft tissue infection: quantitative analysis. *Diagn Imaging.* 1982;51:249–258.

58. Rubin RH, Fischman AJ, Callahan RJ, et al. ^{111}In-Labeled nonspecific immunoglobulin scanning in detection of focal infection. *N Engl J Med.* 1989;321:935–940.

59. Seabold JE, Nepola JV, Conrad GR. Detection of osteomyelitis at fracture non-union sites: comparison of two scintigraphic methods. *AJR.* 1989;152:1021–1027.

60. Spencer RB, Levinson ED, Baldwin RD, Sziklas JJ, Witek JT, Rosenberg R. Diverse bone scan abnormalities in "shin splints." *J Nucl Med.* 1979;20:1271–1272.

61. Subramanian G, McAfee JG. A new complex for skeletal imaging. *Radiology.* 1971;99:192–196.

62. Subramanian G, McAfee JG, Bell EG, Blair RJ, Omara RE, Ralston RH. Tc-99m–Labeled polyphosphate as a skeletal imaging agent. *Radiology.* 1972;102:701–704.

63. Wilcox JR, Moniot AL, Green JP. Bone scanning and the evaluation of exercise-related injuries. *Radiology*. 1977;123:699–703.

Computed Tomography

64. Brant-Zawadzki M, Miller EM, Federle MP. CT in the evaluation of spine trauma. *AJR*. 1981;136:369–375.

65. Brasch RC, Boyd DP, Gooding CA. Computed tomographic scanning in children: comparison of radiation dose and resolving power of commercial CT scanners. *AJR*. 1978;131:95–101.

66. Canale ST, Manugian AH. Irreducible traumatic dislocations of the hip. *J Bone Joint Surg Am*. 1979;61:7–14.

67. Chang W. Slice characteristics of the Imatron cine-CT scanner. *J Comput Assisted Tomogr*. 1987;11:554–557.

68. Coin CG, Pennink M, Ahmad WD, Keranen VJ. Diving type injury to the cervical spine: contribution of computed tomography to management. *J Comput Assisted Tomogr*. 1979;3:362–372.

69. Colley DP, Dunsker SB. Traumatic narrowing of the dorsolumbar spinal canal demonstrated by computed tomography. *Radiology*. 1978; 129:95–98.

70. Destouet JM, Gilula LA, Murphy WA, Sagel SS. Computed tomography of the sterno-clavicular joint and sternum. *Radiology*. 1981; 138:123–128.

71. Dooms GC, Fisher MR, Hricak H, Higgins CB. MR Imaging of intramuscular hemorrhage. *J Comput Assisted Tomogr*. 1985;9:908–913.

72. Drebin RA, Magid D, Robertson DD, Fishman EK. Fidelity of three dimensional CT imaging for detecting fracture gaps. *J Comput Assisted Tomogr*. 1989;13:487–489.

73. Ehman RL, Berquist TH. Magnetic resonance imaging of musculoskeletal trauma. *Radiol Clin North Am*. 1986;24:291–319.

74. Fishman EK, Magid D, Robertson DD, et al. Metallic implants: CT with multiplanar reconstruction. *Radiology*. 1986;160:675–681.

75. Genant HK. Computed tomography. In: Resnick D, Niwayama G, eds. *Diagnosis of Bone and Joint Disorders*. Philadelphia: Saunders; 1981:380–408.

76. Genant HK, Cann CE, Chafetz NI, Helms CA. Advances in computed tomography of the musculoskeletal system. *Radiol Clin North Am*. 1988;19:645–674.

77. Gilula LA, Murphy WA, Chandrakant CT, Patel RB. Computed tomography of the osseous pelvis. *Radiology*. 1979;132:107–114.

78. Griffiths HJ, Hamlin DJ, Kiss S, Lovelock J. Efficacy of CT scanning in a group of 174 patients with orthopedic and musculoskeletal problems. *Skeletal Radiol*. 1981;7:87–98.

79. Handel SF, Lee YY. Computed tomography of spinal fractures. *Radiol Clin North Am*. 1981;19:69–89.

80. Lange TA, Alter AJ. Evaluation of complex acetabular fractures by computed tomography. *J Comput Assisted Tomogr*. 1980;4:849–852.

81. Lasda NA, Levinsohn EM, Yuan HA, Bunnell WP. Computerized tomography in disorders of the hip. *J Bone Joint Surg Am*. 1978;60: 1099–1102.

82. McCullough EC, Payne JT. Patient dosage in computed tomography. *Radiology*. 1978;129:457–463.

83. McLeod RA, Stephens DH, Beabout JW, Sheedy PF III, Hattery RR. Computed tomography in the skeletal system. *Semin Roentgenol*. 1978; 13:235–247.

84. O'Callaghan JP, Ulrich CG, Yuan HA, Kieffer SA. CT of facet distraction in flexion injuries of the thoracolumbar spine: the naked facet. *AJR*. 1980;134:563–568.

85. O'Connor JF, Cohen J. Computerized tomography in orthopedic surgery. *J Bone Joint Surg Am*. 1978;60:1096–1098.

86. Pate D, Resnick D, Andre M, et al. Perspective: three dimensional imaging of the musculoskeletal system. *AJR*. 1986;147:545–551.

87. Toombs BD, Lester RG, Ben-Menachem Y, Sandler CM. Computed tomography in blunt trauma. *Radiol Clin North Am*. 1981;19:17–35.

88. Totty WG, Vannier MW. Complex musculoskeletal anatomy: analysis using three dimensional surface reconstruction. *Radiology*. 1984; 150:173–177.

89. Welch TJ. Computed tomography. In: Berquist TH, ed. *Imaging of Orthopedic Trauma*. 2nd ed. New York: Raven; 1991:26–28.

Magnetic Resonance Imaging

90. Beltran J, Nato AM, Mosure JC, Shaman OM, Weiss KL, Suegler WA. Surface coil imaging at 1.5 T. *Radiology*. 1986;161:203–209.

91. Berquist TH. Magnetic resonance imaging: preliminary experience in orthopedic radiology. *Magn Resonance Imaging*. 1984;2:41–52.

92. Berquist TH. *Magnetic Resonance Imaging of the Musculoskeletal System*. New York: Raven; 1990.

93. Block F. Nuclear induction. *Phys Rev*. 1948;70:7–8.

94. Bydder GM, Steiner RE, Young IR, et al. Clinical NMR images of the brain: 140 cases. *AJR*. 1982;139:215–236.

95. Crooks LE, Ortendahl DA, Kaufman L. Clinical efficacy of nuclear magnetic resonance imaging. *Radiology*. 1983;146:123–128.

96. Crooks LE, Arakawa M, Hoenninger J, et al. Nuclear magnetic resonance whole-body images operating at 3.5 kgauss. *Radiology*. 1982; 143:169–174.

97. Damadian R. Tumor detection by nuclear magnetic resonance. *Science*. 1971;171:1151–1153.

98. Davis PL, Crooks L, Arakawa M, McKee R, Kaufman L, Margulis A. Potential hazards of magnetic resonance imaging. *AJR*. 1981;137: 857–860.

99. Fisher MR, Barker B, Amparo E, et al. MR imaging using specialized coils. *Radiology*. 1985;157:443–447.

100. Fletcher BD, Scoles PV, Nelson DA. Osteomyelitis in children: detection by magnetic resonance imaging. *Radiology*. 1984;150:57–60.

101. Kanal E, Shellock FG, Talagala L. Safety considerations in MR imaging. *Radiology*. 1990;176:593–606.

102. King CL, Henkelman RM, Poon PY, Rubenstein J. MR Imaging of the normal knee. *J Comput Assisted Tomogr*. 1984;8:1147–1154.

103. Lackman RW, Kaufman B, Hans JS. MR Imaging in patients with metallic implants. *Radiology*. 1985;157:711–714.

104. Lauterbur P. Magnetic resonance zeugmatography. *Pure Appl Chem*. 1975;40:40.

105. Moon KL, Genant HK, Helms CA, Chafetz NI, Crooks LE, Kaufman L. Musculoskeletal applications of magnetic resonance imaging. *Radiology*. 1983;147:161–171.

106. New PFJ, Rosen BR, Brady TJ, et al. Potential hazards and artifacts of ferromagnetic and nonferromagnetic surgical and dental materials and devices in magnetic resonance imaging. *Radiology*. 1983;147:139–148.

107. Pavlicek W, Geisinger M, Castle L, et al. The effects of magnetic resonance imaging on patients with cardiac pacemakers. *Radiology*. 1983;147:149–153.

108. Purcell EM, Torrey HC, Pound RV. Resonance absorption by nuclear magnetic moments in a solid. *Phys Rev*. 1946;69:37–38.

109. Pykett I, Newhouse JH, Buonanno FS, et al. Principles of nuclear magnetic resonance imaging. *Radiology*. 1982;143:157–168.

110. Ranade SS, Shah S, Advani SH, Kasturi SR. Pulsed nuclear magnetic resonance studies of human bone marrow. *Physiol Chem Phys*. 1977; 9:297–299.

111. Saunders RD. Biological effects of NMR clinical imaging. *Appl Radiol*. 1982;11:43–46.

112. Schwartz JL, Crooks LE. NMR imaging produces no observable mutation or cytotoxicity on mammalian cells. *AJR*. 1982;139:583–585.

Angiography

113. Conn J, Bergan JJ, Bell JL. Hypothenar hammar syndrome: posttraumatic digital ischemia. *Surgery*. 1970;68:1122–1128.

114. Crossland SG, Slovin AJ. The role of arteriography in diagnosing unsuspected vascular injuries. *Am Surg*. 1978;44:98–103.

115. Fisher RG, Hadlock F, Ben-Menachem Y. Laceration of the thoracic aorta and brachiocephalic arteries by blunt trauma. *Radiol Clin North Am*. 1981;19:91–110.

116. Foley WD, Milde MW. Intra-arterial digital subtraction angiography. *Radiol Clin North Am*. 1985;23:293–319.

117. Hessel SJ. Complications of angiography and other catheter procedures. In: Abrams HL, ed. *Angiography*. Boston: Little, Brown; 1983: 1041–1056.

118. Kam J, Jackson H, Ben-Menachem Y. Vascular injuries in blunt pelvic trauma. *Radiol Clin North Am*. 1981;19:171–186.

119. Lang EK. Pelvic angiography. In: Abrams HL, ed. *Angiography*. Boston: Little, Brown; 1983:1753–1788.

120. Lang EK. Transcatheter embolization of pelvic vessels for control of intractable hemorrhage. *Radiology*. 1981;140:331–339.

121. Lang EK. The role of arteriography in trauma. *Radiol Clin North Am*. 1976;14:353–370.

122. Love L. Arterial trauma. *Semin Roentgenol*. 1970;5:267–283.

123. McDonald EJ, Goodman PC, Winestock DP. The clinical indications for arteriography in trauma to the extremity. *Radiology*. 1975;116:45–47.

124. Reid JDS, Redman HC, Wergelt JA, Thal ER, Frances H III. Value of angiography in detection of arterial injury. *AJR*. 1988;151:1035–1039.

125. Slaney G, Ashton F. Arterial injuries and their management. *Postgrad Med*. 1971;47:257–269.

126. Uflacker R. Transcatheter embolization of arterial aneurysms. *Br J Radiol*. 1986;59:317–324.

Myelography

127. Ahn HS, Rosenbaum AE. Lumbar myelography with metrizamide supplemental techniques. *Am J Neuroradiol*. 1981;136:547–551.

128. DiChiro G, Fisher RL. Contrast radiography of the spinal cord. *Arch Neurol*. 1964;11:125–143.

129. Fox AJ, Venulia F, Debrun G. Complete myelography with metrizamide. *Am J Neuroradiol*. 1981;2:79–84.

130. Genant HK, Chefetz N, Helms CA. *Computed Tomography of the Lumbar Spine. Diagnosis and Therapeutic Implications for the Radiologist, Orthopedist, and Neurosurgeon*. San Francisco: University of California Press; 1982.

131. Kieffer SA, Binet EF, Esquerra JV, Hantman RP, Gross CE. Contrast agents for myelography: clinical and radiographic evaluation of Amipaque and Pantopaque. *Radiology*. 1978;129:695–705.

132. Leo JS, Bergeron RT, Kricheff II, Benjamin MV. Metrizamide myelography for cervical spinal cord injury. *Radiology*. 1978;129:707–711.

133. McClennan BL. Low osmolality contrast media: premises and promises. *Radiology*. 1987;162:1–8.

134. Paling MR, Quindlin EA, DiChiro G. Spinal seizures after metrizamide myelography in a patient with spinal block. *Am J Neuroradiol*. 1980;1:473.

135. Pay NT, George AE, Benjamin MV, Bergeron T, Lin JP, Kricheff II. Positive and negative contrast myelography in spinal trauma. *Radiology*. 1977;123:103–111.

136. Skalpe IO. Adhesive arachnoiditis following lumbar radiculography with water soluble contrast agents. A clinical report with special reference to metrizamide. *Radiology*. 1976;121:647–651.

Arthrography and Tenography

137. Evans GA, Frenyo SD. The stress tenogram in diagnosis of ruptures of the lateral ligament of the ankle. *J Bone Joint Surg Br*. 1979;61:347–351.

138. Freiberger RH, Kaye J. *Arthrography*. New York: Appleton-Century-Crofts; 1979.

139. Gilala LA, Oloff L, Caputi R, Destouet JM, Jacobs A, Solomon MA. Ankle tenography: a key to unexplained symptomatology. *Radiology*. 1984;151:581–587.

140. Hall FM, Rosenthal DI, Goldberg RP, Wyshak G. Morbidity from shoulder arthrography. *AJR*. 1981;136:59–62.

141. Hasselbacher P, Schumacher HR. Synovial fluid eosinophilia following arthrography. *J Rheumatol*. 1978;5:173–176.

142. Johansen JC. Arthrography with Amipaque and other contrast media. *Invest Radiol*. 1976;11:534–540.

143. Katzberg RW. Evaluation of various contrast agents for improved arthrography. *Invest Radiol*. 1976;11;528–533.

144. Lasser EC. Pretreatment with corticosteroids to prevent reactions to IV contrast material: overview and implications. *AJR*. 1988;150:257–259.

Thermography

145. Ash CJ, Shealy CN, Young PA, Beaumont WV. Thermography and the sensory dermatome. *Skeletal Radiol*. 1986;15:40–46.

146. Bagarone A, Colombo G, Garagiola U. Correlation between clinical and thermographic evaluation in overuse injuries treatment. *J Sports Med*. 1987;27:64–69.

147. Bassett LW, Gold RH, Clement PJ, Furst D. Hand thermography in normal subjects and in scleroderma. *Acta Thermogr*. 1980;5:19–27.

148. Collins AJ, Ring F, Bacon PA, Brookshaw JD. Thermography and radiology. Complementary methods for the study of inflammatory disease. *Clin Radiol*. 1976;27:237–243.

149. Edieken J, Wallace AB, Curley BS, Lee S. Thermography and herniated lumbar disks. *AJR*. 1986;102:790–796.

150. Eiker A. Contact thermography in diagnosis of reflex sympathetic dystrophy: a new look at pathogenesis. *Thermography*. 1986;1:106–109.

151. Feldman F, Nickoloff EL. Normal thermographic standards for the cervical spine and upper extremities. *Skeletal Radiol*. 1984;12:235–249.

152. Hubbard JE, Hoyt C. Pain evaluation in 805 studies by infrared imaging. *Thermology*. 1986;1:161–169.

153. Lawson R. Radiology implications of surface temperature in diagnosis of breast cancer. *Can Med Assoc J*. 1956;75:309–310.

154. Milbrath JR. Thermography. In: Bassett LW, Gold RH, eds. *Mammography, Thermography, and Ultrasound in Breast Cancer Detection*. Orlando, FL: Grune & Stratton; 1982:143–149.

155. Pochacyevsky R. Liquid crystal thermography. *Orthop Clin North Am*. 1983;14:271–288.

156. Pulst SM, Haller P. Thermographic assessment of impaired sympathetic function in peripheral nerve injuries. *J Neurol*. 1981;226:35–42.

157. Sandler DA, Martin JF. Liquid crystal thermography in diagnosis of deep venous thrombosis. *Thermology*. 1986;1:92–94.

158. Ulmatsu S, Hendler N, Hungerford D, Long D, Ono N. Thermography and electromyography in the differential diagnosis of chronic pain syndromes and reflex sympathetic dystrophy. *Electromyogr Clin Neurophysiol*. 1981;21:165–182.

Chapter 3

The Spine

INTRODUCTION AND ANATOMY

Severe spinal injury is infrequent during recreational or sporting activities compared to its incidence in high-velocity motor vehicle accidents.[2,21,27] For example, only 4 head and neck injury fatalities in football occurred in 100,000 participants in 1968.[8] Nevertheless, significant spinal injury does occur in contact and high-velocity sports (Tables 3-1 and 3-2). Spine injuries due to sports accounted for 14% of 1,447 cases in a series reported by Reid and Saboe[20] and for 10% of injuries in children in a study by Anderson and Schutt.[2] The incidence of neurologic deficit and the location of injuries vary with the type of activity (Table 3-2). In sports such as diving, rugby, snowmobiling, skiing, and ice hockey, however, the incidence of neurologic deficit is high (42%).[20,27] Reid and Saboe[20] reported a 67% incidence of paralysis due to cervical spine fractures in hockey players. Less significant lower spinal injury is more common with jumping, running, or dancing[6,12,15] (Table 3-2). This chapter discusses the mechanism of injury and imaging approach in sports-related injuries to the cervical, thoracic, and lumbar spine.

Review of the essential osseous and ligamentous anatomy is crucial for proper interpretation and utilization of imaging

Table 3-1 Spine Injury: Etiology and Severity

Etiology	*Incidence of Spine Injury (%)*	*Incidence of Neurologic Deficit (%)*
Motor vehicle accident	53	26
Occupational	15	23
Home injuries	14	6
Sporting injuries	14	42
Other	4	30

Source: O'Leary P and Boiardo R in Nicholas JA and Hershman EB, *The Lower Extremity and Spine in Sports Medicine,* Vol 2, 1986, CV Mosby.

Table 3-2 Spinal Injury in Sports: Location and Frequency

	Location of Spine Injury		
Sport	*Cervical*	*Thoracic*	*Lumbar*
Auto racing[19]	+ + +	+ +*	
Ballet dancing[12]	+	+	+ +
Basketball[9,30,31]	+	+	+ +
Cross-country skiing[15,23]			+
Cycling[13]	+ +	+	+ + +
Diving[19,20]	+ + +	+	+
Equestrian[28]	+ + +	+	+ +
Football[5,8,14,16,18,25–27]	+ + +	+	+ +
Gymnastics[2,19]	+ +	+	+
Hockey[20,24]	+ + +	+	+ +
Jogging[1]	+	+	+ +
Motorcycling[6,19]	+ +	+ +*	
Parachuting[7]	+ + +	+	+ +
Racquet sports[19]	+ +	+	+
Rugby[29]	+ + +	+	+ +
Skiing[17,20]	+	+ + +*	
Snowmobiling[20]	+ +	+ + +*	
Tobogganing[20]	+ +	+ + +*	
Trampolining[22]	+ + +	+	+ +
Water skiing[11]	+	+	+ +
Weight lifting[3]	+	+	+ +
Wrestling[19]	+ + +	+	+ +

Symbols: +, uncommon location; + +, common location; + + +, most common location; *thoracolumbar junction.

techniques. Although a complete review of spinal anatomy is beyond the scope of this chapter, the essential anatomy required for radiographic interpretation is discussed.

Osteology

The vertebral column is composed of 7 cervical, 12 thoracic, 5 lumbar, 5 sacral, and 4 coccygeal segments. The lateral masses of C-1 (atlas) articulate with the occipital condyles at the base of the skull. The sacrum articulates with the innominate bones of the pelvis.[4,10]

The typical vertebral body consists of the anterior body and the vertebral arch, which is composed of two pedicles and two paired laminae. The laminae join posteriorly to form the spinous process. In addition, there are transverse processes bilaterally. Four extensions from the lamina-pedicle junction form the apophyseal or facet joints. The facets articulate with the vertebrae above and below. These apophyseal joints play an important role in determining the range and direction of motion of the vertebral column. Most of the weight-bearing function is provided by the vertebral bodies and interposed elastic vertebral discs. The apophyseal joints are also involved in weight-bearing, however, especially when one changes from the sitting to the standing position.[4,10]

There are several anatomic features that distinguish the regions of the spine. The bodies of the cervical and lumbar vertebrae are wider in transverse than in anteroposterior (AP) diameter (Fig. 3-1A). The thoracic vertebral body is more uniform in AP and lateral diameter. In the upper thoracic region the vertebral bodies are somewhat heart shaped. The spinal canal in the cervical and lumbar region is triangular compared with the smaller, circular configuration in the thoracic region (Fig. 3-1B). The transverse processes in the cervical region contain anterior and posterior tubercles as well as a distinguishing feature, the foramen transversarium (Fig. 3-1A). The vertebral artery traverses this foramen from C-7 to C-1. The transverse processes in the thoracic region are directed dorsally, and T-1 through T-10 contain facets for rib articulation (Fig 3-1B). Transverse processes in the lumbar region project almost straight laterally and increase in size from L-1 to L-3. The L-4 transverse process is shorter and directed more cephalad. The transverse process of L-5 is broader and sturdier and also is directed dorsally (Fig. 3-2).[4,19]

Spinous processes are short and often bifid in the cervical spine (Fig. 3-3A). The spinous process of C-7 is the longest and most prominent, whereas the spinous process of C-2 is short and bulbous (Fig. 3-3B). Spinous processes in the thoracic region are directed sharply caudad; they are long and narrow compared with the broad-based, short spinous processes in the lumbar region.[4]

The articular facets differ significantly in the cervical, thoracic, and lumbar regions. In the cervical spine the articular facets angle approximately 20° in a caudad direction with the facet directed posteriorly (Fig. 3-3B). A similar but steeper angle is present in the thoracic region, and the facets are angled slightly dorsolaterally. The facet joints in the lumbar region change abruptly, with the superior facets being directed dorsally and medially and the inferior facets being directed ventrally and laterally. This results in restricted rotation in the lumbar region.[4,10,12]

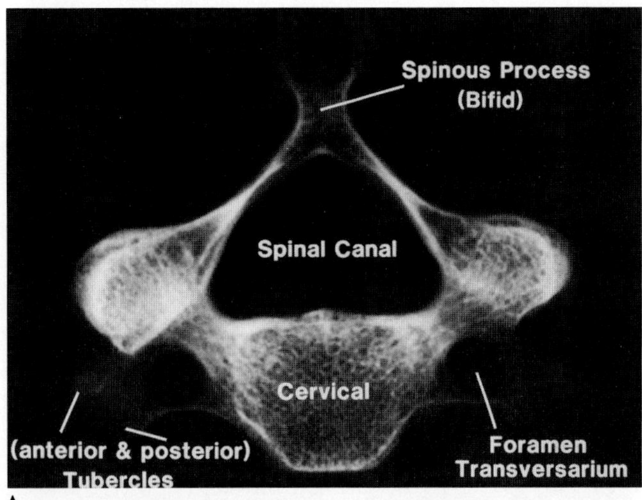

A

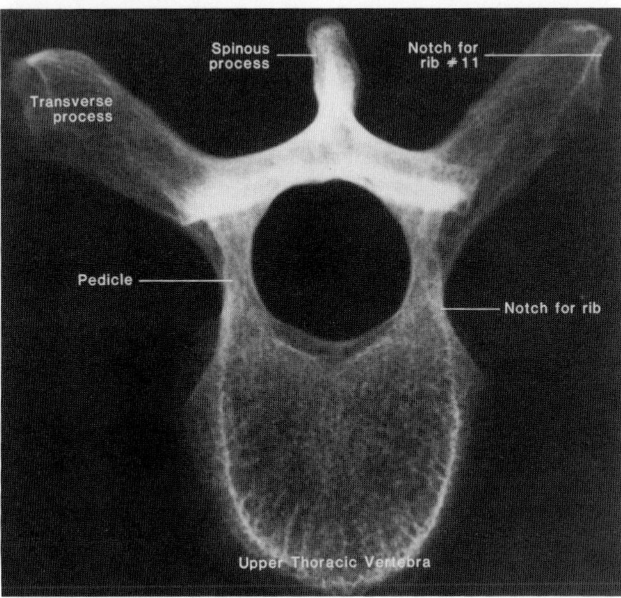

B

Fig. 3-1 Axial view of cervical (**A**) and thoracic (**B**) vertebrae. Note the difference in configuration of the spinal canal and foramen transversarium in the cervical vertebra. *Source:* Reprinted from *Imaging of Orthopedic Trauma* ed 2 by TH Berquist, 1991, Raven Press, © Mayo Foundation.

Cervical Vertebrae

The distinguishing feature of the cervical vertebrae is the foramen transversarium (Fig. 3-1). In addition, there are several significant anatomic differences between C-1, C-2, C-7, and the remaining cervical vertebrae (C-3 to C-6). The atlas has no vertebral body and lacks a true spinous process. C-1 (atlas) is a ringlike structure with a large vertebral foramen bounded by the anterior and posterior arches. There are two

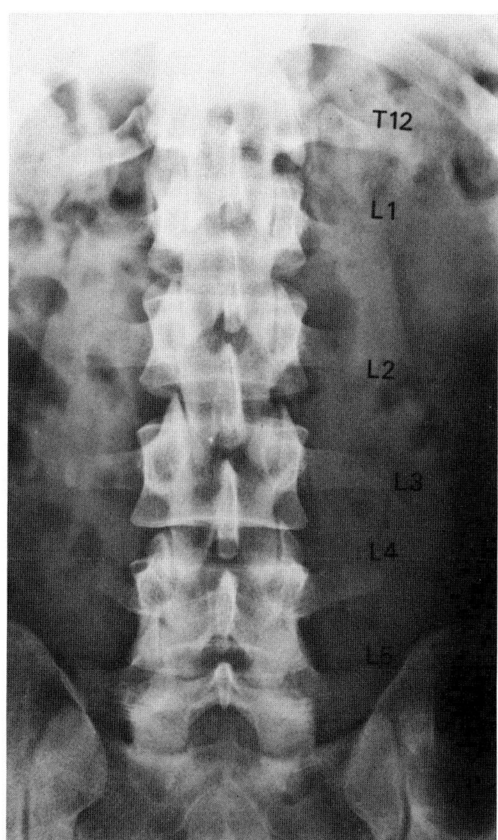

Fig. 3-2 Anteroposterior (AP) view of the lumbar spine demonstrating the configuration of the transverse processes.

large lateral masses that contain a superior articular facet. This facet articulates superiorly and medially with the occipital condyle. The inferior facet is directed medially and articulates with the superior facet of C-2. Medial to the lateral masses are tubercles for the attachment of the strong transverse ligament. The transverse processes of C-1 are also much larger compared with those of the remaining cervical vertebrae.[4,10]

The C-2 vertebra has several distinguishing features. These include a prominent but short spinous process that is helpful in differentiating the level of the upper cervical spine when the entire spine is not included on a radiographic film (Fig. 3-3B). The odontoid or dens projects superiorly from the body of C-2 and articulates with the anterior ring of C-1 (Fig. 3-4). The spinal canal at C-2 is significantly smaller and rounder than that of C-1. The articular facets of C-2 are also atypical compared with those of the remaining cervical spine. The superior facets are directed in a superolateral direction at an angle of approximately 20°.[4,10]

The C-3 through C-6 vertebrae are typical cervical vertebrae (Figs. 3-1 and 3-3) with triangular vertebral foramina, and typically the facet joints are directed inferiorly at approximately 20°. C-7 can be distinguished by its prominent spinous process (Fig. 3-3B).[4,10]

Thoracic Vertebrae

The upper and lower thoracic vertebrae have some features similar to those of the cervical or lumbar vertebrae. Thus the middle four thoracic vertebral bodies are most typical. In the upper thoracic spine the vertebral bodies are more triangular or heart shaped, with the apex of the triangle being directed ventrally (Fig. 3-1B). The vertebral bodies in the thoracic spine are typically larger in AP than in transverse diameter. The thoracic vertebral body is 1.5 to 2.0 mm shorter ventrally than dorsally (Fig. 3-5). This normal feature should not be confused with a compression fracture. Costal facets for rib articulations are a distinguishing feature of thoracic vertebrae. These are located on the inferior or ventral surface of the transverse process from T-1 to T-10 and at the junction of the

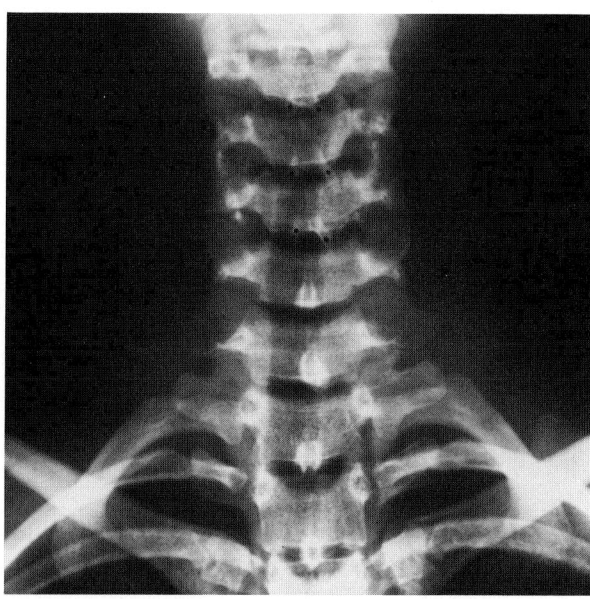

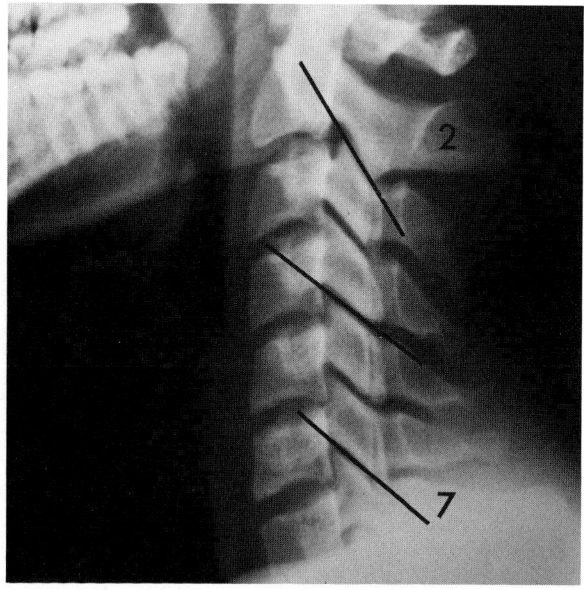

Fig. 3-3 AP (**A**) and lateral (**B**) views of the cervical spine demonstrating the angles of the facet joints (lines in **B**) and bifid spinous processes (dots in **A**). The spinous process of C-2 is bulbous, and the spinous process of C-7 is most prominent in length.

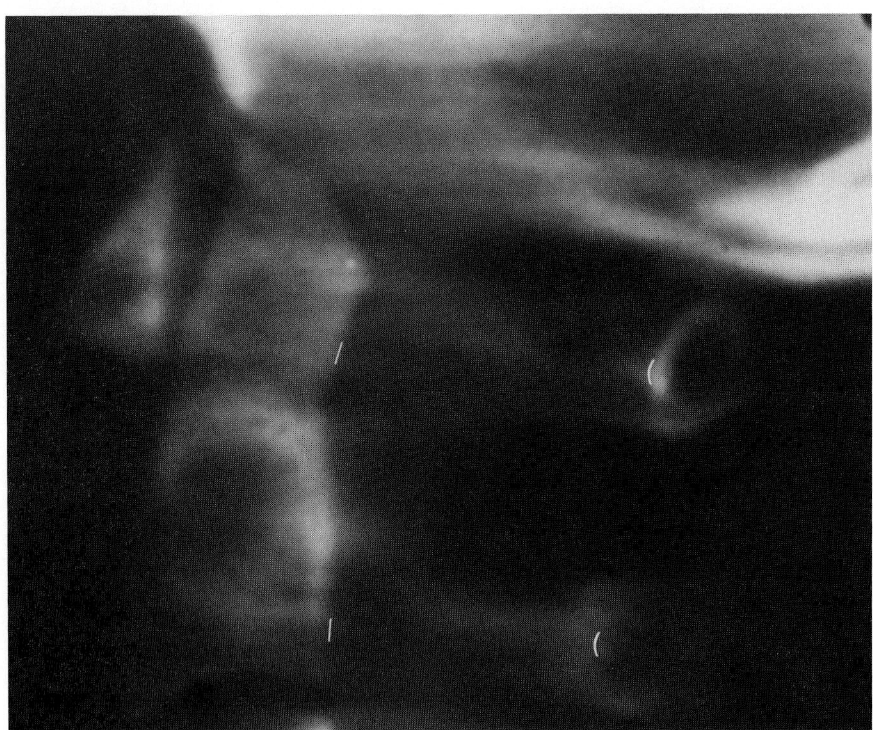

Fig. 3-4 Lateral tomogram of the upper cervical spine demonstrating the articulation of the anterior ring of C-1 with the odontoid. The AP diameter of the spinal canal is greater at C-1 (white lines).

body and pedicle from T-1 to T-12. The last two ribs do not typically articulate with the transverse processes. The pedicles in the thoracic spine are short and thin, and the vertebral foramina are smaller and more circular than those in either the cervical or lumbar region. The transverse processes typically decrease in length as one progresses from T-1 to T-12. Orientation of the facets in the thoracic region is almost vertical.

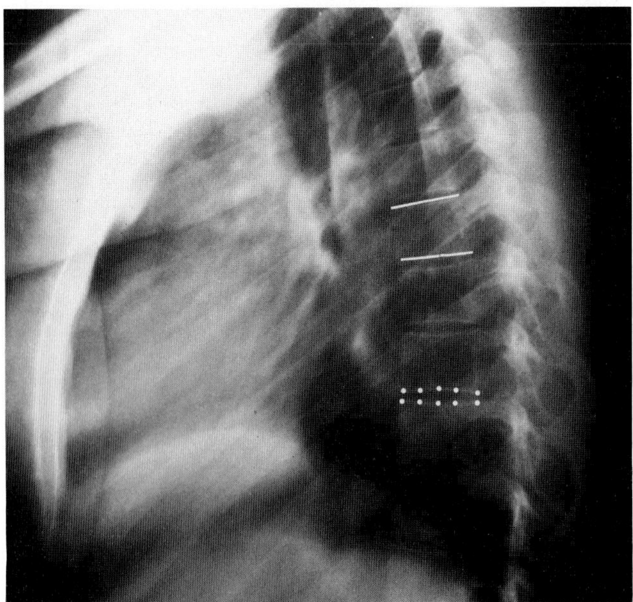

Fig. 3-5 Lateral view of the thoracic spine. The disc spaces (dotted lines) are equal in height anteriorly and posteriorly. The vertebral bodies (solid lines) have 1.5 mm less vertical height anteriorly.

They are directed posteriorly and slightly laterally throughout the thoracic spine except at the T-12 level. Here the inferior facets face laterally to articulate with the superior facets of L-1.[4,10]

Lumbar Vertebrae

The lumbar vertebral bodies are larger than the thoracic vertebrae and typically are kidney shaped, with the transverse diameter being greater than the AP diameter (Fig. 3-6A). The vertical dimension of L-5 is greater anteriorly than posteriorly (Fig. 3-6B). As in the case of the cervical spine, the spinal canal or the vertebral foramen is triangular in the lumbar region. The laminae in the lumbar region are strong and often symmetric. The pedicles are short and thick. The apophyseal joints arise from the lamina-pedicle junction. The superior facets are directed posteriorly and medially, and the inferior facets are directed posteriorly and laterally. The lumbar vertebrae have no costal facets and no foramina transversaria. The transverse processes of the first three lumbar vertebrae are straight and project almost directly laterally, increasing in length from L-1 through L-3. At L-4 and L-5 the transverse processes are shorter, with the transverse process of L-4 being directed somewhat dorsally and superiorly compared with the short, stout transverse process of L-5 (Fig. 3-6).[4,10]

Sacrum

In adults the sacrum is composed of five nonmovable segments. The discs are ossified and fused (Fig. 3-7). The first sacral segment and C-1 are the only vertebrae with true lateral masses. The sacrum articulates with the ilia, forming paired

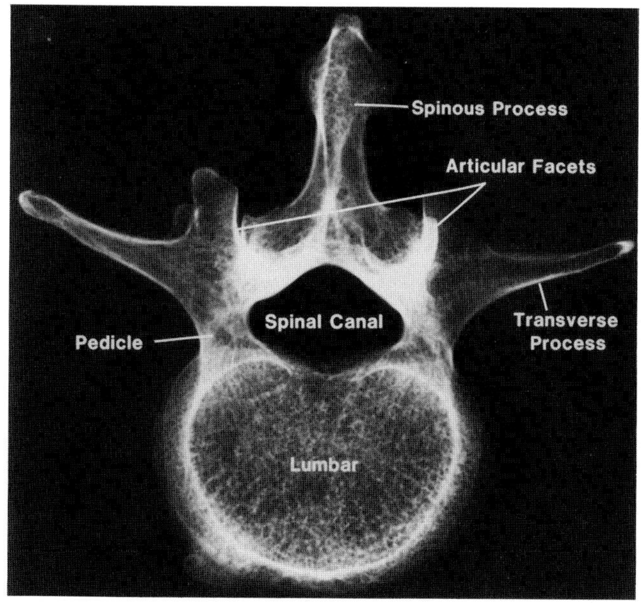

A

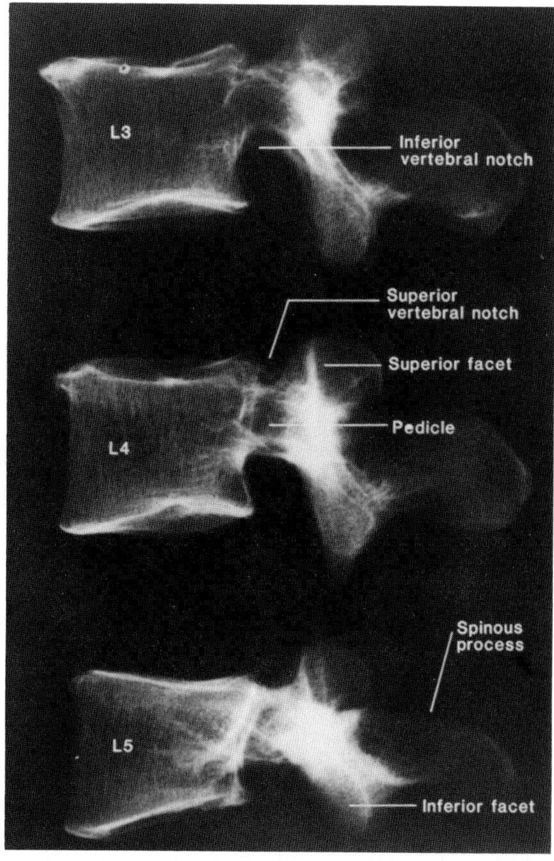

B

Fig. 3-6 Bone specimens of the lumbar vertebrae seen in the axial (**A**) and lateral (**B**) projections. *Source:* Reprinted from *Imaging of Orthopedic Trauma* ed 2 by TH Berquist, 1991, Raven Press, © Mayo Foundation.

synovial sacroiliac joints. Superiorly, two facets articulate with the inferior facets of L-5. Of the five sacral segments, the first is the largest. The size of the segments diminishes as one progresses inferiorly. The costal elements and transverse processes are fused. On the AP or frontal view the ventral sacral foramina (four pairs) can be clearly visualized.[4,10]

Ligamentous Anatomy

The fibrocartilaginous intervertebral discs are the main connecting segments between the vertebral bodies from C-2 through the sacrum. There may be rudimentary discs at the sacral levels, but the sacral segments are usually completely fused.

The nucleus pulposus and anulus fibrosus are derived from the notochord embryologically. The discs, composed of the nucleus pulposus and anulus, contribute approximately one-fourth to one-third of the height of the vertebral column. The configuration of the disc varies somewhat, depending upon the region of the vertebral column in which it is located. In the cervical region the discs are taller ventrally than dorsally (Fig. 3-3B). A similar situation is present in the lumbar region (Fig. 3-5). In the thoracic region the discs are approximately equal in height anteriorly and posteriorly (Fig. 3-5). The thickness of the disc in the lumbar region increases slightly as one progresses from L-1 to L-4, with the disc at the L-4 level being the largest. The L5–S1 disc is triangular and much thicker ventrally. The fibers of the anulus fibrosus develop in concentric rings running obliquely, with the superficial fibers blending into the anterior and posterior longitudinal ligaments.[4,10]

The anterior longitudinal ligament (Fig. 3-8) is stronger and wider than the posterior longitudinal ligament. It is narrowest at its origin at the base of the skull and gradually widens to the level of its insertion on the pelvic surface of the sacrum.[10]

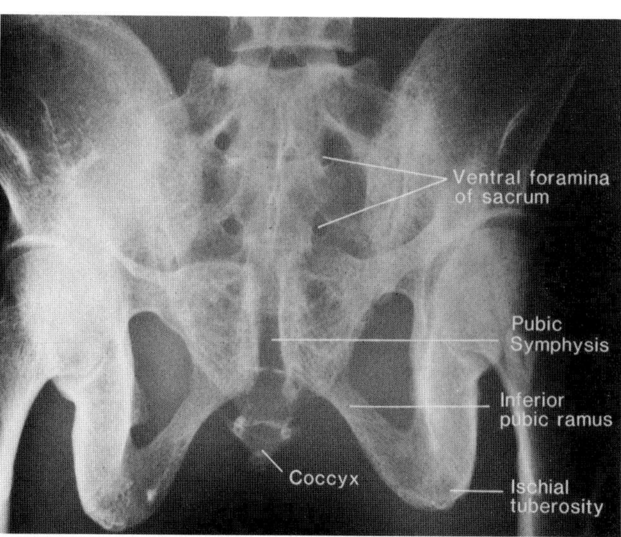

Fig. 3-7 AP angled view of the pelvis demonstrating the sacrum, the coccyx, and their articulations. *Source:* Reprinted from *Imaging of Orthopedic Trauma* ed 2 by TH Berquist, 1991, Raven Press, © Mayo Foundation.

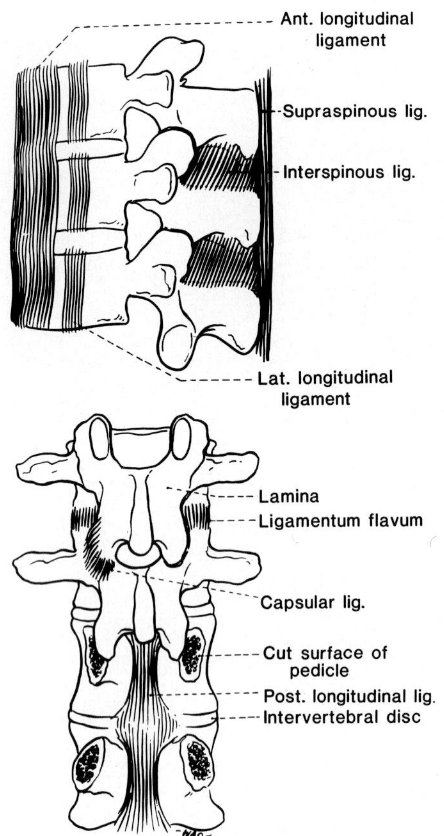

Fig. 3-8 Illustration of anterior and posterior spinal ligaments. *Source:* Reprinted from *Anatomy for Surgeons, Vol 3, The Back and Limbs* ed 3 by HW Hollinshead, 1982, JB Lippincott.

The posterior longitudinal ligament (Fig. 3-8) lies within the vertebral foramen along the posterior surface of the vertebral body. This ligament is contiguous with the tectorial membrane superiorly and extends caudally into the sacral canal. The posterior longitudinal ligament blends with the fibers of the anulus fibrosus but is separated from the vertebral body by a venous plexus.[4,10]

The ligamentum flavum is an elastic, thick, paired ligament that extends between the laminae of adjacent vertebrae (Fig. 3-8). The ligaments blend with the articular capsules of the apophyseal joints. Posterior to the ligamentum flavum is the thinner intraspinous ligament, which joins the spinous processes and blends superficially with the supraspinous ligament. The supraspinous ligament in the cervical region is stronger and is called the ligamentum nuchae. This structure extends from the external occipital protuberance to the spinous process of C-7. Extending between the transverse processes are the intertransverse ligaments, which are best developed in the thoracic and lumbar regions and essentially are nonexistent in the cervical region. Also, in the cervical region the interspinous ligament may be sparse and disappear with age; thus if this ligament were torn secondary to trauma the significance of the injury would be questionable.[4,10]

The apophyseal or facet joints are synovial joints with a fibrous capsule. Internally there are meniscuslike tabs composed primarily of synovium and fatty tissue that project from the capsule into the joints. The articular capsules are more lax in the cervical spine, allowing more motion than in the remainder of the spine.[10]

The ligamentous anatomy in the atlantoaxial region is more complex (Fig. 3-9), requiring more emphasis. The posterior longitudinal ligament is continuous with the tectorial membrane that extends cephalad to the inner aspect of the foramen magnum. The transverse ligament lies ventral to the tectorial membrane. It is a strong fibrous band that connects the tubercles of the lateral masses of C-1 posteriorly and maintains the relationship of the odontoid to the anterior ring of C-1. There are synovial joints between the odontoid and anterior ring at C-1 and between the odontoid and the transverse ligament. In addition, there are three ligaments extending vertically from the tip of the odontoid. The apical ligament extends superiorly and attaches to the occipital bone. The two alar or check ligaments extend from the apex of the odontoid in a dorsilateral direction. The accessory ligament is a significant structure attaching at the base of the odontoid on either side. It is through this ligament that the odontoid receives part of its blood supply.[4,10]

Neuroanatomy

The spinal cord with its meningeal envelope lies within the vertebral foramen and extends in the adult from the foramen magnum to the upper border of L-2. The vertebral foramen is bordered by the body anteriorly, the pedicles laterally, and the lamina posteriorly. The size of the vertebral foramen is largest in the lumbar and cervical regions, which coincides with the nerve distribution to the upper and lower extremities. The spinal cord occupies approximately 50% of the vertebral foramen. The remainder of the space is occupied by the epidural venous plexus, which is intermixed with fat, connective tissue, and the protective meningeal portions of the spinal cord. The dura is a dense fibrous tube contiguous with the foramen magnum that extends to the level of the third sacral segment. The dural sleeves surround each set of spinal nerve roots as they exit the dural sac. The pia mater is the thin innermost layer of the meninges that is applied to the spinal cord and nerve roots as they cross the subarachnoid space. More peripheral to the pia mater is the arachnoid, which encloses the subarachnoid space. The arachnoid, pia, and dura are united by the dentate ligaments that pass from the spinal cord to the dura. In the adult the spinal cord proper terminates at the conus medullaris. The filum terminale continues caudally until it blends with the posterior ligament and sacral canal. Both structures are enveloped in the dural sac to the S-2 level.[4,10]

There are 31 pairs of spinal nerves: 8 cervical, 12 thoracic, 5 lumbar, 5 sacral, and 1 coccygeal. Cervical nerve roots exit above the level of the adjacent vertebral body (C-8 exits between C-7 and T-1). In the remainder of the spine the nerve roots exit below the adjacent bodies (T-1 exits at the intervertebral foramen between T-1 and T-2).[10]

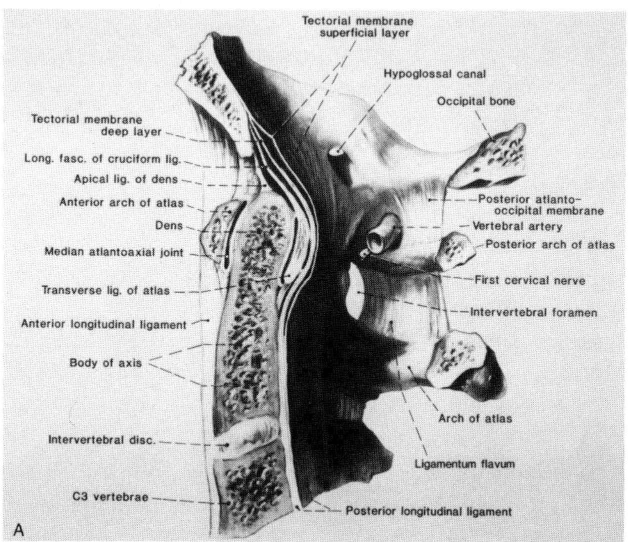

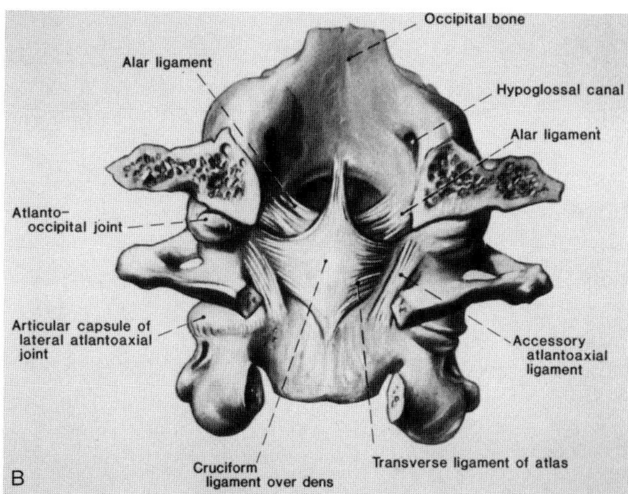

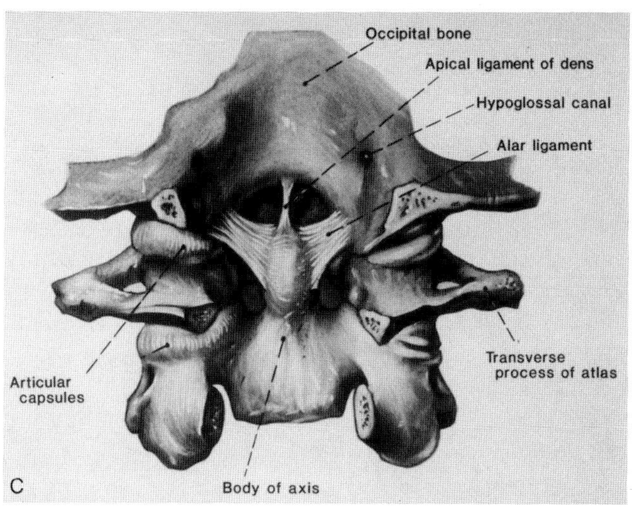

Fig. 3-9 Illustration of the ligamentous anatomy of the upper cervical spine viewed from the side (**A**) and posteriorly (**B** and **C**). *Source:* Reprinted from *Anatomy for Surgeons, Vol 3, The Back and Limbs* ed 3 by HW Hollinshead, 1982, JB Lippincott.

CERVICAL SPINE TRAUMA

Cervical spine fractures, fracture-dislocations, and soft tissue injuries are less common in sports than in high-velocity motor vehicle accidents. Even so, up to 14% of adult and 10% of childhood cervical spine injuries are related to sports injuries.[36,79] Common winter sports associated with cervical spine trauma include snowmobiling, skiing, tobogganing, and ice hockey.[79] Other sports implicated in cervical spine trauma include football, rugby, gymnastics, trampolining, and diving.[79,84,85,88,92,95]

Mechanisms of Injury

Understanding the mechanisms of injury and the structures, both bone and soft tissue, that may be affected is essential for proper selection of imaging techniques. The type and severity of cervical spine injury vary with the sport and mechanism of injury. The literature has provided numerous in-depth discussions of mechanisms of cervical spine injury.[40–42,48,50,55,59,63,80,87,94] Although most of the reports do not deal with sports injuries specifically, the mechanisms described can also frequently be applied to sports injuries.

The mechanism of injury is rarely pure (eg, flexion or extension alone without compression or axial loading). In one series of 420 cervical spine fractures and fracture-dislocations,[40] most injuries could be classified into four groups. Hyperextension occurred in 38% of patients. Hyperflexion injuries were somewhat more common (46%). Most were flexion-compression or disruptive hyperflexion injuries. This group included 12% of the total subjects in the series who had unilateral facet locking or perching. Vertical compression injuries occurred in 4% of the 420 patients. Radiographic classification could not be accomplished in 10% to 12% of the cases. These patients presented with radiographic findings that did not allow exact determination of the mechanism of injury. These injuries included nondisplaced odontoid fractures, in which the radiographic features were insufficient to determine the mechanism of injury even when combined with clinical data. Spinous process fractures may result from flexion, extension, or direct trauma. If there are no associated fractures, classification is difficult in such cases as well.[40]

Daffner[48] and colleagues[49,50] describe similar findings in 646 cervical spine injuries. Radiographic features allowed identification of four basic mechanisms of injury (flexion, extension, shearing, and rotation) in the majority of patients.

Hyperflexion Injuries

There are many descriptive terms in the literature that attempt to define the motion of the cervical spine and the direction of the force that results in injury. Certain of these terms are extremely helpful, and others are confusing. Flexion injuries have been classified as disruptive, compressive, and shearing in nature.[40,48–50,59] Disruptive hyperflexion indicates that the blow was directed upward toward the occipital region, resulting in forward flexion of the head. The major force is applied to the posterior ligaments and spinous processes, resulting in distraction of the spinous processes (Fig. 3-10). If the force is sufficient and the motion of the head continues, the posterior ligaments are interrupted, resulting in an unstable injury. The cervical spine may then return to a nearly normal position, depending upon the extent of force applied. In this case, the lateral radiograph may demonstrate kyphosis with widening of the interspinous distance and facet joints (Fig. 3-11). If the disruptive force continues, however, unilateral or bilateral locking of the facets occurs, depending on the degree of associated rotation. Some authorities prefer to consider unilateral locking a flexion-rotation injury. As mentioned earlier, this type of injury occurred in 12% of 420 patients in one series.[40] Flexion-rotation injuries may be subtle, with only minimal anterior subluxation. On the lateral view the facet joints at the level of the injury rotate, giving a bow-tie appearance (Fig. 3-12). Oblique views will usually demonstrate the injury more clearly.[40]

Compressive hyperflexion injuries (axial loading plus flexion) occur when a force is applied to the top of the head, resulting in forward arching of the head (Fig. 3-13). These injuries are common in contact sports. The main force is distributed along the vertebral bodies. As described earlier,

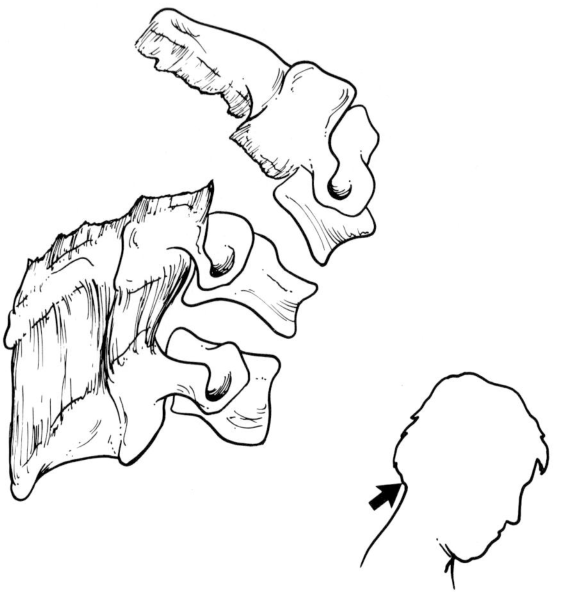

Fig. 3-10 Illustration of disruptive hyperflexion injury. *Source:* Reprinted from *Imaging of Orthopedic Trauma*, ed 2 by TH Berquist, 1991, Raven Press, © Mayo Foundation.

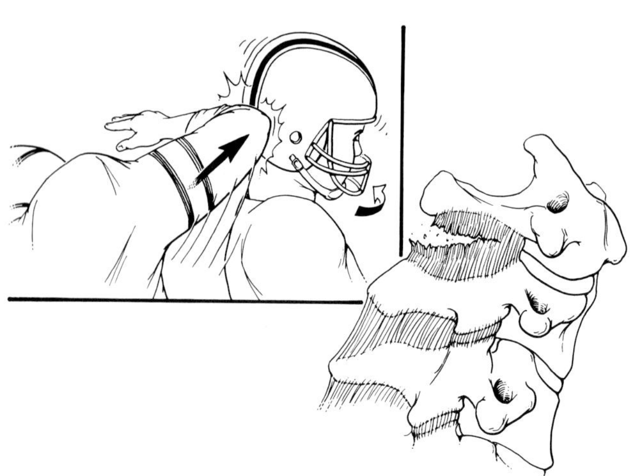

Fig. 3-11 Illustration of flexion-rotation injury.

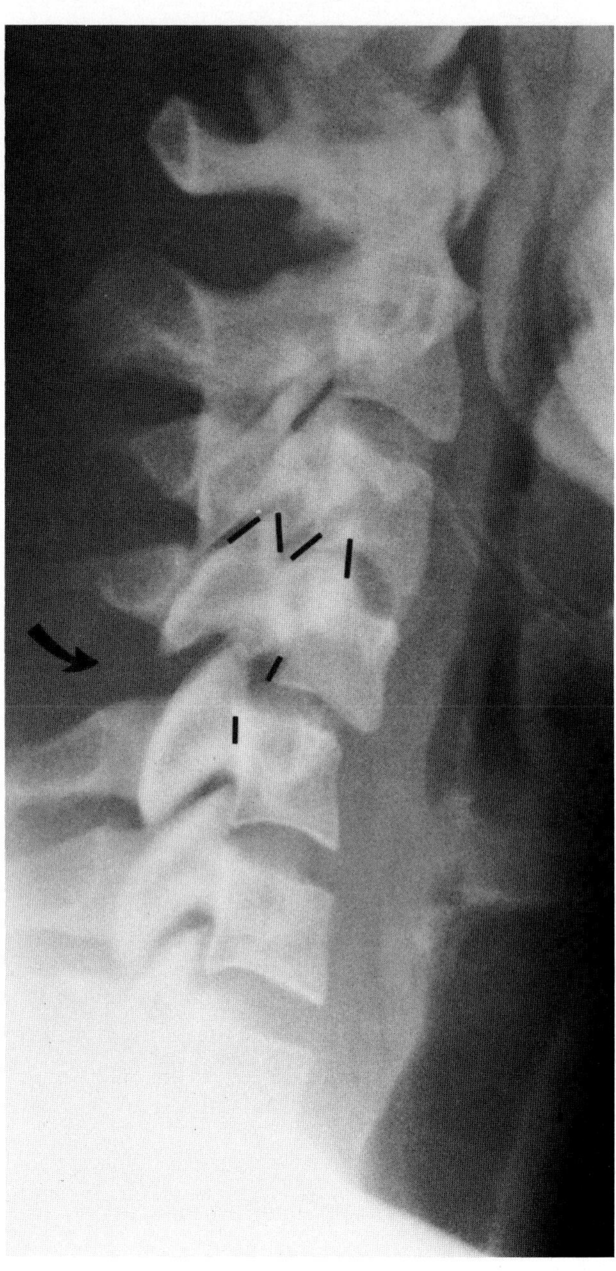

Fig. 3-12 Lateral view of the cervical spine after flexion-rotation injury at C4–5. Note the widened interspinous distance (arrow) and the bow-tie sign (lines) due to rotation of C-4 on C-5.

the force is mainly compressive, and thus the posterior ligaments may remain intact (Fig. 3-14). Wedge fractures of the bodies, teardrop fractures, and fracture-dislocations may result.[62,69] Harris[62] states that the flexion teardrop injury is the most unstable lesion of all. In this situation the vertebrae above the injury move anteriorly and the vertebrae below posteriorly in a circular direction (Fig. 3-15).

Compressive shearing forces result from a force directed to the back of the head with the head moving forward. The end result may be an anteriorly displaced fracture of the odontoid. Atlantoaxial and atlantooccipital dislocations are rare but may also occur in this type of injury. This injury is unusual even in contact sports.

Hyperextension Injuries

Hyperextension injuries may occur when a force is applied to the mandible in an upward direction, leading to disruption of the anterior longitudinal ligament and disc (Fig. 3-16A). The lateral radiograph may be normal or reveal soft tissue swelling with displacement of the prevertebral fat stripe. Widening of the anterior disc space may also be evident.[40,45,59] A small chip fracture, usually from the anteroinferior aspect of the vertebral body, may be noted. The radiographic changes may be very subtle, and further confusion may be added by the presence of significant neurologic deficits. Neurologic damage often is the result of AP compression of the cord, leading to a decrease in the AP diameter of the spinal canal and vascular compromise of the cord (central cord syndrome).[40,50,55] Infolding of the ligamentum flavum may also play a part in the cord impingement.[40,59]

Hyperextension may also result from blows directed to the vertex of the skull, when most of the force is absorbed by the posterior arch. Fractures of the spinous process, lamina, pedicles, and articular pillars may result (Figs. 3-16B and 3-17). Anterior subluxation may occur, which on the lateral radiograph could be mistaken for a flexion injury. Oblique and pillar views will demonstrate the posterior arch fractures and aid in differentiating the mechanism of injury. In these cases, conventional tomography or computed tomography (CT) is often needed to evaluate the neural arch. Facial injuries are also common in patients with hyperextension injuries.[55] Finally, anterior shearing forces result in posterior fracture-dislocations in the upper cervical spine.

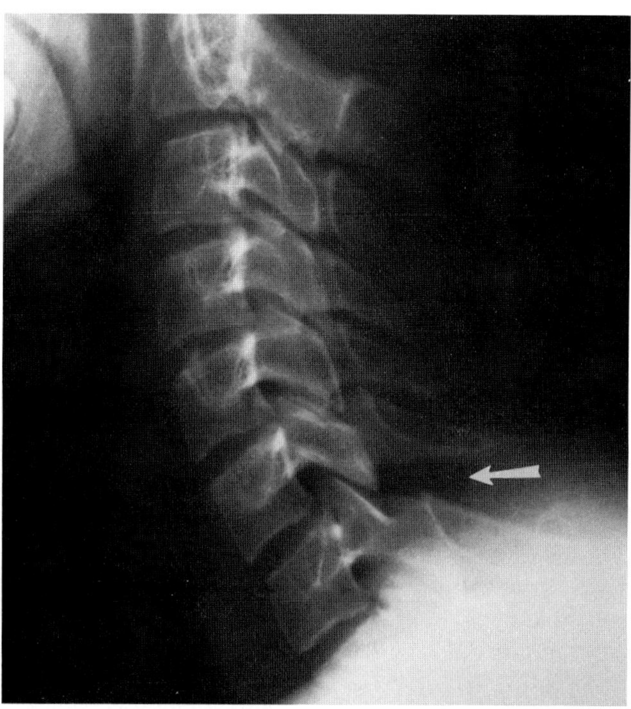

Fig. 3-14 Lateral view of the cervical spine after a compression injury of C-7; this patient slid into the boards while playing ice hockey. Note the chip fracture and anterior wedging of C-7. There is slight widening of the interspinous distance (arrow), indicating some degree of posterior ligament injury.

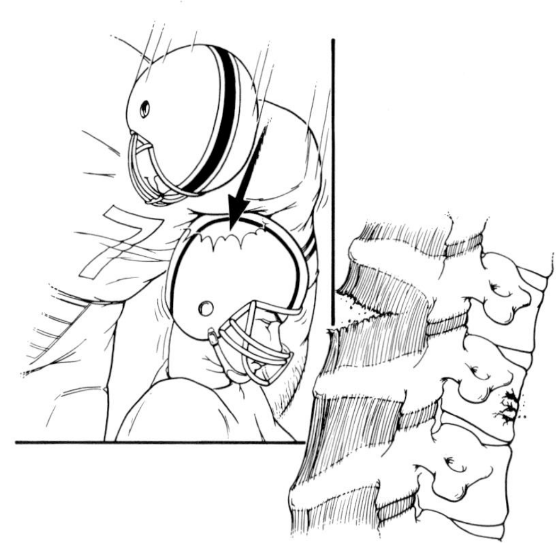

Fig. 3-13 Illustration of flexion-compression injury.

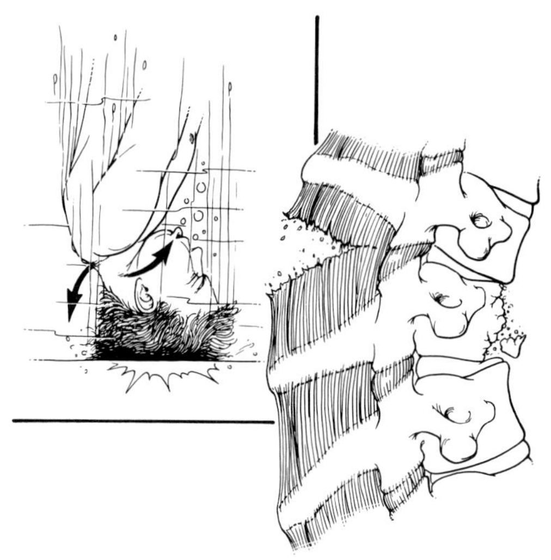

Fig. 3-15 Illustration of teardrop hyperflexion injury in a diver.

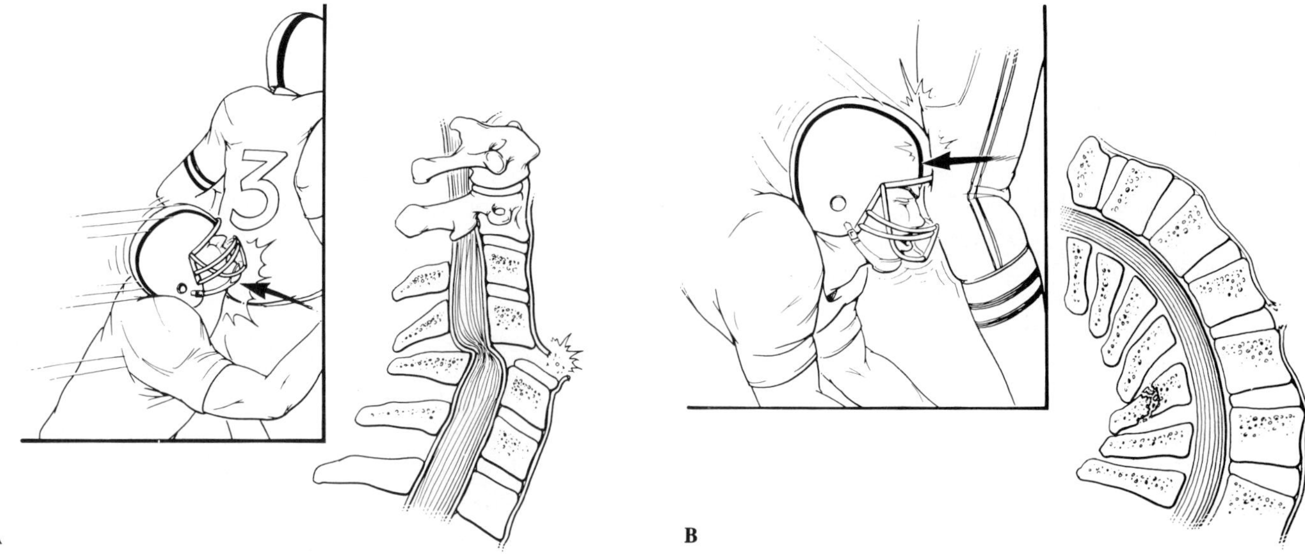

Fig. 3-16 Illustration of hyperextension injury during football with forces applied to the facial region (**A**) and anterior calvarium (**B**).

Vertical Compression (Axial Loading) Injuries

Pure vertical compression or axial loading may result in a typical Jefferson fracture (Fig. 3-18A) or a burst fracture (Fig. 3-18B) in the lower cervical spine. The spine must be in a nearly neutral position when the vertical force is applied. Although axial loading injuries are common in contact sports, some degree of flexion, extension, or rotation is typically present as well. Usually there is an asymmetric vertical compression with lateral flexion (Fig. 3-19). This may result in a compression fracture of one of the lateral masses of C-1, a pillar fracture, or a stinger.[64,78] Fractures of the uncinate process or a transverse process fracture may also occur.[40,59] Axial forces with flexion may also lead to lower cervical burst fractures.[85,88,91]

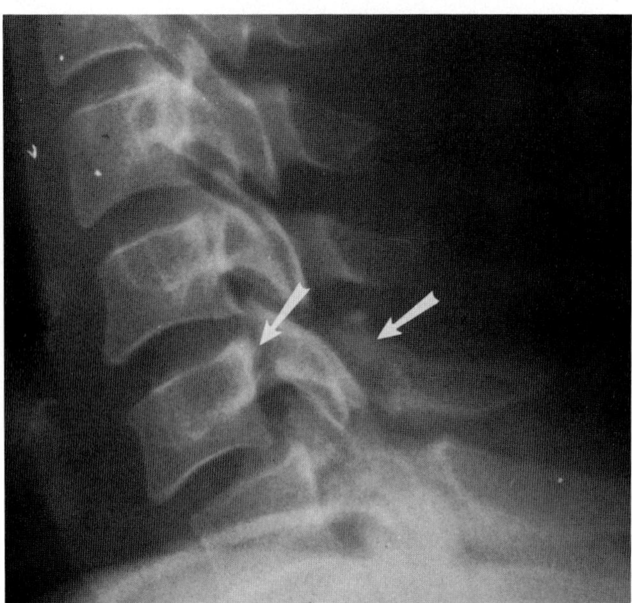

Fig. 3-17 Unstable hyperextension injury with fractures of the pedicle and lamina (arrows) and subluxation of C-6 on C-7.

Minor Injuries

Most sports injuries are due to minor sprains or strains from hyperflexion, hyperextension, or rotary forces.[64] Complete disruption of a muscle or ligament without associated fracture is unusual but can occur. This can lead to an unstable injury with subtle radiographic fingings. Motion studies or magnetic resonance imaging (MRI) may be required for detection and classification of these injuries.

The so-called stinger usually results from lateral flexion but can also occur with flexion and extension injuries.[78] Sudden lateral flexion during tackling or blocking in football is often described (Fig. 3-20).[62] The injury results in traction or impingement of nerves of the brachial plexus, leading to pain, numbness, and tingling that extend down the arm on the involved side. The C5–6 levels are most commonly involved. Usually the symptoms clear in several minutes. With significant or repeated episodes, however, the symptoms may be more severe.

Three grades of stinger injury have been described. Athletes with grade 1 injuries recover in a few minutes. Grade 2 injuries lead to decreased strength in the deltoid, infraspinatus, supraspinatus, and biceps muscles that may last up to 3 weeks. With grade 3 injuries the motor and sensory deficits may last 1 year or more.[64,78] Electromyographic abnormalities may be evident with grade 2 and 3 injuries. Radiographic findings are unusual, however, except in severe or recurrent injuries. In this setting, disc space narrowing or subtle fractures may be noted in up to 25% of cases.[78]

Avulsion injuries are generally stable and do not necessarily require withdrawal from contact sports once they have healed.

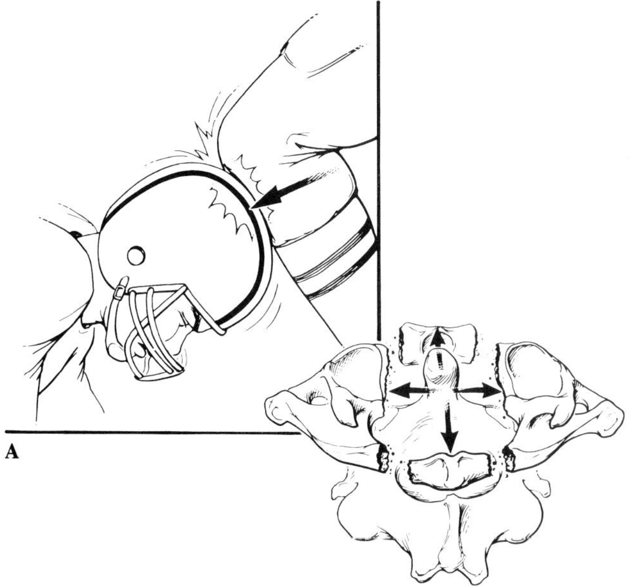

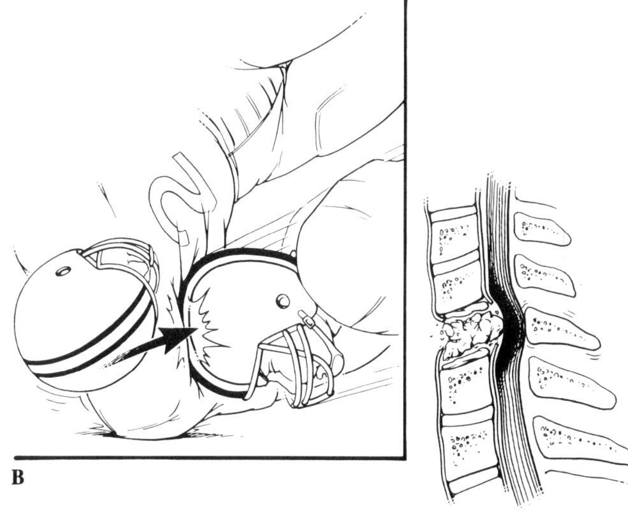

Fig. 3-18 Illustration of mechanisms of injury due to vertical compression. (**A**) Jefferson fracture. (**B**) Burst fracture.

These injuries are most common with hyperextension or hyperflexion.[89] Clay shoveler's fractures (spinous process of C-6, C-7, or T-1) and anteroinferior C-2 body avulsions occur most frequently.[40,89]

Traumatic disc herniations are uncommon but may lead to neurologic symptoms. Herniated cervical discs may present with pain, reduced motion, and sensory changes in the upper extremities. Loss of reflexes in the distribution of the affected nerve root may be noted on physical examination. MRI or CT myelography may be needed if conservative therapy fails.[64]

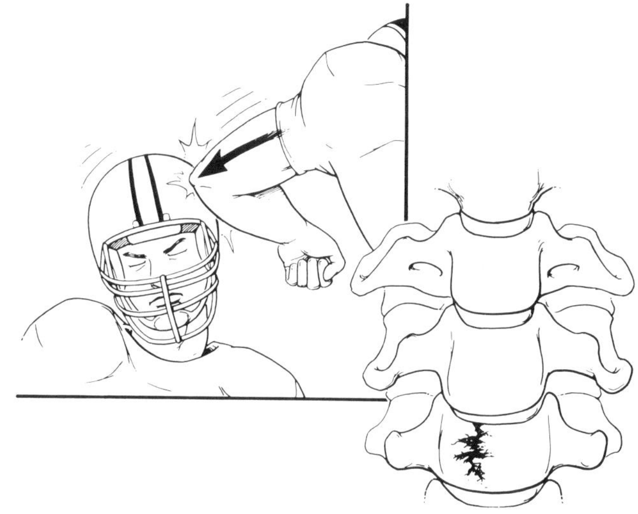

Fig. 3-19 Illustration of lateral flexion injury.

Imaging of Cervical Spine Injuries

Acutely injured patients with suspected spinal trauma must be properly immobilized until the radiographic examination is complete and treatment is instituted. Radiographic evaluation can be accomplished only when close communication between the radiologist and clinicians (orthopaedic surgeons and neurosurgeons) is maintained.[40,59] A well-organized approach will ensure optimal use of routine films, tomography, CT, MRI, and other techniques in determining the extent of injury and stability of the lesion.

A simple radiographic table with an overhead tube capable of being positioned at different angles is sufficient for evaluation of the spine.[40,56] The necessary views for evaluation of the cervical, thoracic, and lumbar spine can be obtained easily. We utilize a C-arm Versigraph, which allows AP, lateral, and oblique views without moving the patient. In addition, tomograms can be obtained in the AP, lateral, oblique, and transaxial projections. Conventional radiographic equipment would require the patient to be placed in the oblique or lateral position to obtain tomograms in these projections.[40]

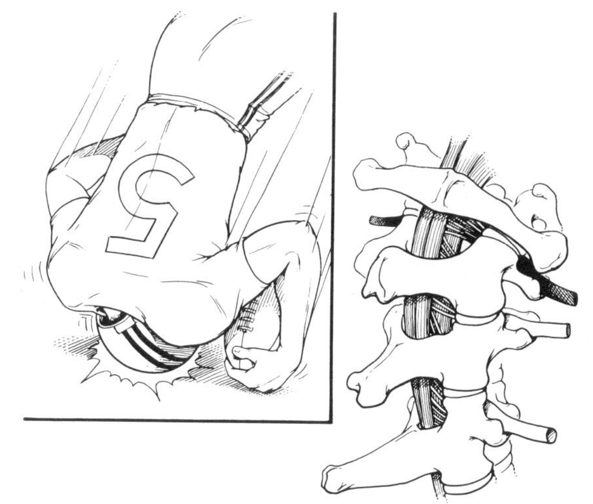

Fig. 3-20 Illustration of mechanism for stinger injury.

Routine Radiography of the Cervical Spine

Routine radiographs remain the most effective screening technique for evaluating spinal trauma.[34,39,40,64,76] Radiographic evaluation of the cervical spine should be thoroughly and completely monitored by the radiologist until the degree of injury has been established. Such an evaluation demands that the examination be tailored to the patient's clinical symptoms. The initial evaluation should include lateral, oblique, AP, and odontoid views. Pillar views may also be indicated. The head must be turned for pillar views, however; therefore, the other views should be studied first to determine whether it is safe or necessary to move the head for pillar views.[37,40]

Lateral view. The lateral view is the most important radiographic view. Ninety percent of significant pathology can be detected on the lateral view.[40,59,62]

There are many features that should be carefully examined on the lateral view. It is essential that all seven cervical vertebrae be well demonstrated. Ideally T-1 should also be visible on the lateral view. The lateral view allows assessment of the following structures: the anterior and posterior arches of C-1, the odontoid, vertebral bodies, disc spaces, facet joints, and spinous processes. The lateral radiograph shows that the body of T-1 is larger than that of C-7, which can give the false impression of subluxation (Fig. 3-21). This fact must be kept in mind when evaluating patients with flexion injuries.

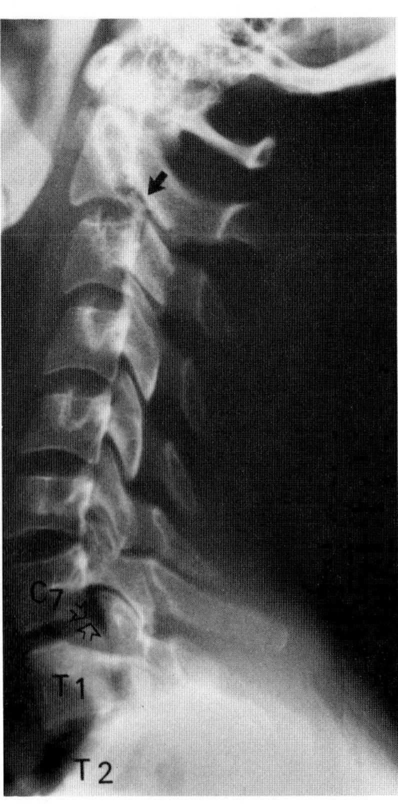

Fig. 3-21 Normal lateral view of the cervical spine including T-1. There is slight subluxation of C-2 on C-3 (upper arrow), which can be normal up to age 20. C-7 is smaller than T-1 (open arrow).

Table 3-3 Cervical Spine Trauma: Lateral Radiographic Evaluation

Upper cervical spine (occipital condyles to C-2)
- Clivoodontoid relationship
- C-1–odontoid measurement
  - 2.0 to 2.5 mm in adults
  - 4.0 to 4.5 mm in children
- Retropharyngeal space
- Posterior pharyngeal wall to anteroinferior body of C-2 (7 mm in adults and children)

Lower cervical spine (C3–7)
- Anteroinferior margin of C-3 to pharyngeal airway (4 to 5 mm)
- Prevertebral fat stripe
- Retrotracheal spaces (posterior tracheal wall to anteroinferior body of C-6)
  - Normal in adults, $\leq$22 mm
  - Normal in children, $\leq$14 mm
- Anterior spinal line
- Posterior spinal line
- Spinolaminar line
- Disc spaces
- Facet joints
- Spinous processes and interspinous distance

Source: Reprinted from *Imaging of Orthopedic Trauma* ed 2 by TH Berquist, 1991, Raven Press, © Mayo Foundation.

The features demonstrated on the lateral view must be studied systematically as shown in Table 3-3. In the upper cervical region there are several relationships and measurements that must be checked routinely. A line drawn along the clivus to the tip of the odontoid should point to the tip of the odontoid at the junction of the anterior and middle thirds (Fig. 3-22). A line drawn tangentially to the lamina of C-1 should intersect the posterior foramen magnum. The space between the odontoid and anterior ring of C-1 measured at its most inferior margin should not exceed 2 mm in adults.[39,40,50,62] This measurement may be as much as 4.5 mm in children.[62]

Careful attention should also be paid to the soft tissues in the prevertebral space. In the adult the measurement of the soft tissue from the anteroinferior margin of C-2 to the retropharyngeal wall should not exceed 7 mm.[40,59,62] The distance from the posterior wall of the trachea to the anteroinferior margin of C-6 should not exceed 14 mm in children and 22 mm in adults.[62] Care must be taken in measuring this distance in young people and children because changes on inspiration can simulate swelling. Nasogastric and endotracheal tubes invalidate measurements of the retropharyngeal space. The posterior portions of the maxillary antra and mandible may also provide a clue to the mechanism of injury. These structures can be partially studied on most lateral views of the cervical spine. Mandibular fractures are often associated with hyperextension injuries.[55]

Perhaps a more useful and readily accessible measurement than these is the prevertebral fat stripe. This can be identified in most adults as it courses along the anterior margin of the

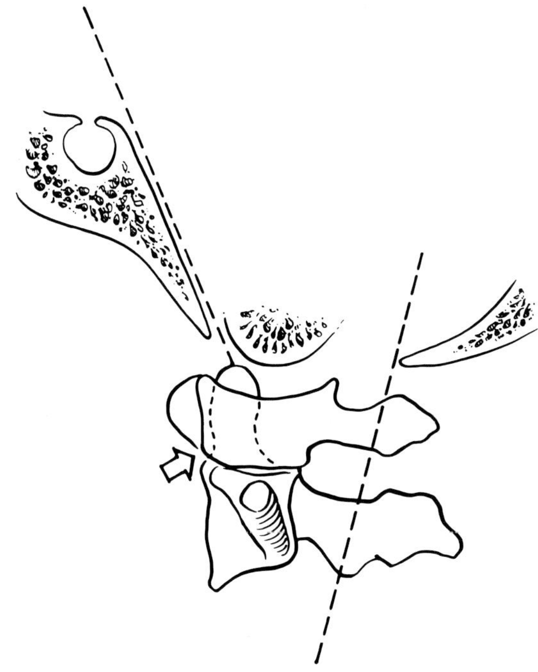

Fig. 3-22 Illustration of upper cervical relationships with the skull base. The upper line indicates clivus to odontoid; the posterior line indicates the lamina to foramen magnum; the arrow indicates the point for C-1–C-2 measurement. *Source:* Reprinted from *Imaging of Orthopedic Trauma* ed 2 by TH Berquist, 1991, Raven Press, © Mayo Foundation.

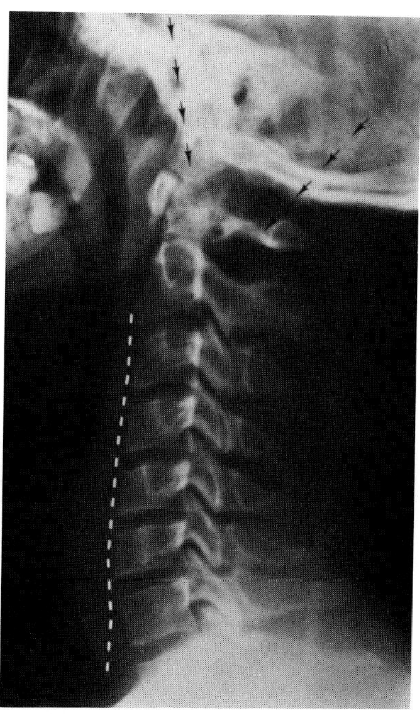

Fig. 3-23 Lateral view of the cervical spine demonstrating the normal upper cervical relationships (arrows) and prevertebral fat stripe (dashed white line).

anterior longitudinal ligament. At the C-6 level it deviates anteriorly over the scalene muscles (Fig. 3-23).[40,59] Hemorrhage from hyperextension injuries will displace the fat stripe anteriorly.[40,55] This may be the only indication of injury. The fat stripe is less frequently seen in children.

Although it is important to evaluate the prevertebral soft tissues, there is obviously overlap between normal and abnormal. Templeton et al[90] demonstrated considerable variation in normal measurements. As a rule, however, if the soft tissues are abnormal one should proceed with further studies, including CT and MRI, to be certain that an injury is not overlooked.[39,40,90] When the prevertebral soft tissue measurements at the anteroinferior margins of C-2, C-3, and C-4 are 7 to 10 mm, further studies should be considered. If the measurement exceeds 10 mm, further imaging evaluation is definitely indicated.[40,90]

The normal lordotic curve of the cervical spine can be followed along the anterior margins of the vertebral bodies (anterior spinal line), the posterior margins of the bodies (posterior spinal line), and the spinolaminar line. Disruption in these lines can indicate instability or ligament injury with resulting subluxation. One must be careful, however, not to confuse normal positional changes with pathology. In the supine position, patients have a tendency to lose the normal cervical lordotic curve, which can be misinterpreted as evidence of a ligament injury. Muscle spasm may result in straightening of the normal cervical lordotic curve. In addition, there is normally slight ligament laxity at C2–3 and C3–4 in children and teenagers (Fig. 3-21). This can result in slight anterior subluxation of C-2 on C-3 or C-3 on C-4 until at least age 18.[39,40]

Evaluation of the disc spaces, facet joints, and spinous processes is an important factor in determining treatment and prognosis of spinal injury.[40,48,50] These areas can be fairly accurately assessed on the lateral view (Figs. 3-21 and 3-23). Lateral radiographs reveal instability, which can be defined as abnormal motion between vertebrae whether or not clinical symptoms are present. Findings indicating instability include narrowing of the disc space, compression of the vertebral body exceeding 25%, subluxation of greater than 3 mm, and an increase in the rotational angle of adjacent vertebrae beyond 11° (Fig. 3-24).[40,41,48,50,62] An additional feature is widening of the interspinous distance, which normally decreases as one progresses caudally from C-1 to C-7 (Fig. 3-14).

The above signs and the location of fractures are useful in accurately predicting lesion instability on the lateral view. Denis[53] popularized the three-column approach for evaluating cervical instability. The spine can be divided into three columns. The anterior column includes the anterior longitudinal ligament, the anterior half of the vertebral body, and the anterior disc. The middle column includes the posterior vertebral body, disc, and posterior longitudinal ligament. The posterior column is made up of the facet joints, posterior osseous structures, and ligaments. Disruption of two adjacent columns indicates instability. Identification of widening of the interspinous distance, subluxation exceeding 3 mm, or widened facet joints as single injuries is also indicative of instability because generally two columns must be involved for these changes to occur.[40,48,50,53]

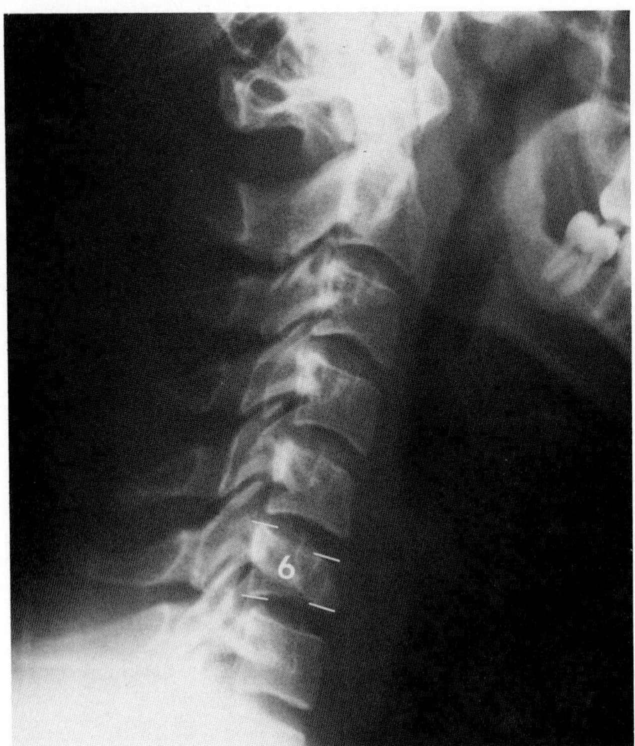

A

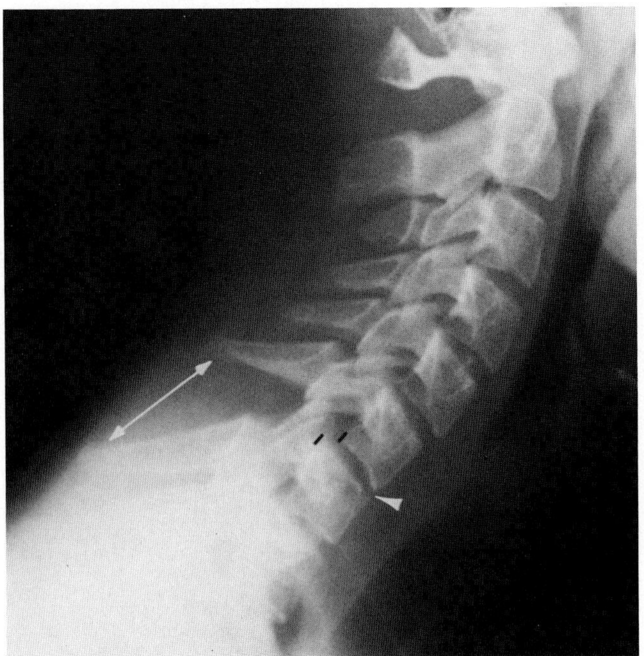

B

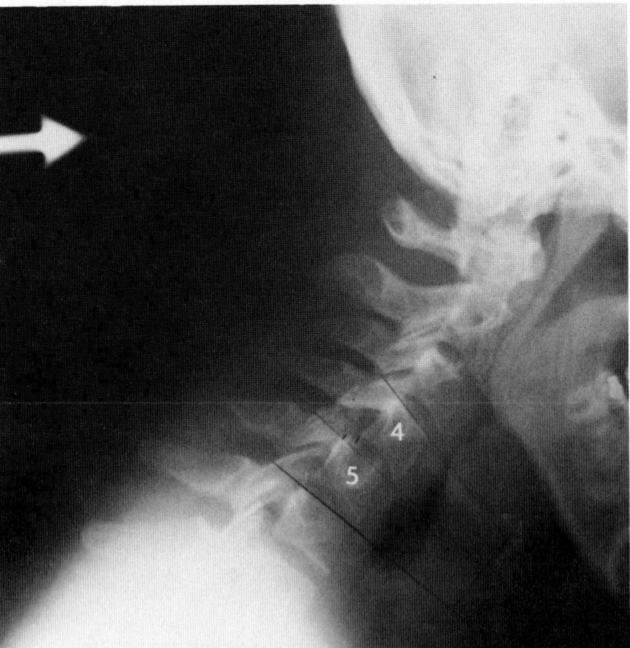

C

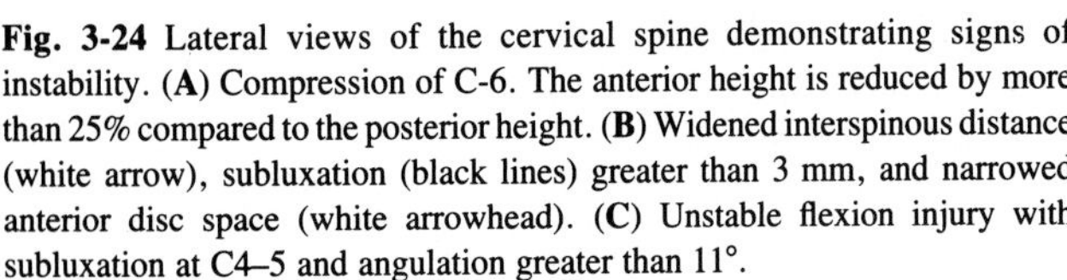

Fig. 3-24 Lateral views of the cervical spine demonstrating signs of instability. (**A**) Compression of C-6. The anterior height is reduced by more than 25% compared to the posterior height. (**B**) Widened interspinous distance (white arrow), subluxation (black lines) greater than 3 mm, and narrowed anterior disc space (white arrowhead). (**C**) Unstable flexion injury with subluxation at C4–5 and angulation greater than 11°.

It may be difficult to obtain a radiograph that includes the entire cervical spine. Penetration of the shoulders may be difficult owing to muscle spasm in the neck or shoulder injuries. The arms can be pulled distally in some patients, however, which may allow better visualization of the lower cervical spine. This requires more attendants in the room and exposes the puller to radiation. This technique should not be used unless there is a low suspicion of injury. Distraction of the arms can cause hyperextension of the cervical spine, thereby exacerbating an existing injury.[40]

At the Mayo Clinic we routinely obtain swimmer's views on all patients if C-7 and T-1 are not visible on the lateral view. This view is taken with the patient supine and the arm closest to the film elevated above the head (Fig. 3-25).[37,40] Occasionally even this technique is inadequate. In such cases lateral tomography can be performed with the Versigraph without moving the patient.

Table 3-4 summarizes injuries that can be identified and those that may be difficult to detect on the lateral view.

AP view. The AP view is obtained by angling the tube 5° to 20° to the head. The beam is centered just below the thyroid cartilage.[37,40] This view allows visualization of the vertebral bodies, uncinate processes, articular pillars, and spinous processes from C-7 to C-3. The upper cervical spine is rarely visualized on this view. In the normal cervical spine, the articular pillars should form a smooth undulating margin bilaterally, and the spinous processes should be centered and equally spaced. Deviation of the spinous process from the midline (Fig. 3-26) may indicate a unilateral locked facet secondary to a flexion-rotation injury. These injuries can be subtle and are frequently missed. Widening of the interspinous distance may indicate subluxation or dislocation. Naidich and colleagues[73] have stated that an interspinous distance

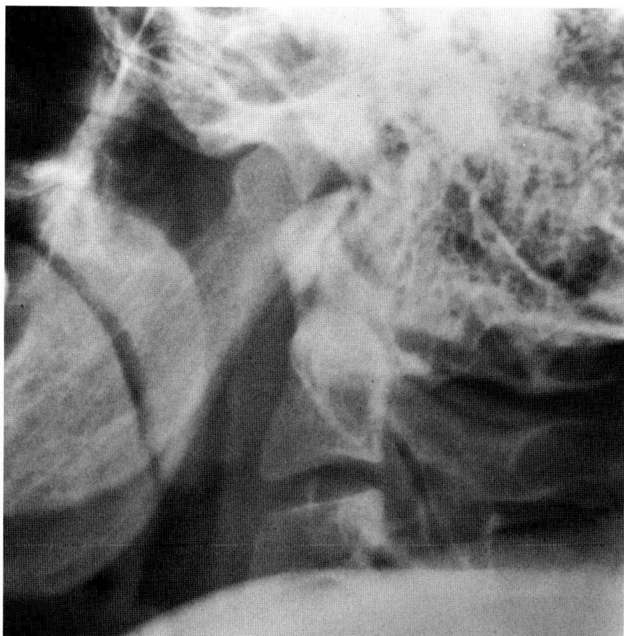

A

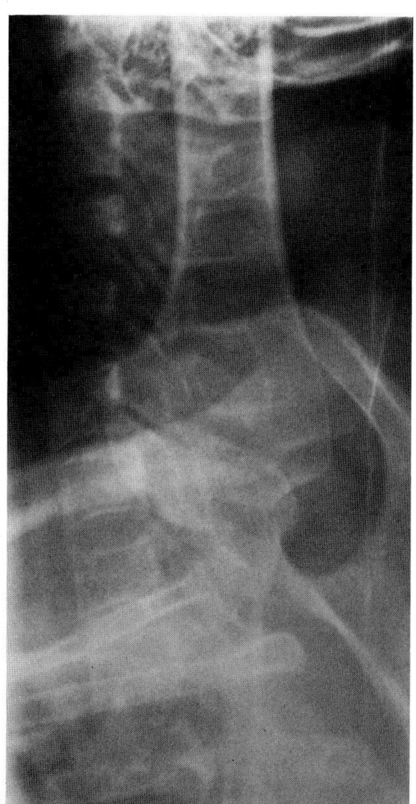

B

Fig. 3-25 Routine lateral (**A**) and swimmer's (**B**) views demonstrating the entire cervical spine.

1.5 times the interspinous distance above and below indicates dislocation. A double spinous process may be seen on the AP view in spinous process fractures.[44]

Careful attention to detail on the AP view of the lower cervical spine may be most helpful. Changes detected may be the only clue to more serious, unstable injuries that may be partially obscured on the lateral view.

Table 3-4 Value of the Lateral Radiograph in Cervical Spine Trauma

Injuries that can be identified

- Upper cervical spine
  - Atlantooccipital dislocation
  - C1–2 dislocation
  - C-1 fractures
    - Anterior arch
    - Posterior arch
  - C-2 fractures
    - Odontoid
    - Vertebral body
    - Hangman's fracture
- Lower cervical spine
  - Compression fracture
  - Burst fracture
  - Spinous process fracture
  - Locked facets
  - Soft tissue injuries
    - Flexion-compression
    - Flexion-distraction
    - Hyperextension

Injuries that are typically not identified

- Upper cervical spine
  - C-1 fractures
    - Jefferson fracture
    - Lateral mass fracture
    - Transverse process fracture
- Lower cervical spine
  - Uncinate process fracture
  - Laminar fracture
  - Pedicle fracture
  - Pillar fracture
  - Transverse process fracture

Sources: Berquist TH, *Imaging of Orthopedic Trauma,* ed 2, 1991, Raven Press; Daffner RH, *Imaging of Vertebral Trauma,* 1988, Aspen Publishers; Gehweiler JH, Osborne RL, and Becker RF, *The Radiology of Vertebral Trauma,* 1980, WB Saunders.

Odontoid view. The odontoid view is obtained with the patient's mouth open as wide as possible. The beam is centered over the open mouth and aligned perpendicularly to the cassette.[37,40] The neck should not be extended or the posterior occiput may obscure the odontoid. This view allows one to study the odontoid, lateral masses, and transverse processes of C-1. If the patient and tube are properly aligned, the spinous process of C-2 will be midline. Spaces between the teeth and the inferior margin of the posterior arch of C-1 may overlap the odontoid and should not be confused with fractures.[37] If the odontoid is not well demonstrated, the tube can be angled (Fig. 3-27) to reduce bony overlap.[37,40]

Oblique views. The oblique views after acute trauma are obtained by angling the C-arm 45° from the horizontal (Fig. 3-28). In the upright position the patient is rotated, so that the side away from the film is demonstrated. Detail is

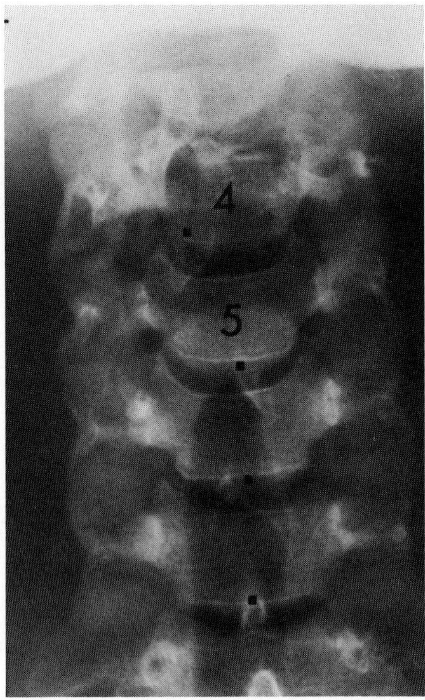

Fig. 3-26 AP view of the cervical spine demonstrating shift of the spinous processes (black dots) due to a C4–5 unilateral facet dislocation.

improved on the Versigraph. Also, magnification caused by the distance between the patient and the film may assist in detecting subtle fractures. With a conventional table, oblique views are obtained by angling the tube 35° to 40° to the horizontal with a 15° cranial angle.[37,40] The oblique views provide excellent detail of the uncinate processes, pedicles, laminae, and alignment of facet joints (Fig. 3-28). These views are particularly important in detecting facet subluxations and dislocations.[32,40,48,50,59]

Pillar views. A significant number of cervical spine fractures (50% in the series reported by Gehweiler et al[59]) involve the posterior arch. Pillar views are useful in evaluation of the articular pillars and laminae. This view is obtained by angling the tube 25° to 30° toward the feet and can be performed with the patient's neck extended or rotated 45°. The AP, lateral, and oblique views must be reviewed first to be certain that there is no unstable or significant injury. Rotation of the head or extension of the neck should be avoided if a significant injury is evident on initial views. Pillar fractures, if present, are almost always stable but can result in significant pain and radiculopathy.[33,40,59,86,93]

Obtaining high-quality pillar views can be difficult. Conventional tomography or CT is more frequently utilized in our practice.

Flexion and extension views. Flexion and extension views of the cervical spine are performed to evaluate stability. The examination is most often indicated to exclude ligament instability after trauma or to determine whether fractures are healed and stable. This examination should be performed fluoroscopically so that a true lateral position can be properly attained and the degree of motion monitored. Some clinicians perform upright lateral views before clearing patients with otherwise normal cervical spine series.[49]

The patient should sit or stand. Physiologic extension and flexion in the lateral position are monitored fluoroscopically. The extension maneuver is performed initially, and alignment of the vertebrae and anterior ligament structures are studied. The patient is then asked to flex the cervical spine slowly so that alignment, subluxation, facet joint widening, and spinous process motion can be carefully observed (Fig. 3-29). The criteria discussed in routine evaluation of the lateral cervical spine (Table 3-3) can be applied (Fig. 3-24). Subtle changes may be important, however, and care must be taken not to

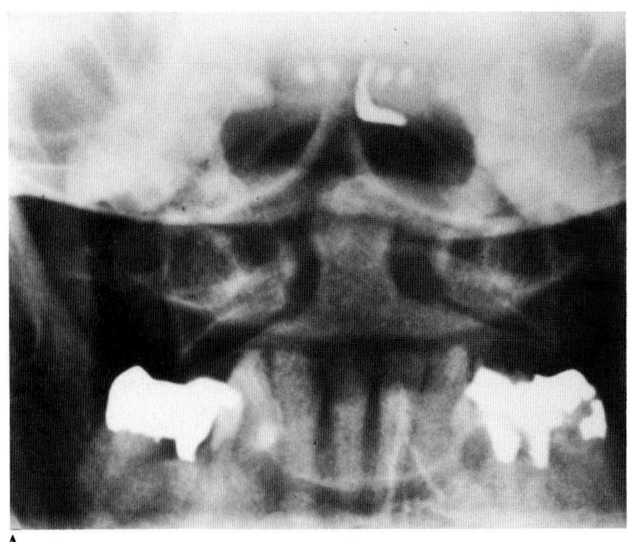

A

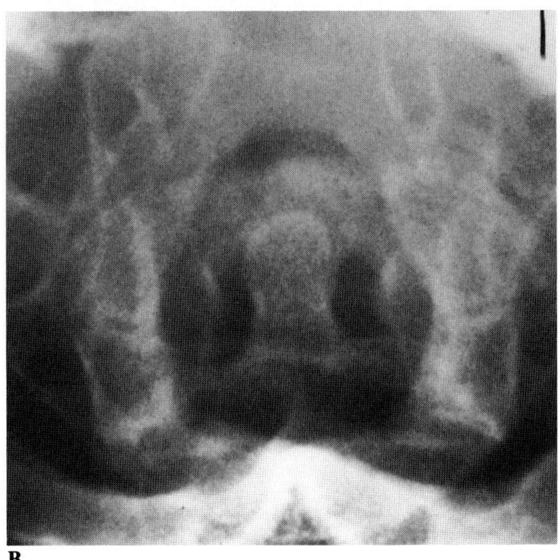

B

Fig. 3-27 Routine (**A**) and angled AP (**B**) views of the odontoid.

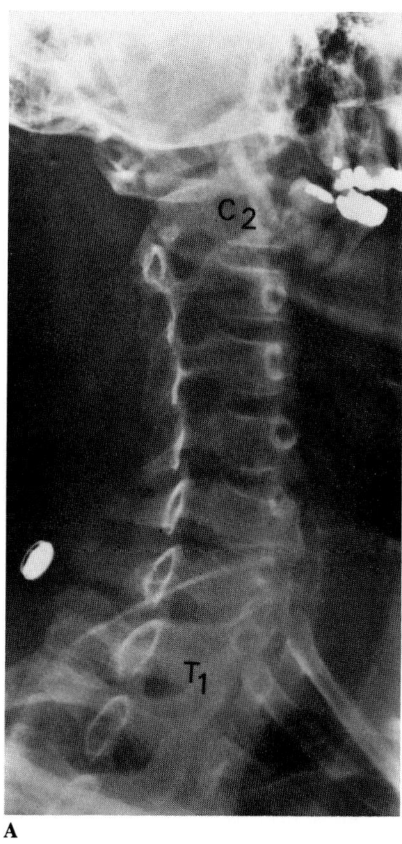

A

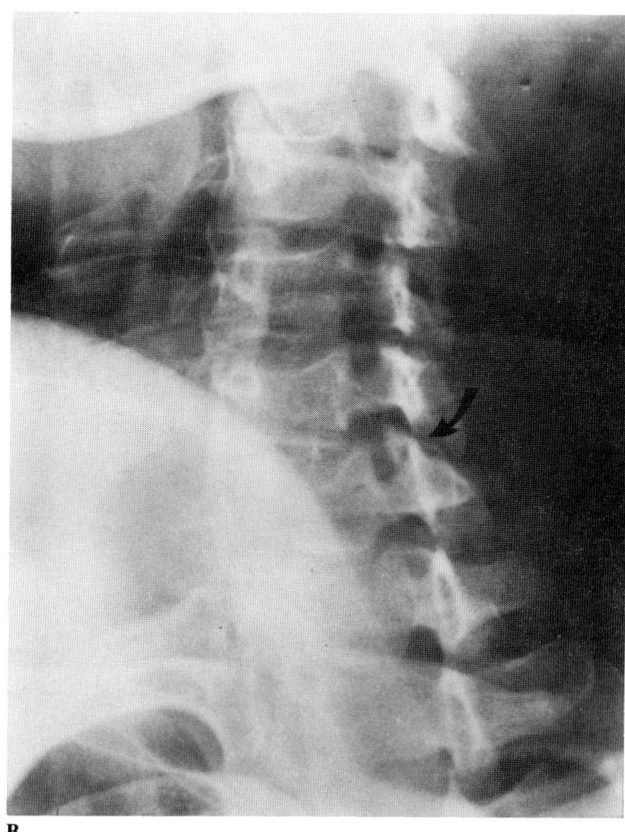

B

Fig. 3-28 (**A**) Normal oblique view demonstrating the laminae and foramina. (**B**) Flexion-rotation injury with a C-6 facet fracture (curved arrow).

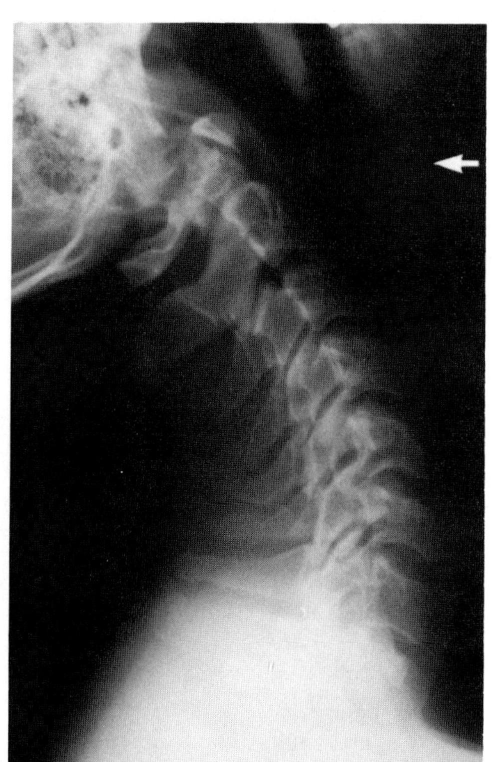

A

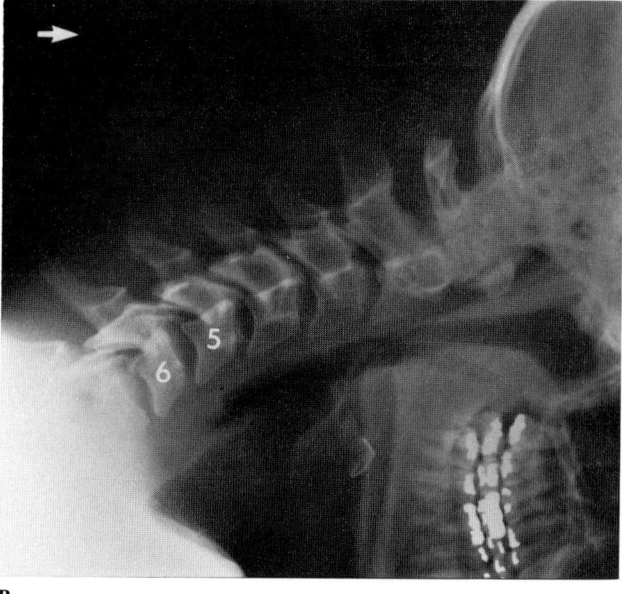

B

Fig. 3-29 Extension (**A**) and flexion (**B**) views of a C5–6 posterior ligament injury with posterior and middle column involvement indicating instability. Arrows indicate direction of motion.

overlook posterior ligament damage. Vertebral body subluxation in flexion should not exceed 1 mm.[40,59,74]

Conventional and Computed Tomography

Tomographic techniques are often helpful in determining the full extent of injury.[34,39,40,47,68,77,96] CT is most frequently selected, but conventional tomography is preferred in patients with suspected odontoid fractures or when the fracture line may be parallel to the CT image plane. In this setting, fractures may be overlooked because of partial volume effects.[39,40]

The choice of examination is based on several factors, including patient status, type of injury suspected, and equipment availability. Most skeletal tomography is performed with complex motion techniques as opposed to linear tomography. This would require moving the patient. The C-arm unit permits linear tomography in the AP, lateral, oblique, and axial planes without moving the patient. We routinely obtain AP and lateral tomograms. Tomography is most useful for evaluating odontoid fractures (Fig. 3-30), fractures in the plane of CT imaging, and fractures of the facet joints (Fig. 3-31) and for demonstrating contiguous segments.[40,97]

CT is most useful for evaluating patients with neurologic deficits, detecting bone fragments in the spinal canal (Fig. 3-32) or neural foramina, and preoperative planning of complex injuries.[34,39,40,47] On occasion, intrathecal contrast medium plus CT is used to evaluate dural tears and nerve root injuries (Fig. 3-33).[40,47,96] Nonionic water-soluble contrast medium can be injected via the lumbar route or by C1–2 puncture. In most patients 5-mm contiguous slices are adequate for evaluating spinal fractures. If reconstruction in the coronal and sagittal planes or three-dimensional processing is required, much thinner slices should be obtained. Three-millimeter slices at 2-mm intervals or 1.5-mm contiguous slices provide superior reconstructed images.[40,96]

Magnetic Resonance Imaging

MRI is an established technique for evaluating the musculoskeletal system.[40,61,70] Soft tissue contrast is superior to that obtained with CT, and images can be obtained in the axial, coronal, oblique, and sagittal planes. Fine bone detail (ie, the thin cortical bone of vertebral bodies) is not as well demonstrated with MRI compared to CT.[39,40] Also, the confining nature of the MR gantry reduces patient access, especially on high-field (>1.0 T) imagers. Therefore, MRI is not as frequently utilized in the acutely injured patient with multiple trauma.

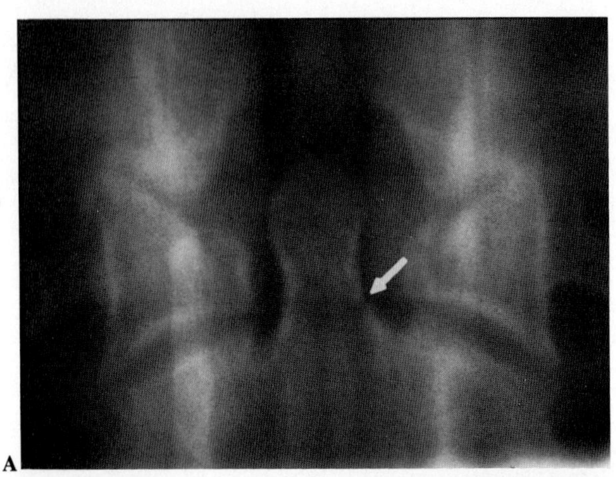

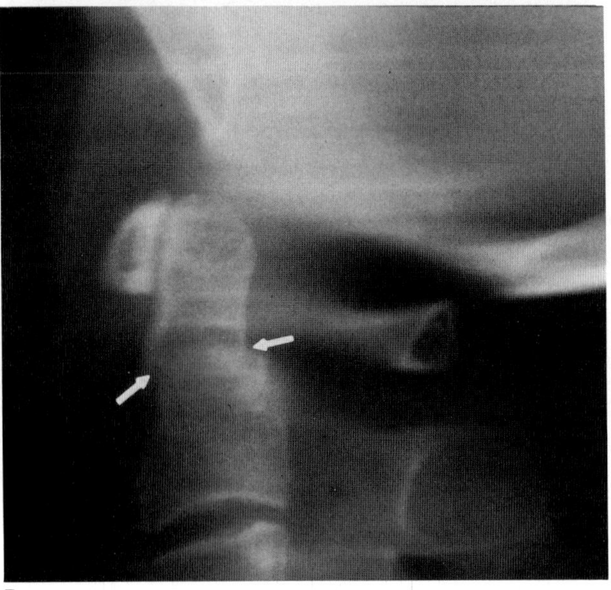

Fig. 3-30 AP (**A**) and lateral (**B**) tomograms of the upper cervical spine demonstrating a slightly displaced odontoid fracture (arrows). Both AP and lateral views are essential. The lesion is most obvious on the lateral tomogram in this patient.

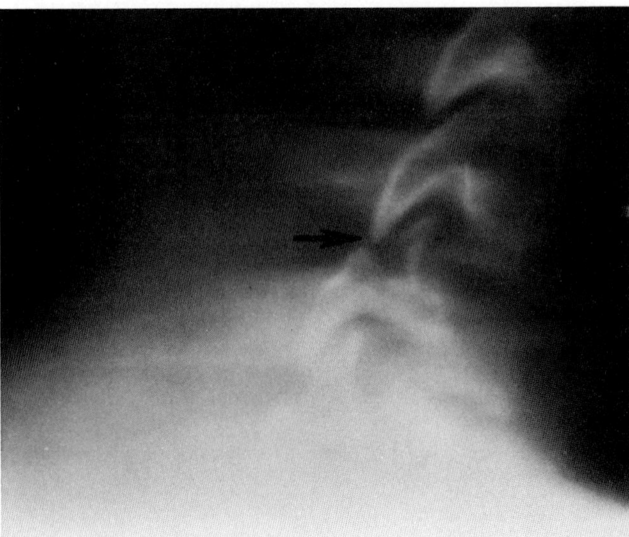

Fig. 3-31 Lateral tomogram of a superior facet fracture (arrow). This was overlooked on computed tomography (CT) because the articular surfaces were not significantly displaced.

MRI techniques have improved significantly over the past several years. Although there are numerous sequences from which to choose, most clinicians utilize both T1- and T2-weighted images to evaluate completely the osseous and soft tissue anatomy.[61,70] Sagittal T1-weighted images (SE 500/20) provide a good screening technique for changes in the vertebral body (Fig. 3-34). T2-Weighted images are more useful for evaluation of the spinal cord and discs. Muscle tears and ligament injuries should also be more easily appreciated on T2-weighted images.[39,40] Spin-echo T2-weighted images (SE $\geq$2000/$\geq$60) require 9 to 16 minutes of imaging time. New gradient-echo techniques with reduced flip angles can provide images with T2-weighting in about 4 minutes, which is advantageous in patients with spinal cord injury. The use of gadolinium DTPA with T1-weighted images is also helpful for more complete evaluation of the spinal cord.

To date, MRI has been most useful for evaluation of the spinal cord and discs.[61,70] Kulkarni et al[70] described patterns of cord abnormality (edema and hemorrhage) that are useful in predicting neurologic recovery. The potential for evaluating posterior muscle and ligament injury also exists, but results are preliminary at this time. Currently, MRI is most often used for evaluating patients with cord injury in the acute and chronic setting.[40,60,61,70]

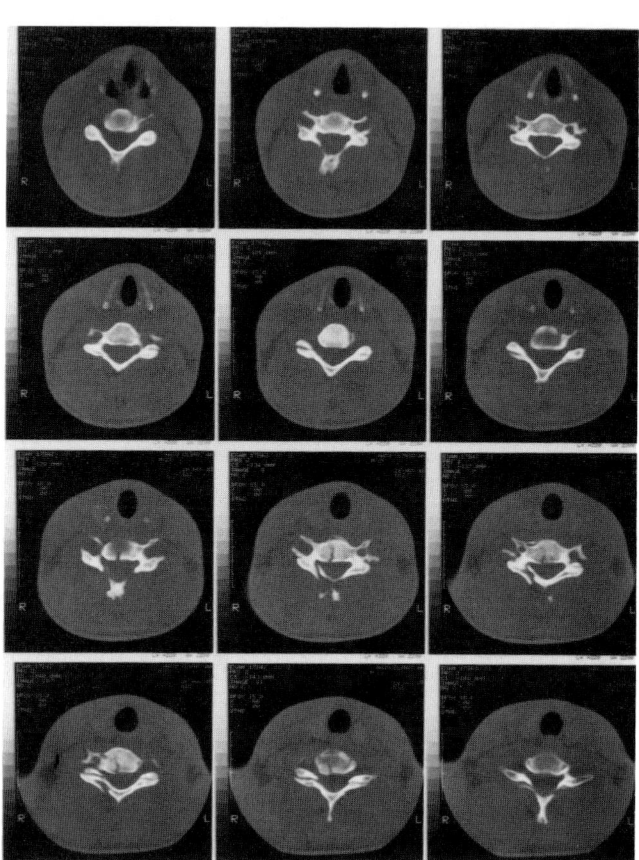

Fig. 3-32 A series of CT sections through the lower cervical spine demonstrating a complex sagittal fracture (lower frames).

Major Cervical Spine Injuries

The anatomic relationships of the upper cervical spine are unique, and the mechanisms of injury differ somewhat from those affecting the lower cervical spine. Therefore, in discussing specific cervical spine injuries the upper and lower seg-

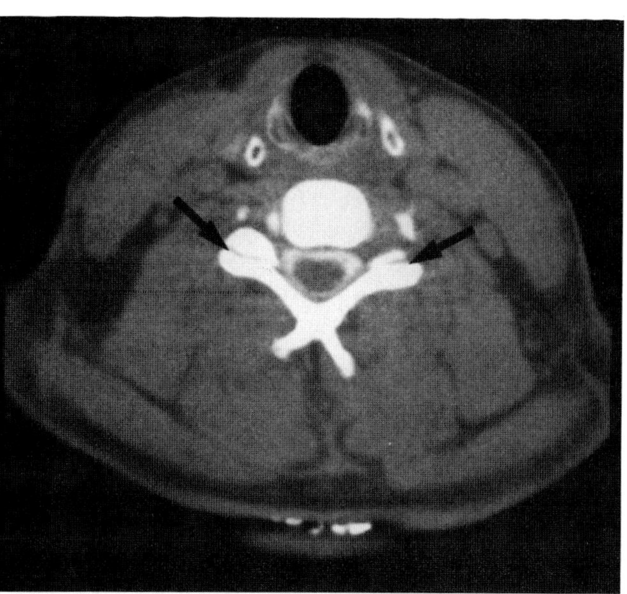

Fig. 3-33 CT image after administration of intrathecal contrast agent. The spinal canal is normal. There are normal facet joints (arrows). Both bone and soft tissue windows must be evaluated.

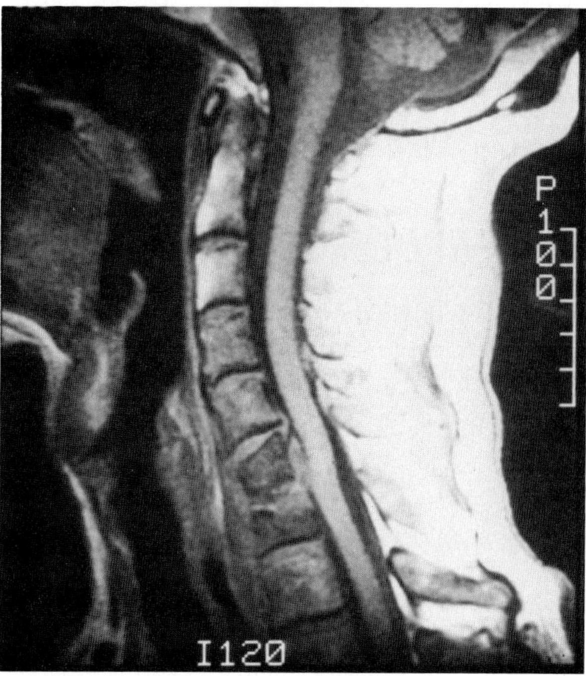

Fig. 3-34 Sagittal (SE 500/20) magnetic resonance (MR) image demonstrating a C6–7 flexion-compression injury. The soft tissue changes narrow the canal slightly.

ments are presented separately. As with injuries incurred in motor vehicle accidents, most sports-related injuries in adults involve the lower cervical spine.[40,54,75,84,85] In children up to 25% of injuries occur above C-4.[36]

Upper Cervical Spine

Injuries involving the occipital condyles and atlantooccipital articulation are rare.[40,59] Fractures of the condyle may result from shearing or rotary forces and blows to the calvarium from above, similar to the mechanism that results in a Jefferson fracture. These injuries may disrupt the hypoglossal canal, injuring the jugular vein and cranial nerves IX, X, and XI. Often, however, the trauma may seem minor with no neurologic deficit. As with other upper cervical spine injuries, tomography (AP and lateral projections) is extremely valuable. Routine radiographs are often normal, and CT may miss this fracture because of partial volume effects.[40,59]

Atlantooccipital dislocations are also rare. This injury usually occurs in high-velocity motor vehicle accidents. Snowmobiling, auto racing, and tobogganing may also lead to this injury. At the Mayo Clinic we noted three atlantooccipital dislocations due to snowmobiling in 1 year. The lesion is usually the result of shearing forces directed either to the face or to the occipital region. Death due to brain stem injury typically follows this injury. Atlantooccipital dislocation is more common in children (Fig. 3-35) owing to their smaller condyles and the more horizontal articular relationship of the condyles with the lateral masses of the atlas.[40]

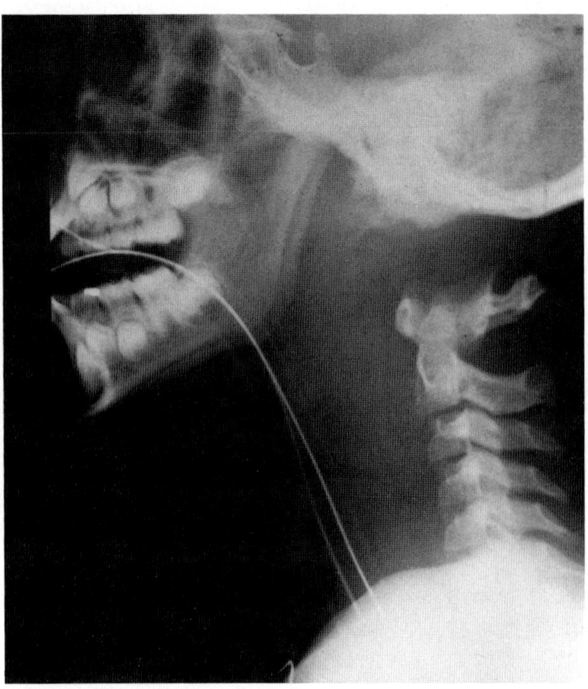

Fig. 3-35 Obvious atlantooccipital dislocation due to a snowmobile accident. The injury was fatal.

Radiographically, the diagnosis is usually obvious on the lateral view of the skull or cervical spine (Fig. 3-35). The occipital condyles lose their normal articular relationship with the atlas, and a large hematoma is present in the retropharyngeal space.[40]

Atlas (C-1). In our experience fractures of the atlas account for approximately 4% of all spinal injuries.[40] Other investigators report a similar incidence.[48,59,65,83] These injuries, although due to axial forces, are infrequent in athletes. Five types of fractures have been described on the basis of the anatomic region affected: fractures of the anterior arch, posterior arch, lateral mass, and transverse process and the Jefferson fracture.[65] Fractures most commonly involve the lateral masses and the posterior arch (Fig. 3-36). Sherk and Nicholson[83] reported that posterior arch fractures account for 67% of fractures of the atlas. Posterior arch fractures are the result of hyperextension injuries in which the arch is compressed between the occiput and spinous process of the axis.[40,59] Associated injuries are common. In one study,[40] spinous process fractures of C-7 were evident in 25% of patients with posterior arch fractures of C-1. Because posterior arch fractures are hyperextension injuries, one should not be surprised by the frequently associated facial injuries.

Pure Jefferson fractures result from a force directed vertically to the skull.[65] The force is transmitted to the occipital condyles, which leads to lateral displacement of the lateral masses of the atlas (Fig. 3-37). The lateral displacement is a result of the anatomic configuration of these articulations. Fractures typically occur in the anterior and posterior arches (Fig. 3-37B). The anterior and, more specifically, the posterior arch are the weak points in the ring of the atlas. Less commonly, horizontal fractures of the anterior arch occur (Fig. 3-38). This injury also results from hyperextension and

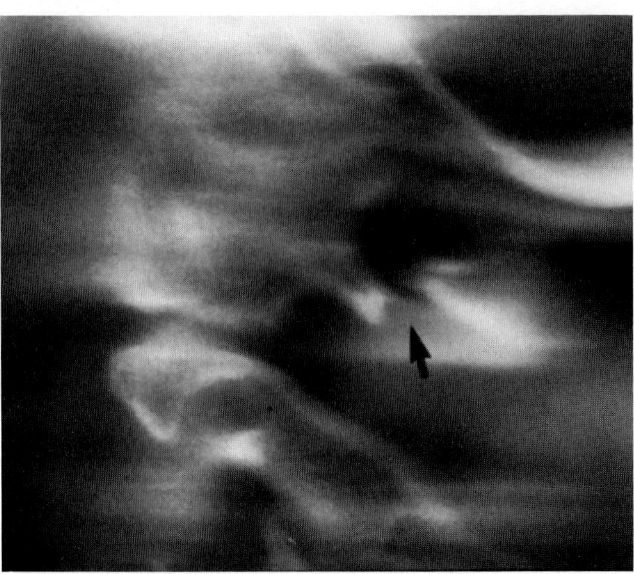

Fig. 3-36 Tomogram demonstrating a posterior arch fracture of C-1 (arrow).

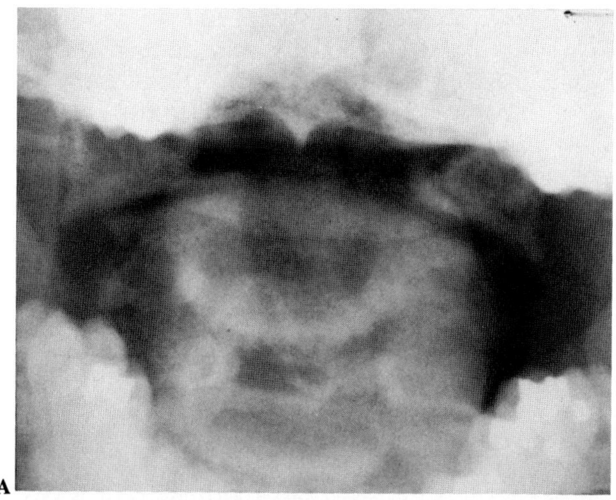

A

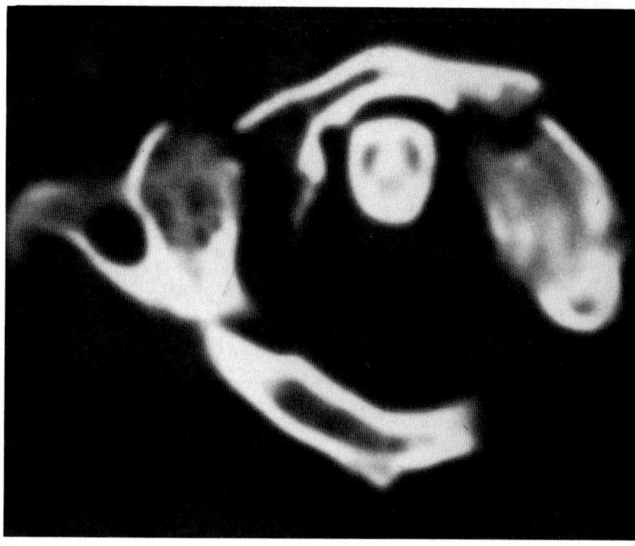

B

Fig. 3-37 Jefferson fracture seen on AP open mouth odontoid view (**A**) and CT (**B**).

avulsion at the insertion of the longus colli.[59,66] It is essential to exclude other associated hyperextension injuries.[66]

Neurologic complications with atlas fractures are rare.[40,59,65] Significant retropharyngeal hemorrhage resulting in difficulty in breathing has been reported, however.

Radiographically, most injuries of C-1 can be detected on the AP odontoid view or on the lateral view of the cervical spine or skull (Figs. 3-36 and 3-37). Several significant features noted on the AP odontoid view (Fig. 3-37A) or AP tomograms should be stressed. Outward displacement of the lateral masses of the atlas of greater than 6.9 mm indicates a tear or avulsion of the transverse ligament.[40,59] Normal features, however, such as the insertion of the transverse ligament and bipartite superior facets should not be confused with fractures. Subtle changes may require conventional tomography or CT for complete evaluation. CT is especially useful in evaluating the ring of the atlas (Fig. 3-37B).[40,50]

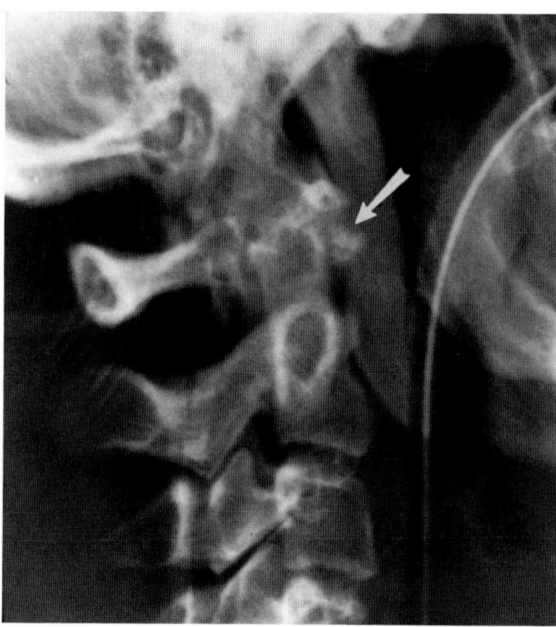

Fig. 3-38 Lateral view of the upper cervical spine demonstrating an avulsion fracture (arrow) of the anterior arch of C-1.

Posterior and rotary dislocations are uncommon and occur more frequently in children and young adults as a result of rotation of the head, which may occur in wrestling or tackling with the arms about the head. Rotary dislocation requires 45° of rotation of C-1 on the axis for locking to occur.[59] This condition differs from the rotary fixation described by Fielding and Hawkins.[58] Sixty-five degrees of rotation is required for fixation to occur if the transverse ligament and odontoid are anatomically normal.[58] If the ligament is interrupted, less rotation is required. Cord injury and vertebral artery injury have been reported with rotary fixation. Fielding and Hawkins[58] defined the following four types of injuries:

- type I: rotary fixation without anterior subluxation of the atlas on the axis (transverse ligament intact)
- type II: rotary fixation with 3 to 5 mm of atlantoaxial subluxation
- type III: rotary fixation with greater than 5 mm of atlantoaxial subluxation
- type IV: rotary fixation with posterior atlantoaxial subluxation (deficient dens required)

Type I is the most common lesion reported.[58] The patient usually presents with the head rotated to the side. Neurologic deficits are rare. The exact etiology is unclear, but fixation may be related to capsular entrapment in the atlantoaxial facets.[58]

Radiographically, the AP and lateral odontoid views may be sufficient for diagnosis. CT is most accurate for evaluation, however, and allows differentiation from torticollis or simple rotation more readily than routine radiographs (Fig. 3-39).

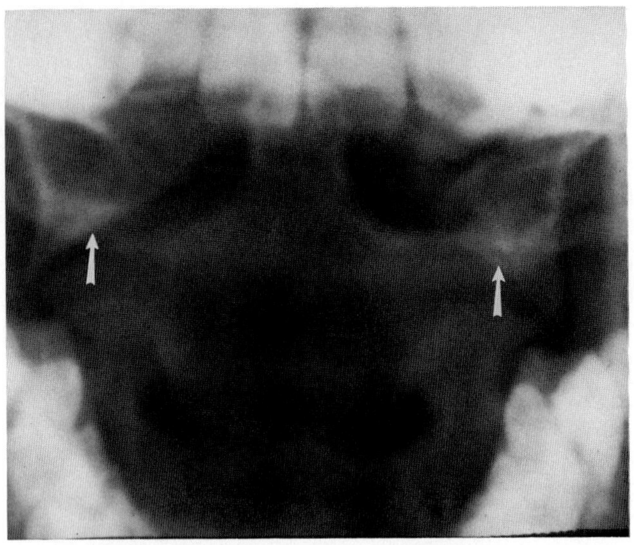

A

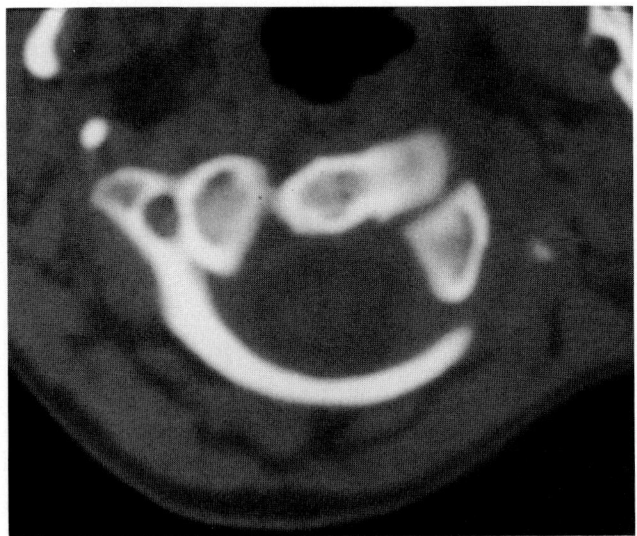

B

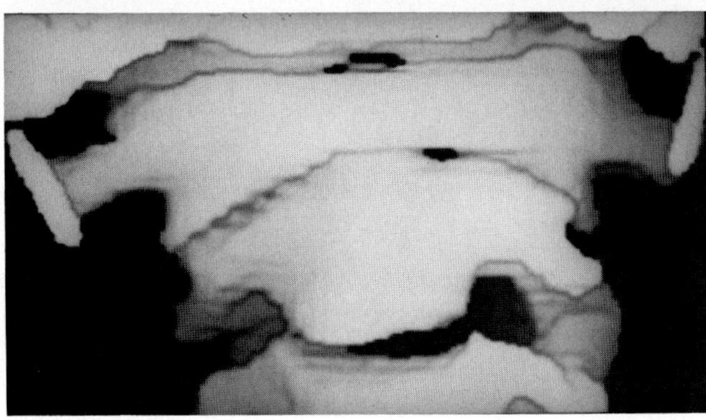

C

Fig. 3-39 Rotary fixation of C-1 on C-2 due to a wrestling injury. (**A**) The open mouth odontoid view shows asymmetry of the lateral masses (arrows). (**B**) CT and (**C**) three-dimensional CT images confirm the injury.

Axis (C-2). Fractures of the odontoid and pedicles account for 80% of injuries to the axis.[43] The vertebral body is involved in about 15% of cases, usually through the antero-inferior chip fracture. The facets, laminae, and spinous processes are less frequently involved.[43,59]

Odontoid fractures may result from anterior shearing (hyperextension), posterior shearing (hyperflexion), or lateral flexion injuries. Obviously, these are most common in contact sports, snowmobiling, auto racing, and the like. Odontoid fractures account for 11% to 13% of all cervical spine fractures.[43] Patients with odontoid fractures usually present with neck pain and rarely have neurologic symptoms.[40] Even if there is displacement of the fractures, there is usually sufficient space to prevent cord injury.

In a significant number of cases, odontoid fractures are undisplaced and subtle, requiring tomography for definitive diagnosis and classification (Fig. 3-30). The mechanism of injury in these cases is often difficult to determine. If the fracture is slightly displaced, the mechanism of injury is more easily established. When the fracture is displaced, the lateral view of the skull or cervical spine and the open mouth odontoid view are usually adequate for diagnosis.

Radiographically, one should check carefully for retropharyngeal soft tissue swelling, which may be the only clue to an odontoid fracture (Fig. 3-40). Tomography is frequently required for diagnosis and classification of the fractures. The classification system of Anderson and D'Alonzo[35] is commonly utilized and is helpful in determining proper management and prognosis of the fracture.[46,59] The classification divides odontoid fractures into three types: type I, oblique fracture of the tip of the odontoid; type II, fracture of the base of the odontoid; and type III, fracture entering the body of the axis (Fig. 3-40).[35,40,59]

A significant number of type II odontoid fractures (59% to 67% of odontoid fractures) will be overlooked on routine radiographs. Also, CT may miss this injury because the fracture line may lie entirely within the image plane. Therefore, AP and lateral tomograms may be the best technique. Tomograms should be considered whenever symptoms are present even if routine views are normal. Both AP and lateral views are necessary because these injuries may be subtle (Fig. 3-30).

Type III fractures account for about 33% of odontoid fractures. These fractures are frequently impacted anteriorly, and anterior displacement can be identified in up to 90% of patients. Undisplaced type III fractures almost always unite with proper treatment.[40,46] Neurologic involvement is slightly less common than with type II fractures. Nonunion is common (40%) if anterior displacement exceeds 5 mm.[46,59]

Fractures of the neural arch of the axis (hangman's fractures) result from hyperextension, and usually anterior subluxation of C-2 on C-3 is evident on the lateral radiograph (Fig. 3-41). The lesion, as originally described, occurred as a

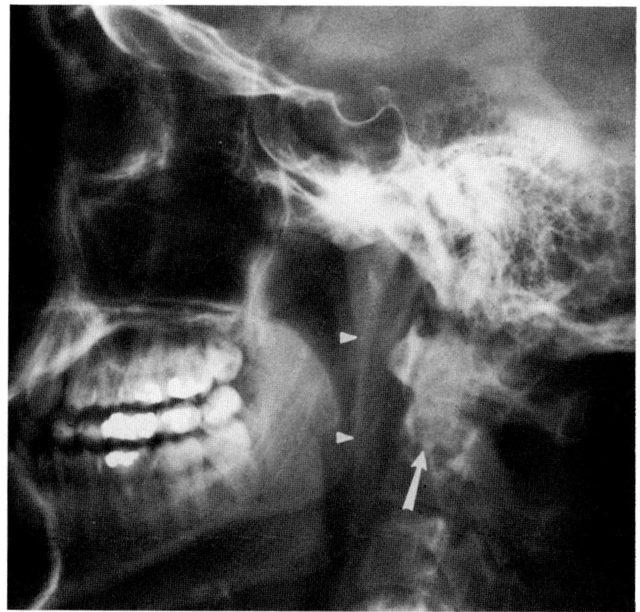

Fig. 3-40 Lateral view of the skull in a patient after a head injury during hockey. There is a subtle type III odontoid fracture (arrow). Note the prevertebral swelling (arrowheads).

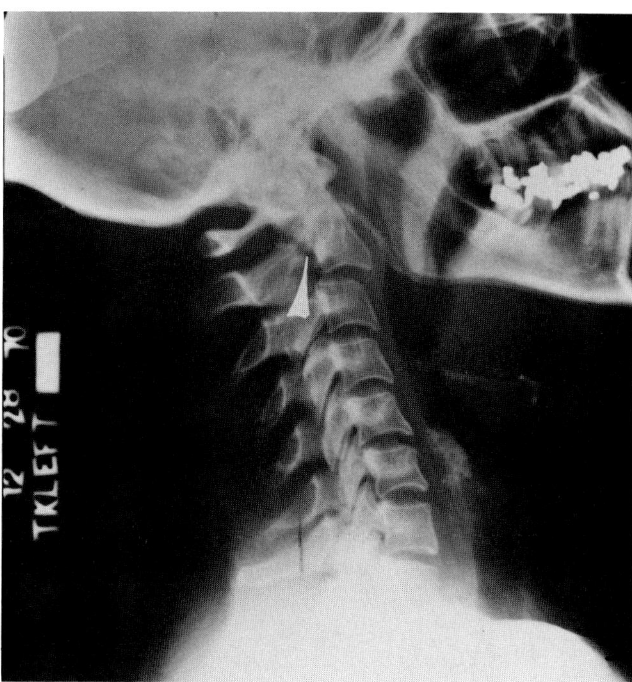

Fig. 3-41 Lateral view of the cervical spine demonstrating a fracture of the C-2 pedicle (hangman's fracture, arrow).

result of judicial hanging.[40,48,59] This mechanism of hyperextension and sustained distraction resulted in death. Flexion-compression and flexion-distraction have also been implicated in hangman's fracture.[59]

Although hangman's fractures have been considered pedicle fractures, this may be anatomically incorrect. Burke and Harris[43] prefer the term *traumatic spondylolisthesis of C-2* because by definition C-2 does not have true pedicles. This may be true, but the terminology will not change quickly; the term *pedicle fracture* will probably continue to be used.

Fractures of the body of the axis occurred in 13% to 15% of patients in the study by Burke and Harris.[43] These fractures were all the result of hyperextension injuries and usually involved the anteroinferior margin of the vertebral body. Soft tissue swelling was common and often marked.

Isolated fractures of the lamina, spinous process, and facets of the axis are uncommon. Facet fractures of the axis are often associated with compression-rotation or lateral compression injuries, which result in associated lateral mass fractures of the atlas.[33]

Lower Cervical Spine (C3–7)

In adults, injuries to the lower cervical spine occur four times more frequently than upper cervical spine fractures.[40,59] Axial loading and flexion are the most common mechanisms of injury in athletes. Also, injuries at the C3–4 level tend to occur more commonly in sports injuries compared to motor vehicle accidents.[91] The location of the fracture varies with the force or mechanism of injury.[40,48,50]

Vertebral Arch Fractures

Fractures of the lamina are usually due to hyperextension injuries. Spinous process fractures are commonly associated with these fractures (Fig. 3-42). Most laminar fractures occur in the C5–7 region. Pillar views and tomography (conventional or CT) are often necessary to detect laminar fractures. CT may also be helpful, but in one study several cases of undisplaced fractures not evident on CT were easily demonstrated with conventional tomography.[68] This is true of any undisplaced fracture in which the fracture is aligned parallel to the slice. The increased utilization of tomography in our practice may be at least partially responsible for the higher incidence of laminar fractures in our series because of a higher rate of detection.[40] Fractures of the lamina frequently extend into the base of the spinous process, resulting in a displaced spinous process. This should not be confused with the more benign clay shoveler's fracture. Laminar fractures with spinous process involvement have been reported frequently with hyperextension injuries of the type V classification (comminuted vertebral arch fracture with hyperextension fracture-dislocation).[59]

Pedicle fractures may be detected in up to 25% of vertebral arch injuries.[40] Most pedicle fractures occur at C-2, but pedicle fractures are also noted in the lower cervical spine with hyperextension injuries.[40,48,55] These injuries may be visible on lateral or oblique views. Conventional tomography or CT is frequently necessary for diagnosis.[40] Acheson et al[34] reported

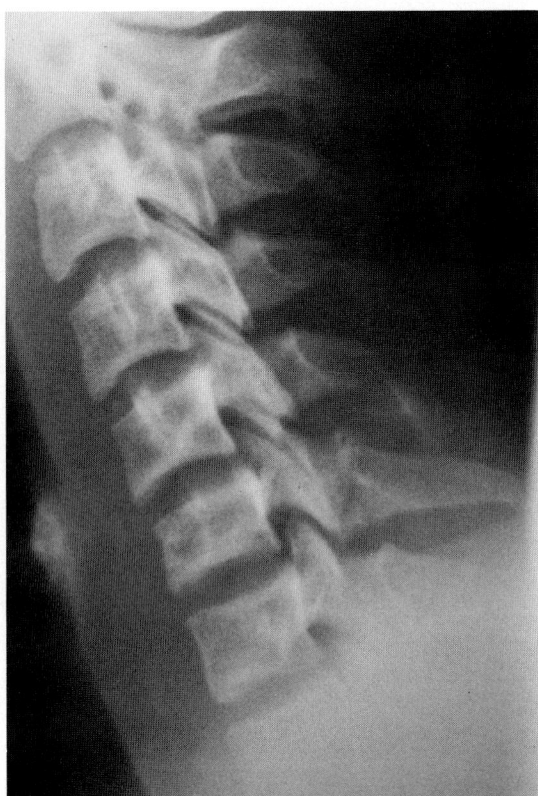

Fig. 3-42 Lateral view of the cervical spine demonstrating C-4 and C-5 spinous process fractures and a C-6 laminar fracture.

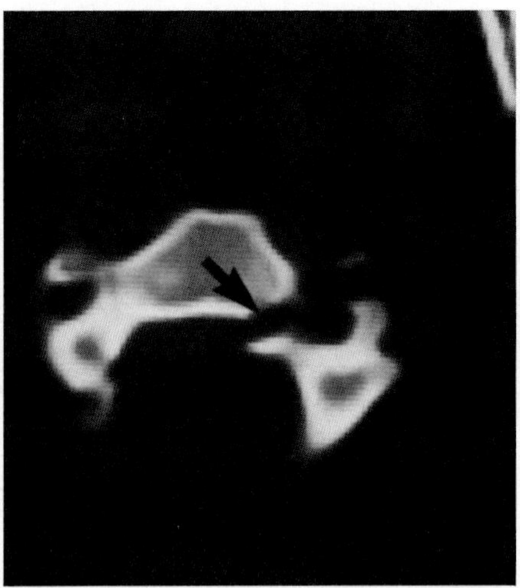

Fig. 3-43 CT section of a lower cervical vertebra demonstrating a pedicle fracture (arrow) on the left.

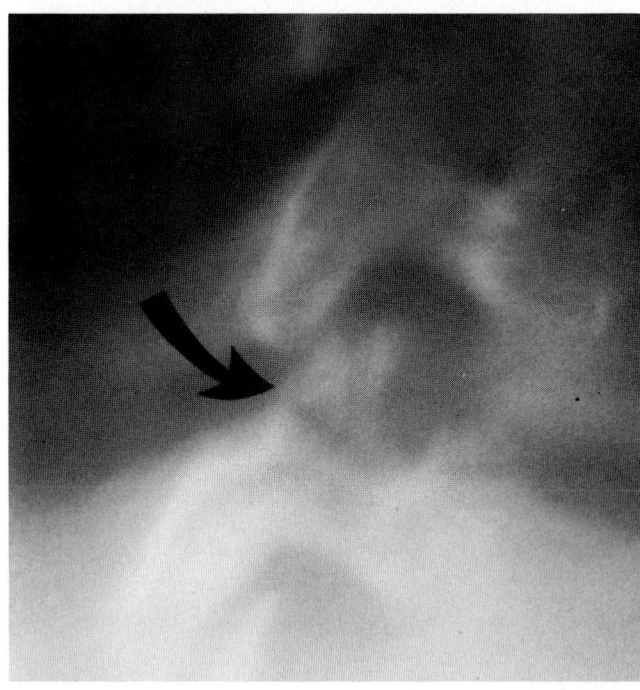

Fig. 3-44 Lateral tomogram demonstrating a superior facet fracture (arrow) in the lower cervical spine.

that 82% of pedicle fractures were overlooked on plain films but were detected with CT (Fig. 3-43).

Spinous process fractures account for 22% of vertebral arch injuries (Fig. 3-32).[40] Most spinous process fractures occur at the C5–T1 level. This fracture may result from direct trauma, hyperextension, or hyperflexion, and it is only through careful evaluation of the remaining vertebral units that the mechanism of injury may be established.[40,50] On the AP view a double spinous process may be the only clue to an unsuspected spinous process fracture.[44] In other cases the lateral view is usually most useful.

Fractures of the articular pillars have been reported to be the most common arch fracture.[59] These injuries usually occur at the C-6 level. In one series pillar fractures occurred in 16% of vertebral arch fractures.[40] The mechanism of injury is usually hyperextension or lateral flexion.[59,86] Occasionally, the AP view will demonstrate the lesion. These fractures are best demonstrated on pillar views or CT.[34,47] Up to 60% will be overlooked on plain film examinations.[40] There is usually no cord injury with a pillar fracture, but radiculopathy may result, especially if proper treatment is not instituted.

Facet fractures represented 9% of vertebral arch fractures in our study.[40] These were most common with hyperflexion and flexion-rotation injuries.[40,82,97] Oblique and lateral views may demonstrate this lesion, but conventional tomography or CT is usually required (Fig. 3-44). Radicular symptoms are common with solitary facet fractures.[97] Facet fractures are usually detected with multiple injuries, including injuries of the posterior ligaments and disc.[39,40,59]

Transverse process fractures are uncommon.[40,59] The injury results from lateral flexion or direct trauma. Associated upper rib fractures are not uncommon.

Vertebral Body Fractures

Vertebral body fractures are common with sports injuries due to axial loading and flexion injuries. Most fractures are in

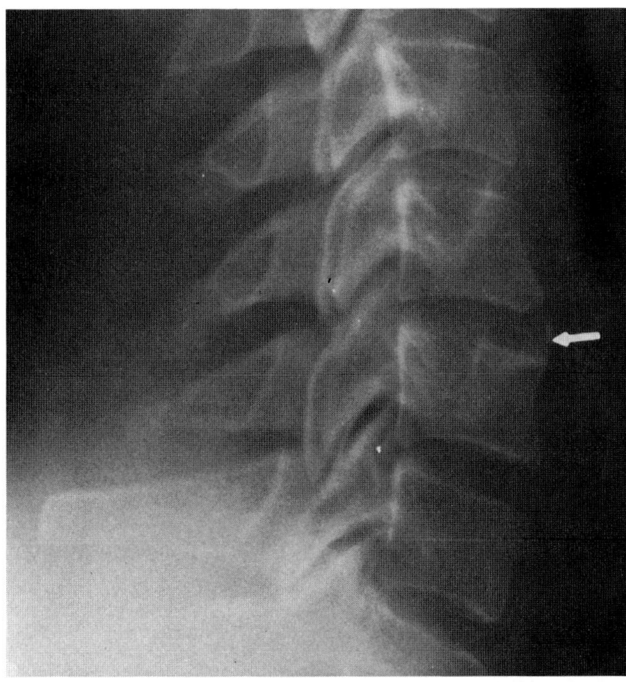

Fig. 3-45 Lateral view of the cervical spine demonstrating an old C-2 pedicle fracture with anterior fusion of C2–3 and a healed anterior ligament injury (arrow) due to hyperextension injury.

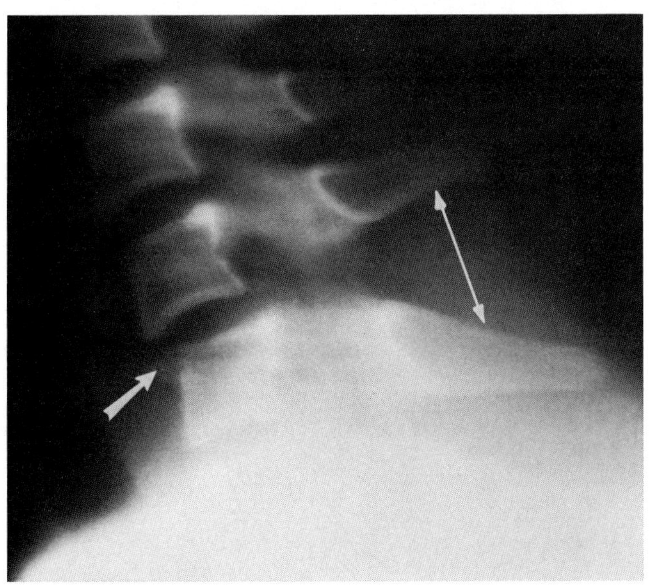

Fig. 3-46 Lateral tomogram of a flexion-compression injury. There is an anterosuperior fracture of C-7 (arrow) with widening of the spinous processes (double arrow) due to ligament injury.

the C5–7 region, but C3–4 lesions are also common in athletes.[91] Fractures are usually evident on the AP and lateral views, with oblique views providing additional information. Tomography and CT are less frequently required for detection of vertebral body fractures, but evaluation of fragment position and classification is aided with CT.[34,40,47,68,77]

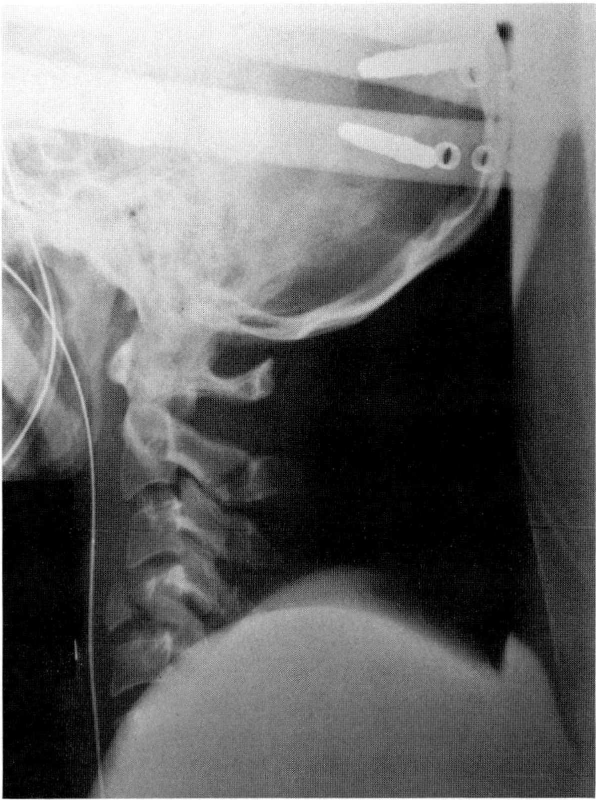

Fig. 3-47 Lateral view of the cervical spine after a C-4 hyperextension fracture-dislocation with a large triangular anterior fragment. There are also arch fractures of C-2 and C-3.

Vertebral body fractures have several radiographic presentations: chip fractures, usually of the anterosuperior or anteroinferior margin; triangular fractures; burst fractures; wedge fractures, usually anterior but also lateral; uncinate process fractures; and sagittal fractures. Care must be taken not to mistake overlying structures for vertebral body fractures.[51]

Chip fractures are commonly due to hyperflexion injuries (anterosuperior margin) and hyperextension injuries (anteroinferior margin). After hyperextension injury, the fracture fragment is avulsed with the anterior longitudinal ligament and in most instances enters the disc space (Fig. 3-45).[40,59,62,67] Hyperflexion injuries are often associated with posterior ligament disruption and are therefore unstable (Fig. 3-46). Hyperextension injuries are usually stable unless the fracture of the body is associated with a posterior arch fracture, in which case the lesion is unstable.[59,71]

Larger triangular or teardrop fractures of the vertebral body are more significant. Most involve the anteroinferior body (Fig. 3-47). The majority of triangular fractures involve the lower cervical spine (67% in one study). Neurologic involvement, usually quadriplegia, occurs in more than 80% of patients.[40,59,62]

Simple compression fractures are most often anterior and result from flexion-compression injuries (Fig. 3-48). The posterior ligaments may be intact, depending upon the degree of

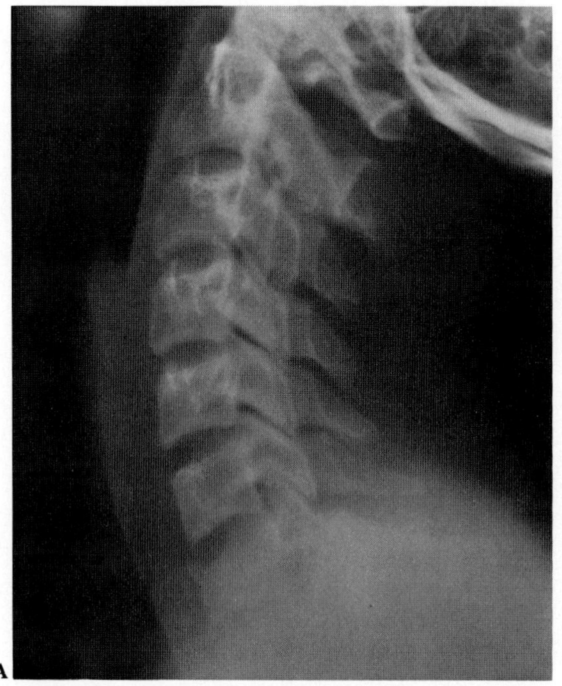

A

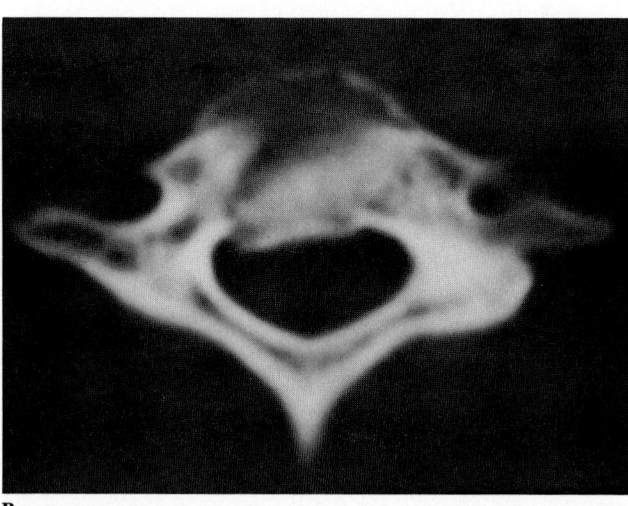

B

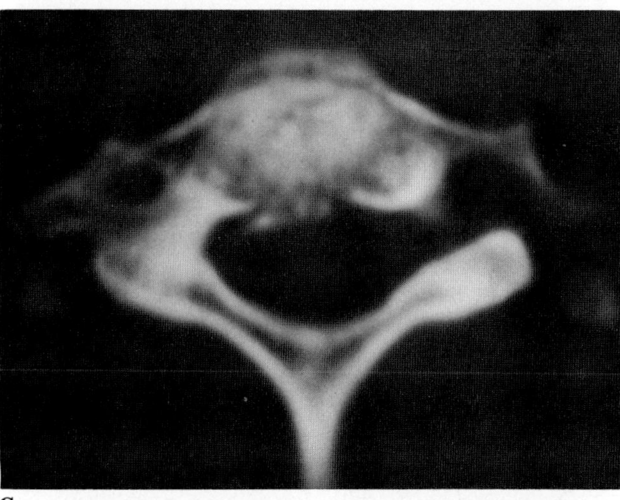

C

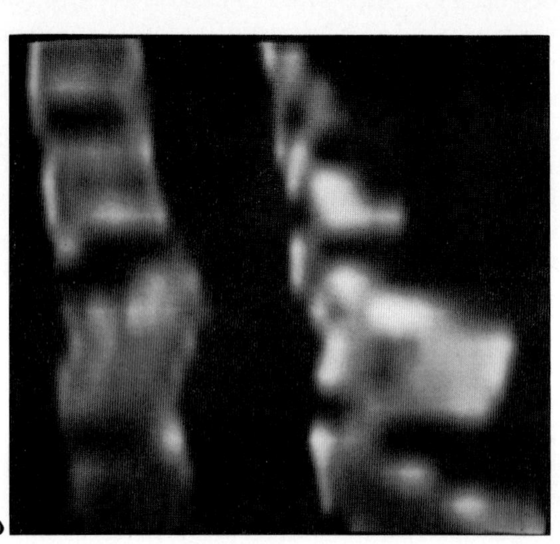

D

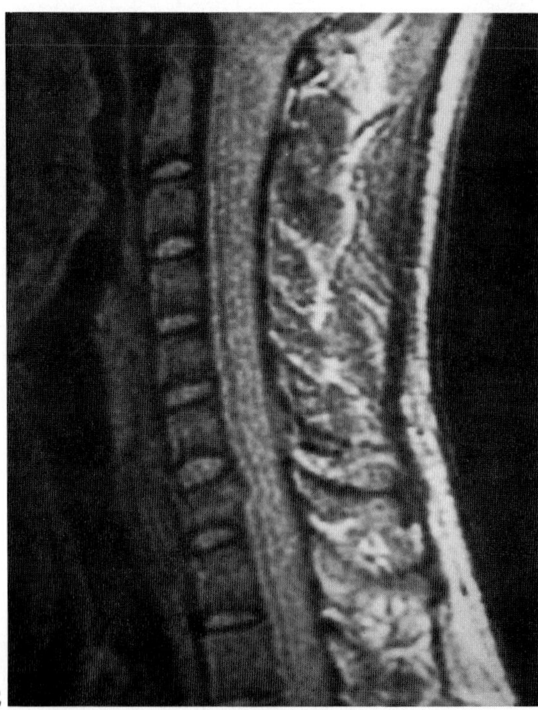

E

Fig. 3-48 Football injury occurring during a tackle. (**A**) Lateral view of the cervical spine shows anterior compression of C-7, suggesting a simple anterior compression fracture. (**B** and **C**) CT images in the axial plain and (**D**) sagittal reconstruction show posterior vertebral involvement due to a burst component. (**E**) Sagittal MR image shows slight narrowing of the canal and an anterior hematoma.

associated posterior element distraction. The posterior ligaments must be evaluated at some point during treatment to be certain that the lesion is stable. This requires fluoroscopically controlled flexion and extension views.

Lateral wedge fractures and uncinate fractures are the result of asymmetric vertical compression or lateral flexion injuries. These fractures are rare.[50,59,62]

Burst fractures in the cervical spine result from vertical compression forces with the spine in neutral position. These injuries are much more common in the thoracolumbar region. The ligaments are intact, and the lesions are usually stable. Fragments in the spinal canal, however, result in neurologic deficits.[59,62] Compression of the vertebral body is often obvious with burst fractures, but subtle changes such as disruption of the posterior vertebral line are useful indicators of a burst fracture. Normally, the posterior vertebral margin is concave or straight. If this line becomes convex, a burst fracture is almost always present.[52] CT (Figs. 3-48 and 3-49) is extremely helpful in evaluating these injuries and in localizing the number and size of intraspinal fragments and epidural hematomas.

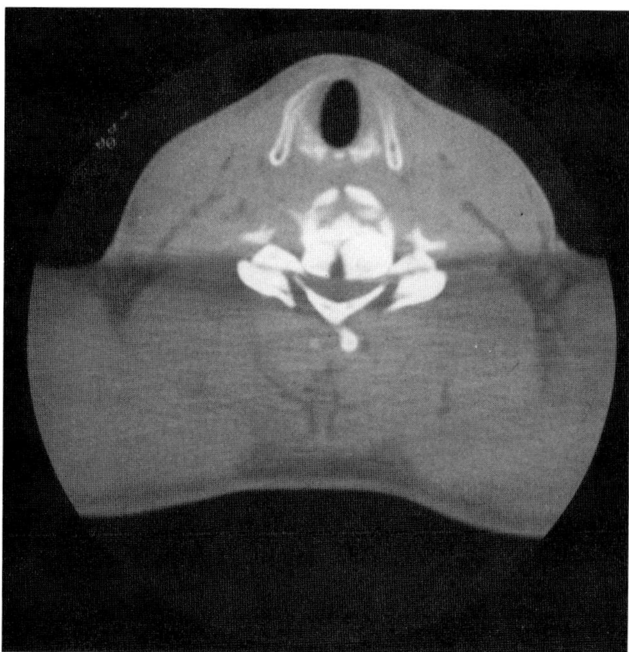

Fig. 3-49 CT scan demonstrating a complex burst fracture of the lower cervical spine with marked narrowing of the spinal canal.

Soft Tissue and Miscellaneous Injuries

Most significant ligament injuries involve the posterior complex. In one series 73% of these injuries occurred at the C5–7 level.[40] Anterior ligament injuries are most common in the C2–4 and C6–7 intervals. Often the changes noted radiographically (body fractures, disc space narrowing or widening, widening of the interspinous distance, and subluxation) will aid in determining whether ligament injury has occurred. Posterior ligament injuries are unstable if complete disruption has occurred, and one must guard against overlooking the often subtle changes associated with this injury (Fig. 3-50).[57,72,81]

The same forces that result in isolated ligament disruption, if continued, may lead to unilateral or bilateral facet dislocation or locking. In athletes these injuries occur infrequently.

Anterior ligament injuries are often associated with anteroinferior chip fractures of the vertebral body (Fig. 3-45). The mechanism of injury is disruptive hyperextension. These injuries are most common at the C2–4 and C6–7 levels. Changes may be subtle, with hematoma or displacement of the prevertebral fat stripe being the only indication of injury.[40,55,59] Facial fractures and central cord syndrome are frequently present.[55] MRI is useful in this setting.[38,40]

Neural injury may be difficult to evaluate with imaging techniques. Brachial plexus injuries are most easily evaluated with MRI.[40] Nerve root avulsion or contusion has been evaluated with CT myelography and MRI.

THORACOLUMBAR SPINE TRAUMA

Anatomic differences in the cervical, thoracic, and lumbar spine must be considered in any discussion of trauma to these regions. In the thoracic spine a slight kyphotic curve is normally present. This is in contrast to the lordotic curves evident in the cervical and lumbar regions. Also, the spinal canal in the thoracic region is circular and smaller in diameter than in the cervical or lumbar portions of the spine. As one progresses inferiorly, the vertebral bodies increase in size and the discs in height, resulting in an increasing resistance to vertical compression forces.[103,113]

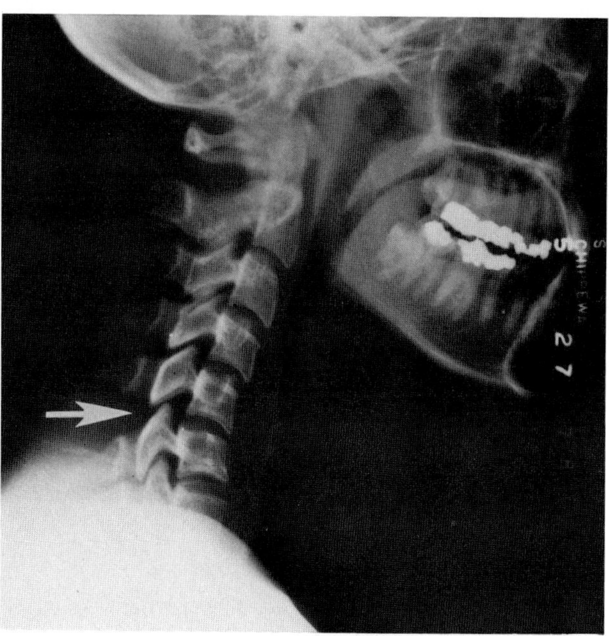

Fig. 3-50 Posterior ligament injury at C5–6 involving the posterior and middle columns. No fracture is present. This injury is unstable.

The lumbar segment is similar to the cervical segment in that both contain a greater potential for motion than the thoracic segment. The large paraspinal muscles in the lumbar region provide more stability than the cervical musculature, however. Owing to differences in range of motion, transition in the facet joints, and other anatomic factors, the thoracolumbar junction is the area most susceptible to injury. Thus the majority of injuries occur at this level.[103,106,108]

Mechanisms of Injury

The majority of athletically related thoracolumbar injuries involve the paraspinal soft tissues. Strains and sprains occur most frequently. Stress injuries to the low back are also common, however, and have been noted in football players, cross-country skiers, and gymnasts.[99,111,117,119–121] Horne et al[116] reported progressive Scheuermann's disease and vertebral wedging in the thoracic spine in water ski jumpers due to repetitive compression forces.

The mechanisms of injury in the thoracolumbar spine are similar to those in the cervical spine, but because of significant anatomic differences the results and presentation may vary.

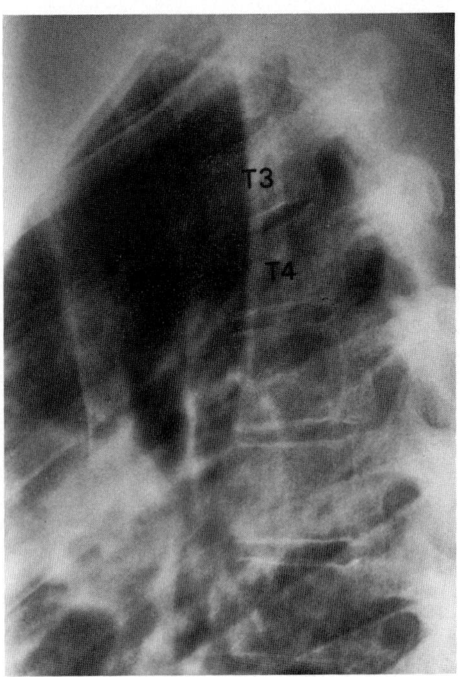

Fig. 3-51 Lateral view of the upper thoracic spine demonstrating typical anterior wedge fractures of T-3 and T-4.

Hyperflexion Injuries

Hyperflexion injuries are by far the most common injury in the thoracic and lumbar spine. Most often the injury is due to flexion-compression forces that result in a simple anterior wedge fracture of the vertebral body. The posterior complex is almost always intact; therefore, this is a stable injury.

The axis of the force in hyperflexion injuries is centered in the nucleus pulposus or in the midportion of the intervertebral disc.[103,105] Thus the appearance of the injury may vary, depending upon the spinal level involved. In the upper thoracic region the discs are narrower, and the fracture is more typically a true anterior wedge fracture (Fig. 3-51). In the thoracic region, especially the upper thoracic spine, the anterior height of the vertebral bodies is normally 1.5 mm less than the posterior height. In the lower thoracic and lumbar regions the discs are larger and more effective as shock absorbers. Thus herniation into the cartilaginous end plates is more likely to occur in the lower thoracic and lumbar regions.[103,113,120]

The degree of compression and changes in the disc space are important in wedge fractures of the vertebral bodies. If compression is greater than 50% and if the disc space is narrowed, the prognosis is less favorable. These findings along with multiple contiguous wedge fractures may lead to delayed instability.[109] Multiple contiguous wedge fractures in the upper thoracic region may lead to cord deficits (Fig. 3-51).[103]

Flexion-Rotation Injuries

Flexion-rotation injuries of the thoracolumbar spine are uncommon.[103,118] When they occur, they are among the most unstable of spinal injuries. The injury usually occurs at the thoracolumbar junction owing to the transition in the facet joints. The incidence of neurologic deficits approaches 70%. This injury is easily overlooked because it is uncommon and, more important, because reduction of the dislocation tends to occur in the supine position.

Radiographic features of the injury are similar to those of a unilateral locked facet in the cervical spine. On the AP view the spinous process may be rotated to the side of the involvement, and a fracture through the upper endplate may be present. The disc space may appear asymmetric or tilted to one side. On the lateral view the disc space is often narrowed and the interspinous distance increased. A slice fracture of the upper vertebral body is usually more obvious on the lateral view. Fractures of the articular processes and laminae frequently require tomography or CT for detection (Fig. 3-52). CT is most useful in evaluating the degree of involvement of the spinal canal.[103,106,108,113]

Vertical Compression Injuries

Vertical compression injuries (axial loading with or without associated flexion) result in burst fractures of the vertebral bodies with outward displacement of fracture fragments, herniation of the disc into the endplates, and posterior extension of the disc and fracture fragments into the spinal canal. Burst fractures are uncommon, accounting for only 1.5% of spinal injuries.[103,113] Most injuries occur at the T12–L2 level. Although these injuries are potentially stable, the incidence of neurologic involvement is high owing to displacement of bone fragments into the spinal canal. Because at least two columns are involved and it may be difficult to evaluate the posterior ligament, these fractures should be considered unstable.

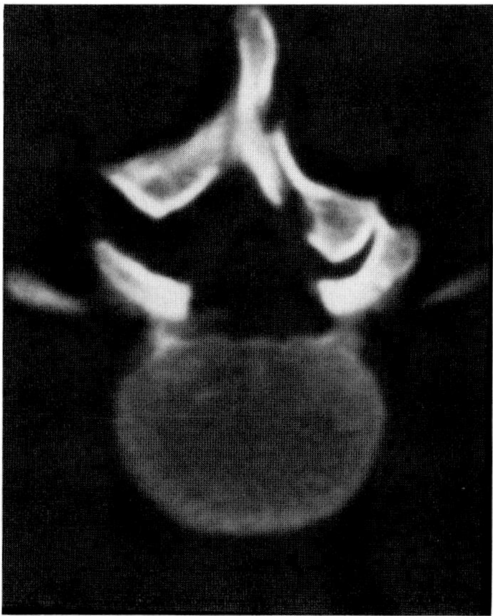

Fig. 3-52 CT section of a lumbar facet dislocation with subluxation of the contralateral facet and laminar fractures.

Burst fractures can usually be seen on the AP and lateral views (Fig. 3-53). Such fractures involve multiple bony fragments and compression of the body and disc space. The interpedicular distance is increased on the AP view, and if tomograms are obtained arch fractures are also common. The posterior vertebral line is usually abnormal on the lateral view.[107] Although the degree of spinal canal involvement can often be appreciated on the lateral view or lateral tomogram, CT is the technique of choice for evaluation of the spinal canal (Fig. 3-54).[101,103,108] Bony fragments, dural tears, and epidural hematomas may be detected with this modality.

Hyperextension Injuries

The majority of hyperextension injuries occur in the midlumbar region and are related to direct blows to the back. Lateral radiographs reveal posterior subluxation of the vertebral body above the level at which the trauma occurred. The incidence of neurologic injury in these patients is not significant, and healing may occur without residual pain.[106,108]

Radiographic findings with hyperextension injuries in the thoracolumbar spine are similar to those noted in the cervical spine. The features are best detected on the lateral view. The disc space may be widened anteriorly, and the posterior structures may be fractured as a result of compression forces. CT is useful in evaluation of the spinal canal and subtle fractures. Mild subluxation or position changes can be difficult to evaluate on axial images.[99,106]

Minor Fractures

Fractures of the posterior arch without an associated fracture-dislocation are uncommon.[122] Fractures of the articular processes may result from twisting injuries and have been described in skiers.[123] Smith et al[126] described posterior arch

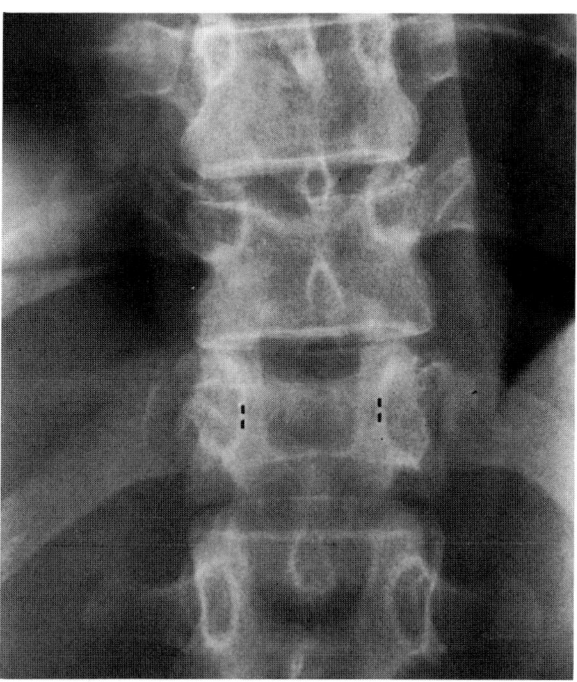

Fig. 3-53 AP view of the thoracolumbar junction with compression of T-12. The pedicles (vertical lines) are displaced laterally as a result of posterior element involvement.

fractures involving the lamina and pars due to jumping injuries; all patients presented with neurologic deficits. Most fractures of the pars interarticularis may actually be stress fractures.[98,99,120,121] Fractures of the transverse processes are most common in the lumbar region and are usually due to direct trauma or muscle contraction (Fig. 3-55).[103] These fractures are usually not significant by themselves, but associated retroperitoneal hematoma and renal injury may result. Fractures of the spinous processes may be due to flexion, extension, or direct trauma. The most common location is the

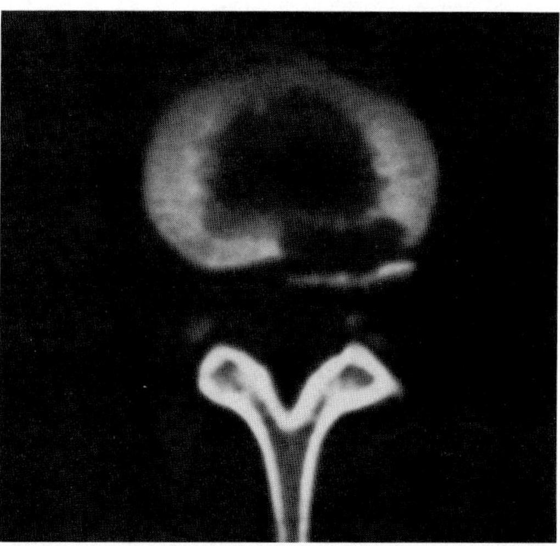

Fig. 3-54 Axial CT image demonstrating a small posterior fragment in the spinal canal.

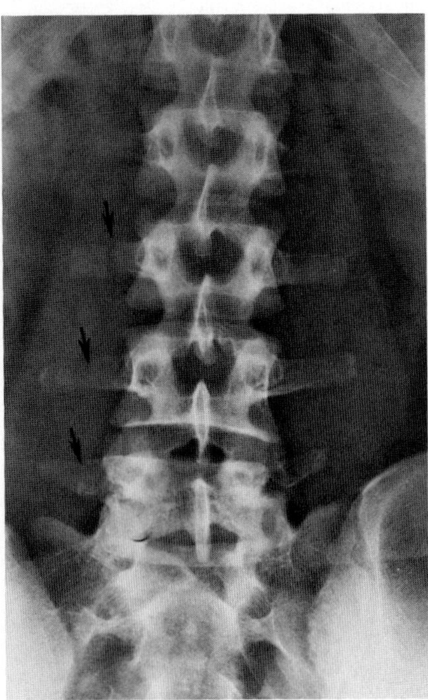

Fig. 3-55 Fractures of the right L-3, L-4, and L-5 transverse processes (arrows) due to a football spearing injury.

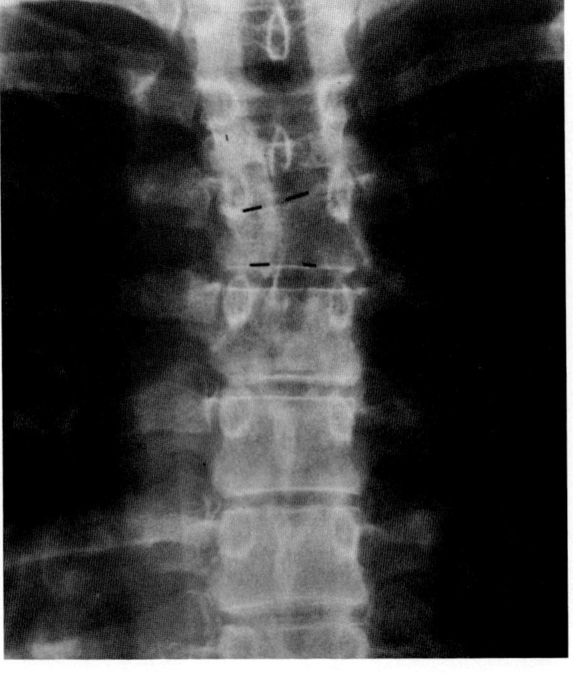

Fig. 3-56 AP view of the thoracic spine demonstrating a lateral compression injury in the upper thoracic spine (black lines).

lower cervical and upper thoracic region. This injury is rare in the lumbar spine.

The most difficult problem in isolated arch fractures is differentiating these findings from congenital clefts and spondylolysis. Clinical history, previous films, and conventional tomography or CT are essential for proper evaluation of these injuries. Congenital clefts and old nonunited fractures have well-defined sclerotic margins. Acute fractures have irregular nonsclerotic margins.

Imaging of Thoracolumbar Trauma

Routine Radiography

AP and lateral views of the thoracic and lumbar spine are routinely obtained. Occasionally, oblique views and tomography are required. The AP thoracic view is obtained with the tube centered over the midthoracic spine. The greater thickness of structures in the lower spine often produces underexposure; overexposure is more common in the upper thoracic spine.[103,106]

In examining the AP view of the thoracic spine, one should pay careful attention to the alignment and configuration of the vertebral bodies. Traumatic compression may be asymmetric. Occasionally lateral wedging can occur, which may be subtle and is best seen on the AP view (Fig. 3-56). Also, changes in the interpedicular distance should be observed (Fig. 3-53) because these may indicate fracture of the posterior elements. The spinous processes can also be seen in the midline posteriorly. The transverse processes in the thoracic spine are best seen on the AP view and normally decrease in length as one progresses caudally. Careful evaluation of the intracostal distances may be helpful, especially in the upper thoracic spine. This may provide the only clue to subluxation in a patient in whom lateral views may be difficult to obtain. Finally, on the AP view the height of each disc space in the thoracic region is usually the same. Evaluation of the paraspinal soft tissues is important. Soft tissue swelling may be the only clue to vertebral fracture.[100,101]

The lateral view of the thoracic spine can be obtained with cross-table technique if rotating the patient is not possible. On the lateral view, one can evaluate the alignment of the vertebral bodies, pedicles, laminae, and spinous processes. The posterior vertebral margin should be straight or concave.[107] The height of the posterior edge of the vertebral body is 1.0 to 1.5 mm greater than that of the anterior edge.[103] This should not be misinterpreted as acute traumatic compression.[100,103]

The AP view of the lumbar spine is usually obtained with the tube centered over the umbilicus. An angled AP view of the lower lumbar spine is useful in evaluating the posterior structures.[99] In the lumbar spine, the interpedicular distance normally widens slightly as one progresses from L-1 to L-5. Careful attention must also be given to the spinous processes and butterfly configuration of the laminae and apophyseal facets. Interruption of these structures may be the only clue to a posterior fracture-dislocation (Fig. 3-53). The transverse

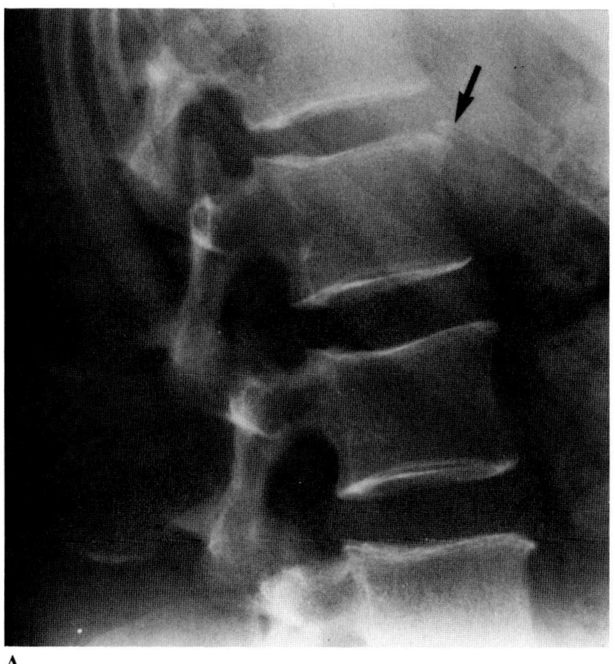

A

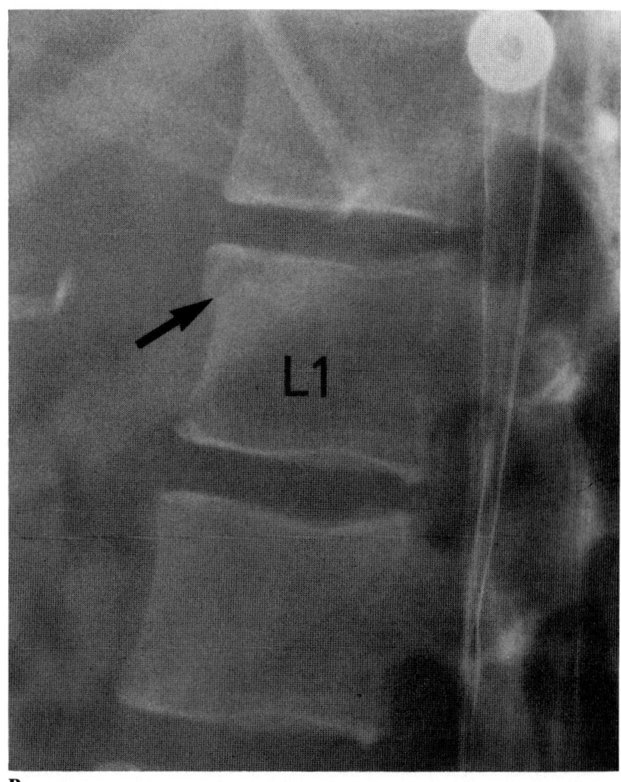

B

Fig. 3-57 (**A**) Normal lateral view of the upper lumbar spine with an ununited ossicle (arrow) and slight anterior wedging. (**B**) Subtle L-1 compression fracture (arrow).

processes are clearly seen and usually increase in length from L-1 to L-3 (Fig. 3-55). The transverse processes of L-4 are directed slightly cephalad; those of L-5 are much shorter and also are directed slightly cephalad. The lateral view of the lumbar spine can be obtained with a cross-table technique, turning the patient (if possible) to the lateral position or utilizing the C-arm Versigraph. The cross-table technique is preferred after trauma.

On the lateral view of the lumbar spine the bodies, pedicles, facet joints, and spinous processes can be clearly demonstrated. It should be noted that the body of L-1 is often slightly wedged anteriorly. On occasion this may be difficult to differentiate from an acute injury (Fig. 3-57). As in the remainder of the spine, alignment of the vertebral bodies is also well demonstrated on the lateral view. A coned lateral view of L5–S1 is also helpful because better detail can be obtained.[99,103] Oblique views are commonly obtained in the lumbar region and are extremely helpful in evaluating the facet joints, laminae, and pars interarticularis.[103] AP and lateral views of the sacrum can be obtained by centering the tube over the sacrum with the central beam perpendicular to the cassette (Fig. 3-7). On the AP view, the arcuate lines and ventral sacral foramina should be carefully studied. Interruption in the arcuate lines may be the only sign of fracture (Fig. 3-7).[103] The lateral view is useful in demonstrating displacement of sacral fractures and in detecting fractures or dislocations of the coccyx (Fig. 3-58).[103,113]

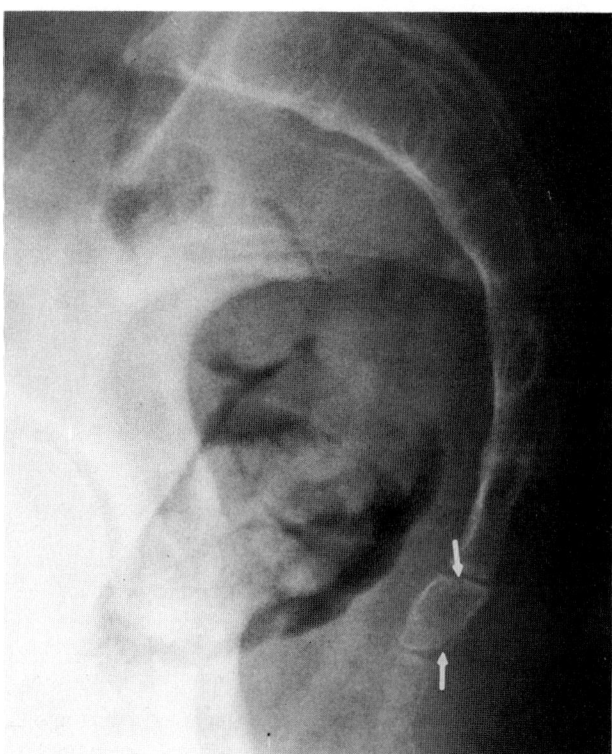

Fig. 3-58 Lateral view of the sacrum and coccyx demonstrating a coccygeal fracture (arrows) in a high jumper who missed the padded landing zone and sustained direct trauma to the region.

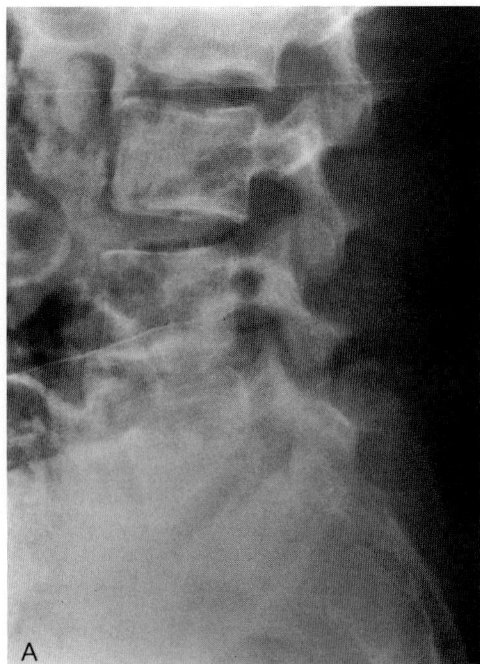

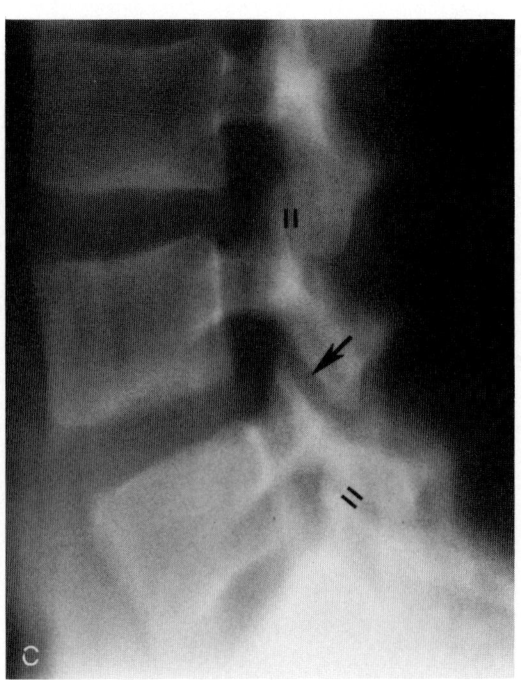

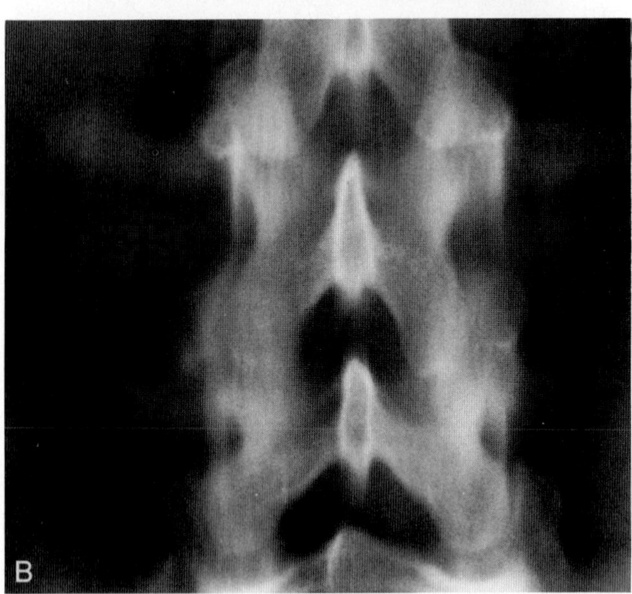

Fig. 3-59 Evaluation of a football player with low back pain after a twisting injury. (**A**) Lateral view of the lumbar spine and (**B**) AP tomogram are inconclusive. (**C**) Lateral tomogram shows widening of the L-4 facet joint (arrow) due to capsular injury. Lines indicate normal joint. *Source:* Reprinted from *Imaging of Orthopedic Trauma* ed 2 by TH Berquist, 1991, Raven Press, © Mayo Foundation.

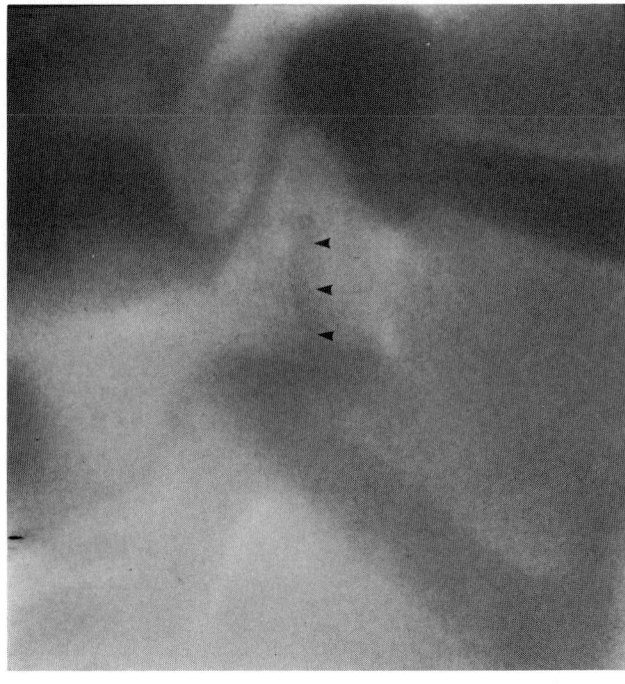

Fig. 3-60 Lateral tomogram demonstrating a subtle fracture (arrowheads) in a gymnast.

Conventional and Computed Tomography

As noted previously, many athletic injuries are due to chronic stress to the posterior elements and result in low back pain.[119,125] Routine views may not be conclusive, so that either conventional tomography or CT is required to clarify subtle or complex injuries.

Conventional thin-slice (3-mm), complex motion tomography is useful in evaluating the facet joints and posterior osseous structures (Fig. 3-59). Typically AP and lateral projections are adequate (Fig. 3-60), but oblique tomograms are useful in classifications of pars defects (Fig. 3-61).[103,125] CT

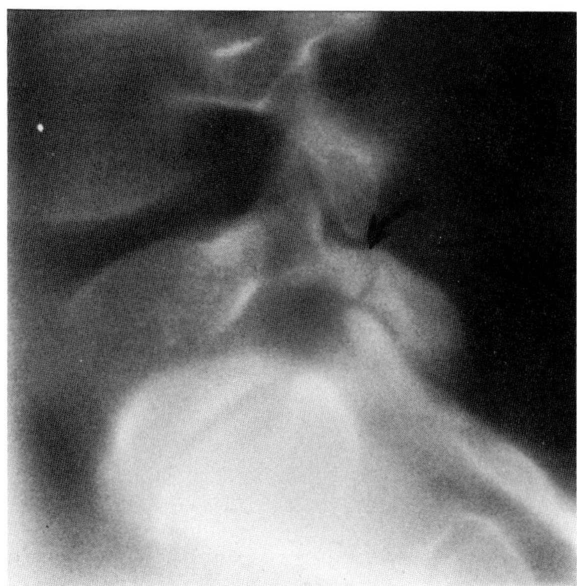

Fig. 3-61 Oblique tomogram demonstrating a pars defect with sclerotic margins.

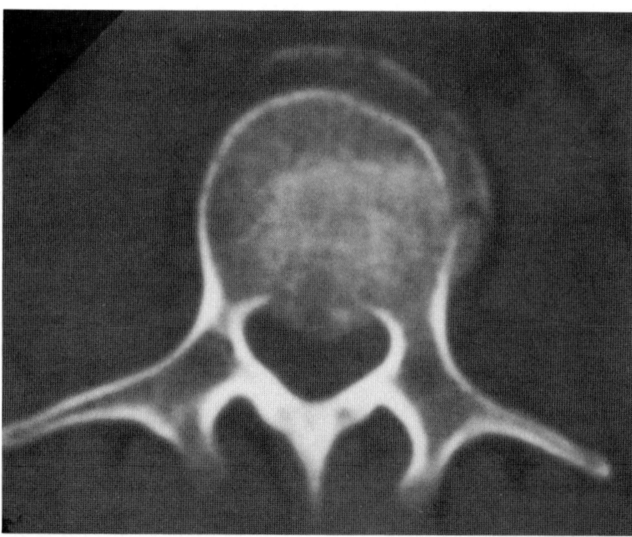

Fig. 3-62 CT of a vertebral burst fracture with posterior bulging and narrowing of the spinal canal.

is also useful for evaluating subtle injuries, but this technique is more commonly reserved for evaluation of the spinal canal (Fig. 3-62).[104,115]

Magnetic Resonance Imaging

MRI is reserved for soft tissue and spinal cord evaluation in most practices.[103,114] This technique is particularly suited for evaluation of muscle tears and nerve root injuries and for differentiating these injuries from disc herniation and other nonosseous causes of low back pain in athletes.[110,112,114] Subtle osseous abnormalities in the posterior elements are more easily evaluated with CT or conventional tomography.[103]

Radionuclide Scintigraphy

Bone scanning is useful for evaluating subtle injuries in athletes with low back pain. A negative bone scan effectively excludes osseous injury. Comparison with radiography is useful in determining the exact nature of these injuries. A negative bone scan in the presence of a well-defined lucent pars defect with sclerotic margins indicates an old or inactive injury. When the radiograph is negative and the bone scan positive, an acute or early stress fracture is probable.[102,111,124,125]

REFERENCES

Introduction and Anatomy

1. Abel MS. Jogger's fracture and other stress fractures of the lumbosacral spine. *Skeletal Radiol.* 1985;13:221–227.
2. Anderson JM, Schutt AH. Spinal injury in children. A review of 156 cases seen from 1950 through 1978. *Mayo Clin Proc.* 1980;55:499–504.
3. Balmasela MT, Wunder JA, Gordon C, Cannell CD. Post-traumatic syringomyelia associated with heavy weight lifting exercises. *Arch Phys Med Rehabil.* 1988;69:970–972.
4. Berquist TH. *Imaging of Orthopedic Trauma.* New York: Raven; 1991.
5. Bruce DA, Schut L, Sutton LW. Brain and cervical spine injuries occurring during organized sports activities in children and adolescents. *Clin Sports Med.* 1982;1:495–514.
6. Daffner RH, Deeb ZL, Rothfus WE. Thoracic fractures and dislocations in motorcyclists. *Skeletal Radiol.* 1987;16:280–284.
7. Ellitsgaard N. Parachuting injuries: a study of 110,000 sport jumps. *Br J Sports Med.* 1987;21:13–17.
8. Feldick HG, Albright JP. Football survey reveals missed neck injury. *Physician Sports Med.* 1976;4:77–81.
9. Henry JH, Lanear B, Niegut D. The injury rate in professional basketball. *Am J Sports Med.* 1982;10:16–19.
10. Hollinshead HW. *Anatomy for Surgeons.* 3rd ed. Philadelphia: Harper & Row; 1982;3.
11. Horne J, Cockshott WP, Shannon HS. Spinal column damage from water ski jumping. *Skeletal Radiol.* 1987;16:612–616.
12. Ireland ML, Michelu LJ. Bilateral stress fractures of the lumbar pedicles in the ballet dancer. *J Bone Joint Surg Am.* 1987;69:140–142.
13. Kilbury D, Jacobs R, Recklung F, Mason J. Bicycle accidents and injuries among adult cyclists. *Am J Sports Med.* 1986;14:416–419.
14. Kraus DR, Shapiro D. The symptomatic lumbar spine in the athlete. *Clin Sports Med.* 1989;8:59–69.
15. Mahlamäki S, Soinakallio S, Michelson JE. Radiological findings in the lumbar spine of 39 young cross-country skiers with low back pain. *Int J Sports Med.* 1988;9:196–197.
16. McCarroll JR, Miller JM, Ritter MA. Lumbar spondylolysis and spondylolisthesis in college football players. *Am J Sports Med.* 1986;14: 404–406.
17. Morrow PL, McQuillen EN, Eaton LH, Berstein CJ. Downhill ski fatalities: the Vermont experience. *J Trauma* 1988;28:95–100.

18. Nicholas JA, Rosenthal PP, Gleim GW. A historical perspective of injuries in professional football. *JAMA*. 1988;260:939–944.

19. O'Leary P, Boiardo R. The diagnosis and treatment of injuries of the spine in athletes. In: Nicholas JA, Hershman EB, eds. *The Lower Extremity and Spine in Sports Medicine*. St Louis, MO: Mosby; 1986;2:1171–1229.

20. Reid DC, Saboe L. Spine fractures in winter sports. *Sports Med*. 1989;7:393–399.

21. Silver JR. Spinal injuries as a result of sporting accidents. *Paraplegia*. 1987;25:16–17.

22. Silver JR, Silver DD, Godfrey JJ. Trampolining injuries of the spine. *Injury*. 1986;17:117–124.

23. Steinbuck K. Frequency and etiology of injury in cross country skiing. *J Sports Sci*. 1987;5:187–196.

24. Tator CH. Neck injuries in ice hockey: a recent unsolved problem with many contributing factors. *Clin Sports Med*. 1987;6:101–114.

25. Thompson RR. A study of the type and cost of football injuries: a single season in a Minnesota high school. *Minn Med*. 1986;69:656–658.

26. Torg JS, Sennett B, Vegro JJ. Spinal injury at the 3rd and 4th cervical vertebrae resulting from axial loading mechanism. *Clin Sports Med*. 1987;6: 159–183.

27. Torg JS, Vegso JJ, Sennett B. The national football head and neck injury registry: 14 year report on cervical quadriplegia. *Clin Sports Med*. 1987;6:61–72.

28. Whitlock MR, Whitlock J, Johnston B. Equestrian injuries: a comparison of professional and amateur injuries in Berkshire. *Br J Sports Med*. 1987;21:25–26.

29. Williams P, McKibbin B. Unstable cervical spine injuries in rugby—a 20 year review. *Injury*. 1987;18:329–332.

30. Yost JG, Ellfeldt HJ. Basketball. In: Nicholas JA, Hershman EB, eds. *The Lower Extremity and Spine in Sports Medicine*. St Louis, MO: Mosby; 1986;2:1440–1446.

31. Zelisko JA, Nobile HB, Porter M. A comparison of men's and women's professional basketball injuries. *Am J Sports Med*. 1982;10: 297–299.

Cervical Spine Trauma

32. Abel MS. The exaggerated supine oblique view of the cervical spine. *Skeletal Radiol*. 1982;8:213–219.

33. Abel MS, Teaque JH. Unilateral lateral mass compression fractures of the axis. *Skeletal Radiol*. 1979;4:92–98.

34. Acheson MB, Livingston RR, Richardson ML, Stimack GK. High-resolution CT scanning in the evaluation of cervical spine fractures: comparison with plain film examination. *AJR*. 1987;148:1179–1185.

35. Anderson LD, D'Alonzo RT. Fractures of the odontoid process of the axis. *J Bone Joint Surg Am*. 1978;56:1663–1674.

36. Anderson JM, Schutt AH. Spinal injury in children. A review of 156 cases from 1950 through 1978. *Mayo Clin Proc*. 1980;55:499–504.

37. Ballinger PW. *Merrill's Atlas of Radiographic Positions and Radiologic Procedures*. 5th ed. St Louis, MO: Mosby; 1982.

38. Beers GJ, Raque GH, Wagner GG, et al. MR Imaging in acute cervical trauma. *J Comput Assisted Tomogr*. 1988;12:755–761.

39. Berquist TH. Imaging of adult cervical spine trauma. *RadioGraphics*. 1988;8:667–694.

40. Berquist TH. *Imaging of Orthopedic Trauma*. 2nd ed. New York: Raven; 1991.

41. Bohrer SP, Chen YM, Sayers DG. Cervical spine flexion patterns. *Skeletal Radiol*. 1990;19:521–525.

42. Brackman R, Penning L. *Injuries of the Cervical Spine*. Amsterdam: Exerpta Medica; 1971.

43. Burke JT, Harris JH. Acute injuries of the axis vertebrae. *Skeletal Radiol*. 1989;18:335–346.

44. Cancelmo JJ. Clay shoveler's fracture. A helpful diagnostic sign. *Am J Roentgenol Radium Ther Nucl Med*. 1972;115:540–543.

45. Cintron E, Gilula LA, Murphy WA, Gehweiler J. The widened disk space. *Contemp Diagn Radiol*. 1981;141:639–644.

46. Clarke CR, White AA. Fractures of the dens. *J Bone Joint Surg Am*. 1985;67:1340–1348.

47. Coin CG, Pennink M, Ahmad WD, Kernanen VJ. Diving type injury of the cervical spine. Contribution of CT to management. *J Comput Assisted Tomogr*. 1979;3:362–372.

48. Daffner RH. *Imaging of Vertebral Trauma*. Gaithersbug, MD: Aspen; 1988.

49. Daffner RH, Deeb ZL, Goldberg AL, Kandabarow WA, Rothfus WE. The radiologic assessment of post-traumatic vertebral instability. *Skeletal Radiol*. 1990;19:103–108.

50. Daffner RH, Deeb ZL, Rothfus WE. "Fingerprints" of vertebral trauma—a unifying concept based on mechanisms. *Skeletal Radiol*. 1986;15: 518–525.

51. Daffner RH, Deeb ZL, Rothfus WE. Pseudofractures of the cervical vertebral body. *Skeletal Radiol*. 1986;15:295–298.

52. Daffner RH, Deeb ZL, Rothfus WE. The posterior vertebral line: importance in detection of burst fractures. *AJR*. 1987;148:93–96.

53. Denis F. Spinal stability as defined by the three column spine concept in acute spinal trauma. *Clin Orthop*. 1984;189:65–76.

54. Distefano S. Neuropathy due to entrapment of the long thoracic nerve. *Ital J Orthop Traumatol*. 1989;15:259–262.

55. Edeiken-Monroe B, Wagner LK, Harris JH. Hyperextension dislocation of the cervical spine. *AJR*. 1986;146:803–808.

56. England AC, Shippel AH, Ray MJ. A simple view for demonstration of fractures of the anterior arch of C1. *AJR*. 1985;144:763–764.

57. Evans DK. Anterior cervical subluxation. *J Bone Joint Surg Br*. 1976;58:318–321.

58. Fielding JW, Hawkins RJ. Atlantoaxial rotary fixation. *J Bone Joint Surg Am*. 1977;59:39–44.

59. Gehweiler JH, Osborne RL, Becker RF. *The Radiology of Vertebral Trauma*. Philadelphia: Saunders; 1980.

60. Goldberg AL, Rothfus WE, Deeb ZL, Frankel DG, Wilberger JE, Daffner RH. Hyperextension injuries of the cervical spine. *Skeletal Radiol*. 1989;18:283–288.

61. Goldberg AL, Rothfus WE, Deeb ZL, et al. The impact of magnetic resonance on the diagnostic evaluation of acute cervicothoracic trauma. *Skeletal Radiol*. 1988;17:89–95.

62. Harris JH. Radiographic evaluation of spinal trauma. *Orthop Clin North Am*. 1986;17:75–86.

63. Holdsworth F. Fractures, dislocations, and fracture-dislocations of the spine. *J Bone Joint Surg Am*. 1970;52:1534–1551.

64. Jackson DW, Lohr FT. Cervical spine injuries. *Clin Sports Med*. 1986;5:373–386.

65. Jefferson G. Fracture of the atlas vertebra. *J Bone Joint Surg Br*. 1920;7:407–422.

66. Jevtich V. Horizontal fracture of the anterior arch of the atlas. *J Bone Joint Surg Am*. 1986;68:1094–1095.

67. Jonsson K, Niklasson J, Josefson PO. Avulsion of the cervical spinal ring apophysis: acute and chronic appearance. *Skeletal Radiol*. 1991; 20:207–210.

68. Keene JS, Galetz TH, Lilleas F. Diagnosis of vertebral fracture: a comparison of conventional radiography, conventional tomography, and computed tomography. *J Bone Joint Surg Am*. 1982;64:586–594.

69. Kim KS, Chen HH, Russell EJ, Rogers LF. Flexion teardrop fracture of the cervical spine. Radiographic characteristics. *AJR*. 1989;152:319–326.

70. Kulkarni MV, Bondurant FJ, Rose SL, Narayama PA. 1.5 Tesla magnetic resonance imaging of acute spinal trauma. *RadioGraphics*. 1988;8:1059–1082.

71. Kurosawa H, Yomonoi T, Yomakoshi K. Radiographic findings of degeneration in cervical spines of middle aged soccer players. *Skeletal Radiol*. 1991;20:437–440.

72. Miles KA, Mairaris C, Finlay D, Barnes MR. The incidence and prognostic significance of radiological abnormalities in soft tissue injuries of the cervical spine. *Skeletal Radiol*. 1988;17:493–496.

73. Naidich JB, Waidich TP, Garfein C. The widened interspinous distance. A useful sign of anterior cervical dislocation in the supine frontal projection. *Radiology*. 1977;123:113–116.

74. Nash CL. Acute cervical soft tissue injury and late deformity. *J Bone Joint Surg Am*. 1979;61:305–307.

75. Nicholas JA, Rosenthal PP, Gleim GW. A historical perspective of injuries in professional football. *JAMA*. 1988;260:939–944.

76. Pavlov H, Torg JS. Roentgen examination of the cervical spine injuries in the athlete. *Clin Sports Med*. 1987;6:751–766.

77. Pech P, Kilgore DP, Pojunas KW, Haughton VM. Cervical spinal fractures: CT detection. *Radiology*. 1985;157:117–120.

78. Poindexter DP, Johnson EW. Football shoulder and neck injury: a study of the stinger. *Arch Phys Med Rehabil*. 1984;65:601–602.

79. Reid DC, Saboe L. Spine fractures in winter sports. *Sports Med*. 1989;7:393–399.

80. Roaf R. A study of the mechanics of spinal injuries. *J Bone Joint Surg Br*. 1960;42:810–823.

81. Scher AT. Anterior subluxation: an unstable position. *AJR*. 1979;133:275–280.

82. Scher AT. Unilateral locked facet in cervical spine injuries. *AJR*. 1977;129:45–48.

83. Sherk HH, Nicholson JT. Lesions of the atlas and axis. *Clin Orthop*. 1975;109:33–41.

84. Silver JR. Spinal injuries as a result of sporting accidents. *Paraplegia*. 1987;25:16–17.

85. Silver JR, Silver DD, Godfrey JJ. Trampolining injuries of the spine. *Injury*. 1986;17:117–124.

86. Smith GR, Beckly DE, Abel MS. Articular mass fracture: a neglected case of post-traumatic neck pain. *Clin Radiol*. 1976;27:335–340.

87. Stauffer ES, Kaufer H, Kling TF. Fractures and dislocations of the spine. In: Rockwood CA, Green DP. *Fractures in Adults*. 2nd ed. Philadelphia: Lippincott; 1984;2:987–1092.

88. Tator CH. Neck injuries in ice hockey: a recent, unsolved problem with many contributing factors. *Clin Sports Med*. 1987;6:101–114.

89. Tehranzadeh J. The spectrum of avulsion and avulsion-like injuries of the musculoskeletal system. *RadioGraphics*. 1987;7:945–974.

90. Templeton PA, Young JWR, Mirvis SE, Buddemeyer EU. The value of retropharyngeal soft tissue measurement in trauma of the adult cervical spine. *Skeletal Radiol*. 1987;16:98–104.

91. Torg JS, Sennett B, Vegso JJ. Spinal injury at the level of the third and fourth cervical vertebrae resulting from axial loading mechanism: an analysis and classification. *Clin Sports Med*. 1987;6:159–183.

92. Torg JS, Vegso JJ, Sennett B. The national football head and neck registry: 14 year report on cervical quadriplegia (1971–1984). *Clin Sports Med*. 1987;6:61–72.

93. Vines FS. The significance of occult fractures of the cervical spine. *Am J Roentgenol Radium Ther Nucl Med*. 1969;107:473–504.

94. White AA, Southwick WO, McSweeney T, Park W. Hidden flexion injury of the cervical spine. *J Bone Joint Surg Br*. 1976;58:322–327.

95. Williams P, McKibbin B. Unstable cervical spine injuries in rugby—a 20 year review. *Injury*. 1987;18:329–332.

96. Wojcik WG, Edieken-Monroe B, Harris JH. Three-dimensional computed tomography in acute cervical spine trauma: a preliminary report. *Skeletal Radiol*. 1987;16:261–269.

97. Woodring JH, Goldstein SJ. Fractures of the articular process of the spine. *AJR*. 1982;139:341–344.

Thoracolumbar Spine Trauma

98. Abel MS. Jogger's fracture and other fractures of the lumbosacral spine. *Skeletal Radiol*. 1985;13:221–227.

99. Amato M, Totty WG, Gilula LA. Spondylolysis of the lumbar spine: demonstration and laminar fragmentation. *Radiology*. 1984;153:627–629.

100. Angtuaco EJC, Binet EF. Radiology of thoracic and lumbar fractures. *Clin Orthop*. 1984;189:43–57.

101. Atlas RW, Regenbogen V, Rogers LF, Kim KS. The radiologic characterization of burst fractures of the spine. *AJR*. 1986;147:575–582.

102. Bellah RD, Summerville DA, Treves ST, Micheli LJ. Low-back pain in adolescent athletes: detection of stress injury to the pars interarticularis with SPECT. *Radiology*. 1991;180:509–512.

103. Berquist TH. *Imaging of Orthopedic Trauma*. 2nd ed. New York: Raven; 1991.

104. Cammesa FB, Eismont FJ, Green BA. Dural laceration occurring with burst fractures and associated laminar fractures. *J Bone Joint Surg Am*. 1989;71:1044–1052.

105. Chance GQ. Note on a type of flexion fracture of the spine. *Br J Radiol*. 1948;21:452–453.

106. Daffner RH, Deeb ZL, Rothfus WE. "Fingerprints" of vertebral trauma—a unifying concept on basic mechanisms. *Skeletal Radiol*. 1988; 15:518–525.

107. Daffner RH, Deeb ZL, Rothfus WE. The posterior vertebral line: importance in detection of burst fractures. *AJR*. 1987;148:93–96.

108. Daffner RH, Deeb ZL, Rothfus WE. Thoracic fractures and dislocations in motorcyclists. *Skeletal Radiol*. 1987;16:280–284.

109. Denis F. The three column spine and its significance on classification of acute thoracolumbar spinal injuries. *Spine*. 1983;8:817–831.

110. DiFazio FM, Barth RA, Frymoyer JW. Acute lumbar paraspinal compartment syndrome. *J Bone Joint Surg Am*. 1991;73:1101–1103.

111. Elliott E, Hutson MA, Wastie ML. Bone scintigraphy in the assessment of spondylolysis in patients attending a sports clinic. *Clin Radiol*. 1988;39:269–272.

112. Freedy MR, Midler KD, Eick JJ, Granke DS. Traumatic lumbosacral nerve root avulsion: evaluation with MR imaging. *J Comput Assisted Tomogr*. 1989;13:1052–1057.

113. Gehweiler JA, Osborne RL, Becker RF. *The Radiology of Vertebral Trauma*. Philadelphia: Saunders; 1980.

114. Goldberg AL, Rothfus WE, Deeb ZL, et al. The impact of magnetic resonance on diagnostic evaluation of acute thoracolumbar trauma. *Skeletal Radiol*. 1988;17:89–95.

115. Guerra J, Garfin SR, Resnick D. Vertebral burst fractures: CT analysis of the retropulsed fragment. *Radiology*. 1984;153:709–772.

116. Horne J, Cockshott WP, Shannon HS. Spinal column damage from water ski jumping. *Skeletal Radiol*. 1987;16:612–616.

117. Ireland ML, Micheli GJ. Bilateral stress fracture of the lumbar pedicles in a ballet dancer. *J Bone Joint Surg Am*. 1987;69:140–142.

118. Kramer KM, Levine AM. Unilateral facet dislocation of the lumbosacral junction. *J Bone Joint Surg Am*. 1989;71:1258–1261.

119. Krause DR, Shapiro D. The symptomatic lumbar spine in athletes. *Clin Sports Med*. 1989;8:59–69.

120. Mahlamaki S, Soimakallio S, Michelsson JE. Radiologic findings in the lumbar spine of 39 young cross-country skiers with low back pain. *Int J Sports Med*. 1988;9:196–197.

121. McCarroll JR, Miller JM, Ritter MA. Lumbar spondylolysis and spondylolisthesis in college football players. *Am J Sports Med*. 1986; 14:404–406.

122. Mitchell LC. Isolated fracture of the articular process of the lumbar vertebra. *J Bone Joint Surg*. 1933;15:608–614.

123. Omar MM, Levinsohn ME. An unusual fracture of the vertebral articular process in a skier. *J Trauma*. 1979;19:212.

124. Papanicolaou N, Wilkenson RH, Emans JB, Treves S, Micheli LJ. Bone scintigraphy and radiography in young athletes with low back pain. *AJR*. 1985;145:1039–1044.

125. Pennell RG, Maurer AH, Burakdapour A. Stress injuries of the pars interarticularis: radiologic classification and indications for scintigraphy. *AJR*. 1985;145:763–766.

126. Smith ER, Northrup CH, Loop JW. Jumper's fractures: pattern of thoracolumbar injuries associated with vertical plunges. *Radiology*. 1977; 122:657–663.

Chapter 4

Pelvis and Hips

Most sports-related injuries to the pelvis and hips involve the soft tissues. Sprains, strains, tendinitis, and bursitis are common, especially in the adult population. Stress fractures and avulsion fractures are also common, but major pelvic fractures are unusual in athletes.

Imaging of these injuries is important in determining the extent of injury and excluding other conditions that may mimic trauma. Diagnostic and therapeutic injections may also be useful in patients with overuse injuries.

ANATOMY

Knowledge of basic bone and soft tissue anatomy is important for understanding sports-related injuries and for selecting the proper imaging or diagnostic injection techniques.

Osseous Anatomy

The innominate bone is composed of the ilium, ischium, and pubis, which during childhood are separated by the triradiate cartilage. During the second decade these three bones fuse, forming the acetabulum.[1,6]

The ilium is composed of the wing and body. The wing is large, with three palpable structures that are helpful in clinical evaluation and radiographic positioning. These structures are the anterosuperior iliac spine, the iliac crest (which extends from the anterosuperior iliac spine to the posterosuperior iliac spine), and the posterosuperior iliac spine.[3] The iliac wing is covered by muscles medially and laterally. Medially the wing serves as the origin of the iliacus, the quadratus lumborum, the erector spinae, and the transversus abdominis.[6] The gluteal muscles originate from the lateral aspect of the ilium, the sartorius from the anterosuperior iliac spine, the rectus femoris from the anteroinferior iliac spine, and the tensor fasciae latae from the anterior iliac crest. The posterosuperior aspect of the ilium contains a large rough area for attachment of the posterior sacroiliac ligaments. This area is termed the iliac tuberosity. Anterior to the tuberosity is the cartilage-covered surface that articulates with the sacrum, forming the sacroiliac joint. The greater sciatic notch is immediately inferior to the articular surface of the iluim.[1,3,6]

The body of the pubic bone articulates with its mate via the pubic symphysis. The superior pubic ramus extends superolaterally to the acetabulum and forms the upper margin of the obturator foramen. The inferior pubic ramus courses posteriorly and laterally and is contiguous with the ischium. The inferior pubic ramus forms the lower margin of the obturator foramen.[2,3,6] The bodies of the pubic bones have small projections anteriorly and superiorly (pubic tubercles), which along with the symphysis are palpable in most patients and are valuable as anatomic landmarks for radiographic positioning. Multiple muscle groups originate from the inferior pubic ramus near the pubic symphysis. These include the muscles of the pelvic floor (deep transversus perinei, levator ani, and sphincter urethrae), adductor longus, adductor brevis, gracilis, adductor magnus, and obturators internus and externus. The pectineus and rectus abdominis are attached to the superior pubic ramus.[6]

The ischium consists of a large body that forms the posteroinferior portion of the acetabulum, a tuberosity (directed

Table 4-1 Pelvis and Hips: Ossification Centers Involved in Sports Injuries

Location	*Muscle Attachments*	*Age of Appearance (years)*	*Age of Fusion (years)*
Ischium	Hamstrings, adductor magnus	14–16	18–25
Anterosuperior iliac spine	Sartorius	13–15	21–25
Anteroinferior iliac spine	Rectus femoris	13–15	16–18
Iliac crest	Anterior: oblique abdominis, tensor fasciae latae, gluteus medius Posterior: latissimus dorsi, gluteus maximus	13–15	21–25
Greater trochanter	Gluteal muscles	4–6	18–20
Lesser trochanter	Iliopsoas	11–12	18–20

Sources: Anderson JE, *Grant's Atlas of Anatomy,* ed 8, 1983, Williams & Wilkins; Berquist TH, *Imaging of Orthopedic Trauma,* ed 2, 1991, Raven Press; Karlin LI in Nicholas JA and Hershman EB, *The Lower Extremity and Spine in Sports Medicine,* 1986, CV Mosby.

inferiorly), and a ramus that is contiguous with the inferior pubic ramus. The ischial spine projects posteromedially and forms the lower margin of the greater sciatic notch. The coccygeus and levator ani attach to the ischial spine. The large ischial tuberosity serves as the origin of the semimembranosus, semitendinosus, biceps femoris, quadratus femoris, and a portion of the adductor magnus.[3,6]

The sacrum consists of five fused vertebral segments, which decrease in size inferiorly. The sacrum articulates with the coccyx inferiorly and with the ilia laterally. Superiorly the sacrum articulates with the body of L-5 via the lumbosacral disc. Posteriorly it articulates with the apophyseal joints of L-5. The surface of the sacrum is concave ventrally and convex dorsally. Four pairs of sacral foramina allow passage of the dorsal and ventral rami of the spine nerves. The large lateral mass of the sacrum is formed by the fused lateral articular processes of the first three sacral segments.[1,3,6,7]

The coccyx consists of four to five rudimentary segments that articulate with the last sacral segment. Four muscles attach to the coccyx. These include a portion of the gluteus maximus, coccygeus, levator ani, and sphincter ani.[1,3,6]

There are several apophyses in the pelvis and hips that are subjected to trauma in sports injuries. It is important to be aware of when these centers appear and at what ages fusion normally occurs. This material is summarized in Table 4-1. Avulsion injuries in these areas are common in young athletes (Fig. 4-1).[3,8]

Ligaments and Articulations

The posterior sacroiliac ligaments have long and short fibers. The anterior sacroiliac ligaments provide much less support and serve as little more than a capsule for the sacroiliac joint. The sacrotuberous and sacrospinous ligaments connect the lower lateral aspects of the sacrum to the ischial tuberosity and ischial spine, respectively. These ligaments prevent posterior displacement of the sacrum. The articular anatomy and surrounding ligaments combine to produce minimal motion at the sacroiliac joints. The iliolumbar and sacrolumbar ligaments restrict the rotary and ventral motion of the lower lumbar spine (Fig. 4-2).[1,3,6]

The articulation of the pubic bones is separated by a fibrocartilaginous disc that is contiguous with the superior and inferior pubic ligaments. The superior and inferior ligaments blend with the stronger anterior pubic ligament. These ligaments allow only slight motion at the pubic symphysis. Although minimal, such motion at the pubic symphysis and

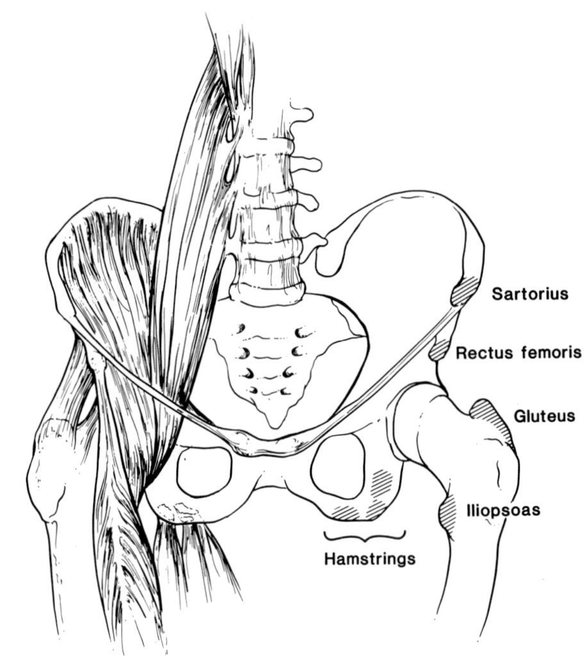

Fig. 4-1 Illustration of ossification centers and muscle attachments in the pelvis and hips commonly involved in avulsion injuries. *Source:* Reprinted from *Imaging of Orthopedic Trauma* ed 2 by TH Berquist, 1991, Raven Press, © Mayo Foundation.

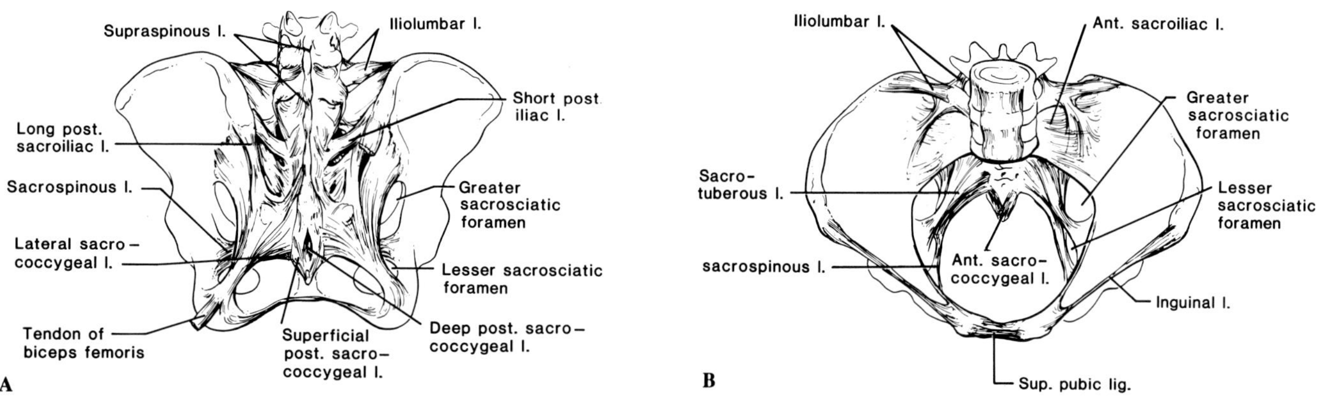

Fig. 4-2 Illustration of the ligaments of the pelvis viewed posteriorly (**A**) and anteriorly (**B**). *Source:* Reprinted from *Imaging of Orthopedic Trauma* ed 2 by TH Berquist, 1991, Raven Press, © Mayo Foundation.

sacroiliac joints allows single undisplaced fractures to occur near these structures. Displaced fractures are usually multiple, as one would expect given the ring configuration of the pelvis (Fig. 4-2).[3,6]

The femoral head articulates with the acetabulum, forming an articulatio spheroidea (ball and socket) joint (Fig. 4-3). The acetabulum is formed by the ischium (45%), the ilium (35%), and the pubic bone (20%) and is directed in an anterior, laterocaudad direction.[6] The bony acetabular rim is incomplete inferiorly (the acetabular notch) and is bridged in this region by the transverse ligament. The transverse ligament is contiguous with the cartilaginous acetabular labrum, which forms a supporting lip around the remainder of the acetabular margin. The synovium-lined capsule is supported by several ligaments as well as by the surrounding muscle groups (Fig. 4-3). The iliofemoral ligament (Figs. 4-3A and 4-3B) is

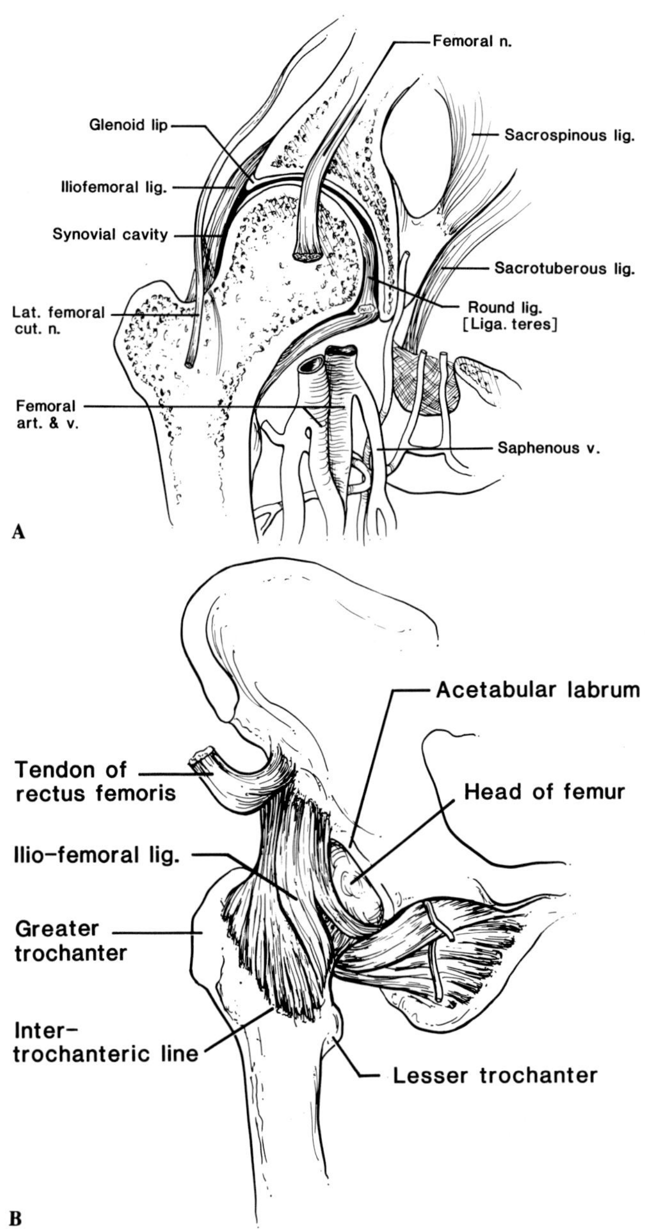

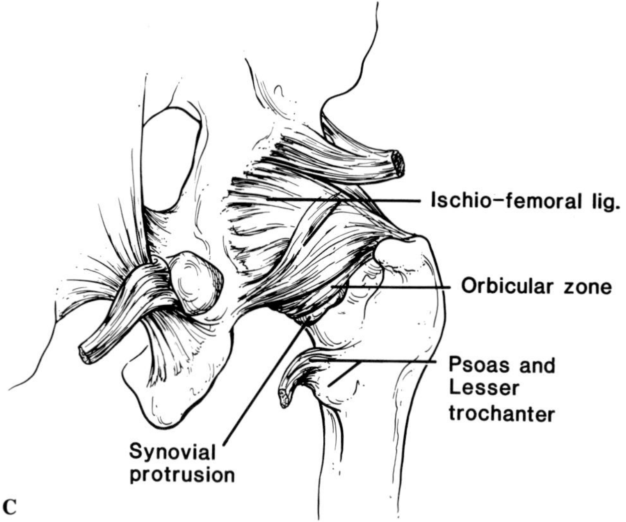

Fig. 4-3 Illustration of the articulations (**A**) and anterior (**B**) and posterior (**C**) ligaments of the hip. *Source:* Reprinted from *Imaging of Orthopedic Trauma* ed 2 by TH Berquist, 1991, Raven Press, © Mayo Foundation.

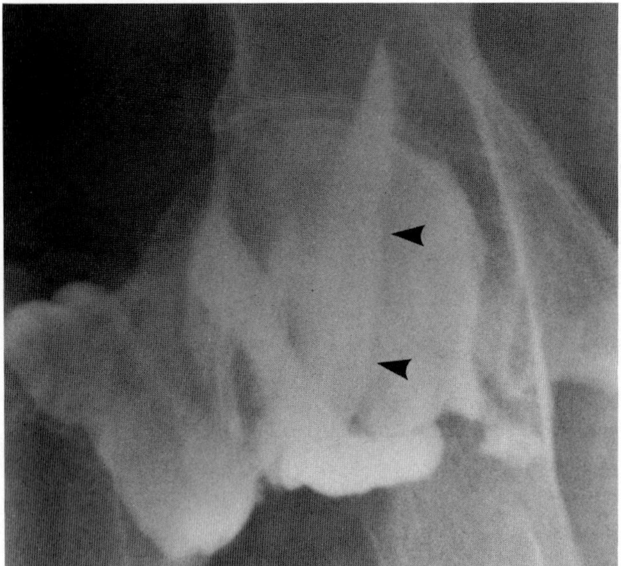

Fig. 4-4 Right hip arthrogram demonstrating communication with the iliopsoas bursa (arrowheads).

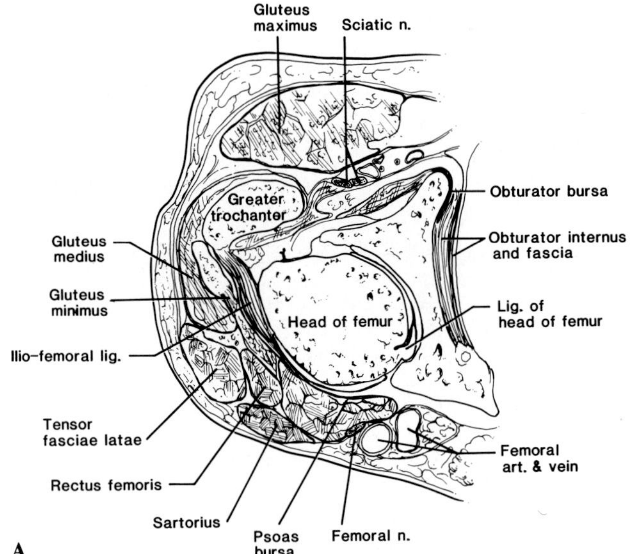

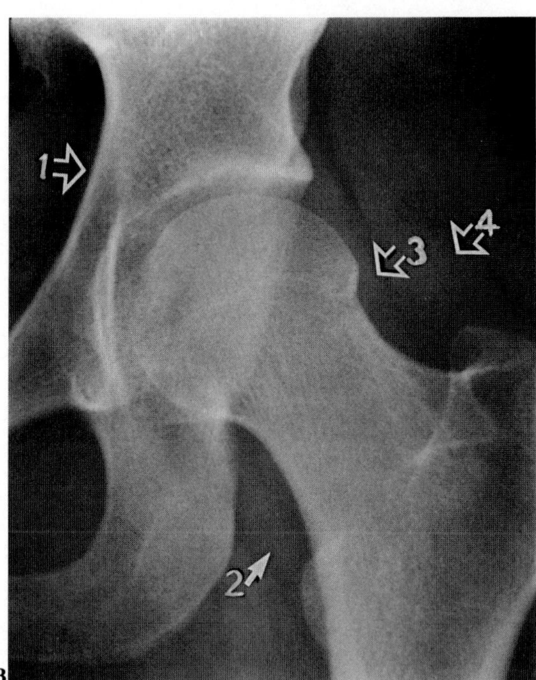

Fig. 4-5 (A) Illustration of the periarticular anatomy of the hip. (B) Anteroposterior (AP) view of the hip demonstrating the obturator internus (1), iliopsoas (2), pericapsular (3), and gluteal (4) fat planes. *Source:* Reprinted from *Imaging of Orthopedic Trauma* ed 2 by TH Berquist, 1991, Raven Press, © Mayo Foundation.

shaped like an inverted Y and lies anterior to the pubofemoral ligament and just inferior to the rectus femoris. A weak area may be present at the crossing point of these two ligaments. This weak area allows communication between the iliopsoas bursa and the hip joint, and arthrography demonstrates such communication in up to 20% of patients (Fig. 4-4).[3] The iliofemoral and ischiofemoral ligaments (Fig. 4-3, B and C) are thicker posteriorly and cross inferiorly, creating the zona orbicularis. The fibers of the capsule and capsular ligaments attach 5 to 6 cm beyond the acetabular labrum posteriorly compared with the perilabral attachment anteriorly.[1,3,6]

The periarticular anatomy of the hip is important to the clinician and radiologist (Fig. 4-5). Knowledge of the various muscle groups and their fat planes and recognition of the relationship between the neurovascular anatomy and the hip joint are of great clinical significance. For example, four fat planes have been identified radiographically, and displacement of these fat planes may indicate intraarticular or periarticular disease (Fig. 4-5).[3–5]

The fat plane of the obturator internus lies medial to this muscle in the bony pelvis. The iliopsoas fat plane is medial and parallel to the iliopsoas muscle as it inserts into the lesser trochanter. The two other fat planes lie lateral to the hip. The more medial of these two was originally thought to be adjacent to the capsule and therefore of great value in detecting joint pathology. Guerra et al,[5] however, demonstrated that the largest portion of this fat plane [the portion demonstrated on the anteroposterior (AP) radiograph] is between the rectus femoris and the tensor fasciae latae and is, in fact, anterior to the capsule of the hip. It is this portion of the fat plane that is visible on the AP radiograph of the hip (Fig. 4-5B). The small juxtacapsular portion of this fat plane, on the other hand, is not visible radiographically. The more lateral of the two fat planes lies between the gluteus medius and gluteus minimus. According to Guerra and colleagues,[5] the two fat planes nearest the hip (Fig. 4-5) are seen in 75% of patients. Other experience indicates that the iliopsoas and pericapsular fat planes are visible in 95% of patients, the obturator internus fat plane in 79%, and the gluteal fat plane in 53%. Significant joint pathology must be present before distortion of the fat planes will be detectable radiographically.[3]

Muscle insertions related to the hip (Fig. 4-1) include the following: The iliopsoas inserts in the lesser trochanter; the gluteus maximus inserts into the tensor fasciae latae over the greater trochanter and into the linea aspera of the upper femur; the gluteus medius, gluteus minimus, and piriformis insert into the greater trochanter; and the quadratus femoris inserts just below the posterior aspect of the greater trochanter.[3,6]

Finally, the sciatic nerve courses posterior to the femoral head, and the femoral artery and veins lie just medial and anterior to the femoral head (Fig. 4-3A).[1,3,6]

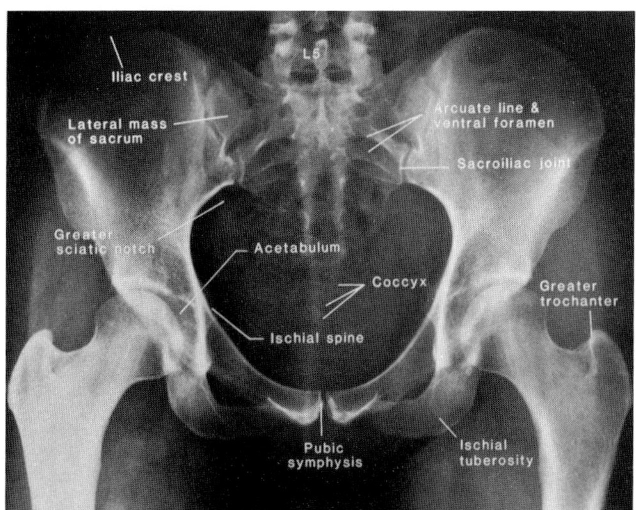

Fig. 4-6 Normal AP view of the pelvis.

IMAGING OF THE PELVIS AND HIPS

Routine Radiography

Multiple imaging techniques are often required to evaluate bone and soft tissue sports injuries. Nevertheless, routine radiography is still an essential technique for initial evaluation. Comparison of other imaging procedures, specifically magnetic resonance imaging (MRI), with radiographs emphasizes the continued importance of routine radiography.[13]

Pelvis

AP view. The AP view of the pelvis and hips should be the initial examination in patients with suspected injury. It provides sufficient information for detection of most significant pelvic fractures. The findings of the AP view can then be applied to decisions regarding further views. The AP view is obtained with the patient in the supine position on the radiographic table. The feet should be internally rotated 15°, so that the medial borders of the great toes are approximated. In certain cases, such as a hip fracture, this may not be possible for the patient. This positioning is important and should be used when possible because it overcomes the natural anteversion of the femoral necks and allows visualization of the neck and greater trochanter. Improper positioning of the feet results in the greater trochanter obscuring the femoral neck and clear demonstration of the lesser trochanter alone.[10–12]

The AP view of the pelvis and hips provides a significant amount of bone and soft tissue information, and the radiograph should be systematically reviewed.[9] When this view is properly obtained, the entire pelvis, sacrum, and proximal fourth of the femurs are included on the film (Fig. 4-6). The integrity of the pubic symphysis and obturator rings (formed by the pubic and ischial rami) should be studied, and any displaced anterior fracture should alert the physician to the possibility of a second fracture (usually posterior to and near the sacroiliac joint or sacrum). The joint space of both hips can also be assessed. The distance from the teardrop (inferomedial acetabular wall) to the medial edge of the femoral head should be symmetric. An increase in distance of 1 mm or more suggests an effusion, subluxation, or intraarticular fragment.[28] The sacroiliac joints should be compared for symmetry, and the arcuate lines of the sacrum should be carefully compared to exclude subtle fractures of the sacrum. The lower lumbar spine is usually also visible on this view, and any transverse process fracture should alert one to the need for more careful study of the anatomy immediately above and below the fracture.[10–12]

Soft tissue structures may be extremely helpful in detecting subtle fractures.[12] Slight displacement of the obturator fat plane may be the only clue to an adjacent fracture. Views of the other fat planes about the hip (iliopsoas, lateral pericapsular, and gluteal fat stripes) may be helpful, but usually a large amount of fluid must be present in the hip joint before these structures are altered on the AP radiograph.[12] The bladder is often visible in the midpelvis near the symphysis, and elevation or deviation of the soft tissue shadow of the bladder may be present with pelvic hematoma or posterior urethral rupture. In complex pelvic fractures large hematomas may obscure the bladder and perivesical fat entirely.[12,29]

AP angled views. Clarification of findings on the AP view of the pelvis may be accomplished with inlet and tangential projections.[10–12] The inlet projection is obtained with the patient in the supine position and the tube angled 40° toward the feet. This view assists in evaluation of the internal architecture of the pelvic ring. Displaced fracture fragments of complex pelvic fractures are more easily assessed with this view.[10,12]

The tangential view is taken with the patient supine and the tube angled 25° (males) or 40° (females) toward the head.[10] This view allows better evaluation of the anterior pelvis, ventral foramina, and margins of the sacrum (Fig. 4-7). Superior or inferior displacement of fracture fragments is evident on this view.[10–12]

Hips

AP and lateral views. AP and lateral views are routinely obtained. Oblique and Judet views may be required to evaluate

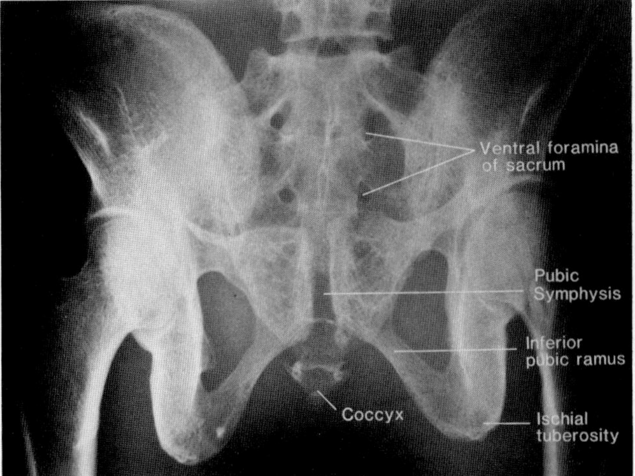

Fig. 4-7 Angled AP view of the pelvis (tube angled 40° to the head). The pubic rami, symphysis, ischial tuberosities, and foramina are well demonstrated. Ischial and pubic avulsion injuries may be more clearly identified on this view.

subtle sports injuries that may be overlooked on routine views, however. The patient is supine on the radiography table for the AP view. The sagittal plane of the central beam should be centered 2 inches medial to a line longitudinal to the anterosuperior iliac spine (palpable). This view provides better visualization of the hip and surrounding structures than the AP view of the pelvis. Table 4-2 summarizes the skeletal, soft tissue, and radiographic angles that should be evaluated on the AP view of the hip (Fig. 4-8).[10–12,28] A single AP view of the hip is inadequate for complete evaluation. This is especially true if a complete evaluation of the acetabulum and anterior and posterior columns is required. Oblique views of the hip are particularly helpful in this regard. These projections were popularized by Judet et al.[19]

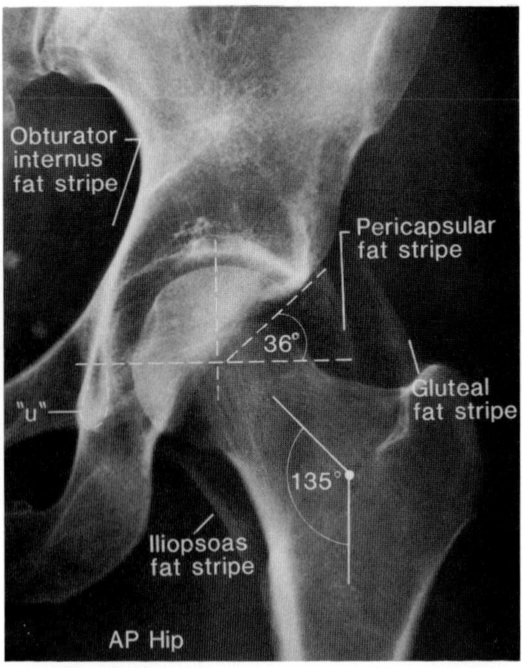

Fig. 4-8 AP view of the hip with key skeletal and soft tissue features. *Source:* Reprinted from *Imaging of Orthopedic Trauma* ed 2 by TH Berquist, 1991, Raven Press, © Mayo Foundation.

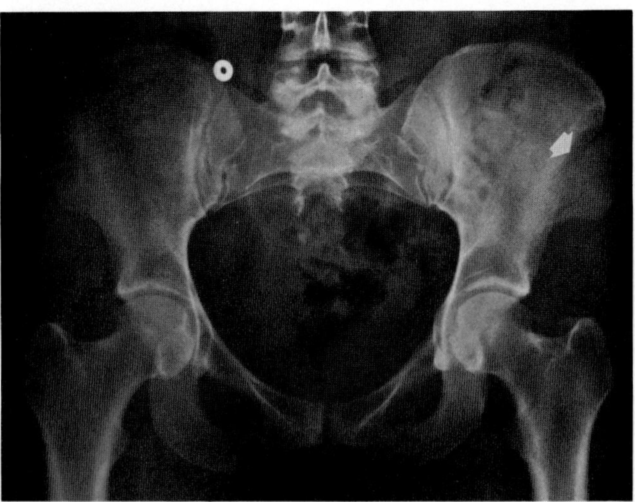

A

Fig. 4-9 (**A**) AP oblique view of the hip.

The first of two Judet views (posterior oblique) is obtained with the involved hip rotated posteriorly 45° toward the film. This view clearly demonstrates the iliac wing (iliac view). The anterior rim of the acetabulum is projected laterally to the posterior rim. The posterior column is also seen to better advantage. The second Judet view (anterior oblique) is obtained with the involved hip rotated 45° away from the film. The anterior oblique view clearly demonstrates the posterior rim of the acetabulum and the anterior column. The obturator foramen is clearly seen. Therefore, this view is often referred to as the obturator oblique (Fig. 4-9).

Evaluation of the upper femur often requires a lateral view to provide a second view to an angle of 90° to the AP view (Fig. 4-10). The lateral view is useful for evaluating the artic-

Table 4-2 Radiographic Evaluation of the Hip: AP View

Skeletal anatomy
- Iliopubic line
- Ilioischial line
- Radiographic U (teardrop)
- Dome of acetabulum
- Posterior rim
- Anterior rim

Angles
- Angle of Wibert (normal, 20° to 40°; average, 36°)
- Neck shaft angle (normal, 135°; coxa valga, >135°; coxa vara, <135°)

Fat planes
- Obturator internus
- Iliopsoas
- Pericapsular
- Gluteal

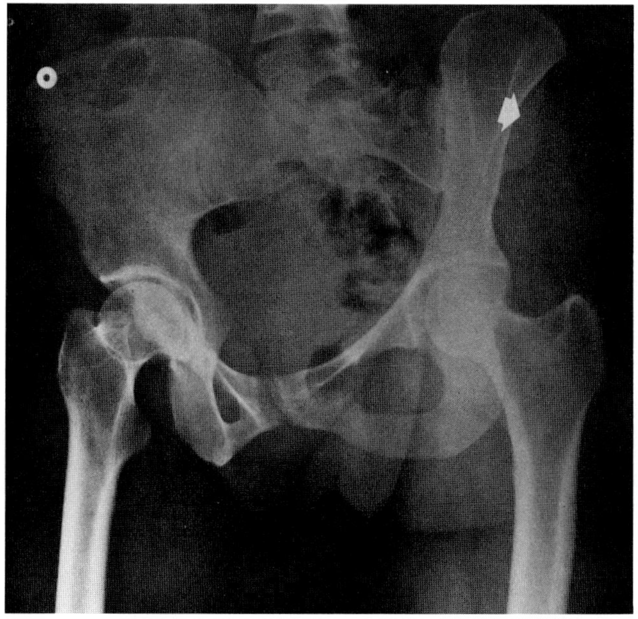
B

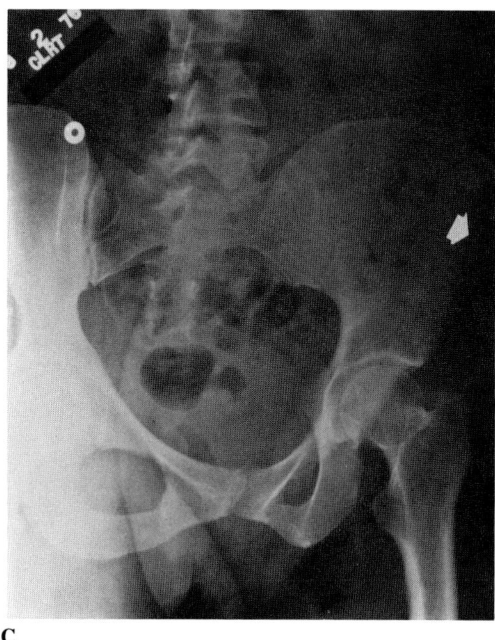
C

Fig. 4-9 contd (**B**) anterior and (**C**) posterior oblique views of the hip (Judet views) demonstrating an anterior iliac wing fracture (arrow in **C**).

ular region, position of fracture fragments (Fig. 4-10), and subtle anterior and posterior acetabular injuries.[12]

Oblique view. The patient is positioned with the affected side of the hip toward the cassette. The opposite hip is elevated approximately 45° and supported by a cushion wedge. The knee and hip on the ipsilateral side are flexed about 45°.[10,12] The beam is centered between the symphysis and anterosuperior iliac spine. This view allows improved visualization of the femoral neck, acetabulum, and lesser trochanter (Fig. 4-11).[11,12]

Conventional and Computed Tomography

Computed tomography (CT) is a proven technique for evaluating complex pelvic and acetabular fractures (Fig. 4-12). Soft tissue injury can also be assessed.[14,16,24] When necessary, three-dimensional images can be obtained (Fig. 4-13).[15]

Typically, sports injuries to the pelvis and hips are subtle. Therefore, conventional tomography in the proper plane (ie,

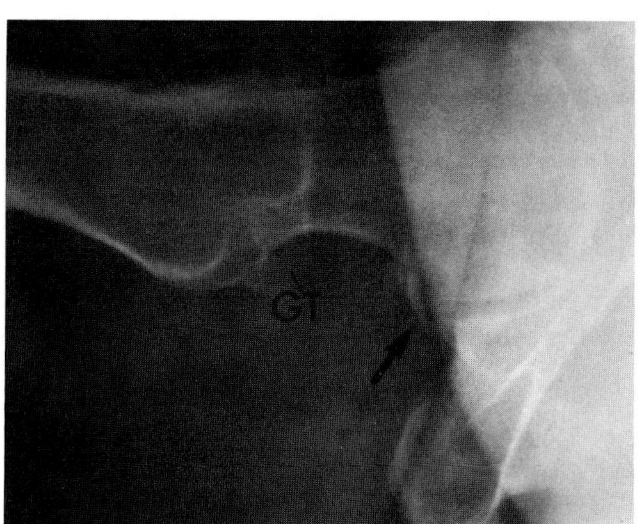

Fig. 4-10 Lateral view of the hip demonstrating subtle posterior neck fragments (arrow) not evident on the AP view. GT, Greater trochanter; AI, anteroinferior iliac spine.

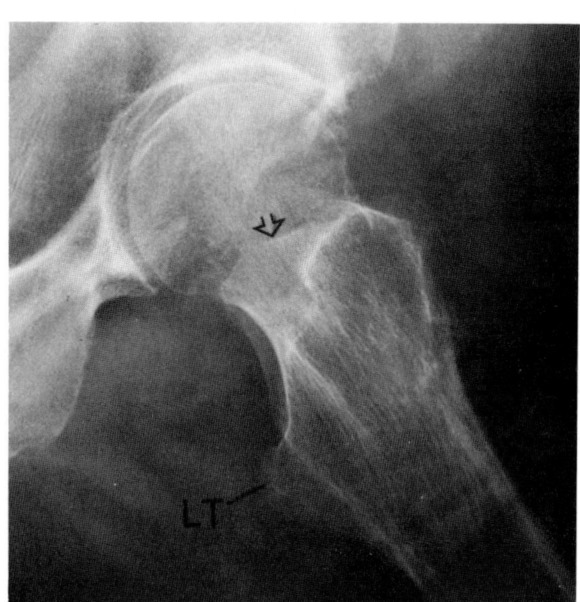

Fig. 4-11 Oblique view of the left hip demonstrating the acetabulum, lesser trochanter (LT), and femoral neck. The greater trochanter (arrow) overlies the neck and should not be confused with a fracture.

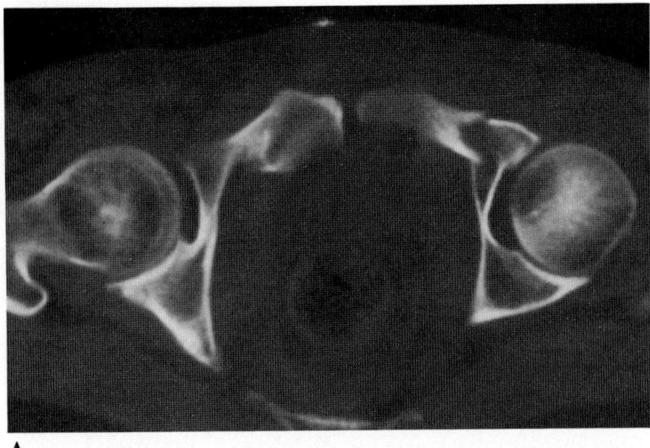
A

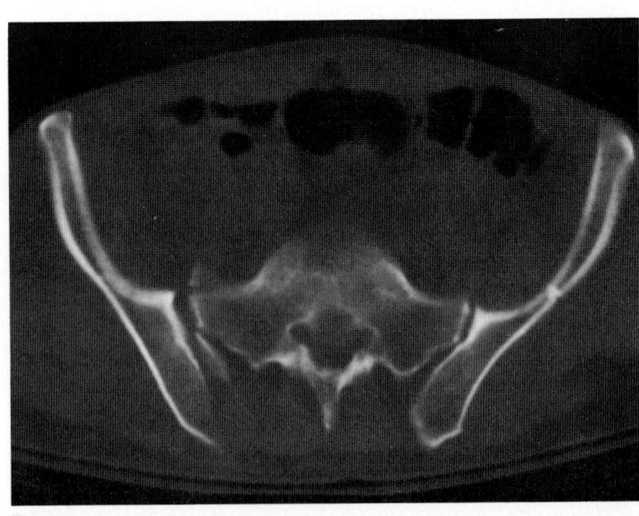
B

Fig. 4-12 CT images demonstrating anterior pubic rami fractures (**A**) and sacral fracture with subluxation of the sacroiliac joint on the right (**B**).

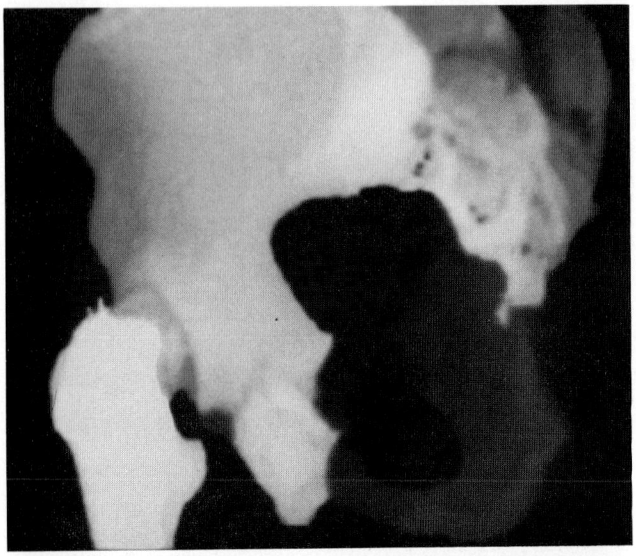

A

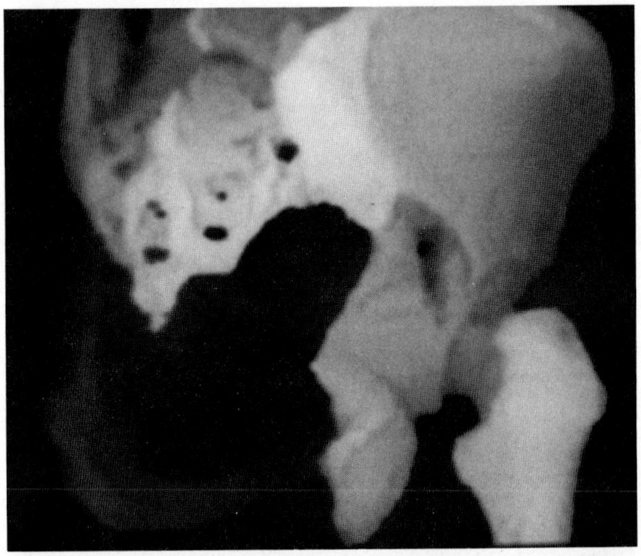

B

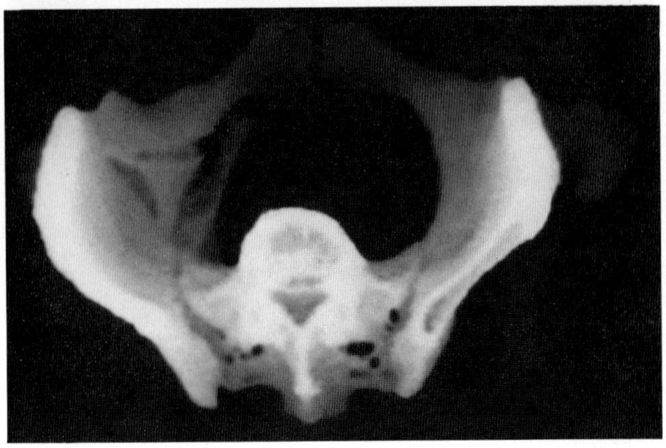

C

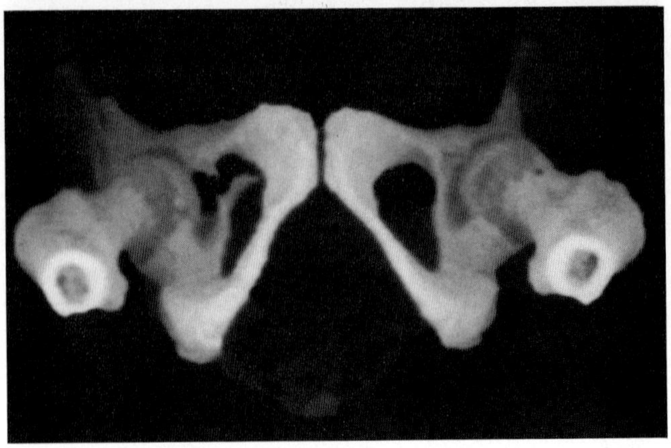

D

Fig. 4-13 Three-dimensional CT images of a complex acetabular fracture. (**A**) Oblique view of normal hip, (**B**) oblique view of abnormal hip, (**C**) view from above, and (**D**) view from below.

right posterior oblique for anterior iliac spines) or CT may be used to detect subtle changes in cortical bone at points of muscle attachment. Both techniques are also of value in association with arthrography to improve evaluation of the hip.[16,18] Other causes of pain may also be detected with tomography or CT (Fig. 4-14).[12,15]

Thin sections through the area of interest are usually superior with either technique. We typically use 10-mm slices of the pelvis and hips for screening, but 3- to 5-mm sections should be obtained through local areas of point tenderness. Trispiral tomograms are likewise performed with 3- to 5-mm sections.[12] Techniques are described more fully below as they apply to specific injuries.

Skeletal Scintigraphy

Radionuclide scans will be positive within 72 hours of skeletal injury. Up to 80% of cases are positive within 24 hours of injury.[12] Subtle injuries are not detectable with routine radiographs (Fig. 4-15). Therefore, bone scans with subsequent localized views, tomography, or CT serve as a useful approach to detection of subtle fractures or avulsion injuries. Early avascular necrosis can also be detected with bone scan.[17] A negative scan effectively excludes osseous injury and suggests that further studies such as MRI be obtained to evaluate the soft tissues.[12,13]

Magnetic Resonance Imaging

MRI is ideally suited for evaluation of soft tissue injuries of the pelvis and hips. Subtle ligament, tendon, and muscle injuries can be detected and classified. Bursal inflammation can also be confirmed.[12,23]

The ability of MRI to detect early avascular necrosis is well established,[13,17,25] but some subtle fractures may be more specifically defined with CT or conventional tomography. Comparison with routine radiographs is also necessary for specific diagnosis (Fig. 4-16).[13]

MR examinations of the pelvis and hips are usually conducted with the body coil. Localized areas, however, such as the hip, may be studied with flat circular or coupled coils to improve image quality.[13] Axial T2-weighted (SE 2000/20,80) and coronal T1-weighted (SE 500/20) images provide an adequate screening examination for the pelvis and hips. In some situations, additional image planes and/or pulse sequences may be required.[13]

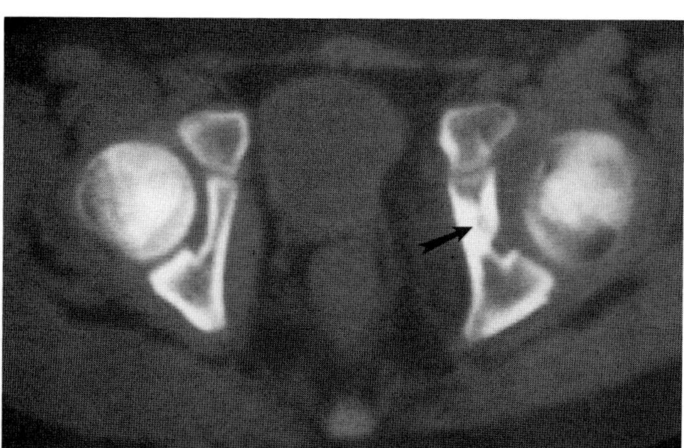

Fig. 4-14 Evaluation of a young soccer player with hip pain after an abduction injury. Routine radiographs taken several weeks later showed a widened joint space on the left. CT scan demonstrates an osteoid osteoma (arrow) with synovial reaction around the ligamentum teres causing the widened joint space.

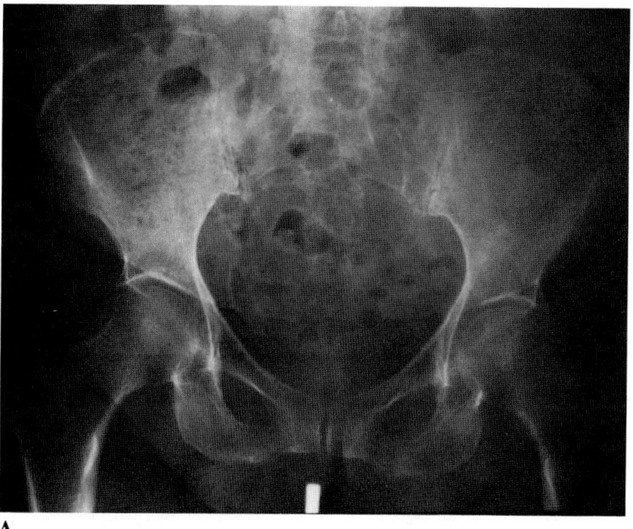

A

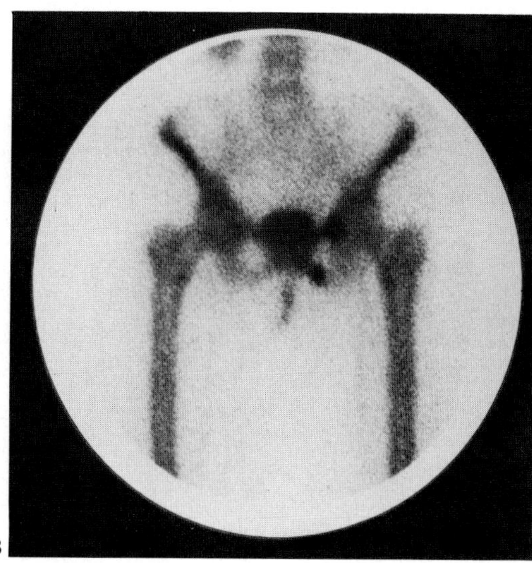

B

Fig. 4-15 (**A**) AP view of the pelvis in a jogger with groin pain. (**B**) Bone scan shows focal increased tracer uptake in the pubic rami on the left due to fracture.

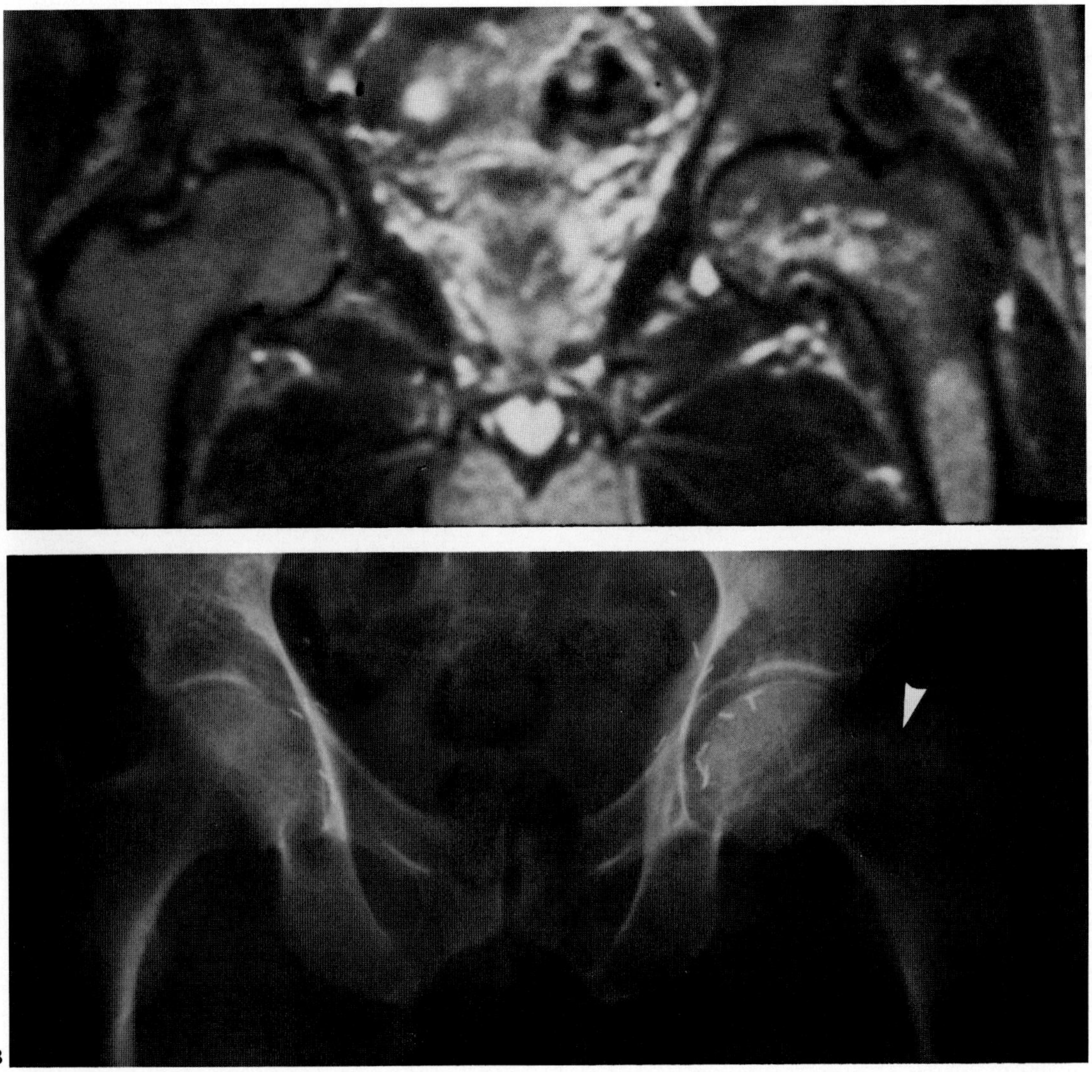

A

B

Fig. 4-16 Evaluation of an elderly jogger with left hip pain. (A) Coronal (SE 2000/60) magnetic resonance (MR) image shows increased signal intensity in the femoral neck. This finding is nonspecific. (B) Routine radiograph shows Paget's disease with a femoral neck fracture (arrowhead).

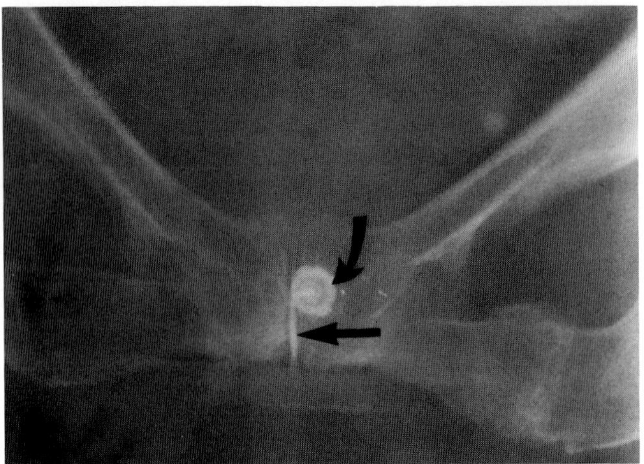

Fig. 4-17 Radiograph taken during diagnostic injection showing contrast medium (straight arrow) and needle (curved arrow). Contrast medium confirms correct needle position. Note the inferior ramus fracture on the left.

Arthrography, Tenography, and Diagnostic Injections

Hip arthrography, tenography, and diagnostic injections are valuable techniques for evaluating athletes with pain, instability, clicking, or snapping and other symptoms.[12,22] Choice of examination or sequence of examinations should be tailored to the symptoms. Variable imaging techniques such as tomography, CT, single- or double-contrast studies, and injection of anesthetic and/or anesthetic-steroid combinations may be required.[12,20,21]

Arthrograms are most commonly performed on the hip. Contrast agent injections in the pubic symphysis (Fig. 4-17) and sacroiliac joint are usually employed to confirm needle position.

Before arthrograms or articular injections are performed, all radiographic studies should be reviewed.[12] Clinical findings and suspected pathology should be thoroughly discussed with the referring clinician. This information is essential for selecting the proper injection and imaging technique.

The injection site for the hip is determined by the fluoroscopic appearance of the hip and the location of the femoral artery. The femoral artery, which must be palpated before injection, generally runs medial to the femoral neck. In patients with significant deformities of the hip as a result of previous surgery or trauma, however, the relationship of the neck of the femoral artery may vary. In making the injection we generally use an anterior or anterolateral approach, with the needle being directed vertically or slightly laterally to medially just lateral to the midline at the junction of the head and neck (Fig. 4-18). The anesthetic needle is positioned over the area, and the skin is infiltrated to form a wheal. After the superficial soft tissues are anesthetized, a 22-gauge, 3½-inch needle is advanced (Fig. 4-18) until it makes contact with the femoral neck. The patient is instructed to flex the hip slightly. This ensures that the bevel of the needle is within the joint capsule.[12,20]

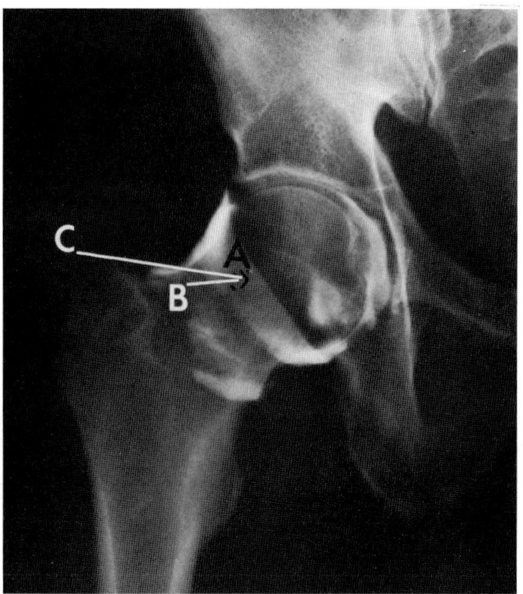

Fig. 4-18 AP view of the hip demonstrating arthrographic approaches. (**A**) Vertical, (**B**) oblique, (**C**) lateral.

Needle position can be confirmed by aspiration of synovial fluid, injection of a small amount of contrast medium (0.5 mL), or injection of air. Aspiration of the joint or saline flush with aspiration is usually performed if synovial fluid analysis for crystals, rheumatoid factor, immunoglobulins, or infection is indicated.[12]

The choice of contrast agent and filming technique varies with the clinical situation (Table 4-3). In routine situations 6 mL or more of contrast medium (meglumine such as Hypaque-M-60 or nonionic agent) is injected. If too much contrast medium is injected, subtle changes will be obscured. Rarely, double-contrast technique (4 mL of contrast material plus 10 mL or more of air) is used. Other cases call for use of air alone.

After the injection of the contrast agent or agents, the hip is exercised and observed fluoroscopically. Any painful motions, clicking, or position changes of intraarticular bodies can be observed. Patients are positioned fluoroscopically for filming. This technique provides added information and ensures proper positioning. Films are taken with the hip in internal and external rotation and in lateral and oblique projections. Depending upon the information obtained fluoroscopically, further views after exercise or additional oblique views are also obtained. If necessary, CT or conventional tomography scans may be obtained. This requires additional planning on the part of the arthrographer. If tomography is contemplated, the injection is usually made on the tomography table to reduce the time required to obtain the films.

Table 4-3 Pelvis and Hips: Arthrography and Injections

Location	*Indication*	*Approach*	*Imaging Technique*
Hip	Labral tear	Anterior, oblique, or lateral (Fig. 4-18)	CT, tomography*
	Capsular abnormality	Anterior, oblique, or lateral (Fig. 4-18)	Routine film with fluoroscopy
	Articular abnormality and/or loose body	Anterior, oblique, or lateral (Fig. 4-18)	Routine film with fluoroscopy
Iliopsoas	Bursitis or snapping tendon	Anterior	Fluoroscopy with routine film and videotape
Pubic symphysis	Pain	Anterior (Fig. 4-17)	Routine film
Greater trochanter	Bursitis	Lateral	Fluoroscopic injection only
Ischial tuberosity	Pain	Posterior	Fluoroscopic injection only
Sacroiliac joint	Pain	Posterior (patient rotated so that involved joint is oriented toward table)	Fluoroscopic injection only

*MRI may prove to be the superior technique.

After the arthrogram bupivacaine (Marcaine) or a combination of bupivacaine and betamethasone (Celestone) is often injected. This is helpful in patients without definitive arthrographic findings. The injection assists in determining whether the pain is intraarticular and in this way facilitates treatment programs.[12,20]

Arthrographic Demonstration of Normal Anatomy

The normal arthrogram demonstrates the articular cartilage, labrum, capsular configuration, and synovial characteristics of the hip joint (Fig. 4-19). The margins of the capsule extend from the acetabular rim to the base of the femoral neck. There are four recesses (Fig. 4-19). Proximally the superior articular recess extends above the cartilaginous labrum. Inferiorly the inferior recess outlines the inferior labrum. The superior recess colli lies above the femoral neck, and the inferior recess colli is found at the lower margin of the neck. The distal insertion of the capsule is irregular and should not be mistaken for synovial inflammation. The acetabular labrum is difficult to visualize in its entirety. Oblique views demonstrate the labrum to best advantage (Fig. 4-19B). A constant extrinsic defect is seen below the femoral head owing to the transverse ligament. With the patient in the supine position, the posterior labrum may be seen as a straight line along the upper portion of the neck. Inferior to the labral line is the orbicular zone, which is caused by thickened ligamentous fibers encircling the capsule. The articular cartilage on the femoral head is well demonstrated and is usually thicker than the acetabular articular surface. Medially the acetabular fossa is well demonstrated, but in normal patients the ligamentum teres is usually not visualized. Communication of the capsule with the iliopsoas bursa occurs in 15% to 20% of patients owing to a defect between the iliofemoral and pubofemoral ligaments.[12,21,26,27]

Indications for Hip Arthrography

Arthritis. Arthrographic evaluation of patients with posttraumatic and inflammatory joint diseases allows one to obtain anatomic and laboratory information. Synovial fluid should always be aspirated. If no fluid can be obtained, a saline flush (nonbacteriostatic sterile saline) with reaspiration can provide information regarding infection. Fluid analysis will vary depending upon the clinical situation (crystals in suspected gout or pseudogout; rheumatoid factor, differential count, and Gram's stain in cases of suspected infection; immunoglobulins in chondrolysis). Grossly bloody fluid may indicate pigmented villonodular synovitis.[12,30]

Evaluation of the articular cartilage is usually adequate with conventional film techniques. Tomography is useful in patients with abnormal routine radiographs or when subtle findings are suspected. For example, in patients with chondrolysis tomography will assist in detection of the subtle erosions in the articular cartilage.[12] Double-contrast technique may provide additional anatomic information.

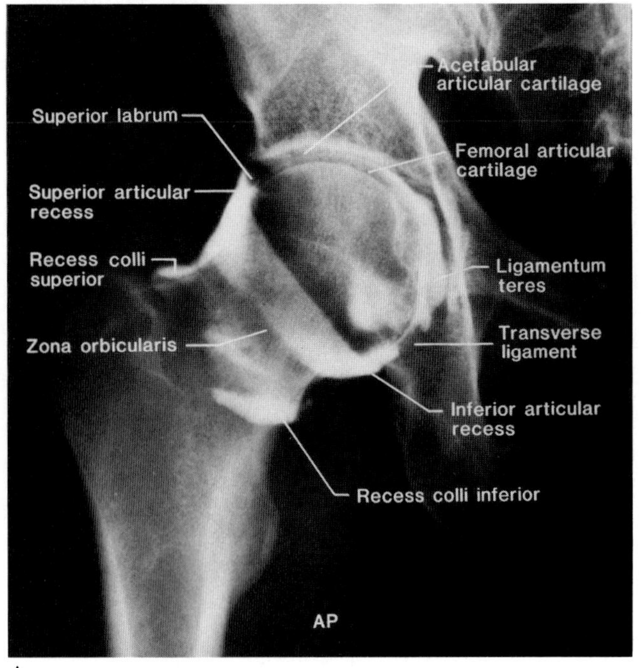

A

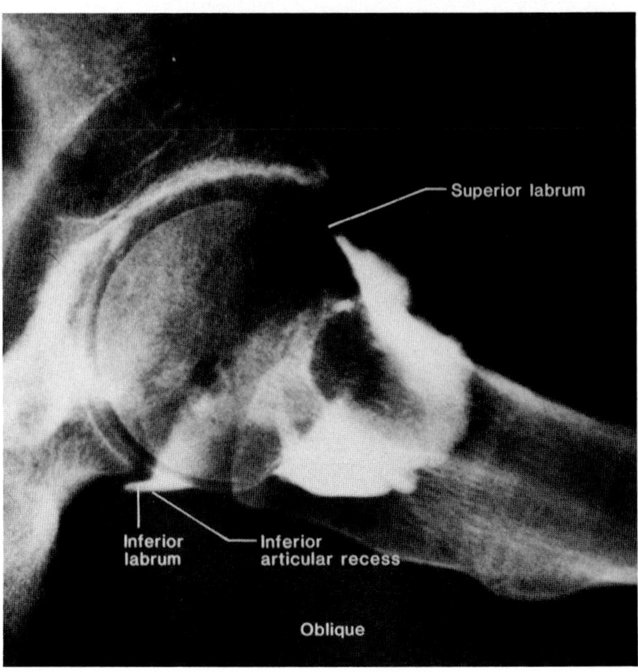

B

Fig. 4-19 (**A**) AP and (**B**) oblique views demonstrating normal arthrographic anatomy of the hip. *Source:* Reprinted from *Imaging of Orthopedic Trauma* ed 2 by TH Berquist, 1991, Raven Press, © Mayo Foundation.

The configuration of the capsule (Fig. 4-19) is also easily defined arthrographically. The normal hip should accommodate at least 10 mL of fluid. In patients with long-standing inflammation or restricted motion for long periods after injury, the capsule may decrease in size with loss of the normal recesses (Fig. 4-20). Symptoms similar to those of adhesive capsulitis in the shoulder may develop. Injection of contrast material may be difficult in patients with advanced capsulitis.

Loose bodies. Arthrography is frequently useful in identification of intraarticular osteocartilaginous bodies. On occasion subtle areas of calcification or more obvious calcifications may be evident on plain films (Fig. 4-21). Arthrography will confirm the location of these densities. The most common cause of intraarticular loose bodies is degenerative arthritis. Fragments of cartilage are nourished by synovial fluid and may actually increase in size over a period of time.[12]

Acetabular labral tears. Evaluation of suspected acetabular labral tears is one of the most frequent indications for hip arthrography in practice at the Mayo Clinic.[12,22] Patients with tears in the labrum present with pain, clicking (especially with flexion and external rotation of the hip), and decreased range of motion.[22] Routine radiographs are of little value. Conventional arthrography (Fig. 4-22) allows partial evaluation of the labrum, although the anterior and posterior portions are difficult to visualize. In this case fluoroscopically positioned oblique views in the frog-leg position allow evaluation of a large portion of the labrum. Tomography or CT is also useful in studying portions of the labrum. Early experience indicates that these methods are not sufficiently accurate, however, and that MRI with radial gradient-echo technique may be most useful for evaluation of the labrum (Fig. 4-23).[12,13]

Iliopsoas bursa or snapping iliopsoas tendon. As mentioned earlier, the joint capsule communicates with the iliopsoas bursa in 15% to 20% of patients.[12,21,26] In long-standing inflammatory arthritis this communication may enlarge, resulting in an inguinal mass (Fig. 4-24). If the bursa

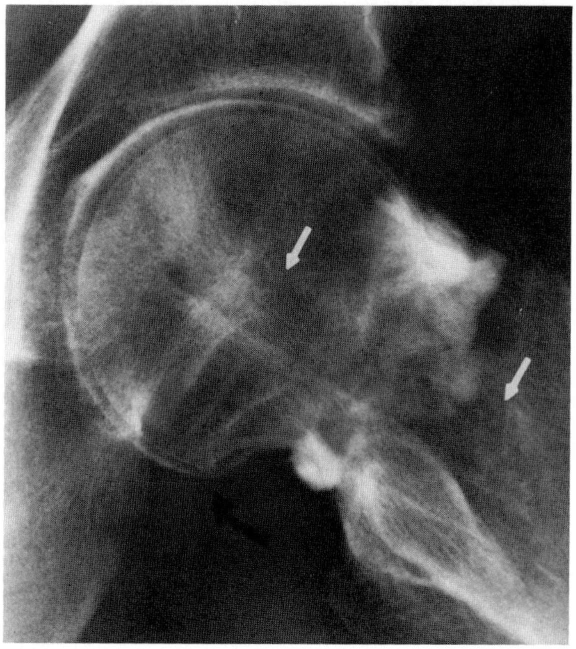

Fig. 4-20 Oblique view after hip fracture. Arthrogram shows reduced capsular volume, early degenerative lipping (curved arrow), and an old sliding screw tract (white arrows).

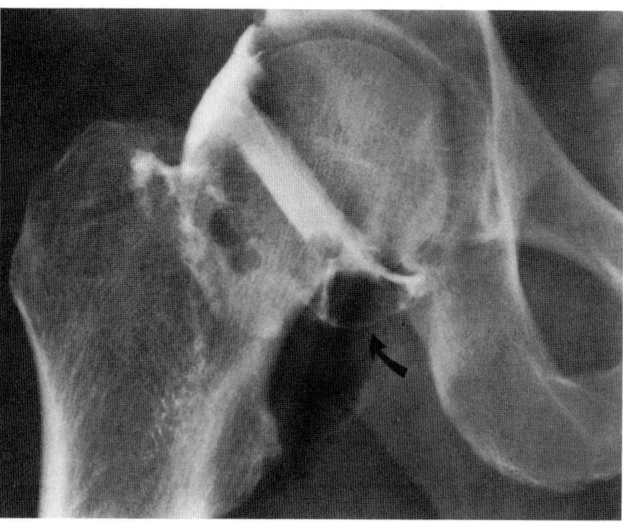

Fig. 4-21 AP arthrogram demonstrating an inferior loose body (arrow).

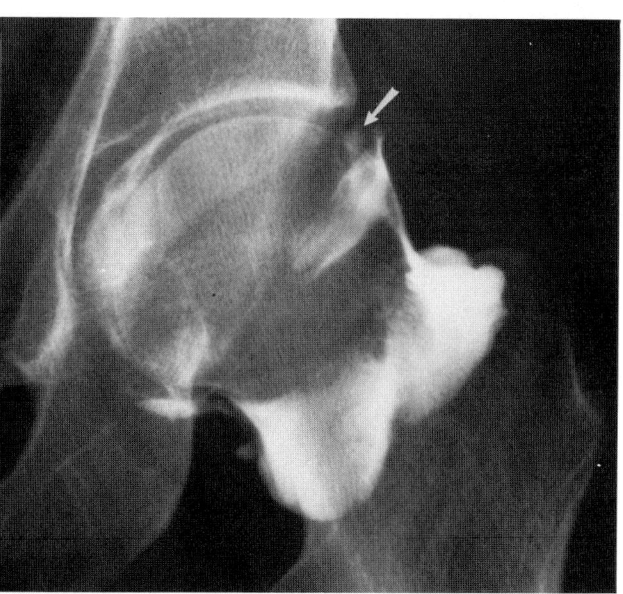

Fig. 4-22 AP arthrogram demonstrating contrast agent in the superior labrum (arrow) due to a tear.

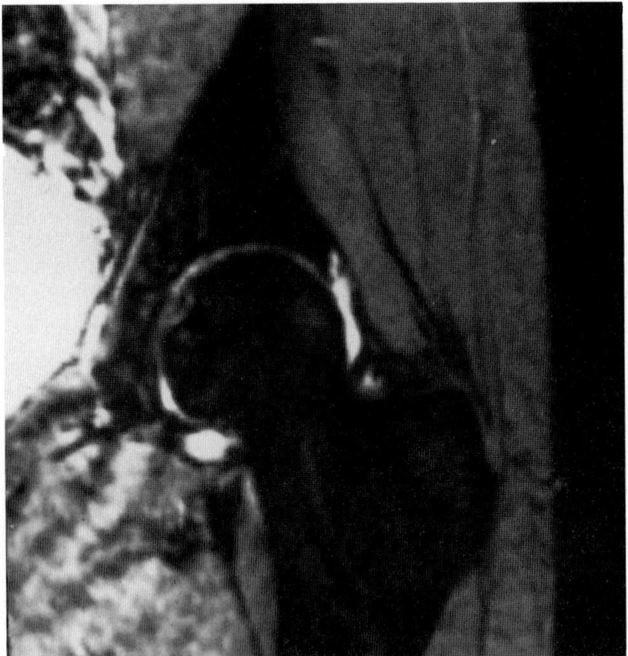

A

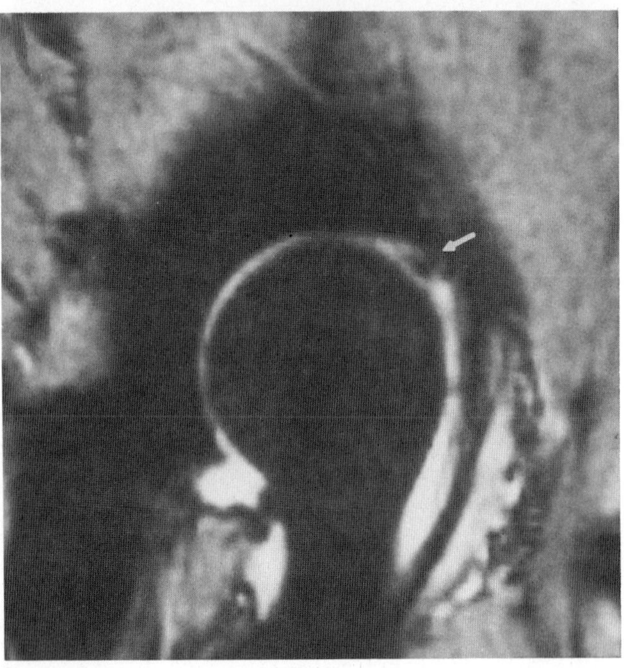

B

Fig. 4-23 Radial MR images of a normal (**A**) and torn (**B**) acetabular labrum (arrow).

extends cephalad, compression of the femoral vessels, bladder, and colon may occur.[12,26]

Injection of the bursa for diagnostic or therapeutic purposes is not uncommon. An anterior approach (Table 4-3) is usually best. CT (Fig. 4-24A) or fluoroscopic guidance can be used. When the bursa is enlarged, the former is more easily accomplished. For normal iliopsoas bursa, however, as in the case of snapping iliopsoas tendon, fluoroscopy is more efficient. This condition is discussed more completely in the soft tissue injury section (below).

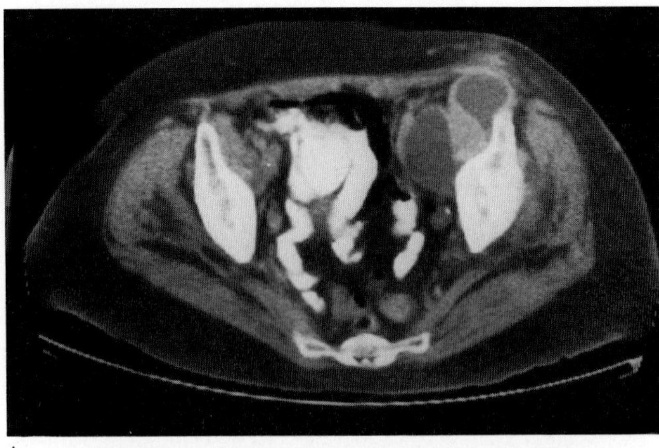

A

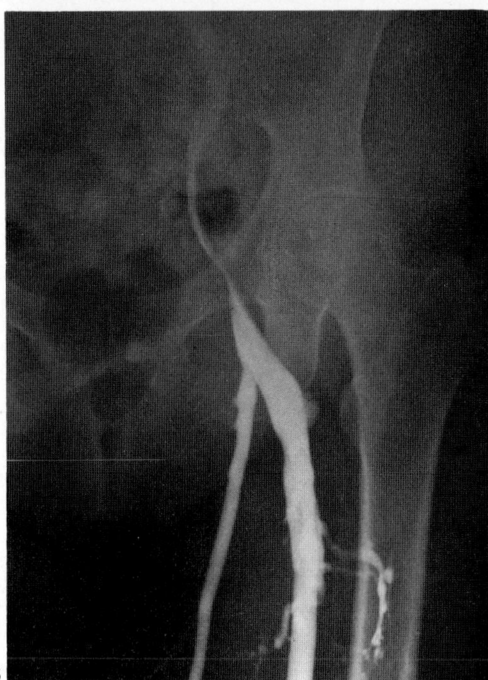

B

Fig. 4-24 Enlarged iliopsoas bursa due to chronic inflammation. (**A**) CT and (**B**) venogram demonstrate the significant size and mass effect.

Injection of other sites in the pelvis and hips is easily accomplished under fluoroscopic guidance (Table 4-3). When appropriate, needle position can be confirmed with injection of a small amount of contrast medium. A mixture of betamethasone and bupivacaine (1:1 ratio) is commonly used. The volume injected varies with location.

FRACTURES

Minor fractures (fractures of individual bones, stress fractures, and avulsion injuries) are common in athletes and also in

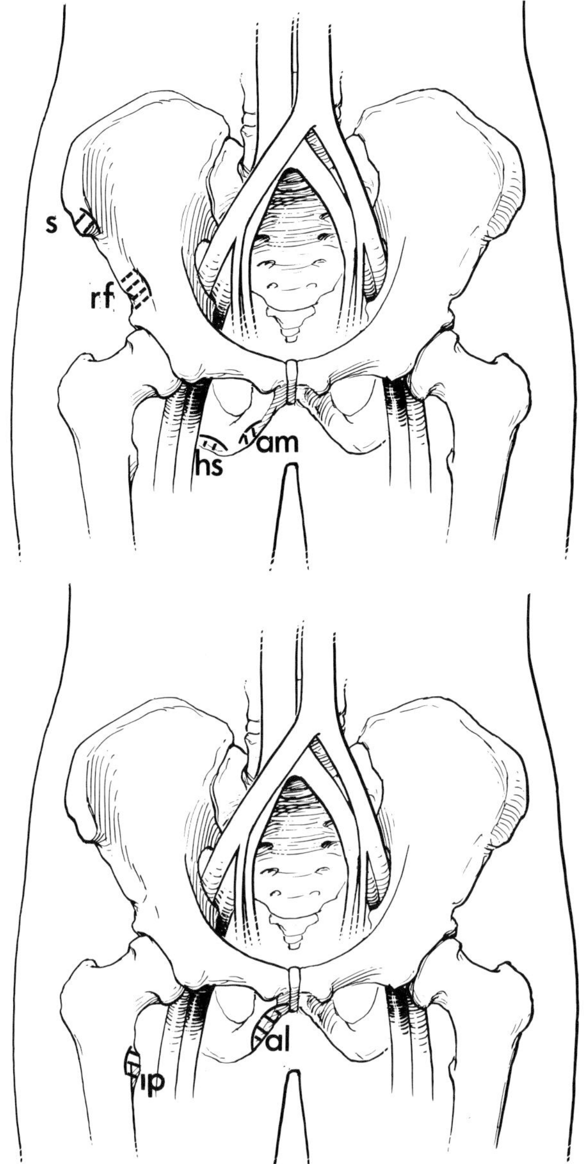

Fig. 4-25 (**A**) Illustration of the origins of the muscles on the ischium (hs, hamstrings; am, adductor magnus), anterosuperior iliac spine (s, sartorius), and anteroinferior iliac spine (rf, rectus femoris). (**B**) Illustration of insertion of the iliopsoas (ip) on the lesser trochanter and origin of the adductor longus (al) on the inferior pubic ramus near the symphysis.

active older individuals.[31,47,58,59] Major fractures of the pelvis and hips are most frequently associated with motor vehicle accidents. Auto racing, snowmobiling, horse racing, skiing, and mountaineering may also result in complex fractures.[63,64]

Minor Fractures

Minor fractures of the pelvis and hips include avulsion injuries, stress fractures, and class I fractures (breaks in individual bones of the pelvis). Osseous overuse injuries could also be included in this category.

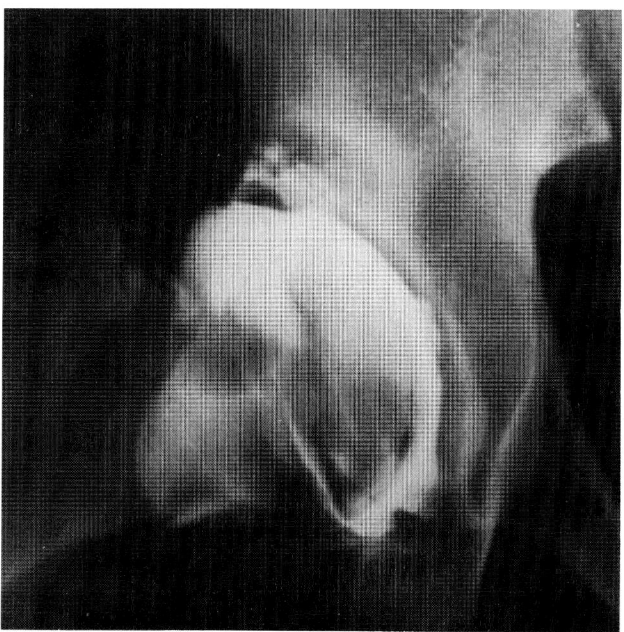

A

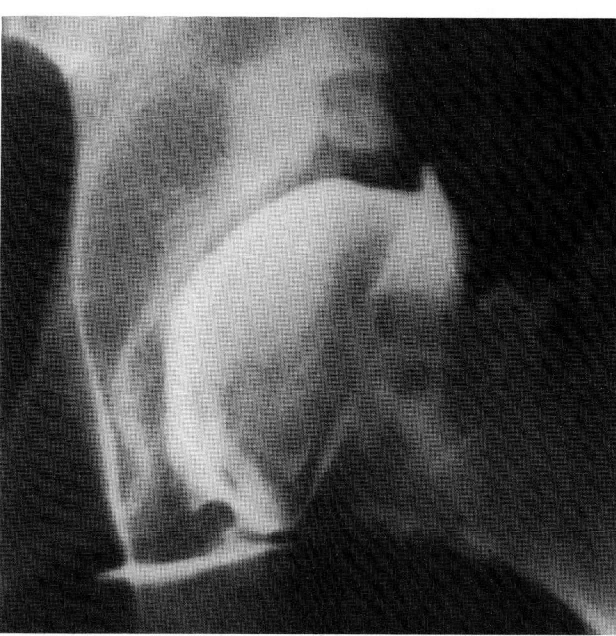

B

Fig. 4-26 Arthrograms of an avulsed os acetabuli (**A**) and a normal os acetabuli (**B**). Contrast medium surrounds or fills in the area of attachment (**A**) when separation occurs. *Source:* Reprinted with permission from *Journal of Bone and Joint Surgery* (1988;70A:1568–1570), Copyright © 1988 Journal of Bone and Joint Surgery.

Avulsion Fractures

Avulsion fractures most commonly occur in adolescents and athletes younger than 25 years of age (Fig. 4-25). Avulsion of the unossified apophysis (Fig. 4-26) may also occur theoretically.[33,34,36,59] Table 4-1 summarizes the appearance and fusion times of commonly injured apophyses in the pelvis and hips.[38]

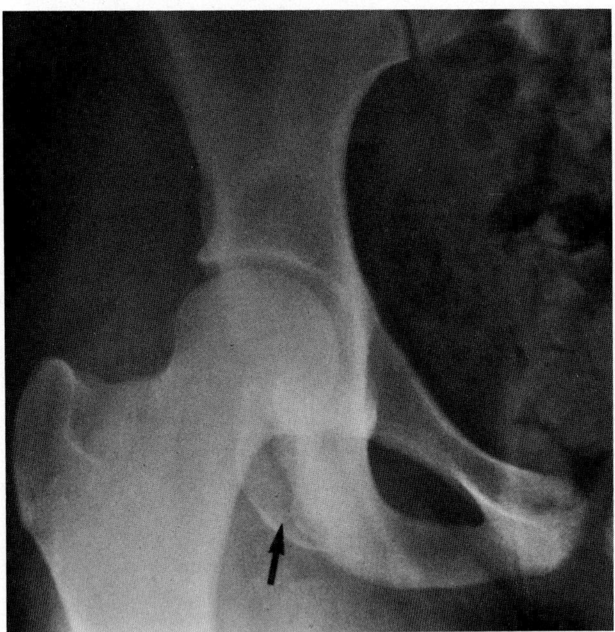

Fig. 4-27 AP view of the hip in a hurdler presenting with acute gluteal pain during a track meet. The ischial avulsion fracture (arrow) is obvious.

Avulsion injuries in the pelvis and hips are usually the result of forceful muscle contraction during acceleration or deceleration. The exact mechanism varies with location and activity.

Ischium. The ischial ossification center appears at age 14 to 16 years and typically fuses by age 18 to 25 years. There are usually two portions (Fig. 4-25A), one for the hamstring and the other for the adductor magnus. Running, jumping, hurdling, and football are most commonly implicated in avulsion injuries. For example, hurdlers most often have hamstring avulsions (Figs. 4-27 and 4-28), and cheerleaders have adductor or anterior ischial avulsions.[47,59] Avulsion of the ischial tuberosity has been associated with sciatic nerve injury. Sciatic nerve injury can also occur with posterior hip fracture or dislocation, myositis ossificans of the biceps femoris, and, of course, herniated lumbar disc.[51]

Anteroinferior iliac spine. Injury to the anteroinferior iliac spine (Fig. 4-29) occurs less commonly than injury to anterosuperior iliac spine. This apophysis appears at age 13 to 15 years and fuses at age 16 to 18 years. Forceful contraction of the rectus femoris leads to this injury (Figs. 4-1 and 4-25A).[31,32] Sports involved include running, soccer, and hockey.[59] In certain cases myositis ossificans occurs, causing a radiographic lesion that can mimic malignancy.[47,59]

Anterosuperior iliac spine. The ossification center for the anterosuperior iliac spine appears at age 13 to 15 years and fuses by 21 to 25 years of age. Sudden contraction of the sartorius (Fig. 4-25A) or hyperextension of the trunk leads to the avulsion fracture. Runners and football players (Fig. 4-30) are most often affected by this injury. Sudden sharp pain usually causes the runner to stop abruptly.

Iliac crest apophysis. The ossification centers appear at age 13 to 15 years and fuse by 25 years of age. Ossification occurs lateral to medial.[38,47] Anterior muscle attachments include the gluteus medius, oblique abdominis, and tensor fasciae latae. The latissimus dorsi and gluteus maximus insert posteriorly. Injuries may be due to avulsion (runners), direct trauma (football), or overuse (twisting forces in middistance runners).[34,47]

Pubic symphysis. Avulsion of the inferior pubic ramus near the symphysis may occur with abrupt contraction of the adductor longus (Fig. 4-25B). As with inferior iliac spine avulsions, the secondary resorptive changes may mimic malignancy.[59]

Lesser trochanter. The lesser trochanter ossifies by age 12 years and fuses by 20 years of age. Avulsion of the lesser trochanter is associated with abrupt iliopsoas contraction (Fig. 4-25B) typically associated with running, football, or basketball (Fig. 4-31).[47,59] Clancy and Foltz[34] reported on 30 lesser trochanteric fractures. Of these, 22 were sports related. Patients experienced sudden sharp pain while running. Inability to flex the hip or climb steps was evident on examination.

Os acetabuli marginalis superior. Rarely, this normal variant (Fig. 4-26) can become separated as a result of

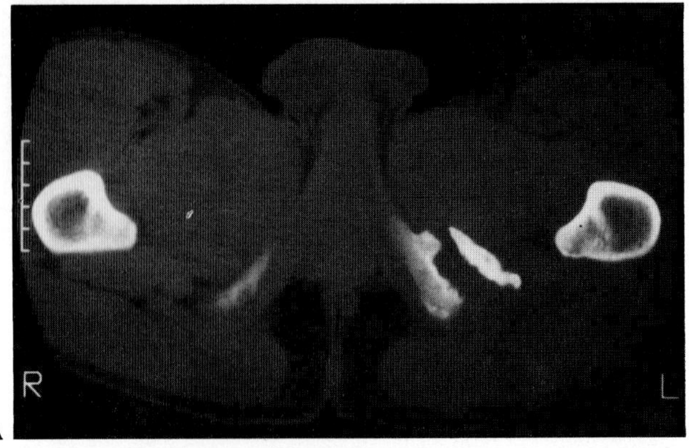

A

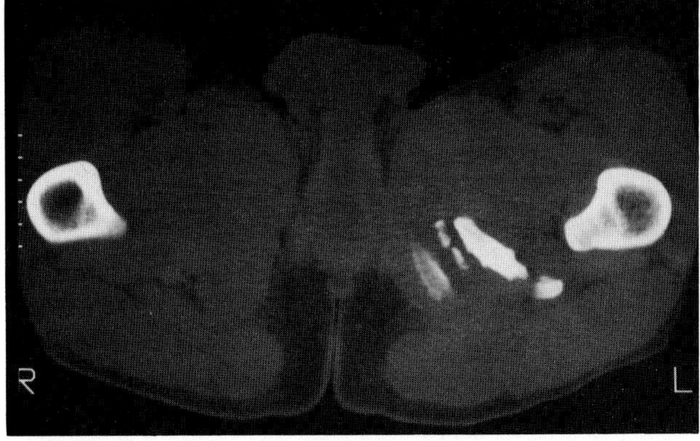

B

Fig. 4-28 CT images of the pelvis in a track athlete presenting with a posterior gluteal mass. Neoplasm was suspected. There is an old displaced avulsion fracture of the ischium.

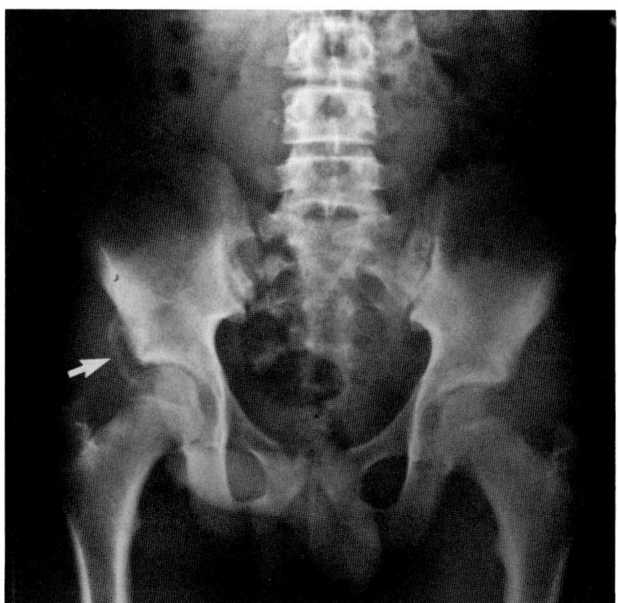

Fig. 4-29 AP view of the pelvis demonstrating an avulsion fracture (arrow) of the anteroinferior iliac spine.

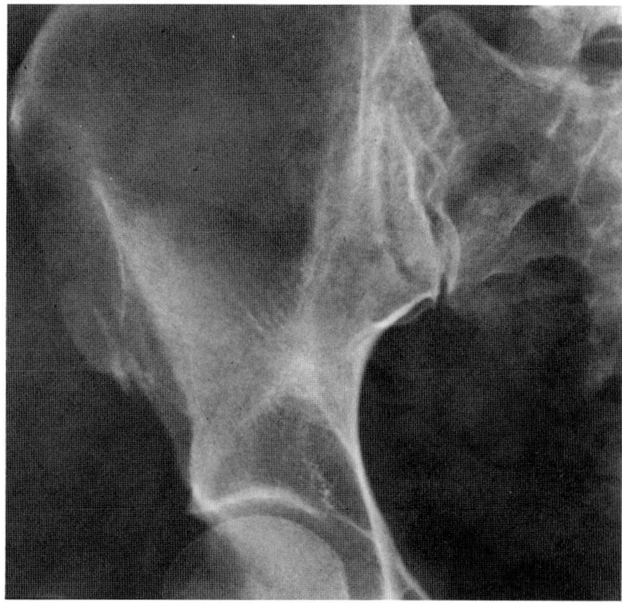

Fig. 4-30 Slightly obliqued view of the right ilium demonstrating a minimally displaced avulsion of the anterosuperior iliac spine in a track athlete.

trauma.[38,46] Routine radiographs may demonstrate asymmetry or obvious displacement on the involved side. Arthrography or MRI may be required to demonstrate subtle separation, however. Avulsion of the anteroinferior iliac spine or peritendinous calcification may have a similar appearance on routine radiographs.[33]

Stress Fractures and Overuse Injuries

Stress fractures of the femoral neck and pubic rami are not uncommon in long distance runners, especially women.[58] Chapter 12 discusses stress fractures more completely. Posttraumatic injury to the apophyses similar in appearance to osteochondritis dissecans can also occur in the pelvis and hips. The ischium and iliac ossification centers are most often involved (Fig. 4-32). Patients present with pain, usually after practice, which may be relieved to some degree by rest and ice applications.[31,34] Radiographs may be normal or reveal fragmentation of the ossification center (Fig. 4-32) similar to changes noted with Osgood-Schlatter disease.

Class I Fractures

Class I pelvic fractures are breaks of individual bones in the pelvis without disruption of the pelvic ring.[31,46] Avulsion fractures and isolated stress fractures are common in athletes

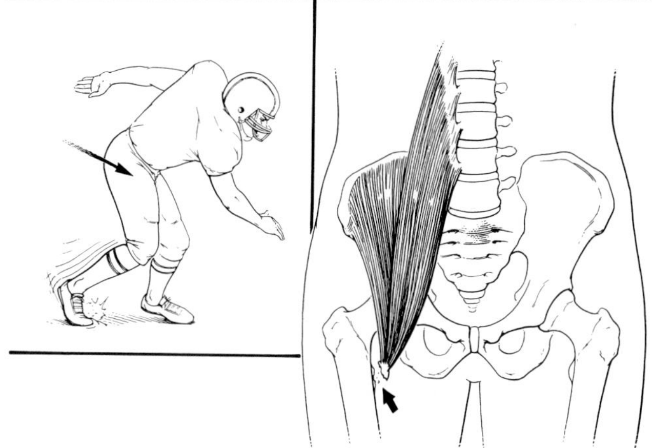

Fig. 4-31 Illustration of the mechanism of lesser trochanteric avulsion.

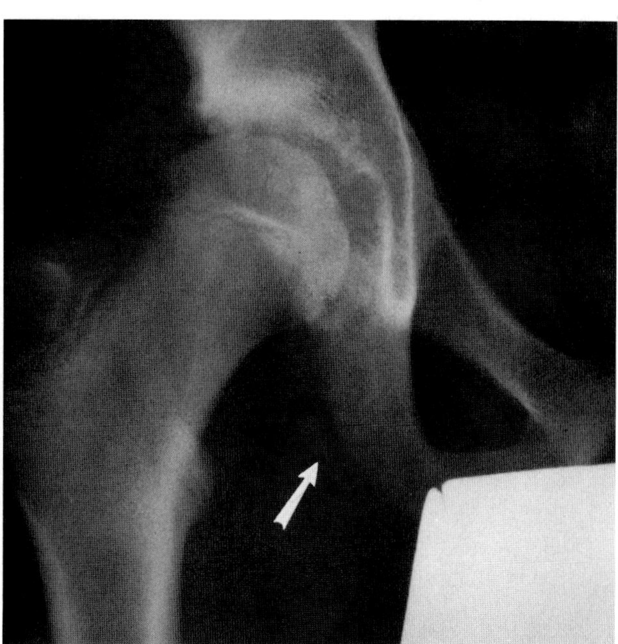

Fig. 4-32 AP view of the pelvis in a football player with chronic hamstring origin pain. Note the fragmentation of the ischium on the right (arrow).

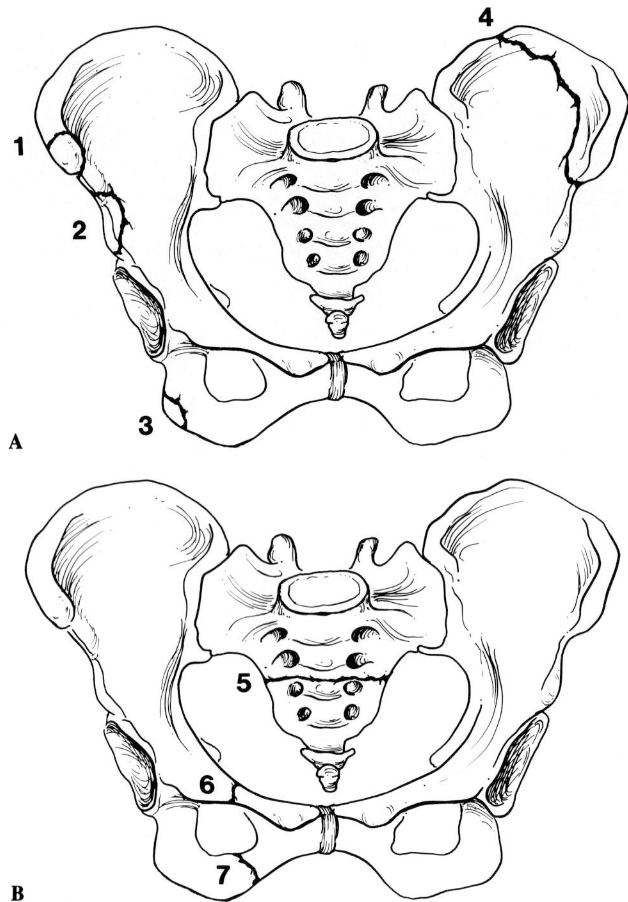

Fig. 4-33 Illustration of class I pelvic fractures.
(A) 1: anterosuperior iliac spine avulsion fracture
2: anteroinferior iliac spine avulsion fracture
3: ischial avulsion fracture
4: DeVerney fracture
(B) 5: transverse sacral fracture
6: superior ramus fracture
7: isolated inferior ramus fracture
There is no disruption of the pelvic ring. *Source:* Reprinted from *Imaging of Orthopedic Trauma* ed 2 by TH Berquist, 1991, Raven Press, © Mayo Foundation.

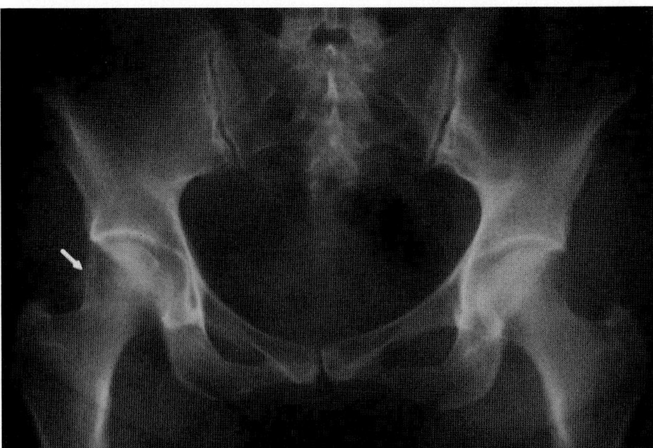

Fig. 4-34 Chronic soft tissue injury of the origin of the rectus femoris with ossification in the proximal tendon (arrow).

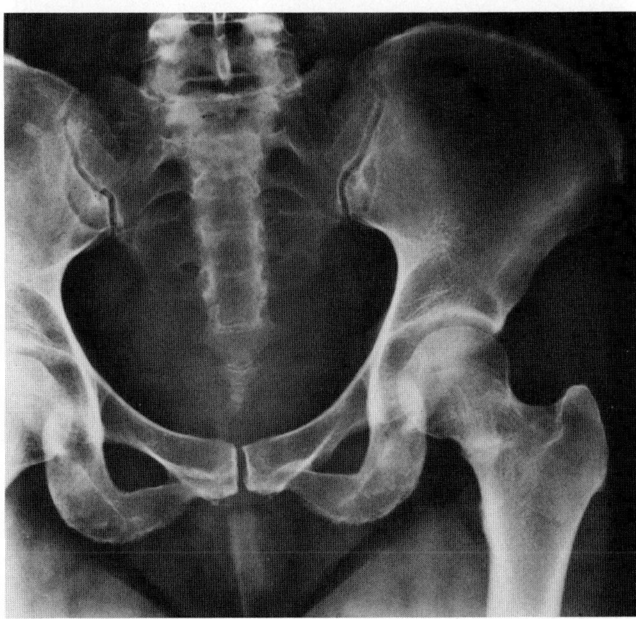

Fig. 4-35 AP view of the pelvis in a long distance runner with a stress fracture in the left femoral neck.

and are included in the category of class I injuries. Other class I fractures occur less frequently. These fractures include isolated acute ischial and pubic rami fractures, fractures of the ilium (DeVerney fracture, Fig. 4-9), and transverse sacral and coccygeal fractures (Fig. 4-33). These injuries are usually the result of direct trauma or falls. Treatment is conservative and complications are minimal compared to more severe pelvic fractures.[31]

Imaging of Minor Fractures

Imaging of minor fractures and osseous overuse syndromes of the pelvis and hips can be accomplished with routine radiographs in most patients if there is good clinical information regarding the symptoms and anatomic location of pain. Routine views including inlet, outlet, and Judet and fluoroscopically positioned spot films are generally sufficient for detection of osseous injury (Figs. 4-29 through 4-35).[31]

Radionuclide scans (Fig. 4-36) are useful for detection of subtle osseous injuries. Stress fractures and injury at muscle, tendon, or ligament origins and insertions can be identified by focal areas of increased tracer uptake at the site of injury. A negative bone scan 72 hours after injury essentially excludes osseous involvement. In this setting, or when more specific information is required, MRI is preferred. This technique (Fig. 4-37) allows one to identify both bone and soft tissue injury. Images should be obtained in two different planes (Fig. 4-37), and T2-weighted sequences should be used. T1-

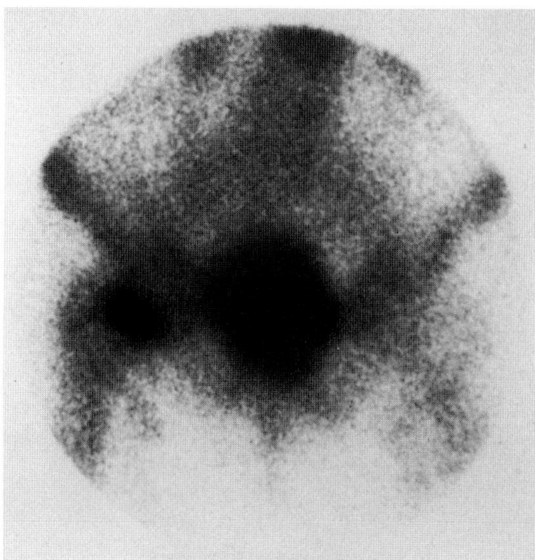

Fig. 4-36 Bone scan in a jogger with hip pain and normal radiographs. There is a linear area of increased tracer uptake in the right femoral neck due to a stress fracture.

weighted sequences are excellent for evaluation of anatomy but not as effective for identification of pathology.[31]

Major Fractures

Major fractures and dislocations of the pelvis and hips are unusual except in sports associated with high velocities or significant falls. These activities would include auto racing, motorcycle racing, horse racing, downhill skiing, snowmobiling, mountain climbing, and the like.[31,47,58]

Pelvic Fractures

There are numerous reports describing classifications and mechanisms of injury for pelvic fractures.[31,35,37,45,52,63,64] Single breaks of a pelvic bone can occur and generally constitute major injuries, as noted above.[31] Radiographic patterns are useful, however, in defining the mechanism of injury of more complex pelvic fractures (class III, double break in the pelvic ring, and class IV, acetabular fractures).[31,35,46,48,63,64]

There are four common patterns noted with pelvic fractures.[35,63,64] Lateral compression injuries represent nearly half of major pelvic fractures.[63,64] Young and Resnick[64] described three patterns of injury due to a lateral blow to the pelvis. Type I injuries are due to forces directed to the posterior pelvis. Minimal distortion of the pelvic ring is noted (Fig. 4-38A). Unilateral or bilateral pubic rami fractures are always present. These fractures are typically oblique or horizontally oriented. There is an associated crush injury of the sacrum or sacroiliac joint. Because the ligaments are intact, the injury is stable.[31,35,64] Central acetabular fractures occur in 19% of cases. Type II injuries occur when the lateral force

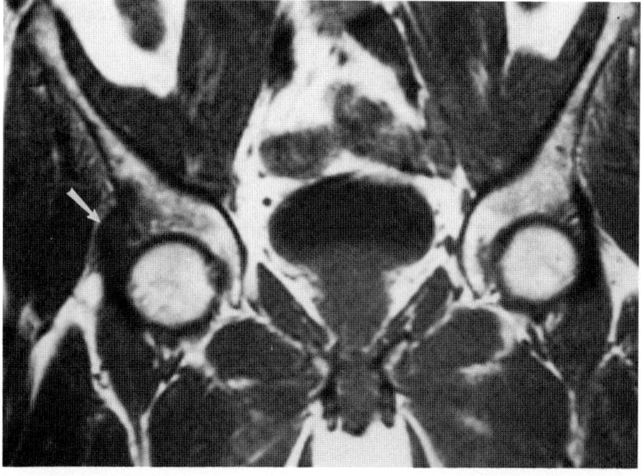

A

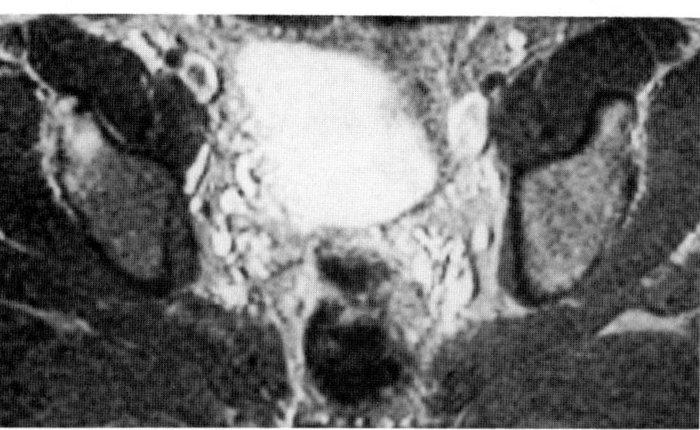

B

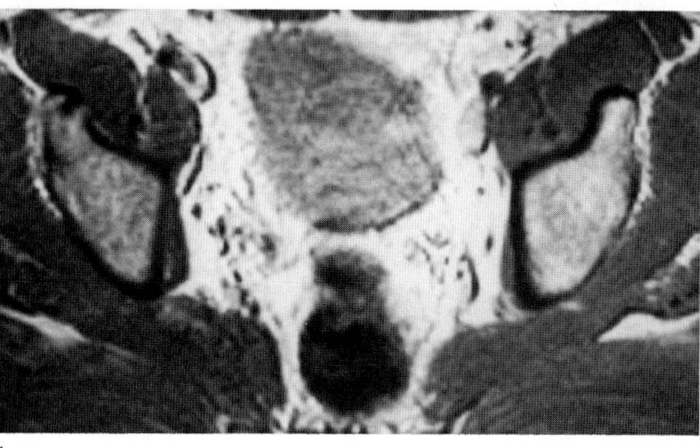

C

Fig. 4-37 Stress fracture of the anteroinferior iliac spine in a runner. Routine films were normal. (**A**) Coronal (SE 500/20) MR image of the pelvis shows low signal intensity near the right acetabular margin (arrow). (**B** and **C**) Axial images (**B**, SE 500/20; **C**, SE 2000/60) demonstrate the anteroinferior iliac spine. The SE 2000/60 image (**C**) allows the injury to be easily identified.

is applied to the anterior pelvis, resulting in medial displacement of the innominate bone on the side of the injury. Rotation of the anterior innominate bone leads to either rupture of the ipsilateral sacroiliac joint (type IIA) or fracture of the iliac wing (type IIB; Fig. 4-38, B and C).[64] Both configurations

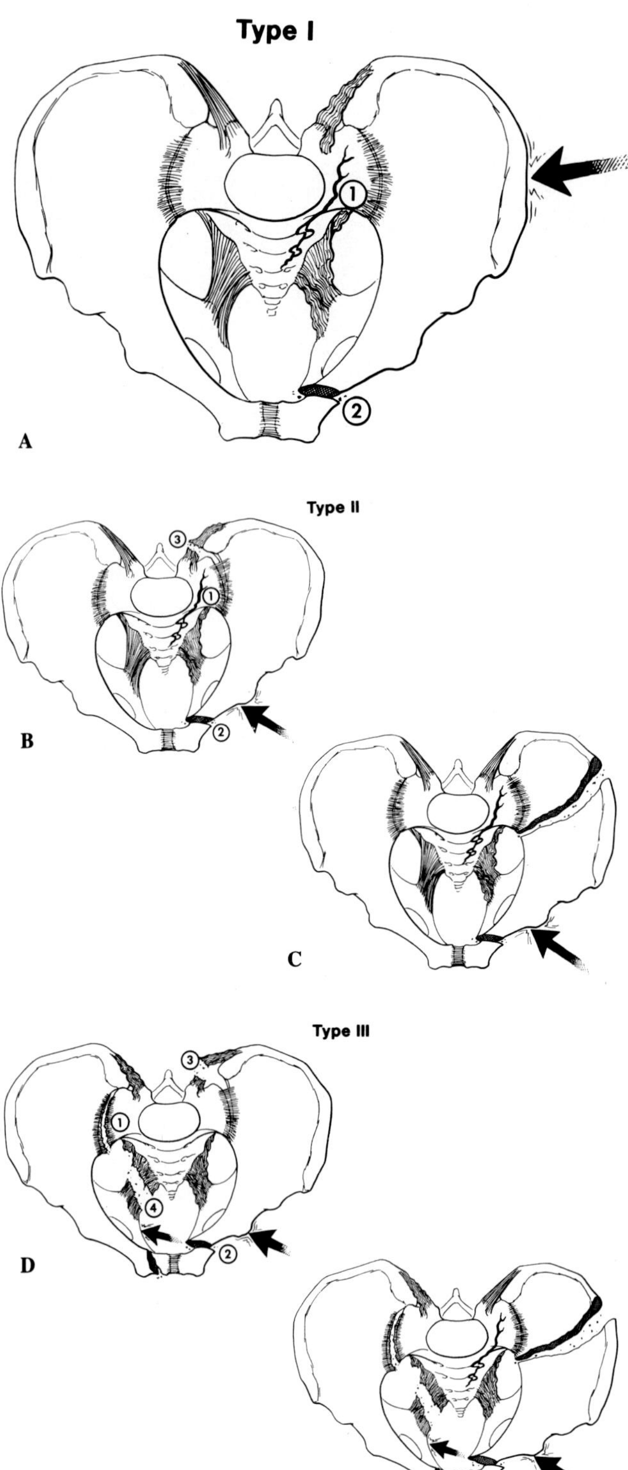

Fig. 4-38 Lateral compression injuries. Arrows indicate direction of force application. (**A**) Type I: pubic rami fractures (2) with crush injury to the sacrum (1), ilium, or sacroiliac joint. (**B**) Type IIA: pubic rami fractures (2) with rupture of the sacroiliac ligaments (1, 3). (**C**) Type IIB: pubic rami fractures with ipsilateral iliac wing fracture. (**D**) Type IIIA: pubic rami fractures (2) with bilateral posterior ligament and sacroiliac joint diastasis (1, 3, 4). (**E**) Type IIIB: pubic rami fractures with contralateral sacroiliac joint and ipsilateral iliac wing injuries. *Source:* Reprinted from *Imaging of Orthopedic Trauma* ed 2 by TH Berquist, 1991, Raven Press, © Mayo Foundation.

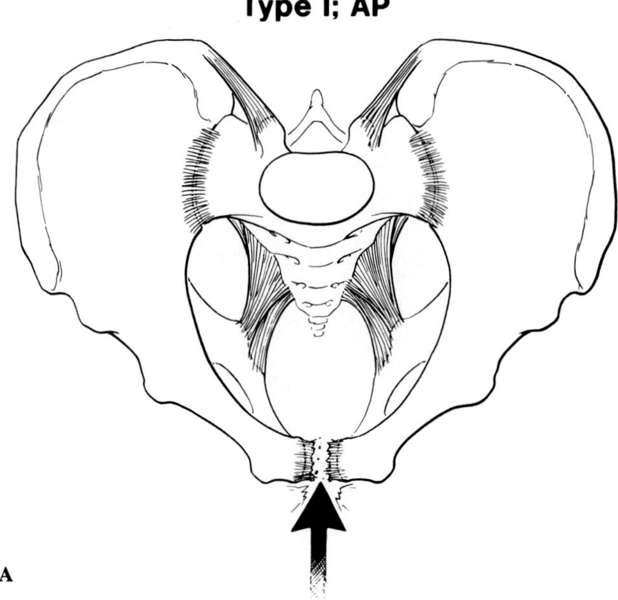

Fig. 4-39 Anterior compression injuries. Arrows indicate direction of force application. (**A**) Type I: pubic rami fractures or mild diastasis of the symphysis.

are unstable. Type III injuries are the most severe and result in bilateral posterior instability. The force is directed more anteriorly, resulting in internal rotation of the innominate bone on the injured side and lateral displacement on the contralateral side. Type IIIA injuries involve the sacroiliac joints and posterior ligament complex (type IIIA) or the ipsilateral iliac wing (type IIIB; Fig. 4-38, D and E).[35,64] Pubic rami fractures associated with lateral compression injuries differ from anterior compression injuries. Fractures are typically oblique, horizontal, or buckling in appearance.[35,63]

Daffner[35] described six radiographic and CT features of lateral compression injuries. These include horizontal obturator ring fractures, vertical sacral buckle fractures (best seen on CT), horizontal iliac fractures, bilateral sacroiliac diastasis, central acetabular fractures, and evidence of rotation on CT images.

Anterior compression injuries account for 21% of major pelvic fractures.[35,63,64] Pubic rami fractures or diastasis of the symphysis with associated posterior injury to the sacroiliac joints, sacrum, or iliac wings occurs. Pubic rami fractures tend to be vertically oriented with anterior compression injuries. Diastases of the pubic symphysis may reach 2.5 cm without disruption of the sacroiliac ligaments. Three fracture patterns have been described (Fig. 4-39). Type I injuries have vertical pubic rami fractures or mild diastasis of the pubic symphysis. The anterior sacroiliac ligaments may be involved (Fig. 4-39A). Type II injuries result when continued force causes further anterior separation (>2.5 cm; Fig. 4-39B) with disruption of the anterior sacroiliac, sacrospinous, and sacrotuberous ligaments. Further widening of both the symphysis and the sacroiliac joint occurs with type III injuries (Fig. 4-39C) as a result of further ligament injury. Common findings of anterior compression injuries include diastases of

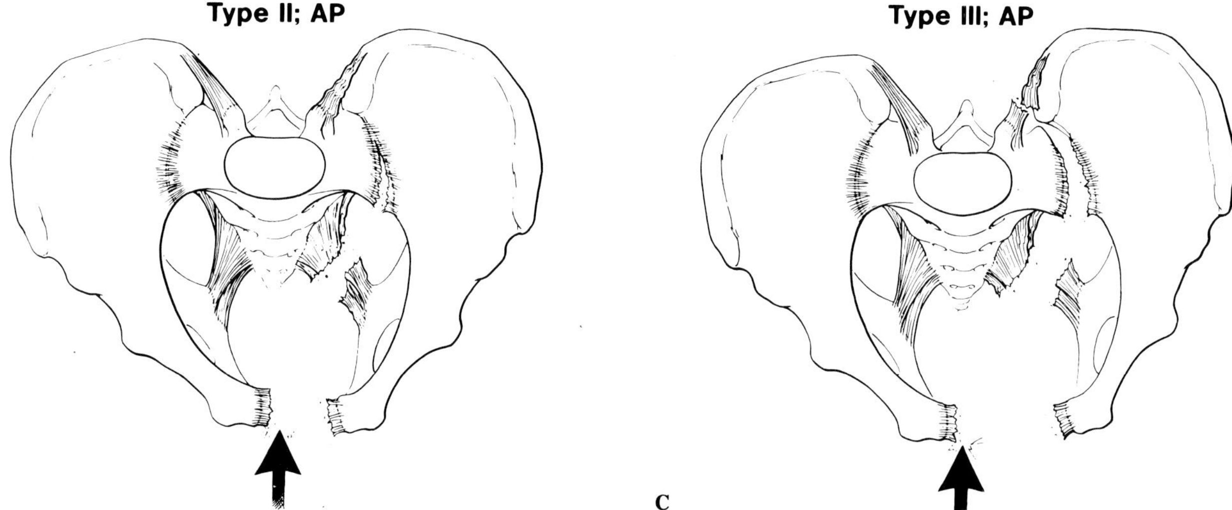

Fig. 4-39 contd (B) Type II: pubic rami fracture or wider diastasis of the symphysis with posterior ligament injuries. **(C)** Type III: wide diastasis of the symphysis with disruption of the anterior and posterior sacroiliac ligaments. *Source:* Reprinted from *Imaging of Orthopedic Trauma* ed 2 by TH Berquist, 1991, Raven Press, © Mayo Foundation.

the symphyses and sacroiliac joints and vertical pubic rami fractures.[35,63]

Vertical shear injuries account for 6% of pelvic fractures.[63,64] These injuries result from vertical forces directed through the femur or lateral to the midline (Fig. 4-40). Disruption of the hemipelvis via the symphysis and sacroiliac joint or iliac and pubic rami fractures result in a definite step-off on AP radiographs.

Complex or combined forces account for 14% of pelvic fractures. Lateral compression with either anterior or shearing forces are most common.[31,35,63,64]

These fracture patterns are useful in determining the mechanism of injury and, therefore, the method of reduction.

Acetabular Fractures

Acetabular fractures deserve more specific mention here because of their increasing frequency in recent years.[31,49,62] In our experience at the Mayo Clinic, acetabular fractures make up 24% of all pelvic fractures. Key and Conwell[48] divide these fractures into undisplaced and displaced, but a more complex and accurate approach is required for the proper evaluation and management of acetabular fractures. We prefer the method of Judet when discussing acetabular fractures.[31,45]

Elementary acetabular fractures. Posterior acetabular fractures may involve a single fragment or multiple fragments and on occasion may result in impaction of the acetabular articular surface.[31,45] The fracture usually results from lower extremity trauma (usually at the knee) with the hip flexed approximately 90° (Figs. 4-41 and 4-42). The size of the fragment is also related to the degree of femoral abduction. The greater the abduction, the larger the fragment.[31]

Fractures of the posterior (ilioischial) column usually begin above the acetabulum, extend through the posterior aspect of the acetabulum, and include the ischial ramus (Fig. 4-43B). The iliopubic line and radiographic U remain intact on the AP radiograph, allowing one to attribute the fracture to the posterior column. The dome of the acetabulum remains intact. This fracture results from a blow to the knee with the hip flexed 90° and abducted about 20°. Posterior dislocation or subluxation of the hip is frequently associated with this fracture, and sciatic nerve injury may result.[31,45,49]

Transverse fractures involve both the anterior and posterior column and frequently the ischial spine (Fig. 4-43A). The mechanism of injury is a blow to the lateral aspect of the greater trochanter or to the posterior aspect of the pelvis with

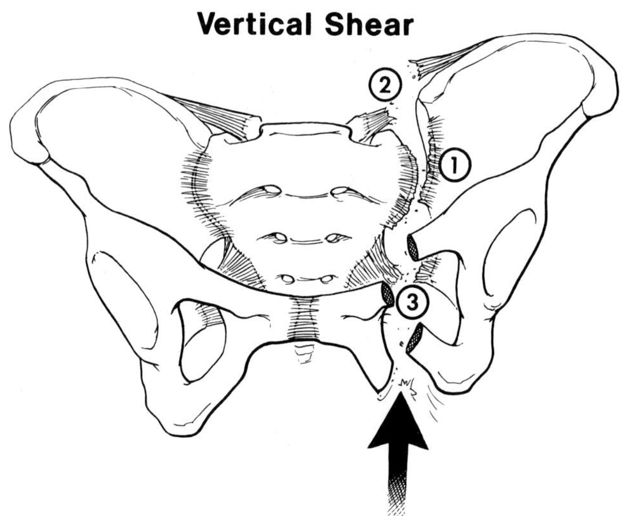

Fig. 4-40 Vertical shearing injury with disruption of the anterior (3) and posterior (1, 2) ring. Arrow indicates direction of force application. *Source:* Reprinted from *Imaging of Orthopedic Trauma* ed 2 by TH Berquist, 1991, Raven Press, © Mayo Foundation.

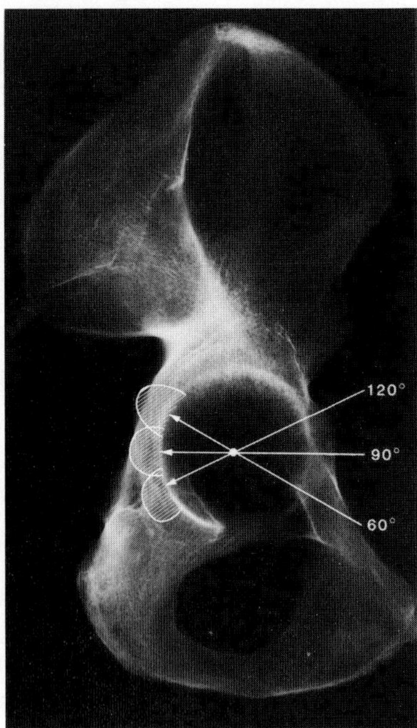

Fig. 4-41 Illustration of how the position of the femur affects the site of posterior acetabular fracture. *Source:* Reprinted from *Imaging of Orthopedic Trauma* ed 2 by TH Berquist, 1991, Raven Press, © Mayo Foundation.

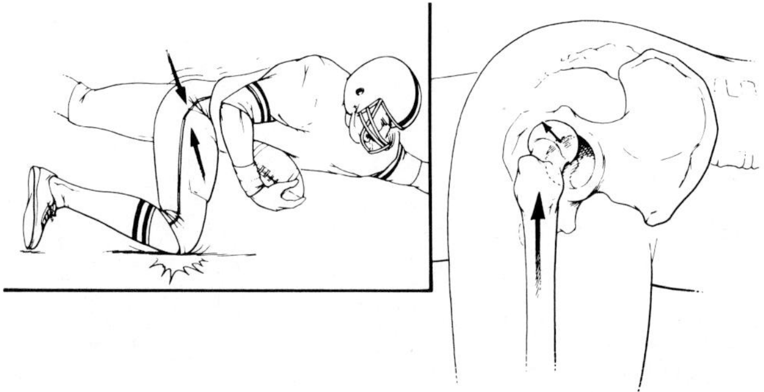

Fig. 4-42 Illustration of mechanism of injury for posterior dislocation or acetabular fracture.

the hip flexed and abducted.[31,37,45] Radiographically these fractures are easily missed on the AP view, especially when no displacement is present (Fig. 4-44).

Fractures of the anterior column (iliopubic column) are less common than posterior column fractures.[31,45] The prognosis with these injuries is reportedly better compared to the prognosis with posterior column fractures. These fractures usually begin just above the anteroinferior iliac spine and extend inferiorly to involve the inferior pubic ramus near the junction with the ischium (Fig. 4-43C). The iliopubic line is disrupted on the AP radiograph, and once again the oblique views will clearly demonstrate the disruption of the anterior column and the intact posterior column. The injury is thought to be the result of a blow to the greater trochanter with the hip externally rotated, an uncommon situation indeed.[31,45,58]

Complex acetabular fractures. Complex acetabular fractures result in multiple fracture lines and increased morbidity. Fractures with significant central displacement of the femoral head and acetabular fragments lead to complications similar to those of other complex pelvic fractures (hemorrhage and instability; Fig. 4-45).[31]

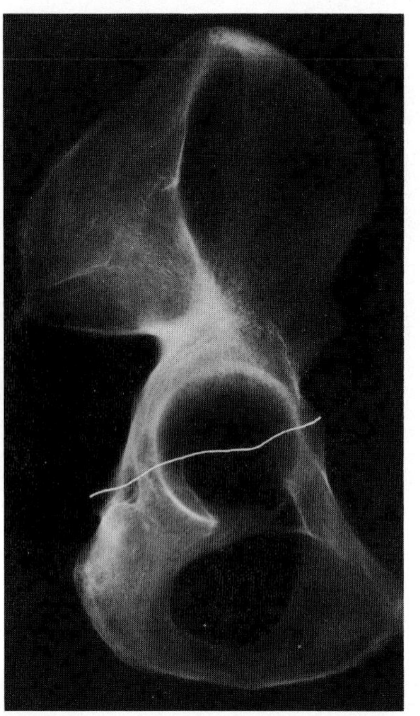

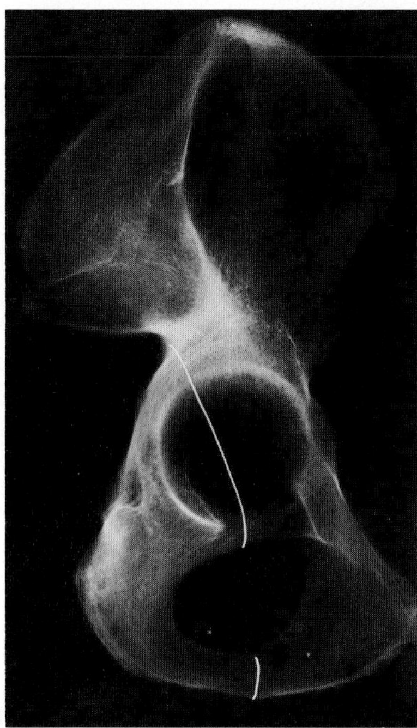

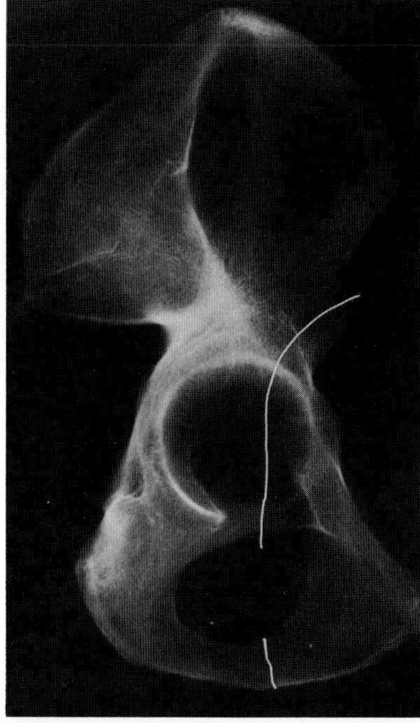

Fig. 4-43 Skeletal specimen demonstrating the planes of transverse (**A**), posterior column (**B**), and anterior column (**C**) acetabular fractures.

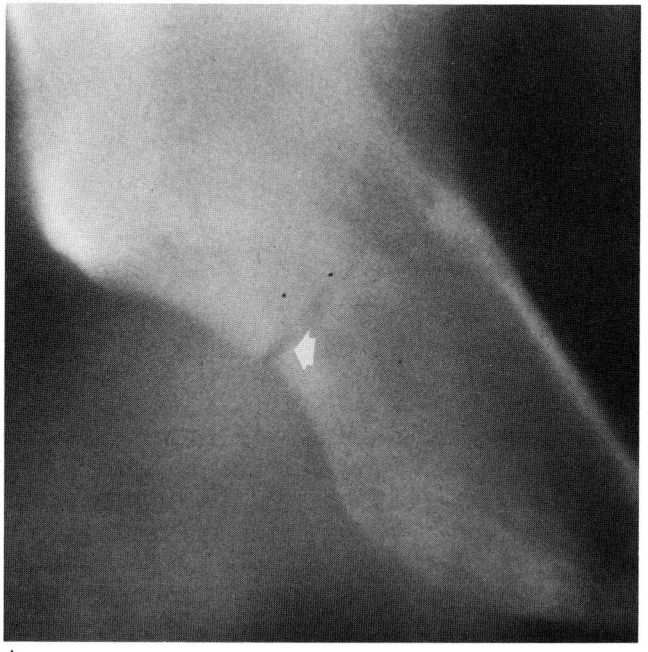

A

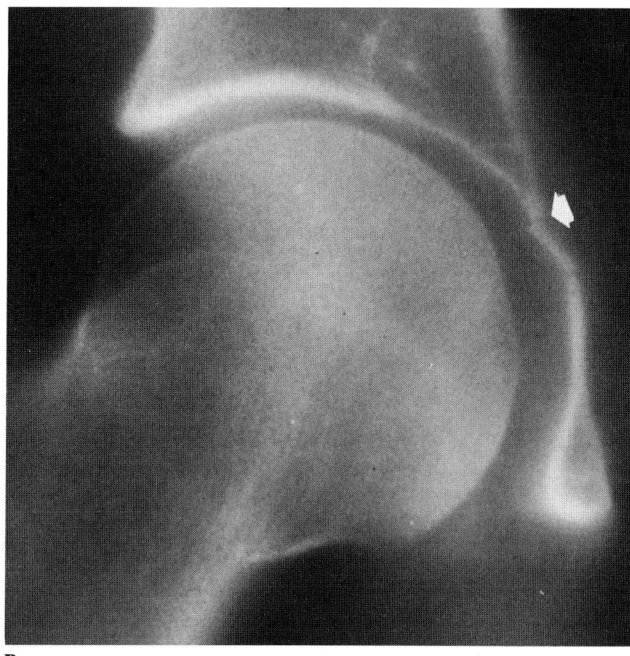

B

Fig. 4-44 AP tomograms demonstrating a subtle transverse acetabular fracture (arrows).

Fragmentation or displacement of the weight-bearing surface of the acetabulum is of particular importance. Any malrotation or comminution of the dome of the acetabulum must be corrected. This may be the most important indication for surgical intervention. Complex fractures with involvement of the iliac wing or adjacent sacroiliac joint also result in a poor prognosis. The sacroiliac joint involvement may be subtle and difficult to detect even with comparison of the joints.[43]

Complications

Complications of major pelvic and acetabular fractures may be significant and affect imaging evaluation in the acute setting. A complete description of these complications is beyond the scope of this text, but certain complications deserve mention.

Pelvic hemorrhage is the most significant local complication. This may require transfusion in up to 71% of cases. In the past, before compression garments were available, mortality from hemorrhage approached 22%.[31] Genitourinary complications (specifically urethral and bladder rupture) may be present in up to 20% of anterior pelvic fractures. Neurologic complications occur in 21% of complex pelvic fractures, usually with posterior involvement.[31,40] Distant fractures and visceral, chest, and head injuries are also frequently associated with complex pelvic fractures.[31]

Dislocations and Fracture-Dislocations of the Hip

Posterior dislocations. Posterior dislocations occur 7 to 10 times more frequently than anterior dislocations.[31,39,60,61] This injury results when a compressive force is applied to the knee or foot with the hip in the flexed position (Fig. 4-42).[31,58] Fractures of the posterior acetabulum are frequently associated with posterior dislocations of the hip. The size of the fragment is dependent upon the position of the femur at the time of injury (Fig. 4-46). If the hip is flexed in a neutral position, a posterior rim fracture may result. With the hip abducted, a larger posterior fragment or comminution is

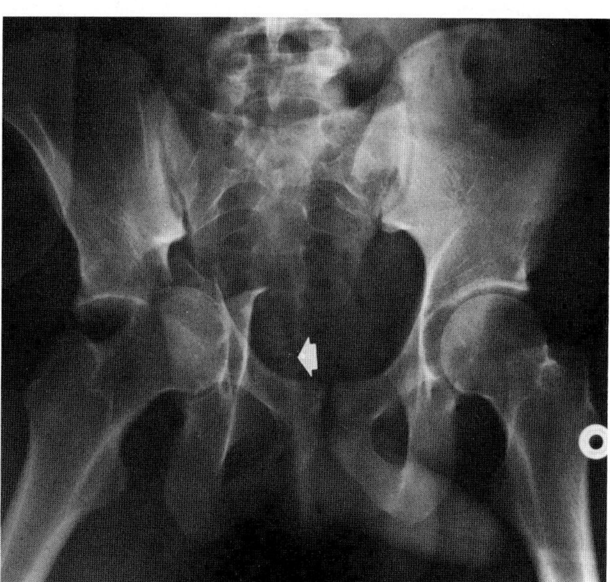

Fig. 4-45 AP view of the pelvis demonstrating a complex pelvic fracture involving both anterior and posterior columns. There is an associated coccygeal dislocation (arrow).

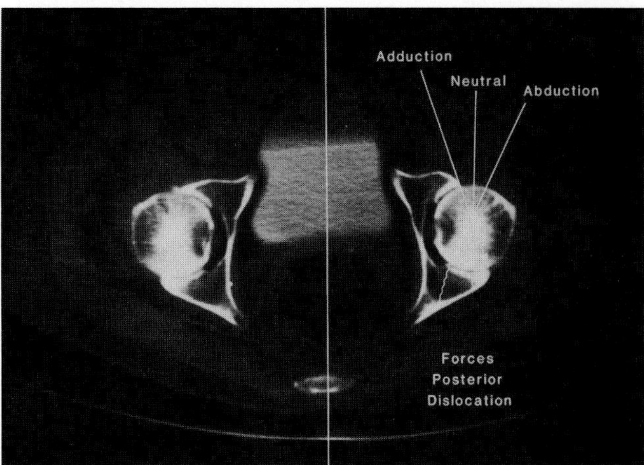

Fig. 4-46 CT scan demonstrating how the position of the femur in posterior dislocations affects the size or likelihood of a posterior acetabular fracture. *Source:* Reprinted from *Imaging of Orthopedic Trauma* ed 2 by TH Berquist, 1991, Raven Press, © Mayo Foundation.

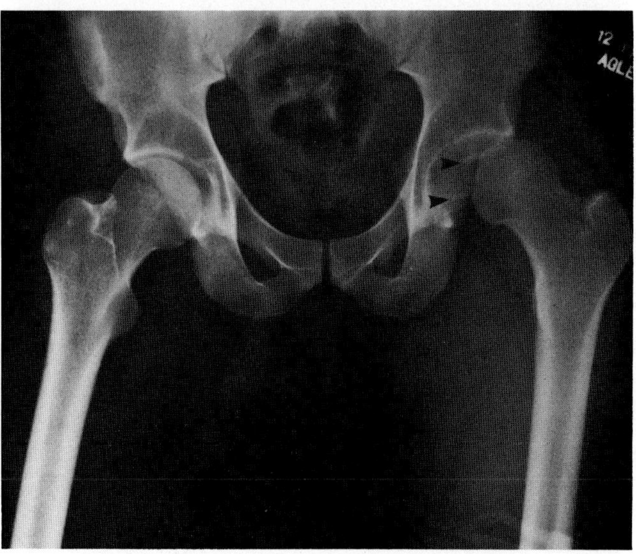

Fig. 4-47 Posterior dislocation of the left femoral head with an associated fracture of the head medially. Note the fragments in the joint space (arrowheads).

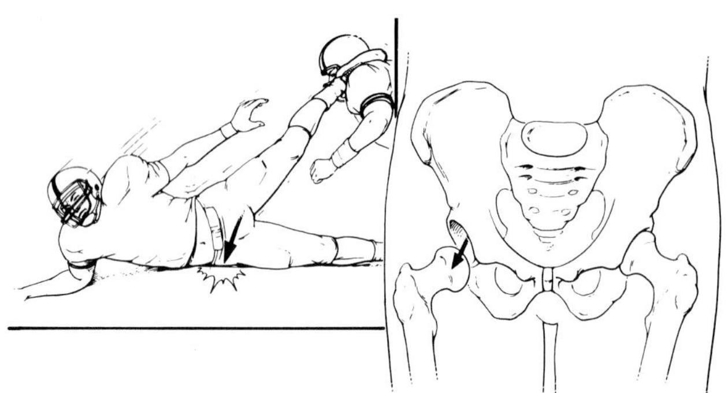

Fig. 4-48 Illustration of mechanism of injury for anterior dislocation of the hip.

more likely to occur. Adduction may result in a tiny chip fracture or pure dislocation of the hip.

Clinically, patients with posterior dislocations usually present with four findings: the hip flexed and externally rotated, elevation of the trochanter, a palpable prominence in the gluteal region, and bruising of the buttock.[31,58]

Femoral head fractures with posterior dislocations of the hip were once considered rare. Recent advances in imaging techniques and increased awareness of this association, however, have resulted in improved detection of femoral head injuries. The incidence of femoral head fractures with posterior dislocations is reported to be up to 63% (Fig. 4-47). Fracture of the femoral head occurs more frequently if the hip is flexed less than 90° (especially at about 60°). This forces the femoral head against the stronger posterosuperior margin of the acetabulum and may result in an osteochondral shearing or impacted fracture.[31,53,54,61]

Anterior dislocations. Anterior dislocations (Fig. 4-48) account for 13% to 18% of hip dislocations.[31,58,60] This injury results from forced abduction and external rotation of the hip. The neck or greater trochanter impinges on the acetabulum and forces the femoral head to dislocate in an anteroinferior direction.[53,54] The type of dislocation is often described by the position of the femoral head on the AP radiograph of the pelvis and hips. With the hip in extension, the head may overlie the pubis or ilium. In flexion the head is seen over the obturator foramen. This is the most common presentation.[31]

Fractures of the femoral head occur frequently with anterior dislocations of the hip (Fig. 4-49). Shearing fractures of the femoral head may result as the femoral head passes the inferior acetabulum. Impaction fractures of the posterosuperior and lateral aspect of the head have an appearance similar to that of a Hill-Sachs defect. This defect may be seen on the AP view if the hip is properly positioned (15° of internal rotation.)[31]

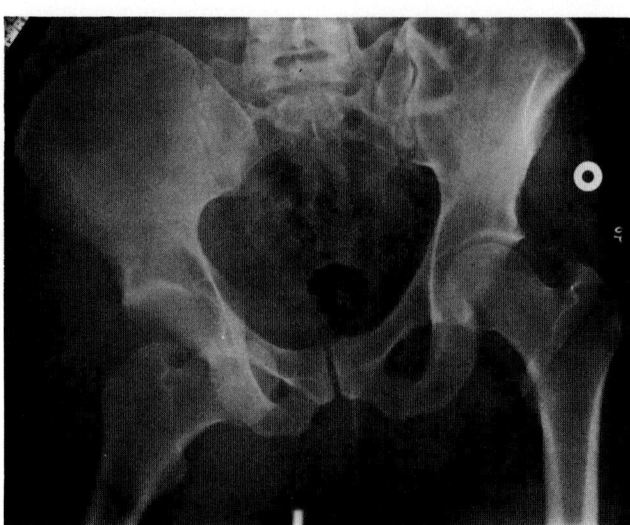

Fig. 4-49 Anterior dislocation of the right hip seen on the AP view.

Femoral Neck Fractures

Femoral neck fractures occur predominantly in the elderly and are more common in women than in men. The femoral neck is frequently demineralized in this patient population. Thus neck fractures have been considered pathologic.[31] Femoral neck fractures in athletes are rare and usually result from high-velocity injuries.

Trochanteric Fractures

Trochanteric fractures generally follow the trochanteric line. These fractures may extend into the subtrochanteric region. Avulsion fractures of the greater and lesser trochanter may occur separately or in association with intertrochanteric and subtrochanteric fractures.[36] Three categories of fractures can be distinguished: intertrochanteric fractures, subtrochanteric fractures, and avulsion fractures. The first group is uncommon in athletes.[31,41,44,50,57] Avulsion fractures are discussed earlier in this chapter. Subtrochanteric fractures involve the cortical bone below the lesser trochanter. Associated involvement of the shaft and intertrochanteric region is common. Fractures tend to occur in young patients after significant trauma (Fig. 4-50).[56]

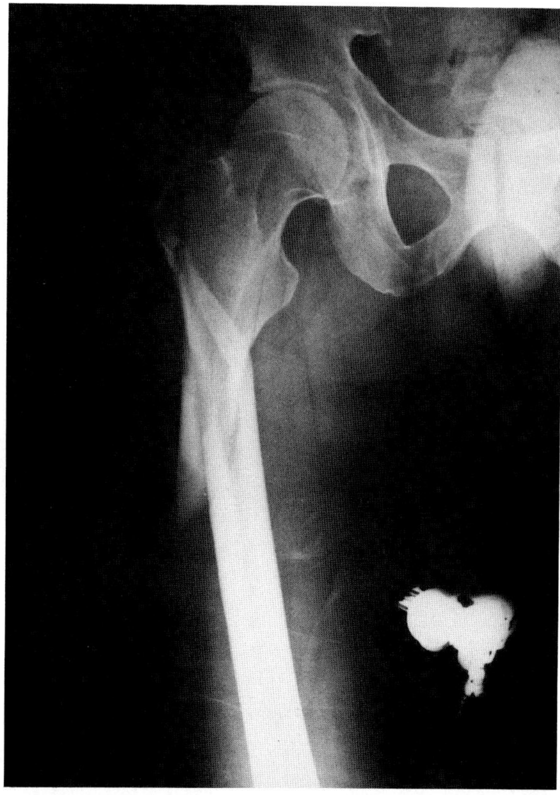

Fig. 4-50 AP view of the right upper femur demonstrating a spiral subtrochanteric fracture.

Imaging of Major Fractures

Complex pelvic fractures can usually be identified and classified on AP, inlet, and outlet views of the pelvis.[31] Subtle posterior fractures, however, especially sacral injuries, may be missed in up to 50% of patients (Fig. 4-12). Therefore, CT is usually performed after conventional radiographs to assess fully the extent of bone and soft tissue injury in patients with pelvic and acetabular fractures.[31,42,43,55]

Fractures and dislocations of the hip can often be detected on routine AP, lateral, or oblique views. Judet views are essential in patients with dislocations or acetabular injuries to determine which portions of the acetabulum are involved and to define clearly the position of the femoral head. Complete assessment of fracture-dislocations of the hip usually requires CT (Fig. 4-51). Other imaging techniques are rarely required for detection of major fractures and fracture-dislocations of the pelvis and hips.

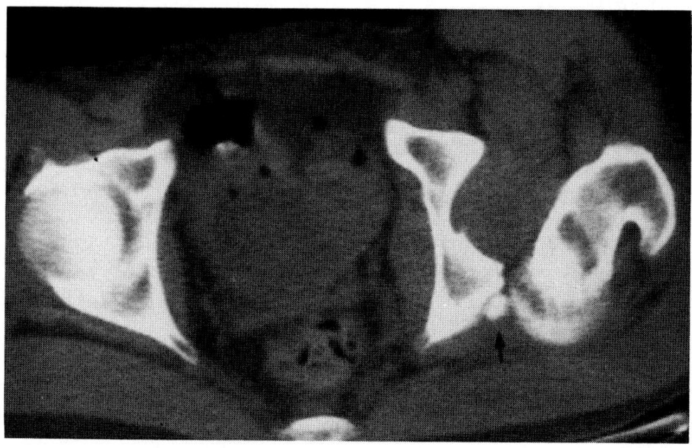

A

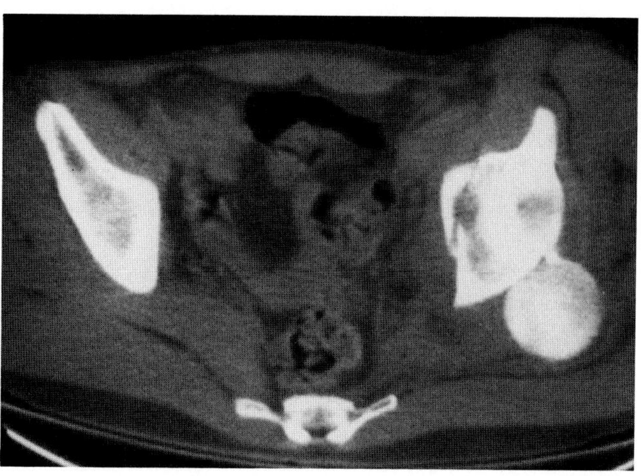

B

Fig. 4-51 Axial CT images after a posterior dislocation of the left femoral head. The femoral head is still dislocated with several small posterior acetabular fragments (arrow).

SOFT TISSUE AND MISCELLANEOUS INJURIES

Soft tissue injuries in the region of the pelvis and hips are usually related to minor sprains and strains. A brief review of the muscles and their functions is important for an understanding of these injuries and which muscle units may be involved with a given symptom complex.

The chief extensors of the hip include the gluteus maximus and the ischial portion of the adductor magnus. Weak extensors include the hamstring, piriformis, and gluteus medius. The gluteus maximus originates from the posterior ilium, dorsolateral sacrum, and coccyx and inserts on the gluteal tuberosity of the femur and iliotibial tract. The other major extensor, the ischial portion of the adductor magnus, arises from the inferior pubic ramus and ischium and inserts on the linea aspera.[72,77] Primary flexors of the hip are the iliopsoas and rectus femoris, with some assistance in flexion being provided by the adductors and tensor fasciae latae. The iliopsoas takes its origin along the lateral margins of T-12 through L-5 and inserts on the lesser trochanter. As discussed previously, the rectus femoris takes its origin in the anteroinferior iliac spine and inserts on the upper patella.[72] The main adductors of the hip include the pectineus, adductor longus, adductor brevis, adductor magnus, and gracilis. The adductor longus takes its origin along the anterior pubic bone and inserts on the medial linea aspera. The adductor brevis originates from the pubic bone and inferior ramus and inserts along the upper linea aspera. The adductor magnus is discussed above. The gracilis originates from the inferior pubic ramus near the symphysis and inserts on the upper anterior tibia medially.

The abductors of the hip include the gluteus medius and minimus, with some weak assistance being provided by the tensor fasciae latae. Both these gluteal muscles take their origin from the posterior ilium below the iliac crest and insert on the greater trochanter.[72,78]

The external rotators of the hip include the piriformis, obturator internus, superior and inferior gemelli, obturator externus, quadriceps femoris, gluteus maximus, and iliopsoas. The internal rotators include the tensor fasciae latae, gluteus medius, and gluteus minimus.[72]

Injuries to these muscle groups result in pain and weakness related to the function of the muscle groups. It is not unusual for adolescents and growing children to have an imbalance, especially between the quadriceps and hamstrings, resulting in increased susceptibility to injury.[67]

Imaging of muscle injury is often not necessary because clinical symptoms and history will confirm the diagnosis. When classification of the extent of injury is important, however, or when treatment does not result in symptomatic improvement, imaging may be necessary. MRI offers the most optimal screening technique for evaluation of soft tissue injury. Images should be obtained in at least two planes. The image planes are selected on the basis of the region of anatomy to be studied. Typically, either axial and sagittal or coronal planes are chosen. T2-Weighted sequences are most useful because the contrast provided by hemorrhage and/or edema is more easily appreciated against the low signal intensity of ligaments and tendons and the intermediate signal intensity of muscle (Fig. 4-52).[66]

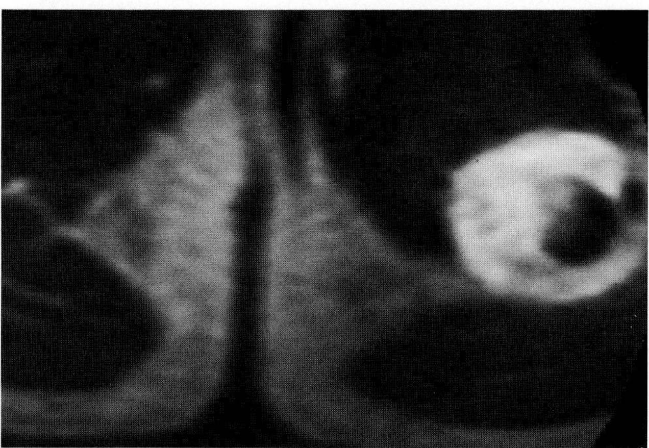

Fig. 4-52 Axial T2-weighted (SE 2000/60) MR image of the ischial regions demonstrating a hamstring tear and hematoma on the left.

A specific soft tissue injury called a hip pointer is common in football (Fig. 4-53). This injury is generally created by a direct blow to the iliac crest, resulting in contusion or hematoma in this region. The patient presents with local pain and difficulty in walking and standing upright due to the spasm in the area. There is frequently local tenderness and ecchymosis. Imaging of this injury is usually not indicated except to exclude a fracture, in which case routine radiography is adequate. When response to therapy is not as expected, MRI may be useful to exclude a tear or other pathology in this region.

Myositis ossificans may be a complication of hip and thigh contusions. This condition may be diagnosed on routine radiography, but CT has the most distinctive features and allows the diagnosis to be made clearly.[69]

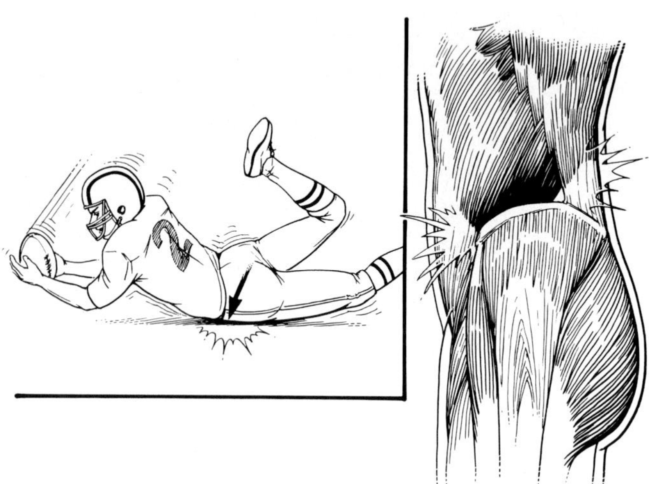

Fig. 4-53 Illustration of mechanism of injury for hip pointer.

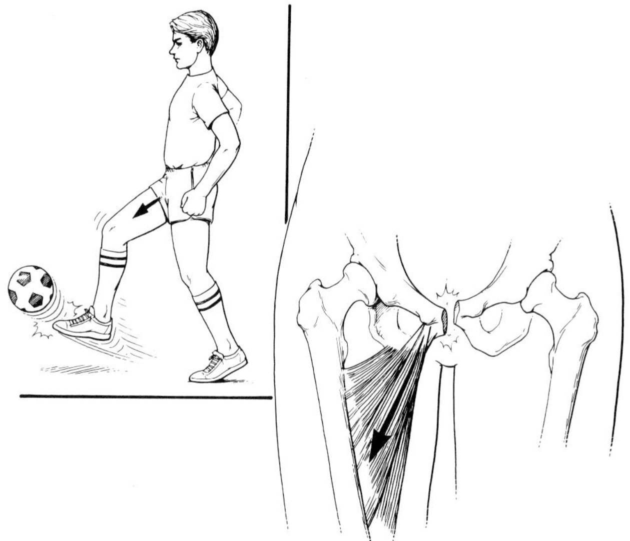

Fig. 4-54 Illustration of a mechanism of symphysis injury or overuse syndrome.

Lesions of the Pubic Symphysis

Sports commonly involved with sprains about the pubic symphysis include football and running.[71] The patients generally present with pain and discomfort about the pubic symphysis. Pain may radiate into both groins or the adductor region of the thigh. Symptoms are brought on by physical exertion and relieved by rest. The pain may also extend into the superpubic region and lower abdomen. Pain tends to be exacerbated by pivoting on the one leg, such as when kicking the ball, sprinting, jumping, climbing, or making sudden changes in direction (Fig. 4-54). History of local injury is usually not obtained.

Radiographic evaluation of this injury may be possible with routine radiographic studies. Irregularity and sclerosis may be noted at the pubic symphysis. Evidence of an articular step-off may also be present in patients with instability. In the acute setting, MRI may provide an earlier diagnosis and also may assist in differentiating this condition from an adductor tear.[66,71,77]

Bursitis

There are numerous bursae about the pelvis and hips that may have clinical significance. The most common is the iliopsoas or iliopectineal bursa, which communicates with the hip joint in 15% to 20% of cases.[65,66,70,74,78,82] This bursa extends for a variable length in the vertical direction but overlies the anteromedial aspect of the hip joint in the axial plane (Fig. 4-55).

Other bursae include the greater trochanteric bursa (Fig. 4-55), which separates the greater trochanter from the gluteal muscles, and the bursa between the tendon of the gluteus maximus and the vastus lateralis. A smaller, frequently inconsistent bursa is located at the ischial tuberosity near the origin of the hamstrings.[72] Repeated microtrauma and inflammation of these bursae can result in chronic, sometimes disabling discomfort that prevents athletes from participating in their sport.

Imaging of these bursae is not generally necessary, but when indicated MRI is the technique of choice. There are two advantages to MRI. The first is that T2-weighted images clearly identify an inflamed bursa as a well-defined area of high signal intensity adjacent to the normally dark ligaments and tendons and intermediate-signal muscle. The second is that MRI provides the advantage of excluding other soft tissue conditions (Fig. 4-56). More frequently, radiologists are

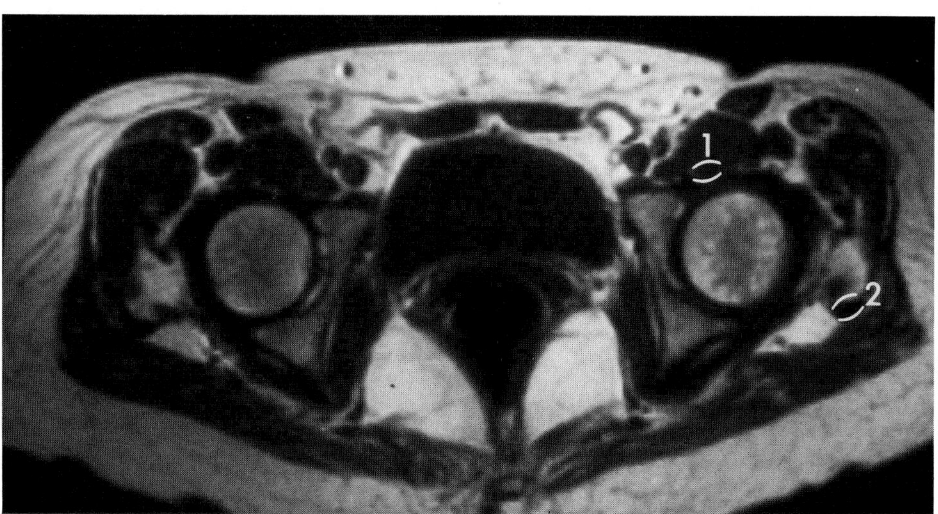

Fig. 4-55 Axial MR image demonstrating the location of the iliopsoas (iliopectineal) bursa (1) and the trochanteric bursa (2).

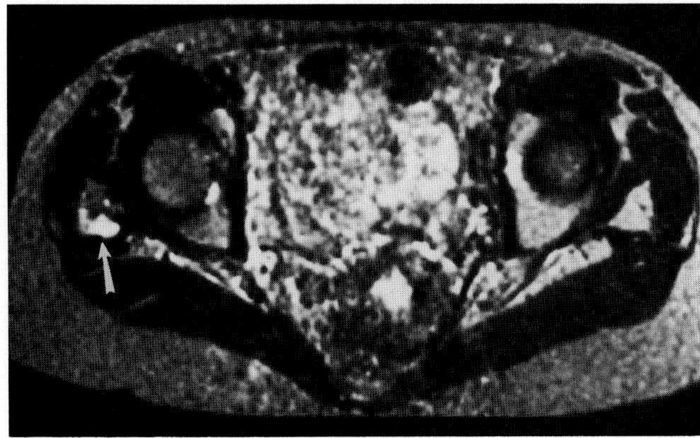

A

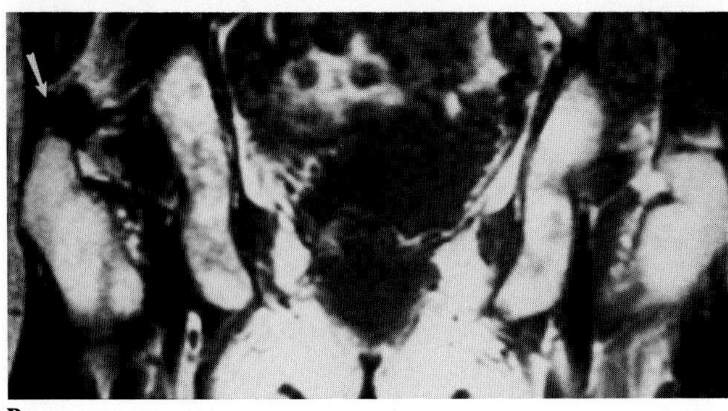

B

Fig. 4-56 (**A**) Axial (SE 2000/60) and (**B**) coronal (SE 500/20) MR images in a patient with greater trochanteric bursitis (arrows).

called upon to localize fluoroscopically and to inject the inflamed bursa. Needle position can be confirmed with a small amount of contrast material or by aspirating a small amount of synovial fluid. Injection of 1 to 2 mL of a 1:1 mixture of bupivacaine and betamethasone can provide significant relief in this setting.

Miscellaneous Conditions

There are numerous other conditions that can result in pain or snapping about the hip. Pain with an audible or palpable click may be caused by extraarticular snapping of the iliotibial band over the greater tuberosity, snapping of the iliopsoas tendon over the iliopectineal eminence or lesser trochanteric ridge (Fig. 4-57), or intraarticular pathology such as tears of the acetabular labrum or loose bodies.[68,73,76,79,80]

Imaging with diagnostic or therapeutic injection is most commonly employed with snapping iliopsoas tendon syndrome. Arthrograms may demonstrate an enlarged iliopsoas bursa (Fig. 4-57, B and C).[75] Changes in the bursa can be observed or videotaped as the patient flexes and extends the hip. There are two problems with using arthrography to make

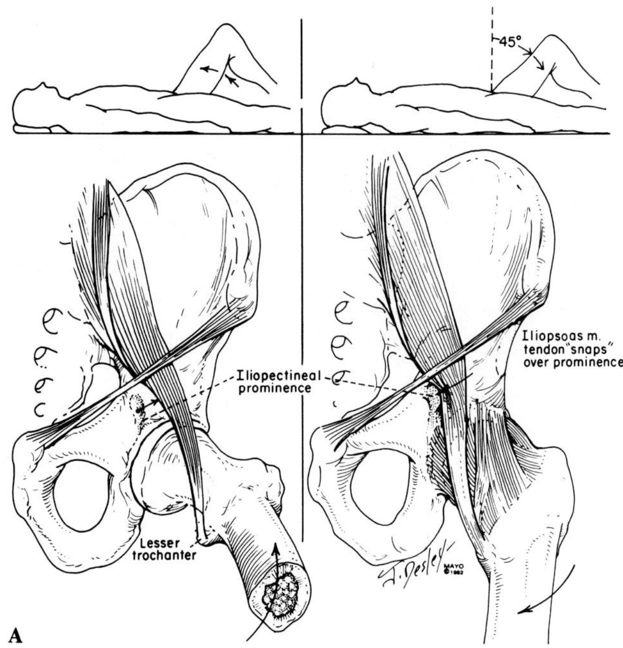

A

Fig. 4-57 Snapping iliopsoas tendon. (**A**) Illustration of maneuver necessary to recreate tendon snapping.

the diagnosis. First, the iliopsoas bursa only communicates with the hip in 15% to 20% of patients. Second, distention of the hip capsule with contrast medium can displace the tendon enough to reduce the snapping. Therefore, direct injection of the tendon sheath is most useful. The tendon passes over the medial aspect of the femoral head (Fig. 4-55) when the hip is in neutral position. The needle can be advanced vertically into the femoral head and contrast material gently injected as the needle is slowly edged back. The contrast material will flow along the tendon or may enter the iliopsoas bursa. At the Mayo Clinic, we typically inject bupivacaine and betamethasone with contrast medium to assist in diagnosis and treatment. A low-osmolality contrast agent is most useful because it is less irritating. The patient is then asked to flex and extend the hip while the tendon movement is documented fluoroscopically or with videotape. The tendon will snap over the iliopectineal eminence or lesser trochanteric ridge when symptoms are related to the iliopsoas tendon. Surgical transfer may be required in patients who do not respond to injection.

Arthrography or MRI may be indicated to evaluate other conditions that may cause snapping in the hip. Arthrography with diagnostic injection is useful in localizing the site of pain and often can define the abnormality. This is especially true in patients with loose bodies (Fig. 4-58), but arthrography is less frequently of value in diagnosis of acetabular labral tears (Fig. 4-59).[66] Although arthrography is still of value for diagnosis of many intraarticular syndromes in the hip, MRI may be most useful as a screening technique for acetabular labral tears and other juxtaarticular capsular pathology (Fig. 4-60).[66]

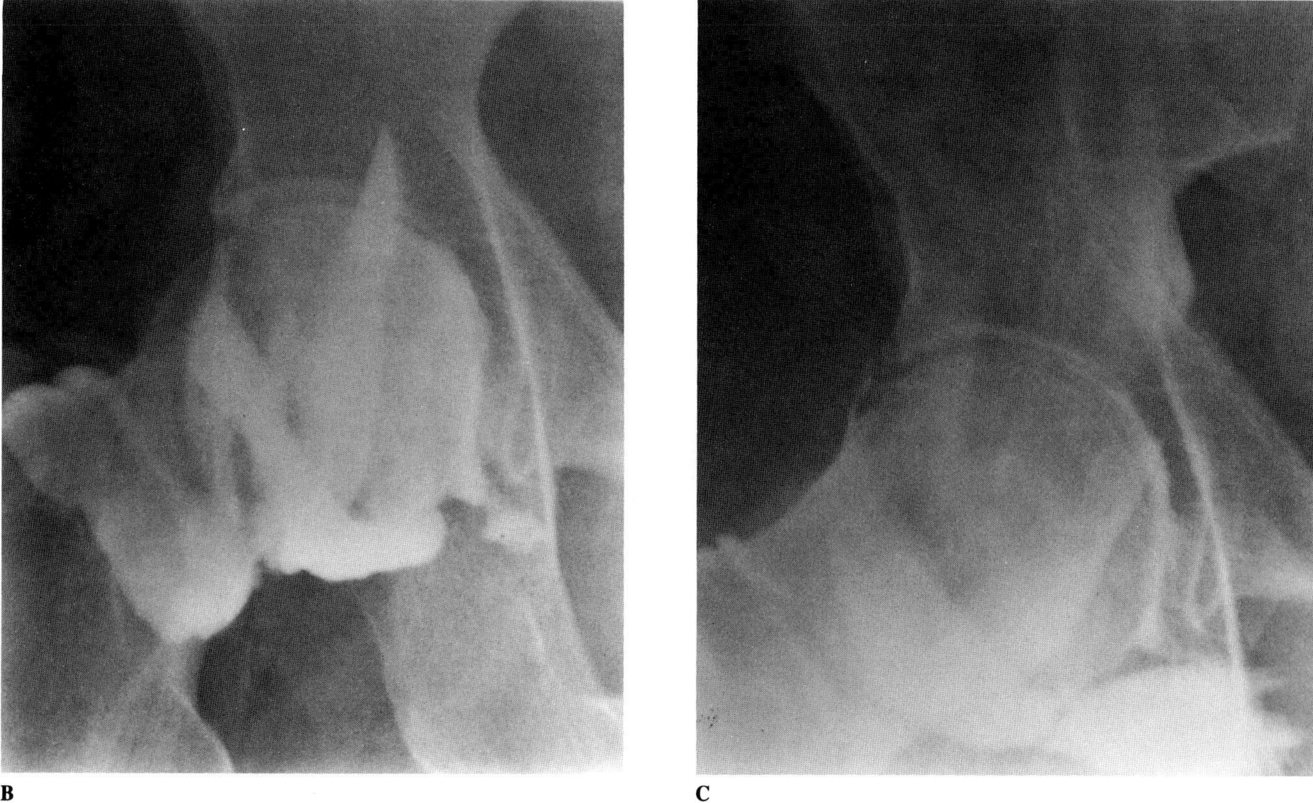

B C

Fig. 4-57 contd (**B** and **C**) The iliopsoas bursa moves with flexion of the hip. This can be recorded on videotape. *Source:* Reprinted with permission from *Mayo Clinic Proceedings* (1984;59:327–329), Copyright © 1984, Mayo Foundation.

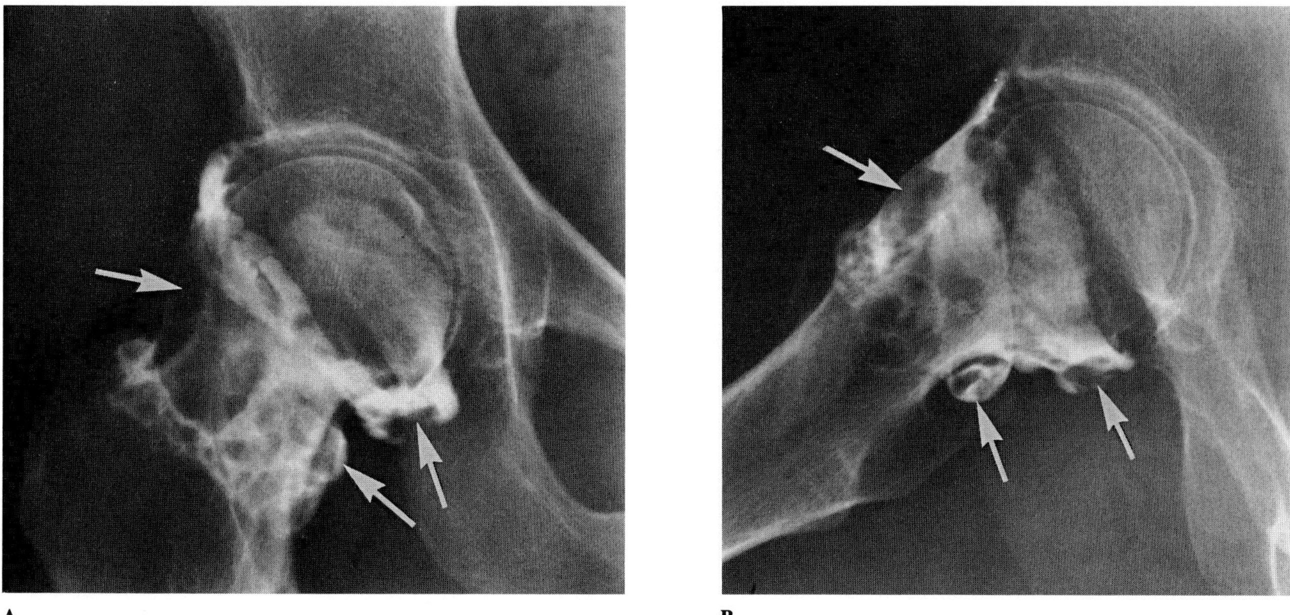

A B

Fig. 4-58 (**A**) AP and (**B**) oblique arthrograms of the right hip in a patient with synovial chonchromatosis (arrows).

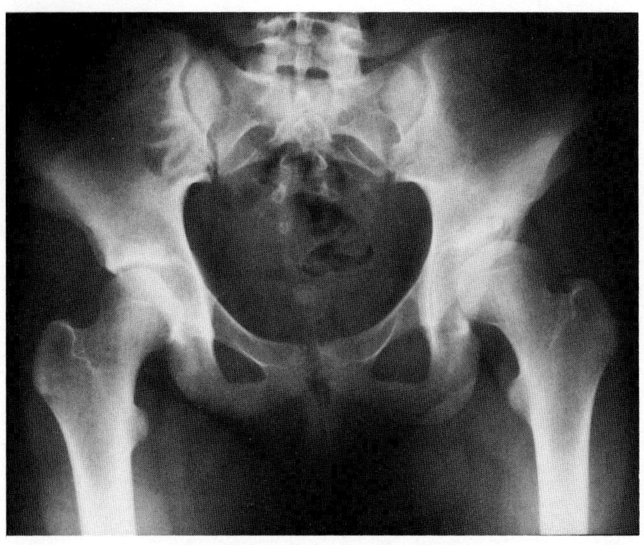

A

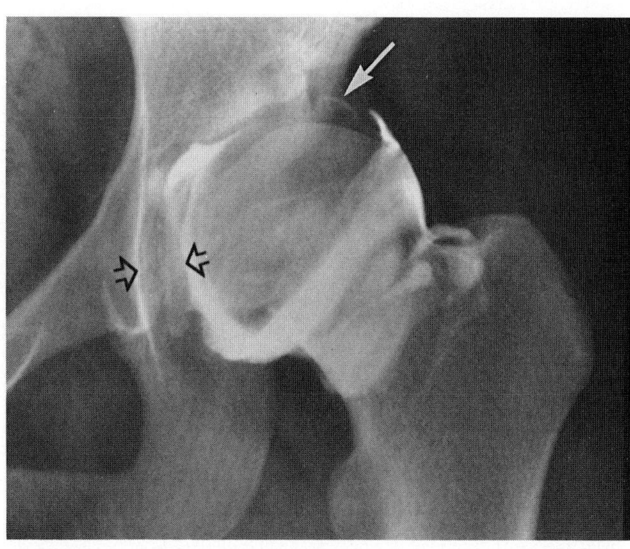

B

Fig. 4-59 (**A**) Routine radiograph demonstrating widening of the hip joint on the left. (**B**) Arthrogram demonstrates a thickened ligamentum teres (open arrows) and a labral tear (closed arrow).

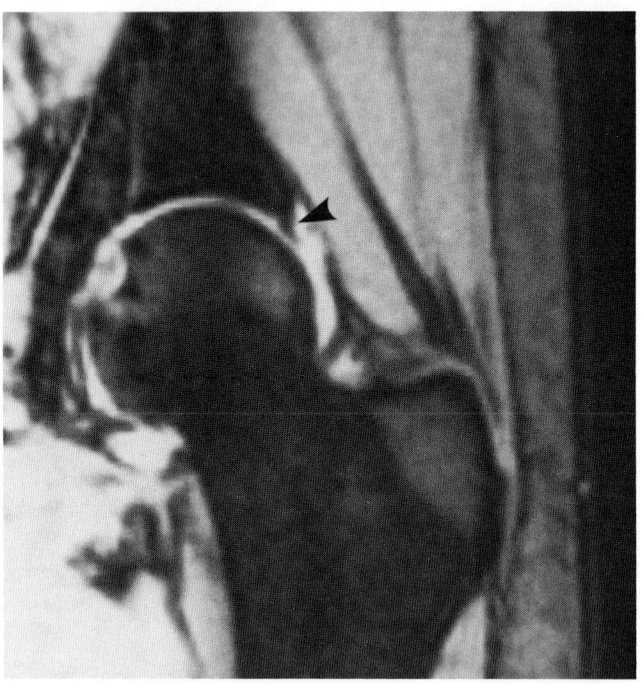

A

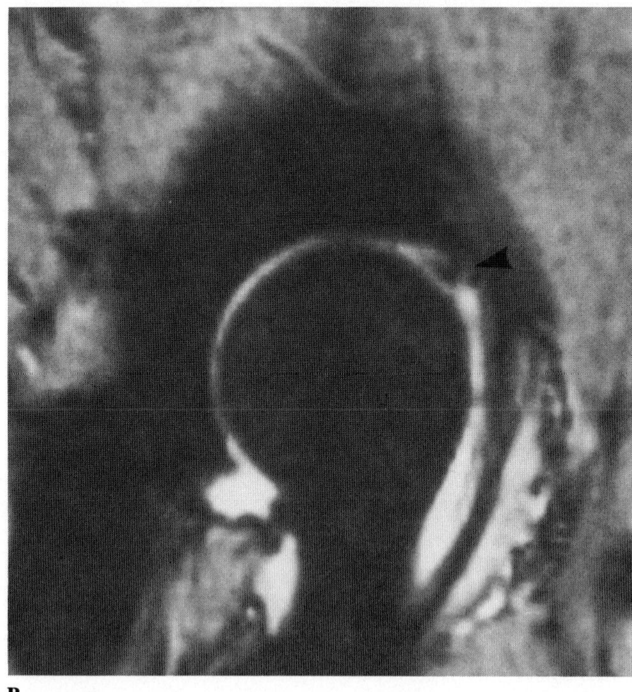

B

Fig. 4-60 Radial MR images of the hip demonstrating a normal (**A**) and torn (**B**) acetabular labrum (arrowheads).

Piriformis Syndrome

Pain in the distribution of the sciatic nerve is most often due to disc disease. Other pelvic or gluteal pathology must also be excluded.

Direct trauma to the gluteal region or sacroiliac joint may lead to inflammation of the piriformis. The sciatic nerve is involved as it exits deep to the piriformis.[72,81] The athlete presents with local pain that is exaggerated by stooping or lifting heavy objects. Walking may also be difficult. Swelling or mass effect may be evident on physical examination. Straight leg raising is usually positive.[81]

Imaging is important to establish the diagnosis and, more importantly, to exclude other causes of sciatic nerve irritation.

MRI is ideal in this setting. Thin-section (3 to 5 mm) axial images with T1-weighted (SE 500/20) and T2-weighted (SE 2000/20,80) sequences are usually adequate. Subtle changes may be more easily appreciated with short T1 inversion-recovery or fat-suppressed T2-weighted images.[66]

Conservative therapy is usually sufficient, but operative resection of the piriformis or evacuation of hematoma may be required.[81]

REFERENCES

Anatomy

1. Anderson JE. *Grant's Atlas of Anatomy*. 8th ed. Baltimore: Williams & Wilkins; 1983.
2. Armbuster TG, Guerra J, Resnick D, et al. The adult hip: an anatomic study. *Radiology*. 1978;128:1–10.
3. Berquist TH. *Imaging of Orthopedic Trauma*. 2nd ed. New York: Raven; 1991.
4. Bowerman JW, Sins JM, Chang R. The teardrop shadow of the pelvis. Anatomy and clinical significance. *Radiology*. 1982;143:659–662.
5. Guerra J, Armbuster TG, Resnick D, et al. The adult hip: an anatomic study. Part II: soft tissue landmarks. *Radiology*. 1978;128:11–20.
6. Hollinshead WH. *Anatomy for Surgeons*. 3rd ed. Philadelphia: Harper & Row; 1982.
7. Jackson H, Burke JT. Sacral foramina. *Skeletal Radiol*. 1984; 11:282–288.
8. Karlin LI. Injuries of the hips and pelvis in the skeletally immature athlete. In: Nicholas JA, Hershman EB, eds. *The Lower Extremity and Spine in Sports Medicine*. St Louis, MO: Mosby; 1986:1292–1329.

Imaging of the Pelvis and Hips

9. Armbuster TG, Guerra J, Resnick D, et al. The adult hip: an anatomic study. *Radiology*. 1978;128:1–10.
10. Ballinger PW. *Merrill's Atlas of Radiographic Positions and Radiologic Procedures*. 5th ed. St Louis, MO: Mosby; 1982.
11. Bernau A, Berquist TH. *Orthopedic Positioning in Diagnostic Radiology*. Baltimore: Urban & Schwarzenberg; 1983.
12. Berquist TH. *Imaging of Orthopedic Trauma*. 2nd ed. New York: Raven; 1991.
13. Berquist TH. *MRI of the Musculoskeletal System*. 2nd ed. New York: Raven; 1990.
14. Burk DL, Mears DC, Herbert DL, Straub WH, Cooperstein LA, Beck EA. Pelvic and acetabular fractures: examined by angled CT scanning. *Radiology*. 1984;153:548.
15. Burk DL, Mears DC, Kennedy WA, Cooperstein LA, Herbert DL. Three dimensional computed tomography of acetabular fractures. *Radiology*. 1985;155:183–186.
16. Dihlmann W, Nebel G. Computed tomography of the hip joint capsule. *J Comput Assisted Tomogr*. 1983;7:278–285.
17. Dodig D, Ugarbovic B, Orlic D. Bone scintigraphy in idiopathic aseptic femoral head necrosis. *Eur J Nucl Med*. 1983;8:23–25.
18. Glynn TP, Kreipke DL, DeRosa GP. Computed tomography arthrography in traumatic hip dislocation. *Skeletal Radiol*. 1989;18:29–31.
19. Judet R, Judet J, Letournel E. Fractures of the acetabulum: classification and surgical approaches to open reduction. *J Bone Joint Surg Am*. 1964;46:1615–1646.
20. Lancaster SJ, Cummings RJ. Hip aspiration. Verification of needle position by air arthrography. *J Pediatr Orthop*. 1982;7:91–92.
21. Lyons JC, Peterson LFA. The snapping iliopsoas tendon. *Mayo Clin Proc*. 1984;59:327–329.
22. Patterson I. Torn acetabular labrum. *J Bone Joint Surg Br*. 1957;39:306–309.
23. Pritchard RS, Shah HR, Nelson CL, Fitzrandolph RL. MR and CT appearance of iliopsoas bursal distention secondary to diseased hips. *J Comput Assisted Tomogr*. 1990;14:797–800.
24. Saks BJ. Normal acetabular anatomy for acetabular fractures assessment: CT and plain film correlation. *Radiology*. 1986;159:139–145.
25. Speer KP, Spritzer CE, Harrelson JM, Numley JA. Magnetic resonance imaging of the femoral head after acute intracapsular fracture of the femoral neck. *J Bone Joint Surg Am*. 1990;72:98–103.
26. Staple TW. Arthrographic demonstration of iliopsoas bursa extension of the hip joint. *Radiology*. 1972;102:515–516.
27. Staple TW, Jung D, Mork A. Snapping tendon syndromes: hip tenography with fluoroscopic monitoring. *Radiology*. 1988;166:873–874.
28. Sweeney JP, Helms CA, Minagi H, Louie RW. The widened teardrop distance: a plain film indicator of hip joint effusion in adults. *AJR*. 1987;149:117–119.
29. Young JWR, Burgess AR, Brumback RT, Poka A. Pelvic fractures: value of plain radiography in early assessment and management. *Radiology*. 1986;160:445–451.
30. Zieger MM, Dorr UL, Schulz RD. Ultrasonography of hip joint effusions. *Skeletal Radiol*. 1987;16:607–611.

Fractures

31. Berquist TH. *Imaging of Orthopedic Trauma*. 2nd ed. New York: Raven; 1991.
32. Bowerman JW. *Radiology and Injury in Sport*. New York: Appleton-Century-Crofts; 1977.
33. Caudle RJ, Crawford AH. Avulsion fracture of the lateral acetabular margin. *J Bone Joint Surg Am*. 1988;70:1568–1570.
34. Clancy WG, Foltz AS. Iliac apophysitis and stress fracture in runners. *Am J Sports Med*. 1976;4:214–218.
35. Daffner RH. Pelvic trauma. In: McCort JJ, ed. *Trauma Radiology*. New York: Churchill Livingstone; 1990:339–380.
36. Dimon JH. Isolated fractures of the lesser trochanter of the femur. *Clin Orthop*. 1972;82:144–148.
37. Dunn W, Morris HD. Fractures and dislocations of the pelvis. *J Bone Joint Surg Am*. 1968;50:1634–1648.
38. Flecher H. Time of appearance and fusion of ossification centers as observed by roentgenographic methods. *Am J Roentgenol Radium Ther Nucl Med*. 1942;47:97–159.
39. Ghormley RK, Sullivan R. Traumatic dislocation of the hip. *Am J Surg*. 1953;85:298–301.
40. Goodill CL. Neurologic deficits associated with pelvic fractures. *J Neurosurg*. 1966;24:837–842.
41. Hafner RHV. Trochanteric fractures of the femur. *J Bone Joint Surg Br*. 1951;33:513–516.
42. Harley JD, Mack LA,Winquist RA. CT of acetabular fractures: comparison with conventional radiography. *AJR*. 1982;138:413–417.
43. Jackson H, Kam J, Harrison JH, et al. The sacral arcuate lines in upper sacral fractures. *Radiology*. 1982;145:35–39.
44. Jensen JS. Classification of trochanteric fractures. *Acta Orthop Scand*. 1980;51:803–810.
45. Judet R, Judet J, Letournel E. Fractures of the acetabulum: classification and surgical approaches to reduction. *J Bone Joint Surg Am*. 1964;46:1615–1646.
46. Kane WJ. Fracture of the pelvis. In: Rockwood CA, Green DP, eds. *Fractures in Adults*. 2nd ed. Philadelphia: Lippincott; 1984:1073–1209.

47. Karlin LI. Injuries to the hip and pelvis in the skeletally immature athlete. In: Nicholas JA, Hershman EB, eds. *The Lower Extremity and Spine in Sports Medicine*. St Louis, MO: Mosby; 1986:1292–1329.

48. Key JA, Conwell HE. *Management of Fractures, Dislocations and Sprains*. 7th ed. St Louis, MO: Mosby; 1961.

49. Knight RA, Smith H. Central acetabular fractures. *J Bone Joint Surg Am*. 1958;49:1–16.

50. Kyle RF, Gustilo RB, Collon DJ. Analysis of 622 intertrochanteric hip fractures. *J Bone Joint Surg Am*. 1979;61:216–221.

51. Miller A, Stedman GH, Beisaw NE, Gross PT. Sciatica caused by an avulsion fracture of the ischial tuberosity. *J Bone Joint Surg Am*. 1987;69:143–147.

52. Pennal GF, Tile M, Waddell JP, Garside H. Pelvic disruption: assessment and classification. *Clin Orthop*. 1980;151:12–21.

53. Reigstad A. Traumatic dislocation of the hip. *J Trauma*. 1980; 20:603–606.

54. Rosenthal RE, Coher WL. Fracture-dislocation of the hip: an epidemiological review. *J Trauma*. 1979;19:572–581.

55. Scott WW, Fishman EK, Magid D. Acetabular fractures: optimal imaging. *Radiology*. 1987;165:537–539.

56. Seinsheimer F. Subtrochanteric fractures of the femur. *J Bone Joint Surg Am*. 1978;60:300–306.

57. Sernito I, Johnell O, Gentz C, Nilsson J. Unstable intertrochanteric fractures of the hip. *J Bone Joint Surg Am*. 1988;70:1297–1303.

58. Sim FH, Scott SG. Injuries to the pelvis and hips in athletes: anatomy and function. In: Nicholas JA, Hershman EB, eds. *The Lower Extremity and Spine in Sports Medicine*. St Louis, MO: Mosby; 1986:1119–1169.

59. Tehranzadeh J. The spectrum of avulsion and avulsion-like injuries of the musculoskeletal system. *RadioGraphics*. 1987;7:945–974.

60. Thaggard A III, Harle TS, Carlson V. Fractures and dislocations of the bony pelvis and hip. *Semin Roentgenol*. 1978;13:117–134.

61. Thompson VP, Epstein HC. Traumatic dislocation of the hip. *J Bone Joint Surg Am*. 1951;33:747–778.

62. Tile M. Fractures of the acetabulum. *Orthop Clin North Am*. 1980;11:481–506.

63. Young JWR, Burgess AR. *Radiologic Management of Pelvic Ring Fractures*. Baltimore: Urban & Schwarzenberg; 1987.

64. Young JWR, Resnick CS. Fractures of the pelvis: current concepts of classification. *AJR*. 1990;155:1169–1175.

Soft Tissue and Miscellaneous Injuries

65. Baker KS, Gilula LA. The current role of tenography and bursography. *AJR*. 1990;154:129–133.

66. Berquist TH. *MRI of the Musculoskeletal System*. New York: Raven; 1990.

67. Burkett LN. Causative factors in hamstring strains. *Med Sci Sports*. 1970;2:39–42.

68. Dameron TB. Bucket handle tear of the acetabular labrum accompanying posterior dislocation of the hip. *J Bone Joint Surg Am*. 1959;41:131–134.

69. Dehlmann W, Nebel G. Computed tomography of the hip joint capsule. *J Comput Assisted Tomogr*. 1983;7:278–285.

70. Harper MC, Schaberg JE. Primary iliopsoas bursography in the diagnosis of hip disorders. *Clin Orthop*. 1987;221:238–241.

71. Harris NH, Murray RO. Lesions of the symphysis in athletes. *Br J Med*. 1974;4:211–214.

72. Hollinshead HW. *Anatomy for Surgeons*. New York: Lippincott; 1982;3.

73. Patterson I. The torn acetabular labrum. *J Bone Joint Surg Br*. 1957;39:306–309.

74. Penkava RR. Iliopsoas bursitis demonstrated by computed tomography. *AJR*. 1980;135:175–176.

75. Pritchard RS, Shah HR, Nelson CL, Fitzrandolph RL. MR and CT appearance of iliopsoas bursal distention secondary to diseased hips. *J Comput Assisted Tomogr*. 1990;14:797–800.

76. Silver SF, Connell DG, Duncan CP. Case report 550. *Skeletal Radiol*. 1989;18:327–328.

77. Sim FH, Scott SG. Injuries to the pelvis and hips in athletes. In: Nicholas JA, Hershman EB, eds. *The Lower Extremity and Spine in Sports Medicine*. St Louis, MO: Mosby; 1986:1119–1169.

78. Staple TW. Arthrographic demonstration of iliopsoas bursa extension of the hip joint. *Radiology*. 1972;102:515–516.

79. Staple TW, Jung D, Mork A. Snapping tendon syndrome: hip tenography with fluoroscopic monitoring. *Radiology*. 1988;166:873–874.

80. Sweeney JP, Helms CA, Minagi H, Louie KW. The widened teardrop distance: a plain film indicator of hip joint effusion in adults. *AJR*. 1987;149:117–119.

81. Vandertop WP, Bosma NJ. The piriformis syndrome. *J Bone Joint Surg Am*. 1991;73:1095–1096.

82. Warren R, Kaye JJ, Salvati EA. Arthrographic demonstration of an enlarged iliopsoas bursa complicating osteoarthritis of the hip. *J Bone Joint Surg Am*. 1975;57:413–415.

Chapter 5

Femur and Thigh

The femur is the largest and strongest bone in the body. Because of its role as a primary weight-bearing bone, it must tolerate the extremes of axial loading and angulatory stresses. Massive musculature envelopes the femur. This musculature provides abundant blood supply to the bone, which also allows great potential for healing. Thus the most significant problem relating to femoral shaft fractures is not healing but restoration of bone length and alignment so that the femoral shaft will tolerate the functional stresses demanded of it.[5,6,18,38]

The soft tissue compartments of the thigh are large and accommodate significant hemorrhage and edema. Isolated soft tissue injury or injury in association with fracture or fracture treatment is not uncommon in the thigh.[1,4,16,23–27]

ANATOMY

The shaft of the femur is tubular in shape (Fig. 5-1). It is generally smooth except for the linea aspera, which is a prominent posterior longitudinal ridge extending from the intertrochanteric crest inferiorly to the middle half of the femur, where it diverges into a medial and lateral lip to become the respective supracondylar lines. The pectineal line extends from the lesser trochanter between the gluteal tuberosity and upper medial lip of linea aspera inferiorly to blend with this lip or the middle part of the linea.[6,18] The body of the femoral shaft is slightly bowed anteriorly. In the standing position, the femoral shaft normally inclines medially about 10°. Structurally the femur can resist angulating forces, but its tubular design is not the best for resisting torsional forces.[18,28]

Multiple muscle groups surround the femoral shaft (Figs. 5-2 and 5-3). Hip flexors, extensors, and abductors and knee flexor and extensor groups provide a bulk of soft tissue protection. The muscles of the thigh are divided into three fascial compartments.[18,30,33] The anterior compartment includes the quadriceps femoris, sartorius, iliopsoas, and pectineal muscles. Neurovascular structures include the femoral artery, vein, and nerve (Fig. 5-2).[18,33] The medial compartment contains the gracilis, adductor group, and obturator externus. The deep femoral artery and vein are also included in the medial compartment. The posterior compartment (Fig. 5-2) contains the sciatic nerve and hamstring muscles. The three compartments are separated by the lateral and medial septa (Fig. 5-2).[6,18,33]

Blood supply to the femoral shaft is through metaphyseal, periosteal, and endosteal vessels. The rich periosteal blood supply is from the large surrounding muscles and is interrupted only in injuries in which extensive stripping has occurred. The nutrient arteries are perforating vessels that originate from the profunda femoris artery. The perforating branches encircle the femur posteriorly and perforate the muscle attachments adjacent to the linea aspera. Usually, there are four perforating branches. The lower part of the femur is supplied by a long descending branch of the nutrient artery in the intramedullary canal.[18] The main femoral artery, which is located medially to the shaft (Fig. 5-3), perforates the adductor hiatus. With distal skeletal injury, this may be the site of vascular injury.

The sciatic nerve, which is well cushioned medially and posteriorly in the thigh (Fig. 5-3), is rarely injured at the shaft level.[18]

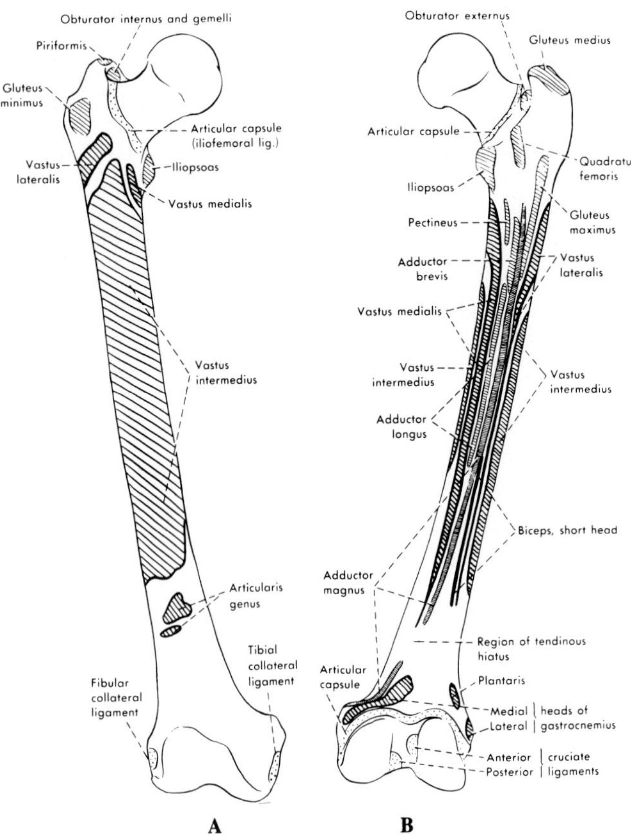

Fig. 5-1 (**A**) Anterior and (**B**) posterior muscle attachments of the femur. *Source:* Reprinted from *Anatomy for Surgeons, Vol 3, The Back and Limbs*, ed 3 by WH Hollinshead, 1982, JB Lippincott.

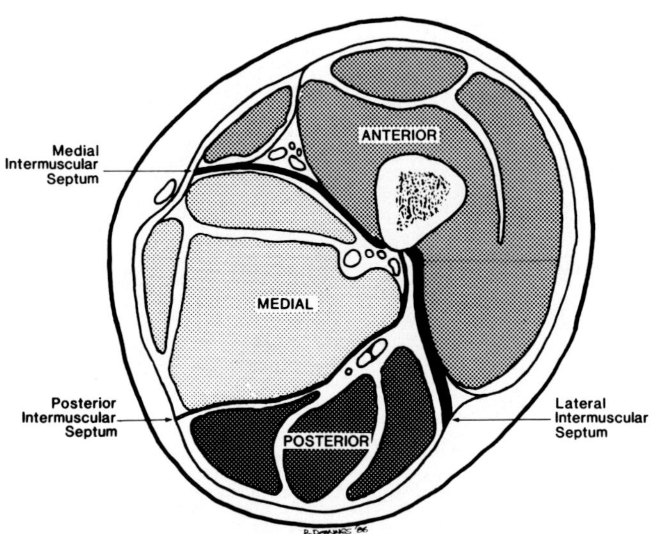

Fig. 5-2 Illustration of the fascial compartments of the thigh. *Source:* Reprinted with permission from *Journal of Bone and Joint Surgery* (1986; 68A:1439–1443), Copyright © 1986, Journal of Bone and Joint Surgery.

FEMORAL SHAFT FRACTURES

Major external violence, as encountered in trauma from motor vehicle or high-velocity sports accidents, is the usual mechanism of injury. Young adults and children are predominantly injured. The metaphyseal areas in the younger population are wider and dissipate stress better than the diaphysis.

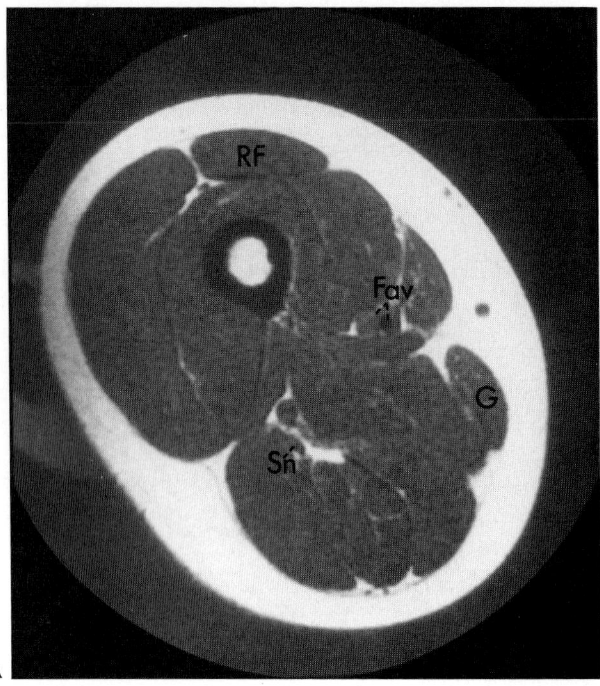

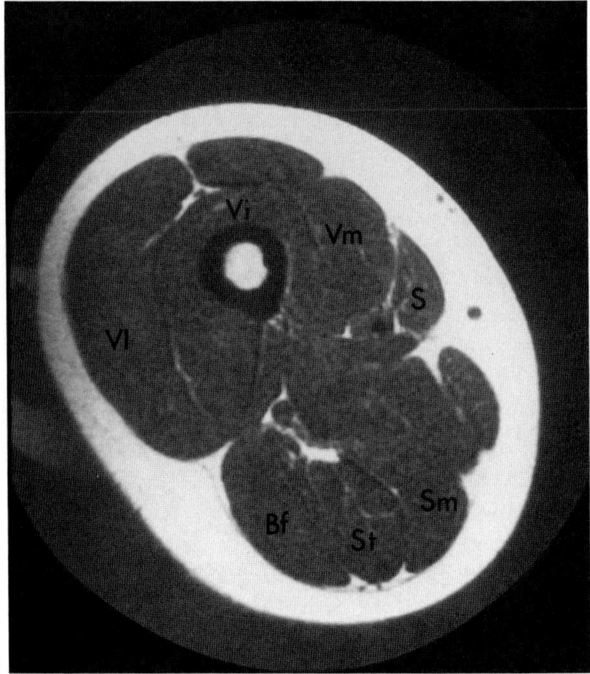

Fig. 5-3 Axial MR images of the thigh demonstrating the muscular and neurovascular anatomy. (**A**) Fav, Femoral artery and vein; RF, rectus femoris; G, gracilis; SN, sciatic nerve. (**B**) Vi, Vastus intermedius; S, sartorius; Bf, biceps femoris; St, semitendinosus; Sm, semimembranosus; Vm, vastus medialis; Vl, vastus lateralis.

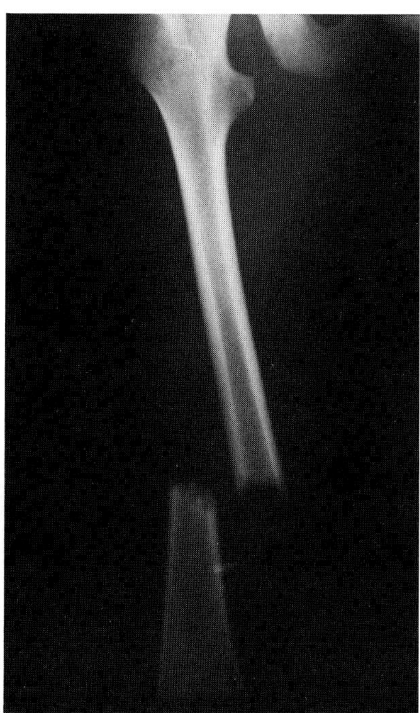

Fig. 5-4 AP view of the femur demonstrating a displaced comminuted fracture sustained in a snowmobile accident.

Thus fracture of the femoral shaft is more likely to occur (Fig. 5-4). In older patients or in patients with metabolic bone disease, however, the metaphyseal areas are more brittle and more susceptible to fracture than the diaphysis. Because of the mechanism of injury, significant soft tissue damage usually occurs with femoral shaft fractures.[6,28,33]

Fractures may be either open or closed. Open fractures suggest greater injury to both bone and soft tissues. Open fractures may result from external damage to the soft tissues or from extrusion of fracture fragments from the inside outward.

Simple fractures may be transverse, oblique, or spiral. With greater injury force, segmental or comminuted fractures may occur. Occasionally, subtle linear fractures along the shaft may be present that are not visible radiographically. These are important to recognize if internal fixation is contemplated.[5,6,28]

Fractures of the femoral shaft may also be classified according to the type of force that produced the fracture. Angulation forces produce transverse fractures, transverse fractures with butterfly fragments and segmental fractures; torsional forces produce oblique and spiral oblique fractures; impaction forces produce comminuted or segmental fractures; and penetrating forces may result in bone loss.[34]

Finally, fractures may be classified according to location. Fractures of the middle third of the shaft are most common. At this level, overriding of fracture fragments and shortening of the limb usually result.[5,6,28] The displacement of the fracture may be the result of muscle pull. The proximal fragment may be rotated outward because of the forces of gravity and the external rotator muscles.[18,21] In fractures of the upper third, the proximal fragment tends to be flexed by the iliopsoas, abducted by the gluteus medius and gluteus maximus, and externally rotated by the short rotators and the forces of gravity. The distal fragment may be adducted by the pull of the adductor muscles. In fractures of the lower third of the shaft, shortening and displacement can occur. Posterior displacement of the distal fragment occurs because of the action of the gastrocnemius, popliteus, and plantaris muscles. Injury to the popliteal vessels may occur.[5,18,21]

Combination injuries involving the ipsilateral femoral neck and tibia are not uncommon.[32,36] Associated femoral neck fractures may be subtle. Swiontkowski et al[32] reviewed 83 patients with femoral shaft fractures. Sixty-two patients had associated femoral neck fractures, and one-third of these were initially overlooked. Combined femoral shaft and tibial fractures are frequently open injuries (58%), requiring extensive surgical reconstruction.

Stress fractures, especially in long distance runners, are not unusual. Stress fractures are more common in the femoral neck and proximal and distal shafts.[6,14] If untreated, these fractures may go on to a complete displaced fracture (see Chapter 12, Stress Fractures).

IMAGING OF FEMORAL SHAFT FRACTURES

The clinical diagnosis of femoral shaft fractures is usually quite easy. Angular deformity, shortening, and pain are readily apparent. An expanding thigh is a sign of hemorrhage and should alert physicians to the possibility of shock and/or compartment syndrome.[6,8,30,31,33]

Standard views of the femoral shaft include anteroposterior (AP) and lateral projections. It is mandatory that the adjacent hip and knee joints be included on the films because of the significant incidence of associated ipsilateral injuries. The tibia, fibula, and foot and ankle should also be examined carefully and radiographs obtained if necessary.[6]

The AP view of the femur is obtained with the patient supine and the legs extended. The unaffected leg should be slightly abducted. The foot is internally rotated approximately 15° to position the patella anteriorly and to minimize anteversion of the femoral neck. The central X-ray beam is directed vertically to the midpoint of the cassette. Soft tissues of the thigh must be included on the film; in this way subcutaneous air and hematomas are readily detected. With larger patients, it is necessary to radiograph the upper and lower femurs separately. The central beam is directed perpendicularly to the film in each case.

The lateral view is obtained with the patient turned onto the affected side. The upper knee is flexed and placed on a large pad in front of the involved extremity. The pelvis is then adjusted for a true lateral position. The involved dependent knee is slightly flexed. The central beam is directed perpendicularly to the midpoint of the film. A severely injured patient is not moved because of the danger of fracture displacement. A grid-front cassette is then placed along the medial or lateral aspect of the thigh and knee with the central beam directed horizontally and perpendicularly to the cassette. The knee is usually included on this film. Proximal femur evaluation is performed with lateral hip views. X-ray examination of the hip is essential; femoral neck fracture or dislocation and acetabular fractures may be present.

Subtle fractures, such as incomplete or stress fractures, may not be visible on routine AP and lateral radiographs.[6] Radionuclide scans are useful to exclude subtle bone injury. When these are negative 72 hours after injury, it is safe to conclude that symptoms are not related to osseous injury.[17] In this situation, magnetic resonance imaging (MRI) or other modalities may be required to exclude soft tissue injury. When a bone scan is positive, further imaging with computed tomography (CT), tomography, or MRI may be required to define more fully the abnormality.[6,7]

SOFT TISSUE INJURIES

Soft tissue injuries may occur alone or in association with femoral fractures.

Vascular injuries may occur at the time of fracture or during treatment. Thrombosis, laceration, false aneurysm formation, and arteriovenous fistula formation are potential complications. Arterial injuries are more common in fractures of the distal third of the shaft and in the supracondylar region.[6,9,30]

Nerve injury is quite rare at the time of initial injury because of the protective role that the large muscle mass provides. Other soft tissue complications such as compartment syndrome may also occur.[30,33]

Isolated injuries include contusion, hematoma, disruption of the muscle and/or tendon units, venous thrombosis, compartment syndrome, and rhabdomyolysis.[7,8,19,20,22–26] Factors affecting soft tissue injury or overuse injury include inappropriate progression of activity, intensity and duration of trauma, anatomic alignment (hip and knee), muscle imbalances, surface, footwear, and type of activity.[21–24] Clinical evaluation of these injuries may be sufficient. Imaging techniques such as ultrasonography, CT, and MRI can provide valuable information regarding the type and extent of injury. MRI is particularly useful for evaluating muscle and neurovascular injuries in the thigh.[7,10–13]

Muscle-tendon injuries may be minor or major. Contusions, mild tears with hemorrhage, and hematomas are most common.[4,7,8,15] Third-degree strains (complete tears of a muscle unit) are unusual.[4,25] The muscle group involved varies with the sport to some degree.[4,26,27]

Hamstring injuries are common in sprinters and soccer players and with deceleration.[8,15] During kicking (soccer and football), 85% of the force is absorbed by the hamstrings.[8,15] Most hamstring injuries are first or second degree (Fig. 5-5; see also discussion in Chapter 1 of soft tissue injuries). These injuries are common (33% of runners), heal slowly, and rein-

Fig. 5-5 (**A**) Illustration of mechanism of hamstring strain. (**B**) Axial and (**C**) sagittal MR images (SE 2000/60) of a first-degree hamstring muscle tear. There is infiltrative high signal in the muscle.

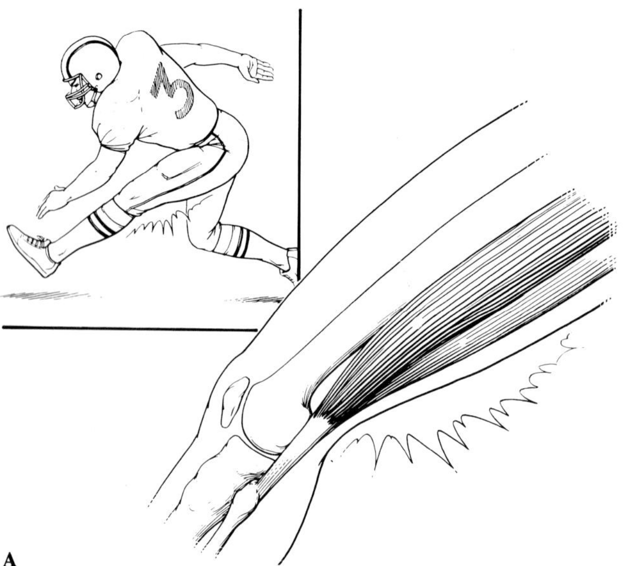

A

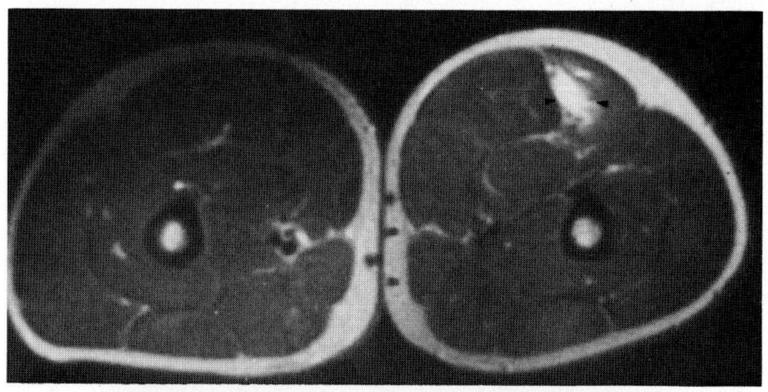

B

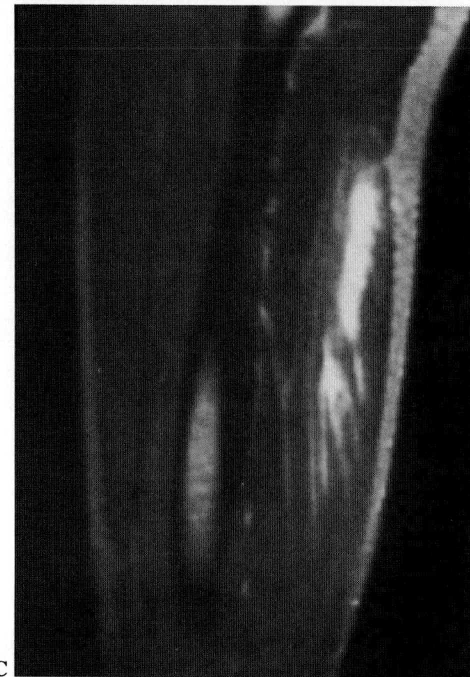

C

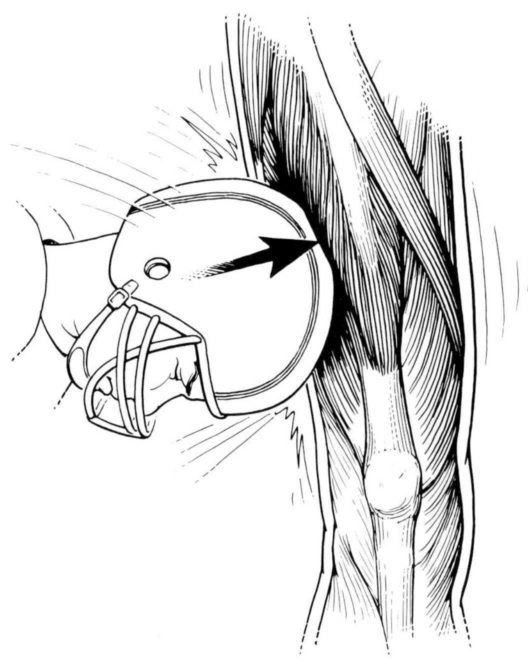

Fig. 5-6 Illustration of mechanism of quadriceps contusion.

jury is frequent.[1,4,16] MRI is most useful for detecting and following the healing process.

Injuries to the quadriceps mechanism are common in contact sports (Fig. 5-6). Contusion, hematoma (Fig. 5-7), and significant hemorrhage can occur. If these injuries are not properly managed, myositis ossificans can develop.[4] Tears of the quadriceps tendon (Fig. 5-8) occur less frequently.

Adductor muscle injuries occur most frequently with running and cutting (change in direction while running). The origins of the muscles (Fig. 5-9) are most commonly involved.[2,6]

Compartment syndrome is uncommon in the thigh compared to the forearm and lower leg. The compartments of the thigh are large (Fig. 5-2) and can accommodate up to 4 L of blood before significant elevations in pressure develop.[2,9,29,33] Compartment syndromes in the thigh have been reported in crush injuries, femoral fractures, overuse syndromes, arterial ischemia, and burns and after external compression for treatment of femoral and pelvic fractures. Sports-related compartment syndromes may be related to chronic microtrauma or a direct blow resulting in intracompartment hemorrhage.[2,9] The pressure required to cause muscle ischemia is not clearly defined, but most reports suggest that intracompartment pressures generally must exceed 30 mmHg before ischemia will occur.[2,33]

Patients with compartment syndrome have pain, swelling, and, on physical examination, a tense thigh. Imaging may not be indicated and in fact may delay treatment when symptoms are obvious and pressures elevated. Fasciotomy should be accomplished as soon as possible when the diagnosis is established. Delays in treatment can result in significant muscle necrosis.[33]

Rhabdomyolysis may occur secondary to overuse and can potentially lead to compartment syndrome (Fig. 5-10). Cell integrity is altered so that intracellular contents escape into extracellular fluid. Elevated enzyme levels (creatine kinase, lactic dehydrogenase, and serum glutamic-oxaloacetic transaminase) and myoglobinuria occur.[3] Enzyme studies are useful in making the diagnosis but are not able to localize the

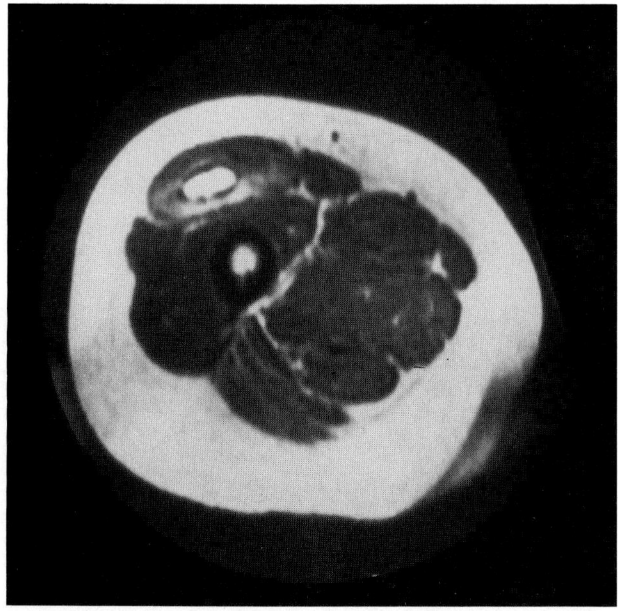

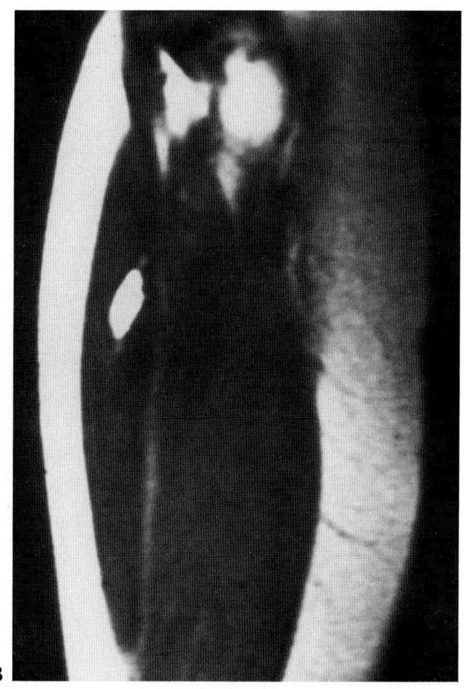

Fig. 5-7 (**A**) Axial (SE 2000/30) and (**B**) sagittal (SE 2000/60) MR images demonstrating a rectus femoris hematoma.

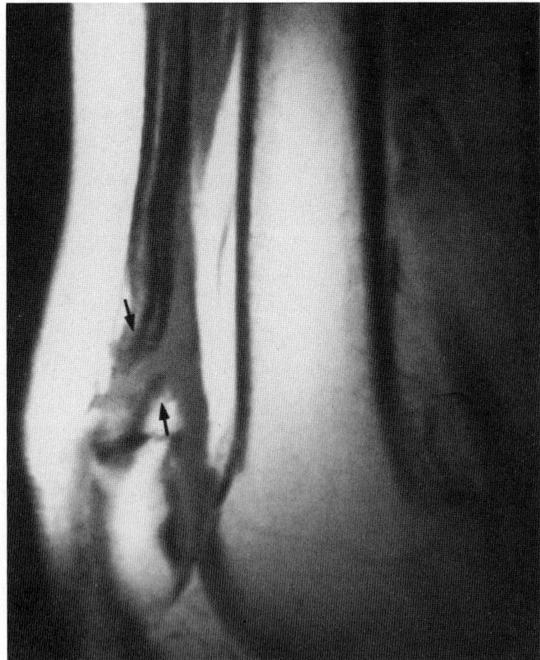

Fig. 5-8 Sagittal (SE 2000/30) MR image demonstrating a complete tear in the quadriceps tendon (arrows).

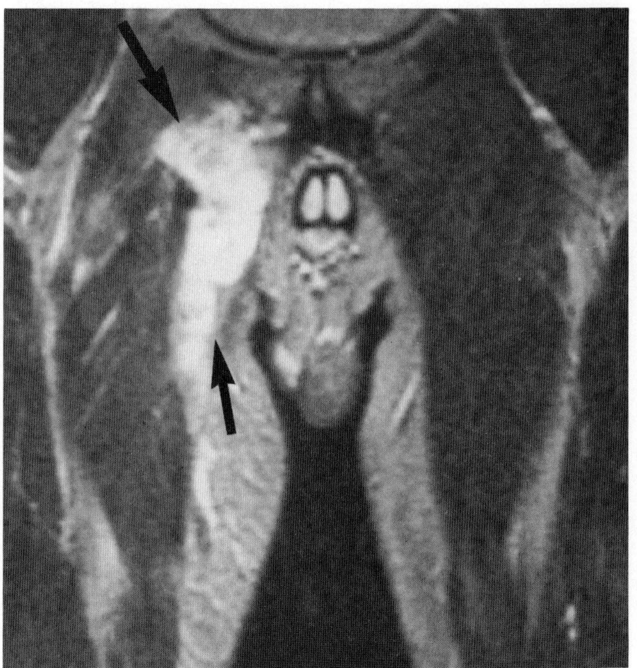

A

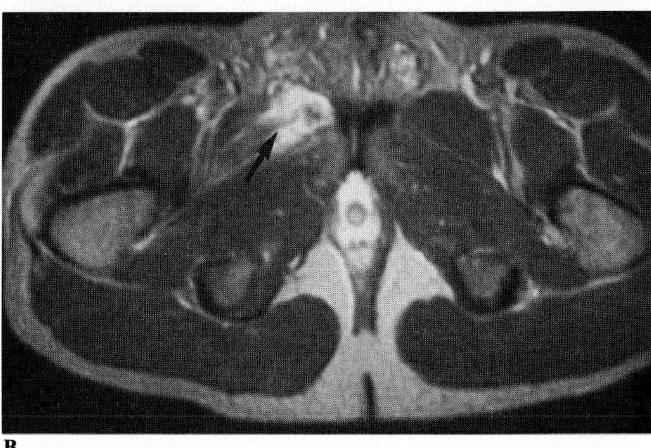

B

Fig. 5-9 (**A**) Coronal (SE 2000/60) and (**B**) axial (SE 2000/60) MR images demonstrating an adductor tear with hematoma (arrows). *Source:* Reprinted from *Magnetic Resonance Imaging of the Musculoskeletal System* by TH Berquist, 1990, Raven Press, © Mayo Foundation.

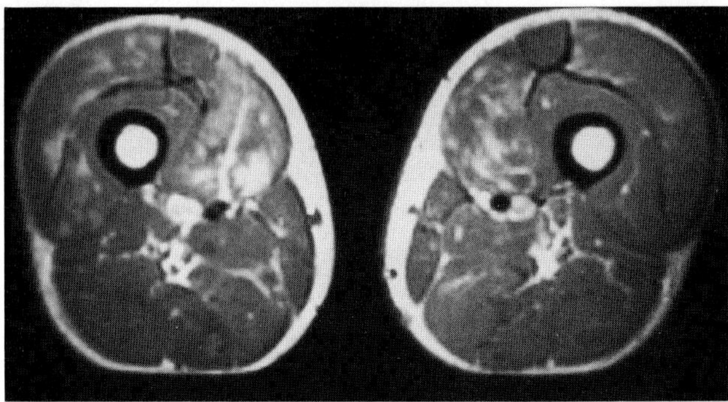

Fig. 5-10 Axial (SE 2000/60) MR image of the thighs demonstrating multiple areas of increased signal intensity due to rhabdomyolysis.

process. Detection of this condition is important to avoid sequelae such as renal failure.[7,35,37,38]

IMAGING OF SOFT TISSUE INJURIES

Soft tissue injuries to the thigh have been evaluated with sonography, MRI, CT, and radionuclide scans. The last may be useful for evaluation of rhabdomyolysis but is not routinely considered a screening tool for soft tissue injury. Radionuclide scans (^{99m}Tc-labeled pyrophosphate) are positive in rhabdomyolysis for several reasons: soft tissue hyperemia, increased capillary permeability, and binding to denatured proteins or enzyme receptors.[35,37]

CT is capable of detecting hemorrhage and hematoma (areas of increased attenuation). It is the technique of choice for evaluation of suspected myositis ossificans.[6,7] Sonography is useful for evaluating superficial muscle and tendon injuries. It is not an effective screening technique for all soft tissue injuries, however.

At the Mayo Clinic we prefer MRI for more complete definition of the location, extent, and type of injury.[6,10,12,13] MRI is also useful to exclude other conditions, such as neoplasm, that may mimic trauma.[7] Venous occlusive disease can also be effectively evaluated with MRI.[12]

MRI should be performed in two planes and with appropriate sequences to identify and stage the injury. Lesions are most conspicuous with long TE/TR (2000/60–80) spin-echo sequences (Fig. 5-11).[7] In some cases short TI inversion

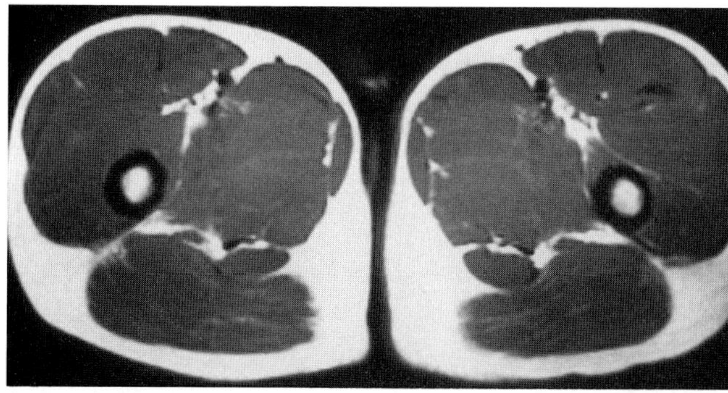

A

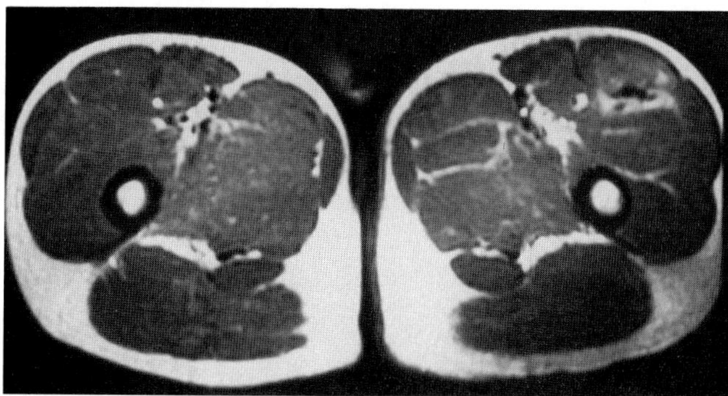

B

Fig. 5-11 Axial (**A**) T1-weighted and (**B**) T2-weighted MR images of the thigh demonstrating a quadriceps hemorrhage after a football spearing injury. The extent of injury is more easily defined on the T2-weighted image (**B**).

recovery (STIR) or (MPGR) multi-planar GRASS (T2*) sequences may be useful.[7] Gadolinium enhancement is rarely necessary.

REFERENCES

1. Agre JC. Hamstring injuries: proposed etiological factors, prevention, and treatment. *Sports Med.* 1985;2:21–33.

2. An HS, Simpson M, Gale S, Jackson WT. Acute anterior compartment syndrome in the thigh: a case report and review of the literature. *J Orthop Trauma.* 1987;1:180–182.

3. Apple FS, Rhodes M. Enzymatic estimation of skeletal muscle damage by analysis of changes in serum creatine kinase. *J Appl Phys.* 1988; 65:2598–2600.

4. Baker BE. Current concepts in the diagnosis and treatment of musculotendinous injuries. *Med Sci Sports Exerc.* 1984;16:323–327.

5. Beam HP Jr, Seligson D. Nine cases of bilateral femoral shaft fractures. A composite view. *J Trauma.* 1980;20:399–402.

6. Berquist TH. *Imaging of Orthopedic Trauma.* 2nd ed. New York: Raven; 1991.

7. Berquist TH. *Magnetic Resonance Imaging of the Musculoskeletal System.* New York: Raven; 1990.

8. Burkett LN. Investigation into hamstring strain. The cause of the hybrid muscle. *Am J Sports Med.* 1975;3(5):228–231.

9. Clancey GJ. Acute posterior compartment syndrome in the thigh. *J Bone Joint Surg Am.* 1985;67:1278–1280.

10. DeSmet AA, Fisher DR, Heiner JB, Keene JS. Magnetic resonance imaging of muscle tears. *Skeletal Radiol.* 1990;19:283–286.

11. Dooms GC, Fisher MR, Hricak H, Higgins CB. MR Imaging of intramuscular hemorrhage. *J Comput Assisted Tomogr.* 1985;9:908–913.

12. Erdman WA, Jayson HT, Redman HC, Miller GL, Parkey RW, Pescholk RW. Deep venous thrombosis of extremities: role of MR imaging in the diagnosis. *Radiology.* 1990;174:425–431.

13. Fleckestein JL, Weatherall PT, Parkey RW, Payne JA, Peshock RM. Sports-related muscle injuries. Evaluation with MR imaging. *Radiology.* 1989;172:793–798.

14. Fox JM. Injuries to the thigh. In: Nicholas JA, Heishman EB, eds. *The Lower Extremity and Spine in Sports Medicine.* St. Louis, MO: Mosby; 1986;2:1087–1117.

15. Gainor BJ, Piotrowski G, Pahl JJ, Allen WC. The kick: biomechanics and collision injuries. *Am J Sports Med.* 1978;6:185–193.

16. Heiser TM, Weber J, Sullivan G, Clare P, Jacobs RR. Prophylaxis and management of hamstring injuries in intercollegiate football players. *Am J Sports Med.* 1984;12:368–370.

17. Holder LE. Clinical radionuclide bone imaging. *Radiology.* 1990; 176:607–614.

18. Hollinshead WH. *Anatomy for Surgeons.* 3rd ed. New York: Harper & Row; 1982;3.

19. Jones DC, James SL. Overuse injuries of the lower extremity. *Clin Sports Med.* 1987;6:273–290.

20. Kellet J. Acute soft tissue injuries—a review of the literature. *Med Sci Sports Exerc.* 1986;18:489–500.

21. Luchini MA, Sarakhan AJ, Micheli LJ. Acute displaced femoral-shaft fractures in long-distance runners. *J Bone Joint Surg Am.* 1983;65:689–691.

22. Maltalino AJ, Deese M, Campbell ED. Office evaluation and treatment of lower extremity injuries in the runner. *Clin Sports Med.* 1989;8: 461–475.

23. McKeag DB. The concept of overuse. *Primary Care.* 1984;11:43–59.

24. McMaster PE. Tendon and muscle ruptures. *J Bone Joint Surg Br.* 1933;15:705–722.

25. Micheli LJ. Lower extremity overuse injuries. *Acta Med Scand.* 1986;711(suppl):171–177.

26. Paty JG. Diagnosis and treatment of musculoskeletal running injuries. *Semin Arthritis Rheum.* 1988;18:48–60.

27. Renstrom P. Swedish research in sports traumatology. *Clin Orthop.* 1984;191:144–158.

28. Rockwood CA, Green DP. *Fractures in Adults.* Philadelphia: Lippincott; 1984.

29. Röőster B. Quadriceps contusion with compartment syndrome. *Acta Orthop Scand.* 1987;58:171–172.

30. Schwartz JT, Brumback RJ, Lakatos R, Poka A, Bathon H, Burgess AR. Acute compartment syndrome of the thigh. *J Bone Joint Surg Am.* 1989; 71:392–400.

31. Styf JR, Korner LM. Chronic anterior compartment syndrome of the leg. *J Bone Joint Surg Am.* 1986;68:1338–1352.

32. Swiontkowski MF, Hansen ST, Kellam J. Ipsilateral fractures of the femoral neck and shaft. *J Bone Joint Surg Am.* 1984;66:260–268.

33. Tarlow SD, Achterman CA, Hayhurst J, Ovadia DN. Acute compartment syndrome in the thigh complicating fracture of the femur. *J Bone Joint Surg Am.* 1986;68:1439–1443.

34. Taylor LW. Principles of treatment of fracture and non-union of the shaft of the femur. *J Bone Joint Surg Am.* 1963;45:191–198.

35. Timmons JH, Hartshorne MF, Peters VJ, Cawthon MA, Bauman JM. Muscle necrosis in the extremities: evaluation with Tc-99m pyrophosphate scanning—a retrospective review. *Radiology.* 1988;167:173–178.

36. Veith RG, Winquist RA, Hansen ST. Ipsilateral fractures of the femur and tibia. *J Bone Joint Surg Am.* 1984;66:991–1002.

37. Walk P. Muscle localization of Tc-99MDP after exertion. *Clin Nucl Med.* 1984;9:493–494.

38. Zagoria RJ, Karstaedt X, Koubek TD. MR imaging of rhabdomyolysis. *J Comput Assisted Tomogr.* 1986;10:268–270.

Chapter 6

The Knee

INTRODUCTION

Lower extremity injuries are among the most common in sports.[4–6,13,14] In one large series of school-age athletes (7468 participants), Backx et al[1] noted 10.6 injuries per 100 participants, with 75% involving the lower extremities. The knee is involved in 22% to 40% of injuries.[1,2,9] Most injuries are minor. For example, 75% of injuries in runners are minor (iliotibial band syndrome, patellofemoral syndrome, quadriceps tendinitis, or patellar tendinitis).[8,10,13] Injuries in high-velocity sports (downhill skiing) and contact sports tend to be more significant.[7,9,12] Up to 33% of ligament injuries to the knee in football players require surgical treatment.[9,11]

Clinical features may be sufficient for diagnosis of certain injuries. Physical findings and history, however, are not always accurate.[3] Therefore, imaging plays a significant role in detection and staging of knee injuries. The introduction of magnetic resonance imaging (MRI) has played a particularly important role in evaluating bone and soft tissue injuries.

ANATOMY

Review of certain aspects of osseous and soft tissue anatomy is essential in understanding knee injuries and determining optimal imaging techniques.[17,27]

Bone and Articular Anatomy

The knee is formed by the femoral and tibial condylar articulations.[17,20,22,23] The tibiofibular articulation (Fig. 6-1, A and B), although often considered a part of the knee, is in fact a separate articulation.[27] The knee is primarily a hinge joint that is protected anteriorly and posteriorly by muscles with special ligamentous attachments to the capsule. The articular surfaces of both the femoral condyles and the tibial condyles are covered with hyaline cartilage. The femoral condyles are oval anteriorly and rounded posteriorly to provide increased stability in extension and increased motion and rotation in flexion. The medial femoral condyle is larger and important in load transmission across the knee. Medial and lateral tibial condyles form the expanded articular portion of the tibia. These condyles are separated by the intracondylar area, which serves for cruciate ligament attachment and restricts translation. Between the tibial condyles are raised areas known as the intercondylar eminences, which have medial and lateral tubercles (Fig. 6-1A). The weight-bearing surfaces of the tibial and femoral condyles are separated by the fibrocartilaginous menisci, which are triangular when viewed tangentially and are thicker laterally than medially (Figs. 6-1C and 6-2).[20–22]

The patella is the largest sesamoid bone in the body and develops in the tendon of the quadriceps (extensor mechanism; Fig. 6-1C). The patellar retinacula, which are formed by expansions in the quadriceps tendon and fascia lata, extend from the sides of the patella to the femoral and tibial condyles. The patella is divided into several Wiberg types. The medial and lateral facets are of equal size in type I. Type II, the most common (57%) configuration, has a smaller medial than lateral facet (Fig. 6-1C). Type III has a small medial facet that is convex and a large concave lateral facet.[29]

The capsule of the knee is lined by synovial membrane that is subdivided into several communicating compart-

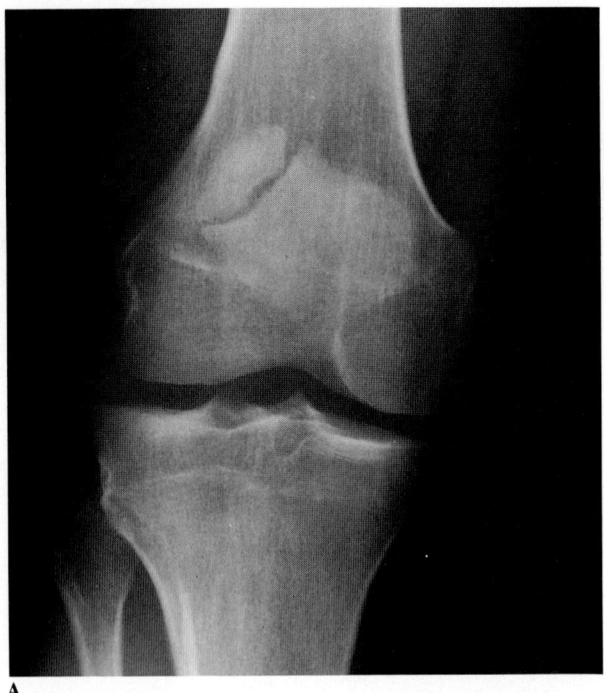

A

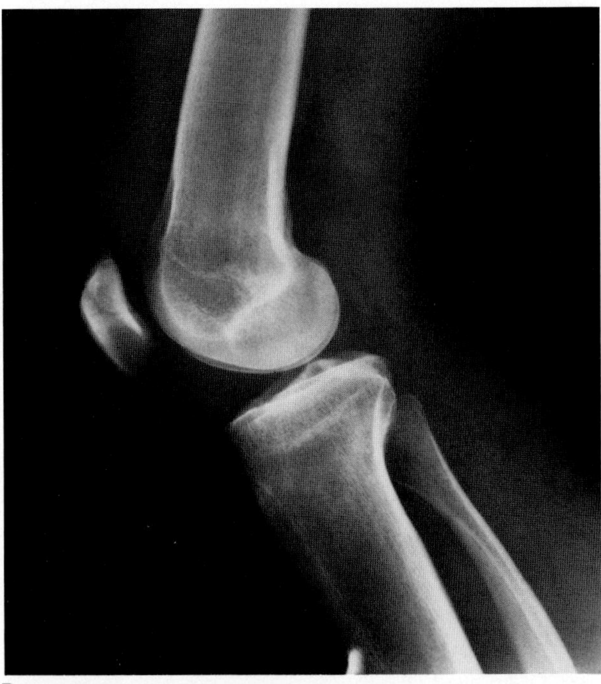

B

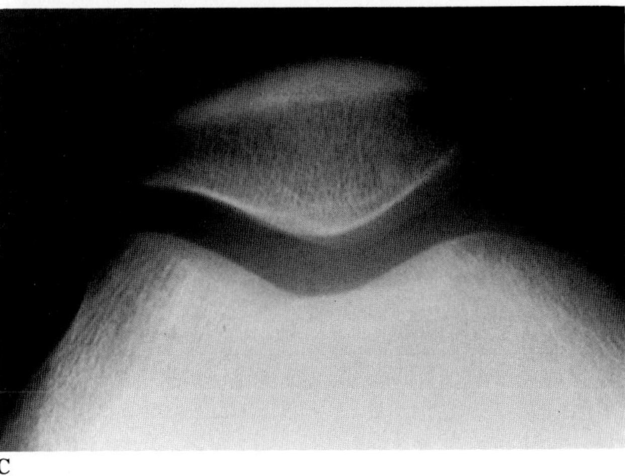

C

Fig. 6-1 (**A**) Normal anteroposterior (AP), (**B**) lateral, and (**C**) patellar views of the knee. Note the bipartite patella, which is a normal variant. The lateral facet of the patella (**C**) is larger than the medial facet (Wiberg II).

ments.[17,23,27] Anteriorly, the synovial membrane is attached to the articular margins of the patella. From the medial and lateral sides, the synovium extends circumferentially and is in contact with the retinacula (Fig. 6-3). From the inferior aspect of the patella, the synovial membrane extends downward and backward and is separated from the patellar ligament by the infrapatellar fat pad (Fig. 6-3A).[17,20]

The synovial membrane extends superiorly from the upper margin of the patella for a variable distance and is closely applied to the quadriceps muscle (Fig. 6-3A). It then reflects onto the anterior aspect of the femur. This forms the suprapatellar bursa, which lies between the quadriceps and the front of the femur. Along the medial, lateral, and posterior aspects of the capsule, the synovial membrane attaches to the femur at the edges of the articular surfaces posteriorly (Fig. 6-3B). Medially and laterally it passes from the articular margins inferiorly to attach to the articular margins of the tibial condyles. The intrasynovial space, which extends from the intracondylar fossa superiorly to the intracondylar area of the tibia inferiorly, houses the cruciate ligaments. The cruciate ligaments are, therefore, covered superiorly, medially, laterally, and anteriorly, but not posteriorly, by synovial membrane. Posterolaterally, the synovial membrane is separated from the fibrous capsule by the popliteus tendon (Fig. 6-3). It is not unusual to identify a bursa along the popliteus tendon that communicates with the joint space posterolaterally. The other common bursae about the knee are discussed more fully later.[17,23,27]

The fibrous capsule and periarticular ligaments of the knee provide passive support for the knee. The musculotendinous units provide active support.[15,16,18,19,24–28] Anteriorly the knee capsule is essentially replaced by the quadriceps and its tendon, the patella, and the patellar ligament and retinacula (Fig. 6-3A). Medially and laterally the capsule is attached to the femur just outside the synovial membrane and extends from the articular margin of the femoral condyles to the articular margin of the tibial condyles. Laterally the main ligamentous support is provided by the fibular or lateral collateral ligament (LCL), which is clearly separated from the capsule (Fig. 6-4). The medial capsule is supported by the tibial or medial collateral ligament (MCL). Unique medial

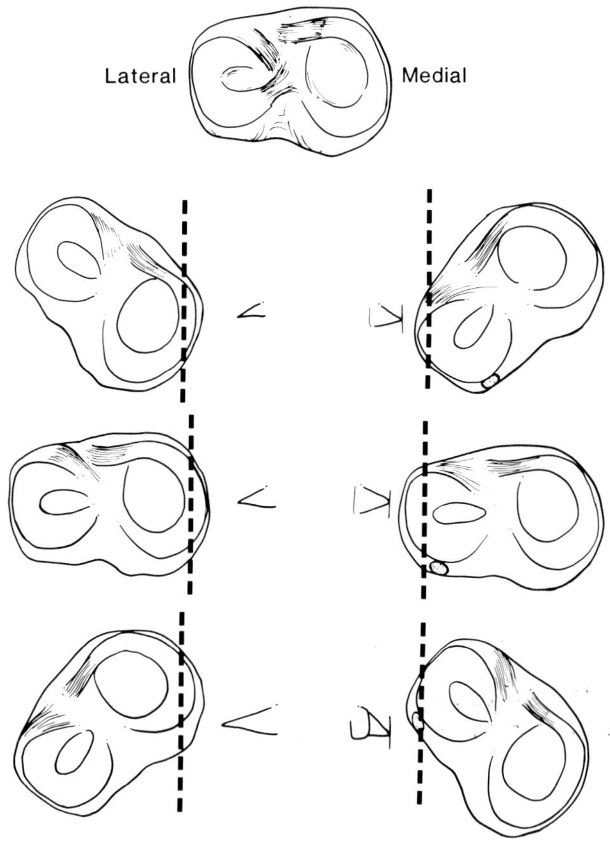

Fig. 6-2 Illustration of the medial and lateral menisci viewed from above (top) and tangentially. Note that the medial meniscus is wider posteriorly. There is a defect at the margin of the posterior lateral meniscus (lower right) for the popliteus tendon.

features include the fact that the MCL blends with the capsule and that the medial meniscus is attached to the capsule (Fig. 6-4). The posterior capsule is supported by the oblique popliteal ligament and arcuate ligament. The oblique popliteal ligament is formed by an expansion from the semimembranosus tendon that turns superiorly and laterally to run across the joint of the lateral condyle of the femur. This ligament helps resist extreme hyperextension of the knee. The arcuate popliteal ligament extends laterally and inferiorly, where it is attached to the head of the fibula (Figs. 6-3 and 6-4).[17,21,24–28]

The coronary ligament is the portion of the capsule to which the meniscus is attached to the tibia. This ligament has some laxity, which allows slight motion of the menisci on the tibia.[18]

The cruciate ligaments are intraarticular but lie outside the synovial compartment of the knee. The anterior cruciate ligament (ACL) arises from the anterior nonarticular surface of the intracondylar area of the tibia adjacent to the medial condyle. It extends obliquely, superiorly, and posteriorly to attach the medial side of the lateral femoral condyle. The ACL has significant variability in its appearance and is typically longer and more slender than the posterior cruciate ligament (PCL). This and its oblique course account for some of the difficulty encountered in evaluating this structure with MRI (Fig. 6-4).[17,18,21]

The PCL arises from the posterior intercondylar area and passes obliquely upward and forward in a nearly sagittal plane to attach to the anterior intercondylar fossa of the lateral surface of the medial femoral condyle (Figs. 6-3 and 6-4). The PCL, because of its larger transverse diameter and straighter sagittal course, is more consistently identified than the ACL on sagittal MR images.[17,20]

The fibrocartilaginous menisci differ in shape, with the medial meniscus being larger and thicker in transverse diameter posteriorly than anteriorly (Figs. 6-2 and 6-4B). The lateral meniscus is more C shaped and uniform in width (Fig. 6-2). There are several ligamentous attachments that may cause confusion on images, particularly MR images.[17] For example, the posterior horn of the lateral meniscus is closely applied to the PCL and may give off a band of fibers, termed the menisco-

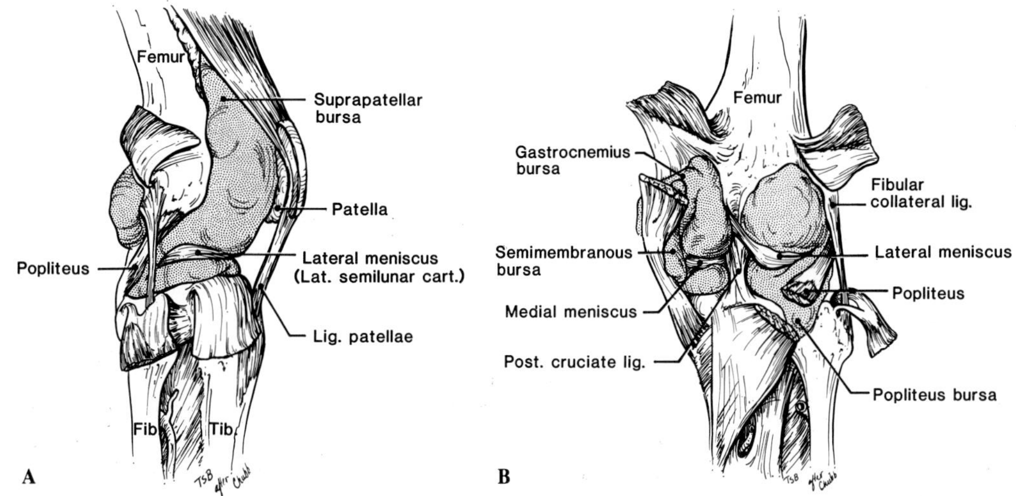

Fig. 6-3 (**A**) Lateral and (**B**) posterior illustrations of the ligaments, capsule, and major bursae of the knee. *Source:* Reprinted from *Imaging of Orthopedic Trauma* ed 2 by TH Berquist, 1991, Raven Press, © Mayo Foundation.

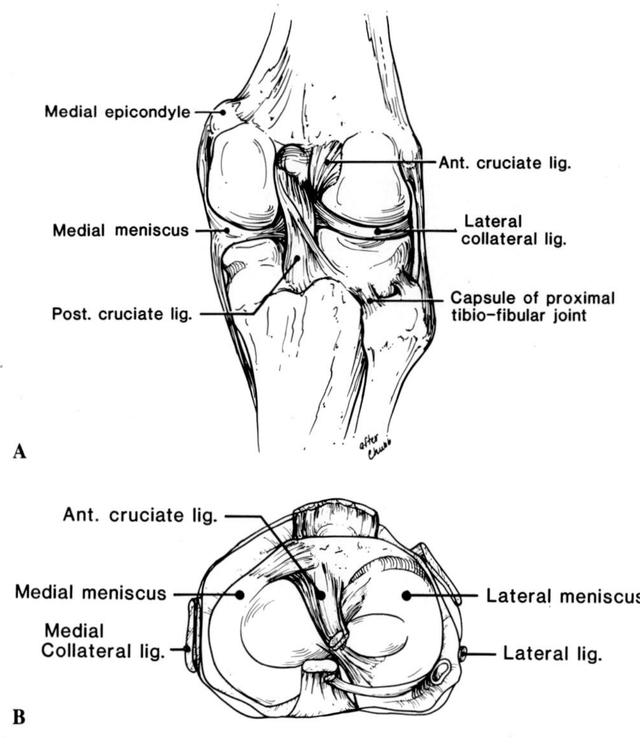

Fig. 6-4 (**A**) Posterior and (**B**) axial illustrations of the ligamentous anatomy of the knee and menisci. *Source:* Reprinted from *Imaging of Orthopedic Trauma* ed 2 by TH Berquist, 1991, Raven Press, © Mayo Foundation.

femoral ligament, that follows the PCL to its attachment on the femur. Between the anterior horns of the medial and lateral menisci there is a transverse band of fibers termed the transverse ligament of the knee. This can easily be confused with an anterior meniscal tear, especially on the medial side.[17,20,23]

Muscles about the Knee

The muscles about the knee provide active restraints.[17,26] Chief movements at the knee are those of flexion and extension. Mild rotation, however, can occur. If one starts from the flexed position, the posterior condyles of the femur are in contact with the posterior horns of both menisci. The MCL and LCL are also relaxed in this position. In full flexion, both the ACL and the PCL are taut. In this flexed position more rotary motion is allowed. As one goes from the flexed to the extended position, the femoral condyles shift such that the more anterior parts of the menisci and tibial condyles are now in contact.[17,18,22,27]

The primary flexors of the knee are the hamstring muscle group (semimembranosus, semitendinosus, and biceps femoris) along with the gracilis and sartorius. The popliteus muscle (Fig. 6-3) has some significance in the early phases of flexion because of its rotary action upon the femur or tibia. In the non–weight-bearing state, the gastrocnemius muscle is also utilized in flexion of the knee. The quadriceps group is the chief extensor of the knee (Fig. 6-3A).[17,26]

Neurovascular Supply of the Knee

The arterial supply about the knee is primarily via branch vessels of the distal superficial femoral and popliteal arteries. Superiorly there are medial and lateral genicular arteries as well as muscular branches at the level of the knee joint. Inferiorly, medial and lateral inferior genicular arteries supply the knee. There are numerous anastomoses that interconnect this vascular supply.[20,23]

Innervation of the knee is primarily by branches of the femoral, obturator, and sciatic nerves. Posterolaterally, recurrent branches of the peroneal nerve also supply the knee.[17,20,23] More specific anatomic information is provided later in discussion of specific injuries.

IMAGING OF THE KNEE

This section provides basic background information about techniques required for evaluating most athletic injuries. Specific variations in techniques may be required for certain injuries. Certain approaches are discussed more completely as they apply to specific injuries discussed in later sections of the chapter.

Routine Radiography

Anteroposterior (AP) and lateral radiographs fulfill the minimum requirements for evaluating knee trauma. In addition, at the Mayo Clinic we routinely obtain both oblique views.[32,47] The AP view may be obtained with the patient supine, the leg extended, and the patella positioned anteriorly (Fig. 6-5).[32] Upright standing views, however, are required to access accurately the femorotibial joint. Several techniques can be used in patients who are able to bear weight for this procedure. Typically, a 14 × 17 cassette is positioned posterior to the knee so that the lower femurs and upper tibias and fibulas are included on the film. The tube is parallel to the floor or angled slightly (tibial plateau, 10° caudad posteriorly) toward the feet.[32] More recently, a 45° weight-bearing view has been described by Rosenberg et al.[55] The knees are flexed 45°, and the tube is angled 10° off the horizontal (Fig. 6-6). The tube is positioned 40 inches from the cassette. This method was found to be more accurate than conventional extension weight-bearing views in evaluating cartilage lesions.[55]

The lateral view may be obtained with routine positioning or with cross-table technique.[32,45,61] In most situations the lateral projection is obtained by positioning the patient on the side with the involved knee adjacent to the table top. The knee should be flexed about 30°. This permits more accurate assessment of the patellofemoral space and patellar position. The

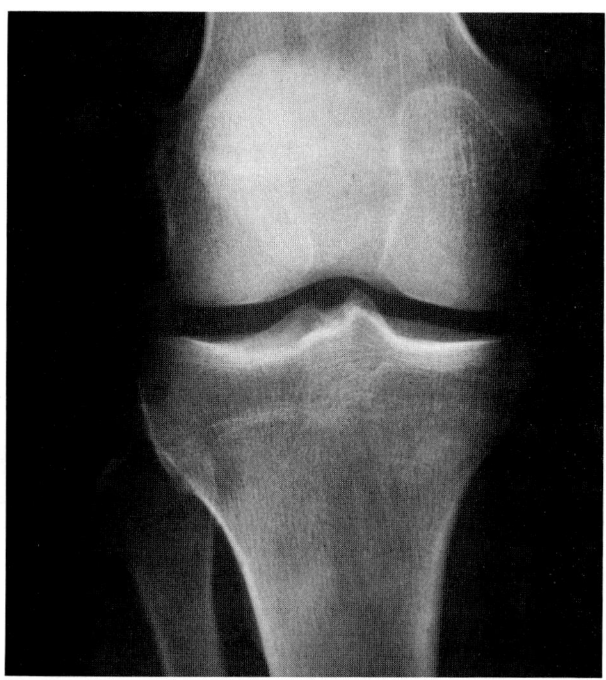

Fig. 6-5 Normal anteroposterior (AP) view of the knee taken with the patient supine. The patella is obscured.

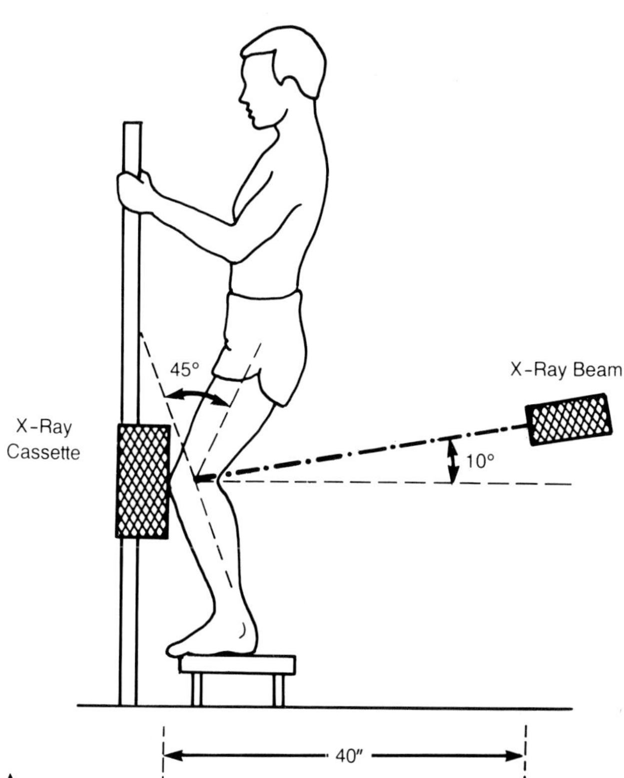

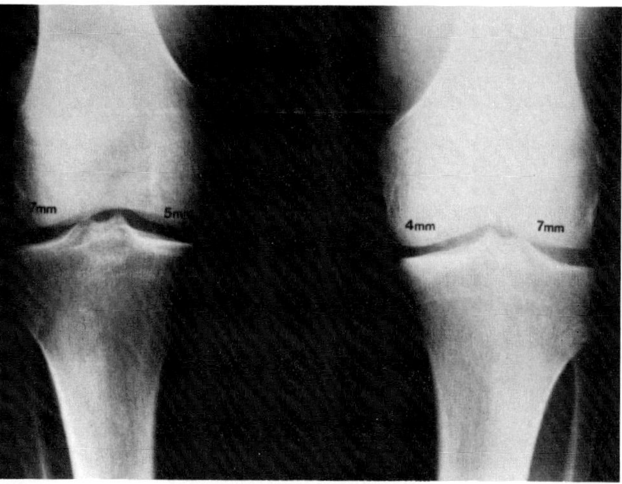

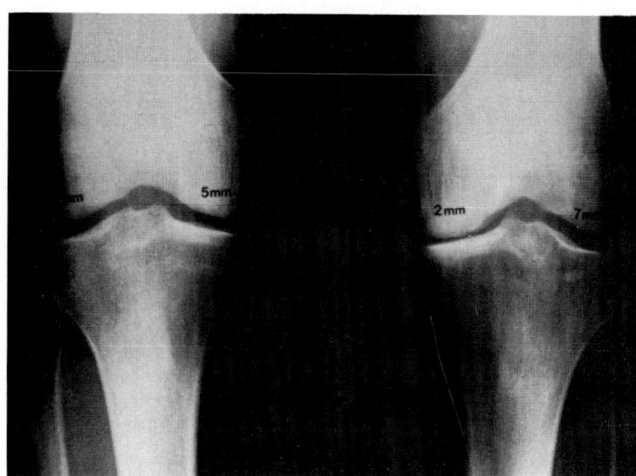

Fig. 6-6 (**A**) Illustration of patient positioned for 45° PA view of the knees. (**B**) Routine standing view shows only minimal medial compartment narrowing medially. (**C**) Forty-five degree PA flexion weight-bearing view demonstrates the joint space changes more clearly. *Source:* Reprinted with permission from *Journal of Bone and Joint Surgery* (1988;70A:1479–1483), Copyright © 1988, Journal of Bone and Joint Surgery.

8 × 10 cassette is centered under the joint with the beam angled 5° to the head. This prevents the magnified medial condyle from obscuring the joint space (Fig. 6-7A).[32]

Effusions may also be detected on the lateral view. Detection of effusions on the lateral view is approximately 77% accurate.[32,45,61] In the presence of an effusion, the posterior quadriceps tendon may be indistinct, the suprapatellar and prefemoral fat pads may be separated by 5 mm or more, or a suprapatellar soft tissue density larger than 10 mm may appear (Fig. 6-7B). The patella may also be displaced more anteriorly in relationship to the femur. An uncommon sign is displacement of the fabella. This displacement requires a large effusion.[32,61]

An alternative method for the lateral view, the cross-table technique, is useful in patients who cannot be moved or in patients with subtle fractures. The cassette is positioned perpendicular to the table and may be held between the knees for support. A small cushion under the knee will ensure that the entire structure is included in the film. The beam is centered on the joint and directed perpendicular to the cassette. This view will demonstrate a lipohemarthrosis, which may be the only indication of an intraarticular fracture (Fig. 6-7C).

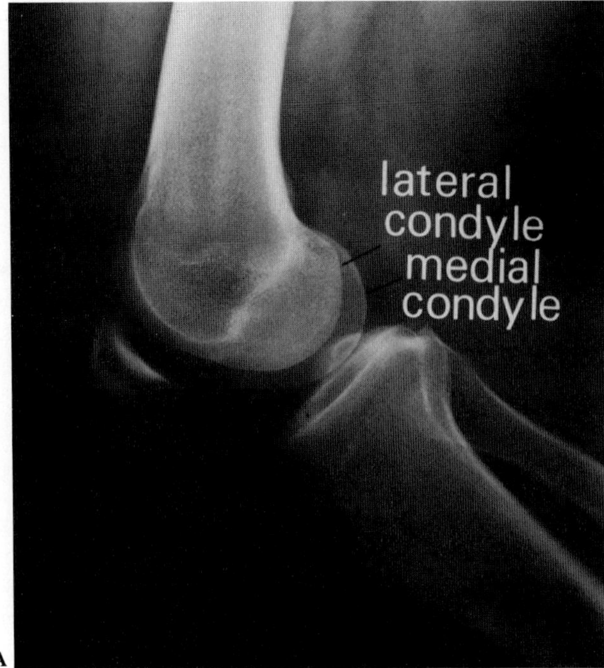

A

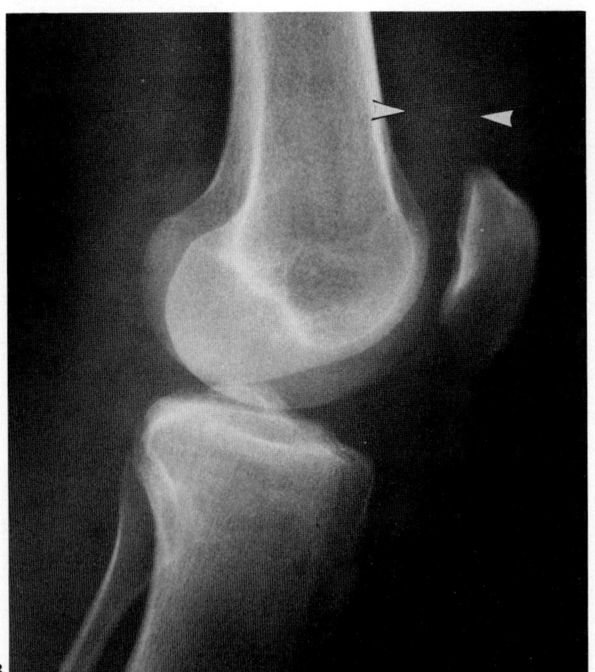

B

Fig. 6-7 (A) Normal lateral view of the knee. (B) Routine lateral view demonstrating fluid in the suprapatellar bursa (arrowheads). (C) Cross-table lateral view demonstrating a lipohemarthrosis (arrows).

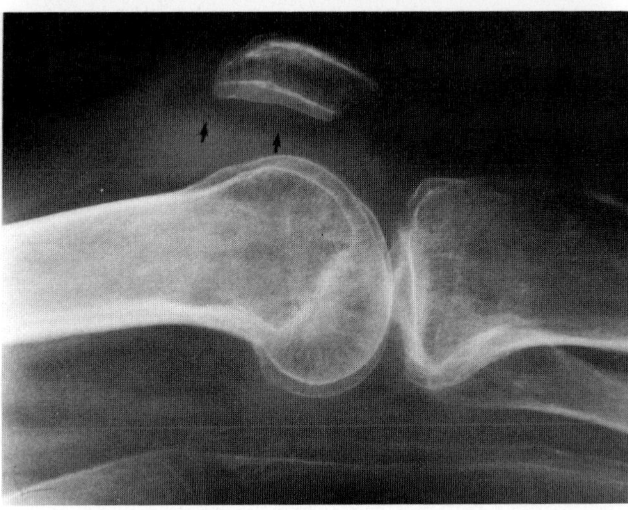

C

Both oblique views can be obtained with the patient supine. For the internal oblique view, the leg is internally rotated about 45°. The cassette is centered under the joint space with the central beam perpendicular to the cassette. This view provides excellent detail of the upper fibula and tibiofibular articulation. The lateral femoral condyle is also seen to better advantage (Fig. 6-8A). The external oblique view is obtained with the same parameters but with the leg rotated externally 45° (Fig. 6-8B). The fibula is projected behind the upper tibia. The medial tibial plateau and femoral condyle are clearly demonstrated.[32]

An alternative method for oblique views is available for patients who cannot be moved. The tube can be angled 45° medially and laterally with the cassette positioned flat on the table and opposite the tube.[38]

These four views (AP, lateral, and both obliques) are usually sufficient for evaluation of the acutely injured patient. The clinical setting, however, may dictate that views of the patella or intercondylar notch be obtained.

Notch View

This view is obtained with the patient prone on the table. The knee is flexed 40°, and the foot is supported on a bolster. The 8 × 10 cassette is placed under the knee with the tube centered on the cassette and angled 40° toward the feet. Simultaneous views of both knees can also be obtained.

The notch view is particularly useful for evaluating patients with osteochondritis dissecans because it visualizes the tibial spines and detects osteochondral fragments in the joint space (Fig. 6-9). An alternative method has been described by Holmblad.[47]

Patellar Views

Tangential views of the patella are frequently required to evaluate position, fractures, and the patellofemoral joint space. Numerous techniques have been described for patellar evaluation.[32,41,50,57] The two most commonly used techniques at the Mayo Clinic are the Merchant and Settegast methods.[32,57]

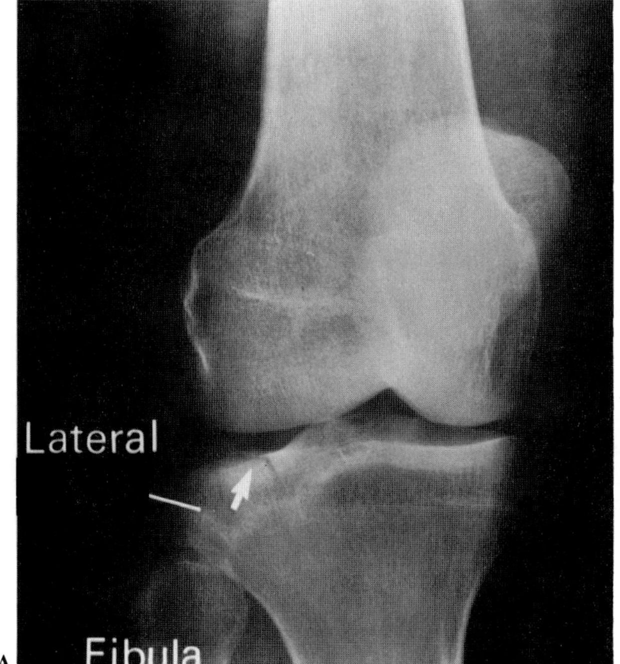

A

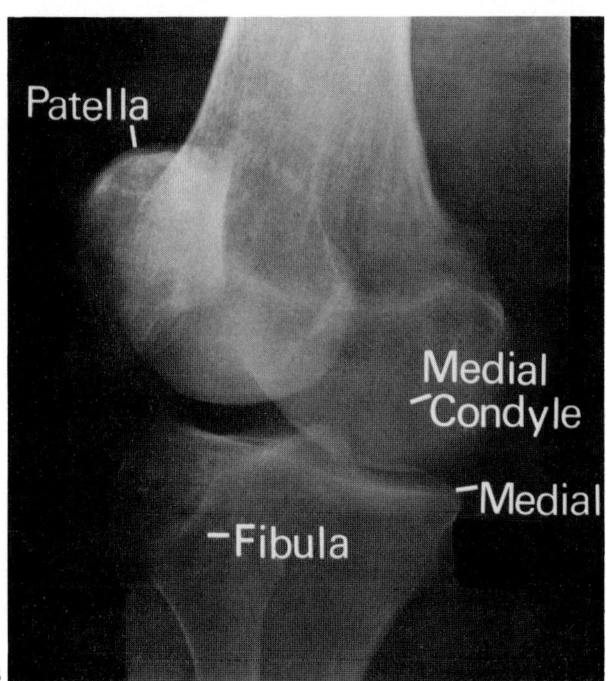

B

Fig. 6-8 (**A**) Internal oblique view. There is a subtle fracture of the lateral plateau (arrow) that was not evident on the other routine views. (**B**) External oblique view.

Consistency is obtained more readily with the Merchant view (Fig. 6-10). The knees are flexed 45° over the table with the cassette perpendicular to the legs. The beam is angled 30° to the horizontal and centered on the cassette. The resulting view clearly demonstrates the patella and patellofemoral relationship (Fig. 6-10).[32]

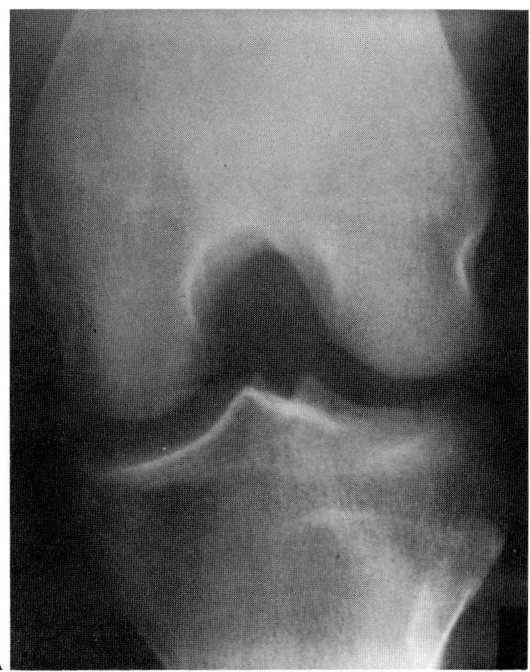

A

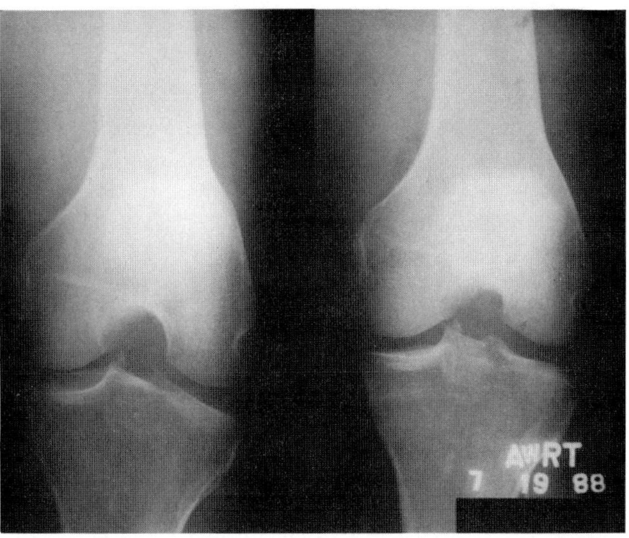

B

Fig. 6-9 (**A**) Normal notch view of the knee. (**B**) Notch view demonstrating a subtle tibial spine fracture.

Stress Views

Initial assessment of suspected ligament injury can be accomplished with stress views. Accuracy of stress views depends upon the experience of the examining physician and the patient's symptoms. Pain and swelling make it difficult to perform this technique in the acutely injured knee. MRI is valuable in this setting and is discussed more fully later. Stress views in patients with acute injuries usually require anesthetic injection, general anesthesia, or spinal anesthesia. The examination is most commonly performed manually by fixing the

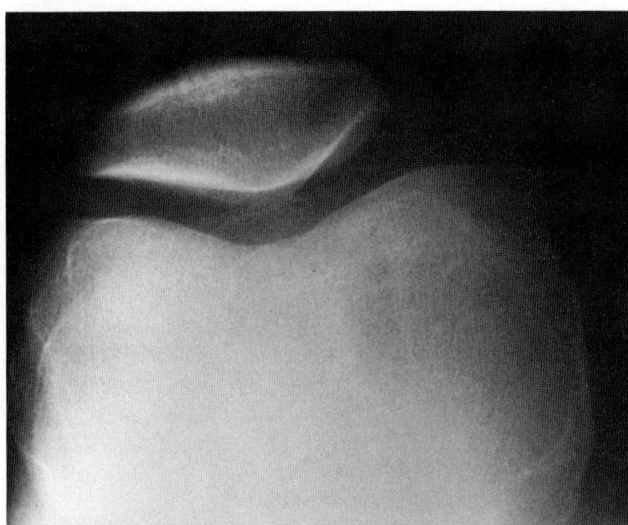

Fig. 6-10 Normal patellar view (Merchant view). The lateral facet is usually larger than the medial.

extremity with a bolster or strap and applying force in the opposite direction (Fig. 6-11). Commercially manufactured devices are now available to obtain more consistency for both AP and varus-valgus stress views (Fig. 6-12).[54,55,62]

Positioning of the joint to assess for both mediolateral and AP instability is best done fluoroscopically. This allows proper angulation of the tube to ensure that the beam is tangential to the joint surfaces.

The measurement can be calculated from the films with the normal knee used for comparison. In the normal knee, minimal motion is possible with stress. On the AP view lines are constructed along the inferior margin of the femoral condyles and lower cortical margins of the tibial plateaus. The angle formed by these lines, as well as the vertical distance in the joint space, is then measured during varus and valgus stress (Fig. 6-11). A difference of more than 5 mm or an angle increase of approximately 10° compared to the normal knee is significant.[32]

Measuring AP instability is much more difficult with radiographic techniques. Positioning is more difficult, and consistency in measurement is difficult to obtain.[32,62] Clinical examination is probably as accurate in most situations of suspected capsular or cruciate ligament injury. If AP stress views are to be performed, the knee is flexed 90° with anterior and posterior forces applied to the tibia just below the knee (Fig. 6-13). Lateral views should be obtained on both the injured and uninvolved knee during these maneuvers. A difference of 3 mm or more is significant.[32]

Conventional and Computed Tomography

Subtle osseous injuries may be overlooked on routine radiographs. In this setting radionuclide scans may be useful. Definitive diagnosis of the type and extent of injury, however, may require conventional tomography or computed tomography (CT).[31,32,52] Conventional tomograms should be obtained in the AP and lateral projections with 3- to 5-mm

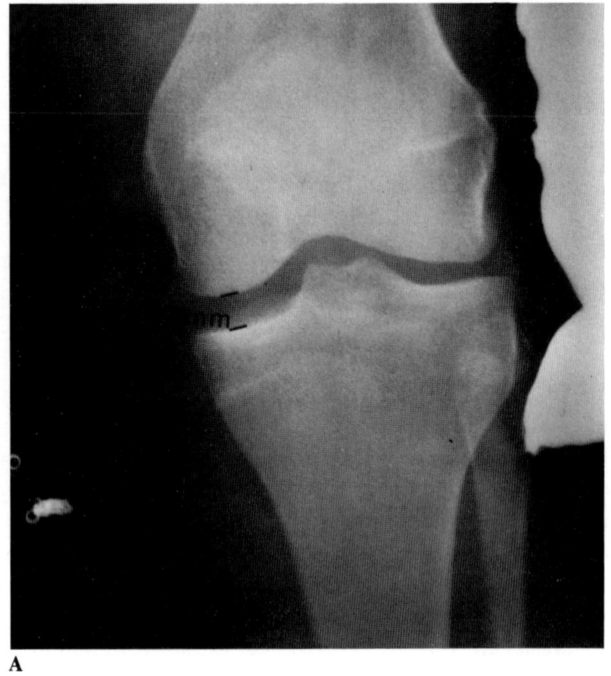

A

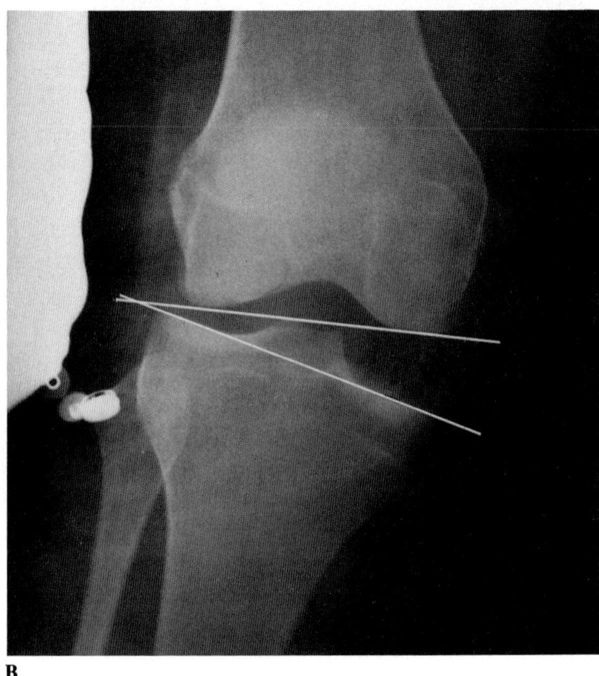

B

Fig. 6-11 Manually positioned stress views of the normal (**A**) and injured (**B**) knee. There is marked widening of the medial joint space in the injured knee (lines in **B**) due to medial collateral ligament (MCL) and capsular injury.

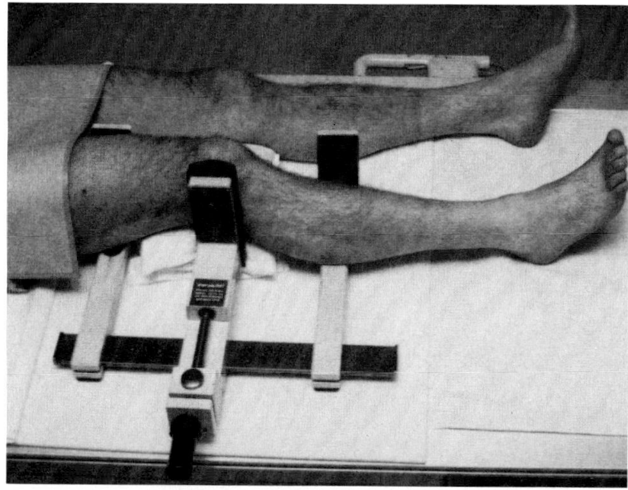

Fig. 6-12 Device for valgus stress view of the knee. *Source:* Reprinted with permission from Tegtmeyer CJ, Weiland DJ and McCue PC, Stress examination of the cruciate ligaments in *Radiology* (1987;165:867–869), Copyright © 1987, Radiological Society of North America.

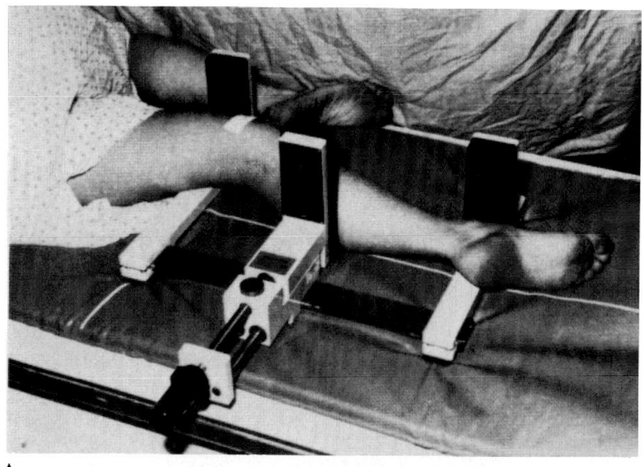

A

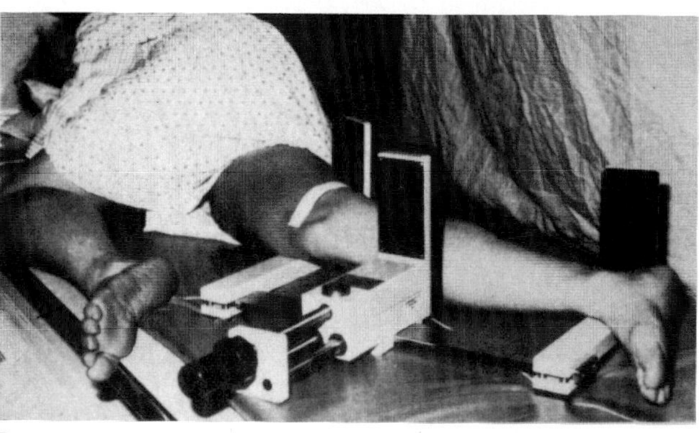

B

Fig. 6-13 Commercial device for AP stress radiographs. *Source:* Reprinted with permission from *Skeletal Radiology* (1987;12:617–620), Copyright © 1987, Springer-Verlag.

sections (Fig. 6-14). CT is less frequently used in our practice. AP, lateral, or fast-scan techniques with flexion and extension, however, may be useful for certain bone and soft tissue injuries and for evaluating patellar tracking disorders.[51,52,56,60] Thin sections (3 mm) are usually required.

Ultrasonography

Since the advent of MRI, ultrasonography has not been used frequently to evaluate knee injuries. Certain superficial ligament and tendon injuries can be studied effectively with ultrasound.[44,49] For example, the patellar ligament, quadriceps tendon, MCL, and LCL can be evaluated effectively with real-time scanning.[32,51] Meniscal cysts and articular cartilage have also been evaluated with ultrasound.[30,39] MRI is such an effective screening technique, however, that ultrasound is rarely used in our practice.[33]

Magnetic Resonance Imaging

The techniques used for evaluating the knee should be tailored to the clinical indication and the imaging system that is employed.[33–37] Although many techniques and image planes may be used, the following discussion is oriented toward the routine screening examination that is commonly used to evaluate most articular and periarticular disorders of the knee. More specific techniques are discussed later in the applications sections as they apply to particular clinical settings.

Typically, the patient is placed in the supine position with the knee placed in a closely coupled extremity coil (Fig. 6-15). The knee is externally rotated 15° to 20° to facilitate visualization of the ACL on sagittal images.[33,37,43]

In choosing pulse sequences, the physician now has many options, ranging from spin-echo sequences to various gradient-echo sequences.[33,36] The contrast requirements in knee imaging are mixed. Meniscal tears are best imaged with MR sequences that are neither purely T1 weighted nor purely T2 weighted. Other structures such as ligaments are best evaluated with T2-weighted images.[37]

A technical requirement that should not be underestimated is the need to use an adequate image geometry. The menisci and the cruciate ligaments are complex structures, and it is unreasonable to expect to be able to evaluate them reliably with a single slice orientation.

The pulse sequences that are now widely available for knee imaging are spin-echo techniques and gradient-echo techniques, both slice selective and three-dimensional Fourier transformation (3DFT) versions.[33]

In the spin-echo category, short TR/TE sequences and long TR multiecho sequences are typically used (TR, repetition time; TE, echo time). We rarely recommend the sole use of

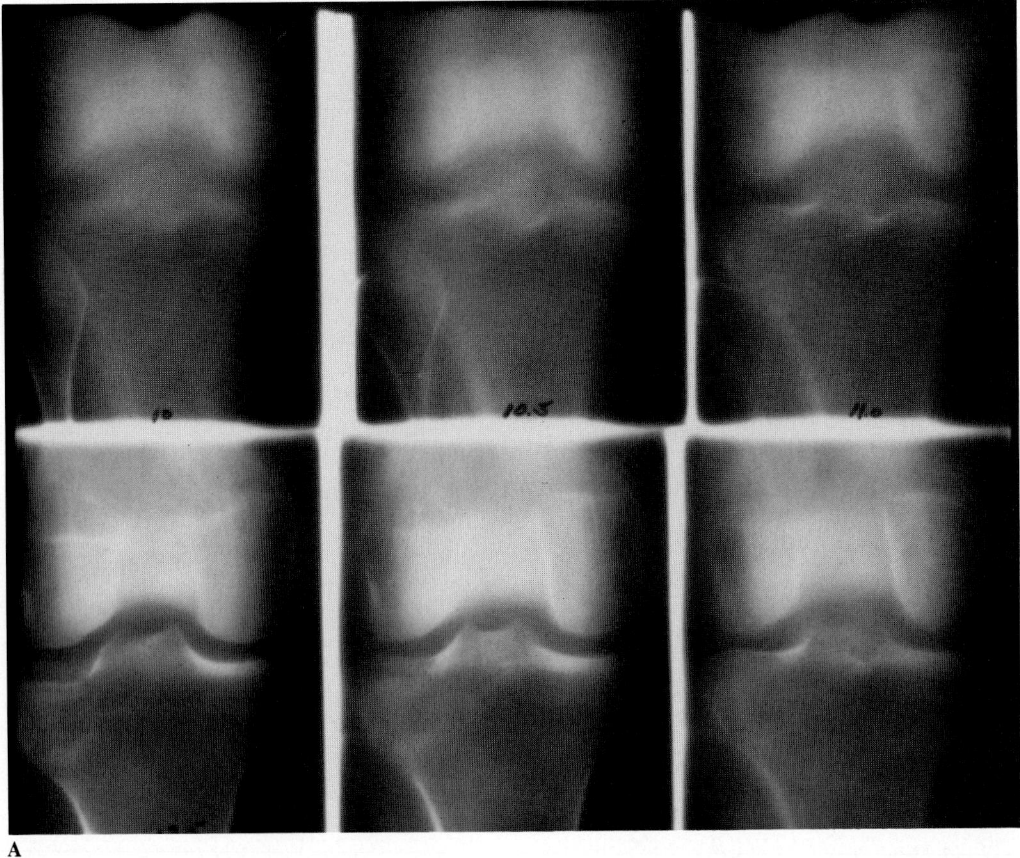

A

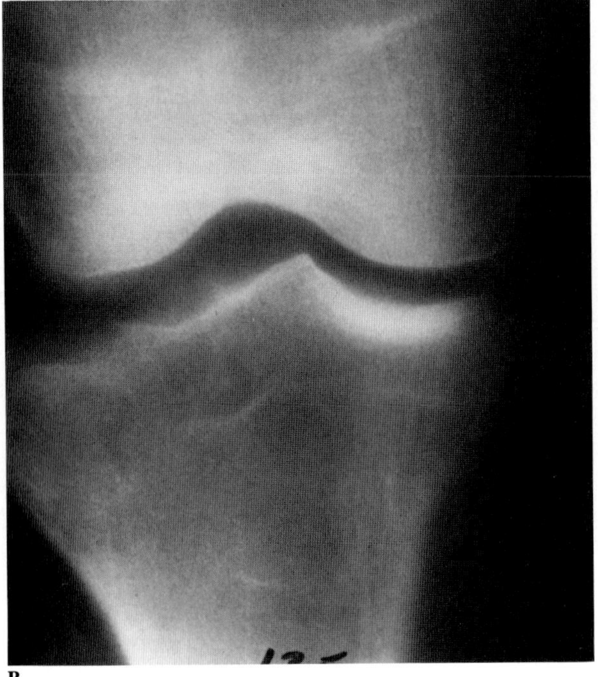

B

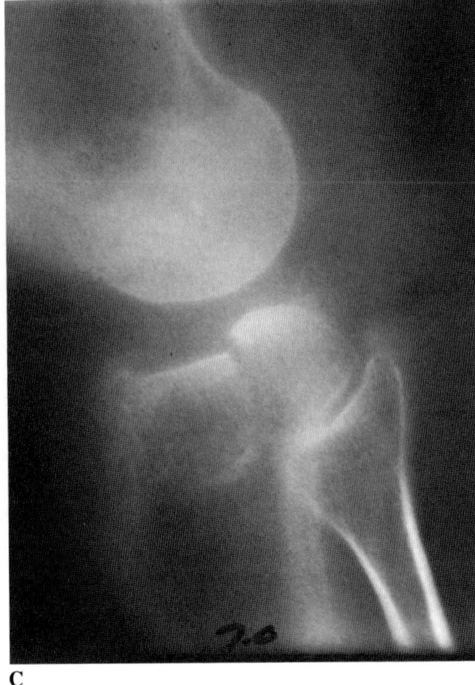

C

Fig. 6-14 Conventional tomography of a lateral plateau fracture. (**A**) Serial AP, (**B**) selected AP, and (**C**) lateral sections clearly demonstrate the extent of fracture and articular depression.

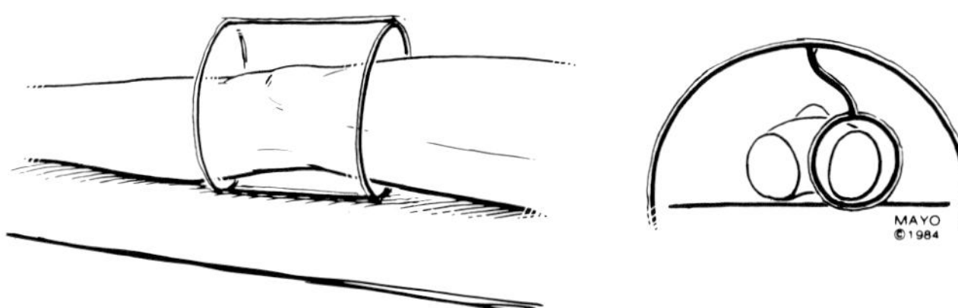

Fig. 6-15 Illustration of a patient positioned for magnetic resonance imaging (MRI) of the knee with the knee in a circumferential extremity coil. *Source:* Reprinted from *Magnetic Resonance Imaging of the Musculoskeletal System* by TH Berquist, 1990, Raven Press, © Mayo Foundation.

short TR/TE spin-echo sequences for knee imaging. Although they are technically undemanding, rapidly acquired, and sensitive for medullary bone lesions, they provide low contrast for meniscal lesions, acute ligamentous injuries, and the interface between joint fluid and articular cartilage.

Long TR multiecho spin-echo sequences are effective for knee imaging. The short first echo provides intermediate contrast, which is excellent for identifying meniscal lesions, and the long second echo provides T2-weighted contrast, which is crucial for evaluation of the cruciate ligaments and other normally low-signal structures.[33,37]

An adequate approach for knee imaging is to perform sagittal and coronal spin-echo acquisitions.[37,43] The exact technical approach will depend on the imaging hardware utilized. We have found the following parameters to be efficient and reliable with a 1.5-T imager: TE 20/60, or 80 msec, TR 2000 msec, 1 number of excitations (NEX), 192 views, 3-mm slices with 1.5-mm gaps, and 16-cm field of view. These acquisitions require only 7.3 minutes each.

Long TR multiecho sequences have the advantages of high slice throughput and excellent contrast characteristics. They require longer acquisition times, however.

Gradient-echo techniques have seen increasing use for musculoskeletal imaging in the last several years. They provide interesting capabilities in terms of contrast and speed. These techniques can be broadly divided into steady-state sequences, such as gradient recalled steady-state (GRASS) and fast imaging with steady-state free precision (FISP), and spoiled sequences, such as fast low-angled single-shot imaging (FLASH) and spoiled GRASS.[33,58,59]

Multislice gradient-echo acquisitions can be performed in two ways: Each slice is acquired individually and sequentially, or the slices are acquired in an interleaved fashion similar to that for multislice spin-echo imaging. For the first alternative, the TR must be short so that the total imaging time to acquire the entire set of slices will not be excessively long.[33] For knee imaging, the longer TR interleaved approach improves contrast and signal-to-noise characteristics of the images compared with short TR gradient-echo sequences.[33]

These long TR, medium TE gradient-echo sequences provide excellent contrast for delineating meniscal tears. Long TR gradient-echo sequences can provide pronounced T2-weighted contrast for depicting ligamentous lesions. Long TR gradient-echo images are also effective for depicting chondral and osteochondral lesions.[33]

We prefer multislice gradient-echo technique with radial imaging. The structure of the meniscus is such that a radially oriented set of slices placed at the center of each semicircular meniscus is a geometrically advantageous imaging approach. The slices in a conventional spin-echo acquisition cannot be crossed for a good reason: There would be severe signal loss in the region of intersection. The special properties of gradient-echo sequences allow them not to have this limitation. In other words, a long TR multislice gradient-echo acquisition with this kind of geometry can have little signal loss in the region where the slices intersect (Fig. 6-16).[33]

It is possible to set up an acquisition of 18 or 20 images that are radially oriented about both menisci and to perform the acquisition in 8 minutes or less. The starting point is a transverse scout image at the joint line. The center of each tibial plateau is identified, and a set of radial images is graphically prescribed. Initially, we utilized separate radial acquisitions for medial and lateral menisci (Fig. 6-16, B and C). These each consisted of double-echo interleaved GRASS sequences (GRIL; TE 12/31 msec, TR 600 to 700 msec, 2 NEX, flip angle 25°, 192 views, 5-mm slice thickness, 16-cm field of view, 10 sections at 18° rotational increments radiating from the central point). These acquisitions require about 5 minutes each.

More recently, we have used a single acquisition to obtain both sets of radial images. The acquisition is graphically prescribed from a transverse scout. A single-echo GRIL sequence with a TE of 15 msec provides excellent results (TR 600 msec, 2 NEX, flip angle 15°, 192 views, 5-mm slice thickness, 16-cm field of view, two radially oriented sets of 9 sections at 20° rotational increments). This complete radial acquisition sequence for both menisci takes less than 4 minutes.[33]

The radial geometry is not suitable for delineation of the cruciate ligaments. Because spin-echo images seem to provide slightly better depiction of ligamentous injuries, we follow the radial examination of the menisci with a sagittal spin-echo acquisition as described earlier. This yields a high-quality examination of the knee with a total imaging time of 12 to 14 minutes. When indicated (eg, patellar tracking, chondromalacia, or plica syndrome), additional images are obtained in the axial plane. T2-Weighted spin-echo or gradient-echo sequences can be selected.[58,59]

Arthrography and Diagnostic and Therapeutic Injections

MRI has essentially replaced knee arthrography, especially for evaluating acute athletic injuries.[33,48] MRI is capable of

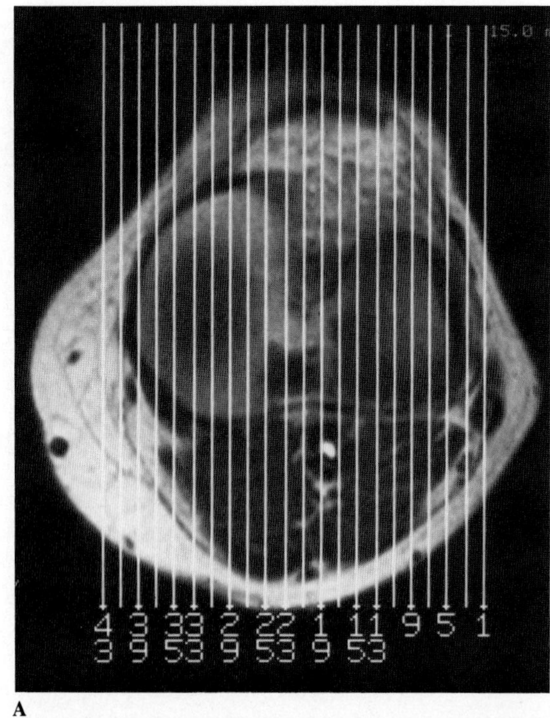

A

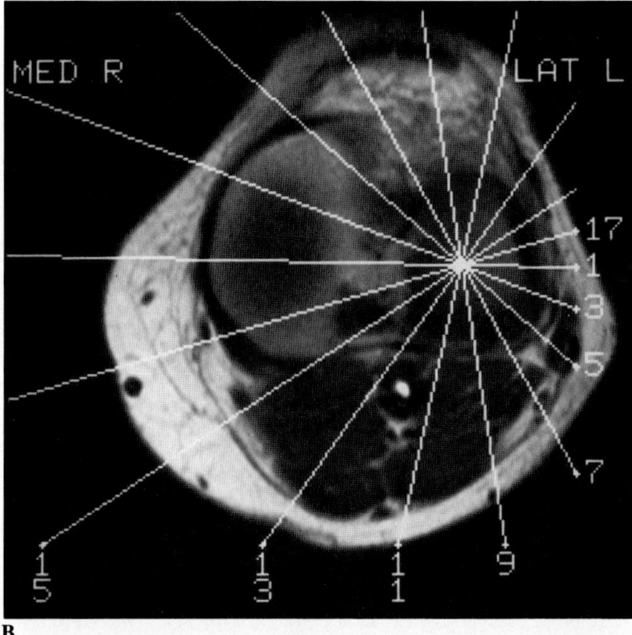

B

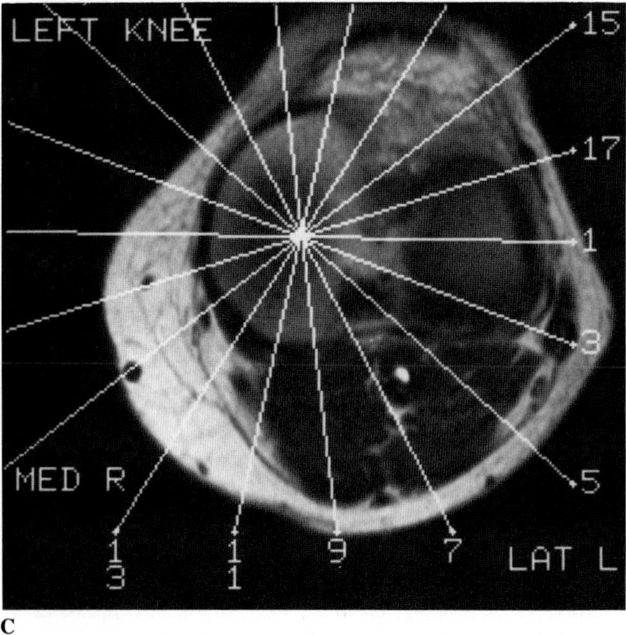

C

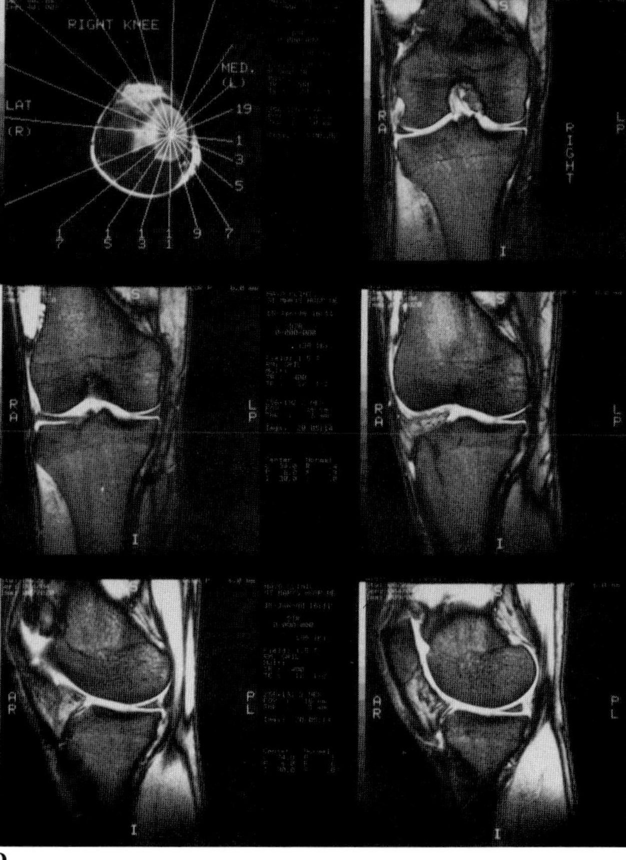

D

Fig. 6-16 MRI technique for screening knee examination. (**A**) Scout axial image with sections for sagittal images selected. (**B** and **C**) Radial sections selected for the lateral (**B**) and medial (**C**) menisci. (**D**) Series of radial images demonstrating tangential meniscal anatomy.

detecting lesions in bone, cartilage, menisci, ligaments, and surrounding soft tissues.[33] Arthrography is less expensive generally and still accurate for evaluating meniscal lesions. Accuracy for detection of meniscal tears is about 93%.[40] Nevertheless, other injuries, specifically of the cruciate ligaments, are less effectively evaluated with arthrography, even when stress views and double-contrast techniques are employed.[32,42,46,48]

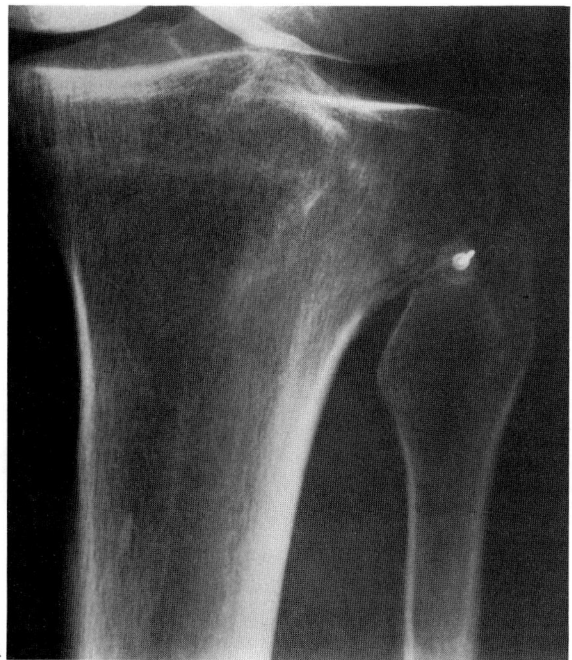

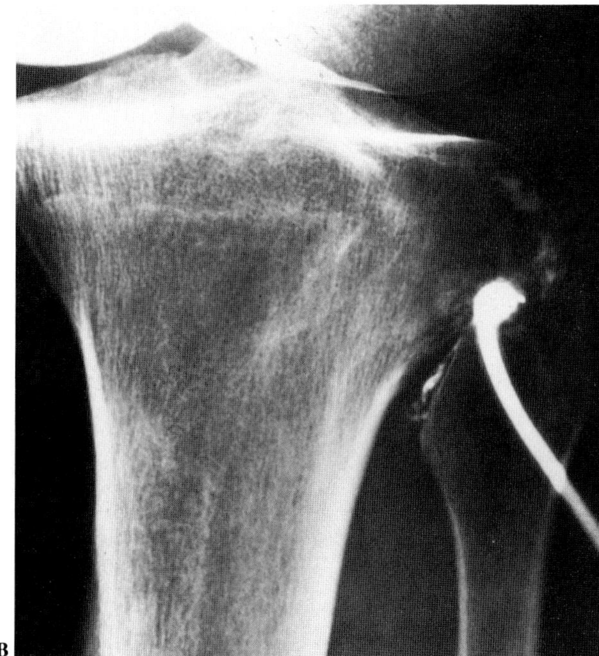

Fig. 6-17 Proximal tibiofibular injection. (**A**) Knee fluoroscopically positioned in internal rotation to align the tibiofibular articulation. (**B**) Contrast injection confirms needle position before injection of 1:1 bupivacaine and betamethasone.

Arthrography and injection techniques may still be useful in certain situations, specifically when needle access is required for fluid aspiration or when injection of anesthetic and/or steroid is indicated for diagnostic or therapeutic purposes. The knee is typically entered laterally just posterior to the patella.[32] Medial and superior approaches are infrequently used. Injection of the proximal tibiofibular articulation may also be indicated in patients with suspected subluxation or local pain (Fig. 6-17). Relief of symptoms following diagnostic injection confirms the location of the symptoms and may provide significant long-term improvement.[32]

Arthroscopy

The role of arthroscopy for diagnostic and therapeutic purposes is well defined for athletic injuries.[32,53] Although arthroscopy is not an imaging technique, the above techniques have affected the role and utilization of arthroscopy in athletes.

Arthroscopy allows early evaluation of menisci, cruciate ligaments, articular surfaces, and capsule. Early assessment and treatment permit earlier return to activity. Athletic participation may be resumed as early as 4 weeks after arthroscopic surgery.[53]

Despite the usefulness of arthroscopy, the need for early intervention can be accurately assessed with MRI. In this manner, conservative therapy may be selected over arthroscopic intervention when MR findings do not indicate an injury that can be managed arthroscopically. Arthroscopy is indicated for management of cruciate ligament, meniscal, articular, or osteochondral injuries and plicae.[32,53]

PATELLAR DISORDERS

Disorders of the patellofemoral joint are common in athletes. Patellofemoral arthralgia, instability, and fractures are frequent. A review of the anatomic features of this region is useful before considering specific injuries and imaging of patellar disorders.

Anatomy

The triangular patella is divided on its articular surface by a vertical median ridge into medial and lateral facets. The medial facet is convex, and the lateral facet is concave. The thickest articular cartilage, which may measure up to 4 to 5 mm in thickness, is present on the median ridge.[92] The trochlear surface of the femur may be divided into convex medial and lateral facets. The lateral trochlear facet is larger and extends more proximally than the medial facet.[112] The superior aspect of the lateral trochlear facet has a smooth transition with the anterior femoral cortex, and the superior medial trochlear facet has a prominent bony and cartilaginous ridge 3 to 8 mm in height.[71,102]

Patellar stabilizers on the medial side are the patellofemoral ligament superiorly and the meniscopatellar ligament inferiorly.[78] The lateral stabilizers are the patellofemoral liga-

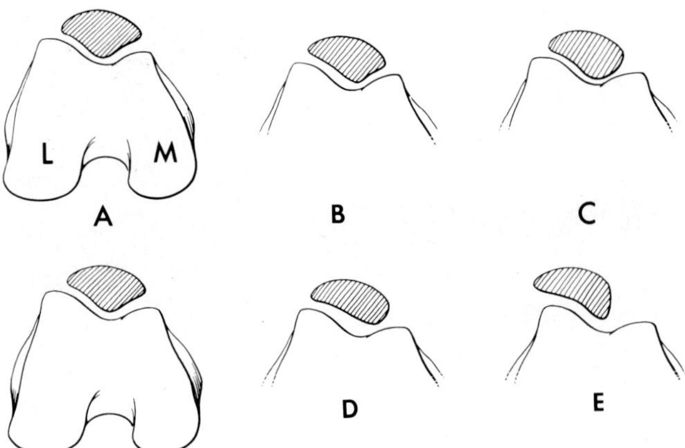

Fig. 6-18 Variations in patellar and condylar anatomy.[68,112] (**A**) I: medial (M) and lateral (L) facets equal. (**B**) II: lateral facet larger than the medial facet. (**C**) III: small medial facet and hypoplastic medial condyle. (**D**) IV: absent medial facet. (**E**) V: no medial facet and lateral subluxation.

ment superiorly and the meniscopatellar ligament inferiorly. The fascia lata also has an attachment laterally to the patella. The lateral stabilizers are stronger than the medial stabilizers. The dynamic stabilizers consist of the four components of the quadriceps muscle. The patellar ligament extends from the inferior part of the patella to the tibial tubercle and has a slight lateral orientation.[68,78,83]

Various patellar shapes and configurations of the trochlea may be present (Fig. 6-18). Wiberg[112] reported on the major patellar types. In type I the medial and lateral patellar facets are equal in size. In type II the medial facet is slightly smaller than the lateral facet (Fig. 6-10). In type III the medial patellar facet is small, and there may be hypoplasia of the medial trochlear facet of the femur. A Wiberg type II patella is the most frequent type.[79,112] The flattened patella or hemipatella with one facet (alpine hunter's cap) is frequently associated with symptoms of patellar instability.[79] Patellar fragmentation (Fig. 6-1) is a common finding, with a bipartite patella being present in 0.05% to 1.66% of knees.[68,79] A bipartite patella may be distinguished from a fracture by a clearly defined radiolucency with rounded margins separating the fragments, sclerosis of the margins, and bilaterality of the lesion (Fig. 6-1).

In the extended position, the patella lies above the trochlear surface of the femur and rests on a layer of subsynovial fat.[108] In this position the patella lies laterally in 87% of knees, with contact being made between the crest of the patella or lateral facet and the lateral trochlear facet.[76] Contact between the patella and trochlea begins with 10° to 20° of flexion. In 20° to 30° of flexion, about 30% of patellas are centered in the trochlear groove.[76,84,86] Hence lateral radiographs are usually obtained with 30% of flexion (see Figs. 6-1 and 6-7). With increasing flexion, the area of contact moves proximally on the patella, and only the articular surface of the patella contacts the trochlea between 30° and 80° of flexion.[76,86] With increasing flexion, the patella also becomes more centered in the trochlear groove, and 96% of the patella is centered with 90° of flexion.[89] Beyond 80° to 90° of knee flexion, the patellar tendon begins to articulate with the femur.[84,86]

The screw-home mechanism of the knee with external rotation of the tibia in the terminal 30° of extension rotates the tibia laterally. This external rotation produces the Q angle, a valgus vector between the quadriceps tendon and the patellar ligament.[86] This valgus vector tends toward lateral displacement of the patella and must be resisted by the static and dynamic medial stabilizers, which consist of the vastus medialis, the medial retinaculum, and the bony architecture of the femur and patella. As knee flexion progresses, the patella is drawn from its superolateral position onto the trochlear surface of the femur and gradually into the intercondylar notch, resulting in a C-shaped tracking that is open laterally.[86]

The patella facilitates knee extension by increasing the distance between the extensor mechanism and the rotational axis of the femur.[78,86] The patella also centralizes the action of the quadriceps muscle, allowing transmission of its force around an angle during knee flexion with minimal loss due to friction.[86] In full extension, the patella is responsible for almost 30% of the quadriceps moment arm.[68,78]

Patellofemoral Pain Syndrome

The clinical syndromes related to the patellofemoral joint are typically due to pain and/or instability. The term *chondromalacia patellae* was initially used by Aleman[64] in 1928 to describe episodes of crepitus and synovitis associated with softening and fissuring of the articular surface of the patella. Since the initial description, the term *chondromalacia patellae* has been used for a number of disorders. To avoid confusion, the term *patellofemoral pain syndrome* is reserved for the description of patients with patellofemoral pain without instability.[78,79,83] The term *chondromalacia* is best restricted to cases involving description of a pathologic entity.[67,68,79]

Patients with patellofemoral pain syndrome present with retropatellar pain and crepitation associated with sitting and ascending or descending stairs.[78,92] Symptoms of giving way, pseudolocking, and swelling are also frequent.[82,92,99] On physical examination there is crepitation, pain on compression of the patella, facet tenderness, effusion, and occasionally abnormal patellar tracking.[78,92,93] Other conditions such as prepatellar bursitis, painful retropatellar fat pad, pes anserinus bursitis, plica syndrome, meniscal lesions, generalized synovitis, and ligamentous instability must be considered in the differential diagnosis.[68,78,99] The excessive lateral pressure syndrome is a clinical radiologic entity characterized by pain and radiographic evidence of tilting of the patella laterally without lateral subluxation.[78] Physical examination reveals a tight lateral retinaculum. Radiographs reveal narrowing of cartilage, increased density in the subchondral bone layer with a change in alignment of the trabeculae from their normal orientation perpendicular to the equator of the patella to a position perpendicular to the lateral facet, and a tight and thickened lateral retinaculum.[68,78]

The pathologic changes of chondromalacia patellae frequently accompany these syndromes. These lesions have been classified with several systems. Outerbridge[102,103] and Outerbridge and Dunlop[104] divided the changes in the articular cartilage into four grades: softening and swelling of the articular cartilage, fragmentation and fissuring in an area 0.5 inch in diameter or less, fragmentation and fissuring in an area greater than 0.5 inch in diameter, and erosion of cartilage down to bone. An arthroscopic grading system for chondromalacia has also been suggested.[78] These arthroscopic grades include early fibrillation or softening of the articular cartilage involving one or more facets of the patella without involvement of the femur, fragmentation or erosion of the articular surface limited to the patella, and articular cartilage changes involving the femur as well as the patella. Goodfellow et al[83] have suggested that there are two distinct pathologic processes affecting the patella: basal degeneration and surface degeneration. Surface degeneration is present in youth, becomes more frequent with age, and primarily affects the odd facet. This process is not associated with patellofemoral pain in youth but may lead to degenerative arthritis in later years. Basal degeneration is a fasciculation of collagen in the middle and deep zones of cartilage that later affects the surface. Basal degeneration is associated with patellofemoral pain in the young individual. It may be divided into three stages: fasciculation of the deep collagen layers with an intact surface, blister formation, and fasciculation extending through the surface of the articular cartilage. Basal degeneration may be the result of excessive pressure and trauma to the patella in this area.[83]

Chondromalacia may also be classified by its anatomic location. Five groups have been established.[79] Group 1 involves the lateral patellar facet, usually just lateral to the median ridge. Group 2 involves the medial facet, usually the odd facet. Group 3 is central chondromalacia affecting the median ridge and extending onto both facets. Group 4 is bipolar chondromalacia involving the central portion of the two facets separated by a normal median ridge. Group 5 is global or total chondromalacia involving the totality of both facets.[79]

The etiology of chondromalacia and patellofemoral pain has remained controversial.[75] Chondromalacia patellae may be related to biomechanical or biochemical causes.[92] Biomechanical causes can be divided into acute and chronic. Acute injuries include dislocation (Fig. 6-19), direct trauma, and fracture. Chronic symptoms may be related to recurrent subluxation, patellar malalignment, excessive lateral pressure syndromes, and meniscal injury leading to loss of synchronous joint motion.[92] Biochemical etiologies include rheumatoid arthritis, recurrent hemarthrosis, and crystal synovitis.[92] Another etiologic classification system that is more easily applied to sports injuries uses six major categories: trauma; dislocation; malalignment with patellar subluxation; normal alignment with osteochondral ridge; increased cartilage vulnerability, as is typical after surgery or immobilization; and occupational hazards.[104]

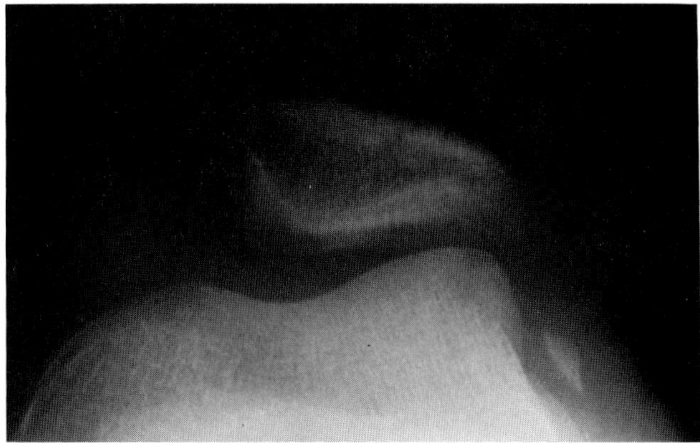

Fig. 6-19 Axial view of the patella after acute lateral dislocation with an associated femoral shearing injury. The patella is still subluxed laterally.

Clinically, patients with chondromalacia patellae or patellofemoral pain syndrome present with symptoms of instability, pain, or crepitation.[68] Physical examination may demonstrate abnormal position and effusion. During flexion, the knee of a patient with subluxation may show the patella in a more lateral position.[66,68]

The Q angle is a useful clinical tool (Fig. 6-20). When the Q angle (formed by a line from the tibial tuberosity to the midpatella and a second line along the quadriceps muscle plane) is 20° or greater, there is an increased incidence of patellar instability and degenerative arthritis.[68,89] The normal Q angle is 14°.[63,91]

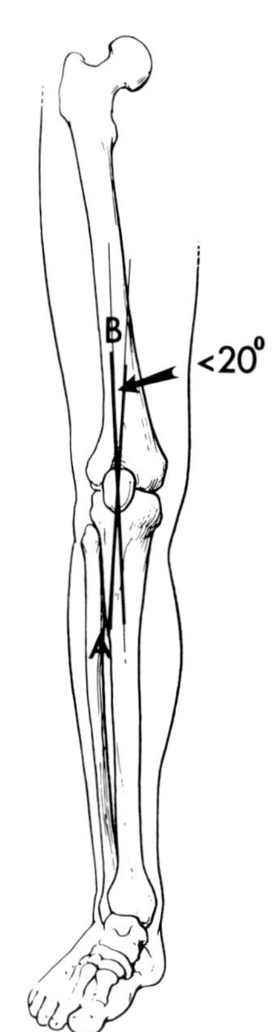

Fig. 6-20 Illustration of Q angle measurement. A line is drawn from the tibial tuberosity to the center of the patella (line A). A second line (B) is drawn along the plane of the quadriceps muscles. The angle should not exceed 20°.

Palpation and pressure on the patella during flexion and extension of the knee may demonstrate crepitation. Symmetry of muscles should be evaluated to exclude atrophy, especially in the quadriceps group.[68,89]

Patellar Instability

Patellar subluxation and dislocation represent problems related to more significant extensor malalignment than that present with chondromalacia. Subluxation and dislocation may follow a significant traumatic incident, or malalignment and trauma may both be etiologic factors (Fig. 6-19). Certain investigators hold that recurrent patellar subluxation and dislocation may be congenital.[66,72,89] In one series, 73% of knees with subluxation of the patella had at least one congenital deficiency.[89] Although the patella may be dislocated by a direct blow to the medial aspect of the knee, an indirect mechanism of injury is more frequent.[66,89] The normal Q angle results in a lateral vector to the extensor mechanism that tends to displace the patella laterally (Fig. 6-21).[78] The patella subluxes or dislocates when a strong quadriceps contraction is combined with external rotation of the tibia, genu valgum, and slight knee flexion, such as during the acceleration phase of activity when the quadriceps is contracting and the extremity is bearing weight (Fig. 6-21).[66,70,73,74]

Recurrent patellar subluxation may be considered of two types: major and minor.[78,87,88,90] In a major subluxation, the patella tracks laterally over the trochlear facet and returns to the patellofemoral groove with an audible snap on the beginning of knee flexion. In a minor subluxation, the patella deviates laterally without clinically apparent relocation. Acute patellar dislocation is usually lateral but may be medial, intra-articular, or superior.[78]

The pathologic changes associated with recurrent dislocation or subluxation include damage to the articular cartilage and the soft tissues. Tearing of the medial retinaculum, either from damage to the medial border of the patella or from rupture of the origin of the vastus medialis, may occur (Fig. 6-22).[66] Tears of the medial capsule of the knee, the cruciate ligaments, and the menisci may also occur. A hemarthrosis is a frequent finding.[68] The pathologic changes that appear in the articular cartilage are a result of trauma to the medial patellar facet and lateral trochlear facet during relocation of the patella.[68] Trauma may lead to such pathologic changes as chondromalacia, osteochondritis dissecans, osteochondral fracture, loose bodies, and late patellofemoral arthritis.[68,78]

Factors predisposing to chondromalacia and the patellar pain syndrome have been reviewed. These same anatomic abnormalities have been implicated in the pathogenesis of recurrent subluxation and dislocation.[66,78,89] The physical examination and history of symptoms are crucial in the recognition of these abnormalities and have been reviewed.

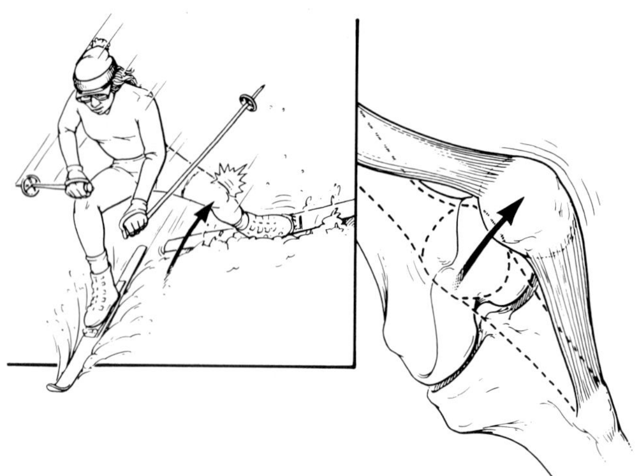

Fig. 6-21 Illustration of mechanism of lateral patellar dislocation.

Patellar Fractures

Although major and minor fractures of the knee are discussed in a later section, patellar fractures are discussed here to avoid redundancy in describing imaging techniques for evaluation of patellar disorders. Fractures of the patella may result from either direct or indirect blows such as shearing forces. Osteochondral fractures involving the patella are particularly common and often associated with patellar dislocation. With lateral dislocation, damage to the lateral patellar facet and lateral trochlear facet of the femur result from shearing forces during the injury.[68] With relocation, the medial patellar facet

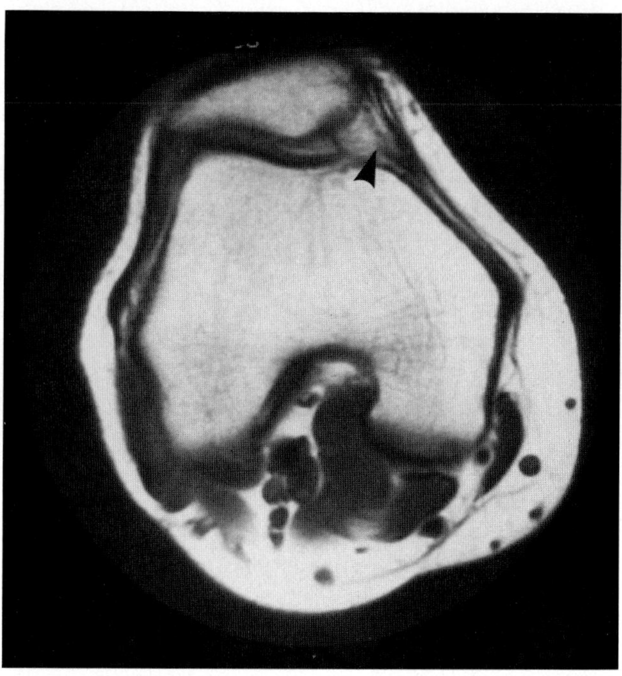

Fig. 6-22 Axial (SE 500/20) MR image demonstrating lateral subluxation with disruption of the posterior medial retinaculum (arrowhead) in a skier with recurrent subluxation.

may sustain cartilaginous injury as it strikes the lateral femoral condyle. Patellar fractures complicate dislocation in up to 28% of patients.[68]

Avulsion fractures of the patella are also common. Avulsion of the superior patellar pole occurs with forceful hyperflexion or hyperextension injury, with traction of the quadriceps tendon avulsing a small fragment of bone from the superior aspect of the patella. A portion of the tendon is also usually torn as it envelopes the upper part of the patella (Fig. 6-23). Other associated injuries (Osgood-Schlatter disease and/or patellar tendinitis) are not uncommon.[106]

The same mechanisms that result in superior pole avulsions can lead to avulsion fractures of the lower pole of the patella. In this setting the intact quadriceps mechanism retracts the patella superiorly, resulting in patella alta (Fig. 6-24).

Stress fractures of the patella have also been reported in athletes participating in running and jumping sports (eg, basketball and volleyball). Most fractures are transverse. Patients present with pain over the midpatella. On occasion, this injury is confused with a painful bipartite patella (Fig. 6-1). Conservative therapy is generally satisfactory in either case.[106]

Fractures of the body of the patella represent approximately 1% of all fractures. These fractures may result from direct trauma or indirect trauma due to forced quadriceps contraction with the knee partially flexed. Because of the mechanism and muscle and ligamentous attachments, there is generally considerable separation of the fragments (Fig. 6-25).

Patellar fractures are transverse in 34% of cases, comminuted in 16%, and longitudinal in 28%, with avulsion fractures making up the remainder. Indirect violence typically results in transverse fractures, and direct violence more often results in comminuted fractures.

Miscellaneous Peripatellar Conditions

Several other entities can result in anterior or peripatellar pain.[65,71,106] Quadriceps tendinitis may mimic proximal pole avulsion or tendon rupture and is, therefore, a diagnosis of exclusion. Patellar tendinitis (Sinding-Larsen disease and Johnsson's disease) is particularly common in jumping sports and represents the second most common extensor injury.[106] The etiology is probably chondroosseous failure, which may lead to calcification or ossification at the distal patellar pole.[106]

Osgood-Schlatter disease is the most common extensor stress injury in adolescents. The injury is generally considered secondary to tendon stress on the anterior tibial tubercle. The tuberosity normally fuses by age 13 years. The athlete presents with pain, swelling, and tenderness over the upper anterior tibia. The diagnosis is usually established clinically, but radiographs do demonstrate swelling and irregularity of the tuberosity (Fig. 6-26).[65,106]

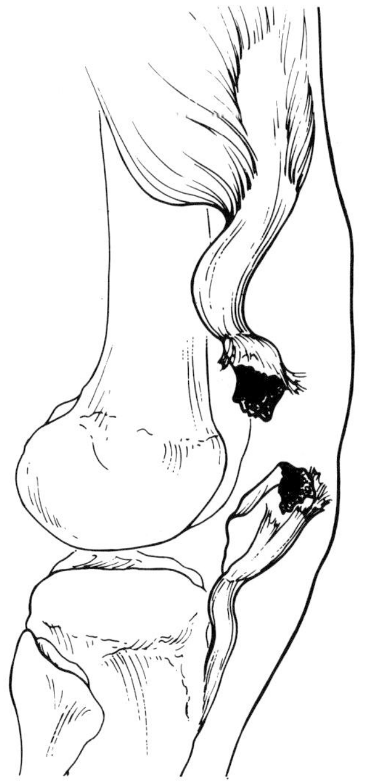

Fig. 6-23 Illustration of avulsion fracture of the superior patellar pole. Note the low position of the main fragment. *Source:* Reprinted with permission from Tehranzadeh J, The spectrum of avulsion and avulsion-like injuries of the musculoskeletal system in *RadioGraphics* (1987;7:945–974), Copyright © 1987, Radiological Society of North America.

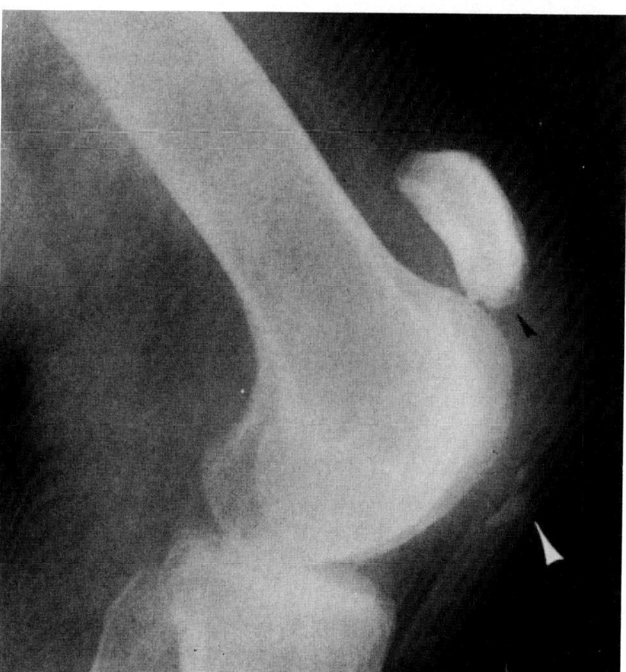

Fig. 6-24 Lateral radiograph after inferior patellar avulsion fracture (white arrowhead). Note the inferior patellar irregularity (black arrowhead) and patella alta. *Source:* Reprinted with permission from Tehranzadeh J, The spectrum of avulsion and avulsion-like injuries of the musculoskeletal system in *RadioGraphics* (1987;7:945–974), Copyright © 1987, Radiological Society of North America.

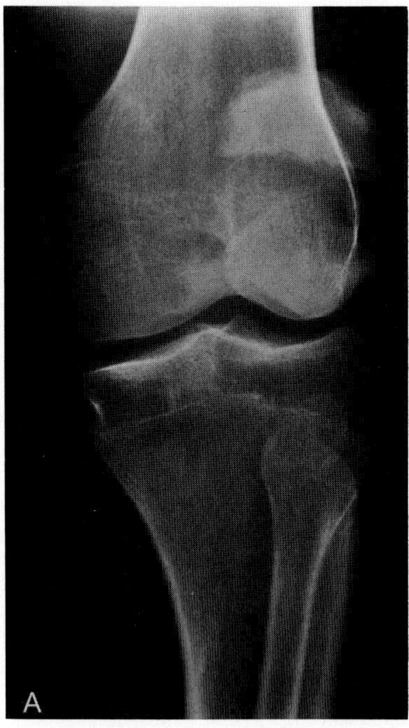

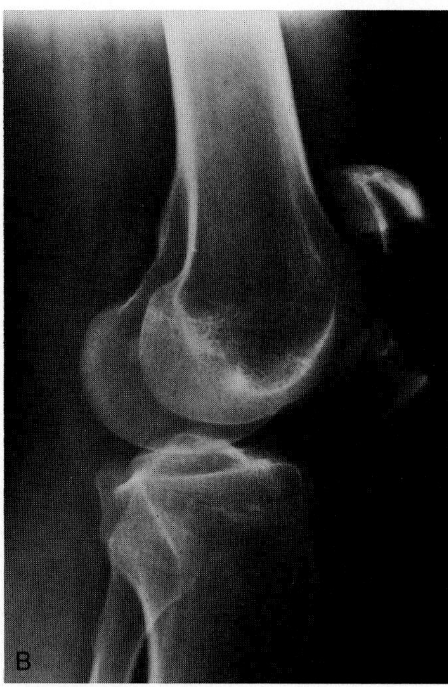

Fig. 6-25 (**A**) AP and (**B**) lateral radiographs of a transverse patellar fracture. There is significant distraction of the fragments. *Source:* Reprinted from *Imaging of Orthopedic Trauma* ed 2 by TH Berquist, 1991, Raven Press, © Mayo Foundation.

Imaging of Patellofemoral Disorders and Fractures

Routine radiographs allow diagnosis of most significant bony injuries and are also useful for evaluating patients with suspected patellar instability or patellofemoral pain syndrome (Fig. 6-27). AP, lateral, and axial patellar views are the minimum requirement. The lateral radiograph, as described previously, must be taken in 30° of flexion to place the patellar tendon under some tension (Fig. 6-27).[65,74] Additional lateral views with 60° and 90° of flexion may be useful in evaluating patellar contact. Position of the patella as noted on the lateral view is important. A high-riding patella or patella alta is

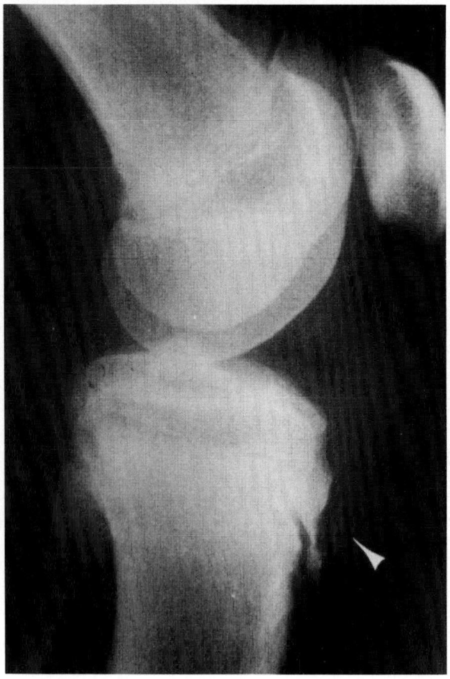

Fig. 6-26 Lateral view of the knee demonstrating fragmentation of the tibial tuberosity (arrowhead) due to Osgood-Schlatter disease. *Source:* Reprinted with permission from Tehranzadeh J, The spectrum of avulsion and avulsion-like injuries of the musculoskeletal system in *RadioGraphics* (1987; 7:945–974), Copyright © 1987, Radiological Society of North America.

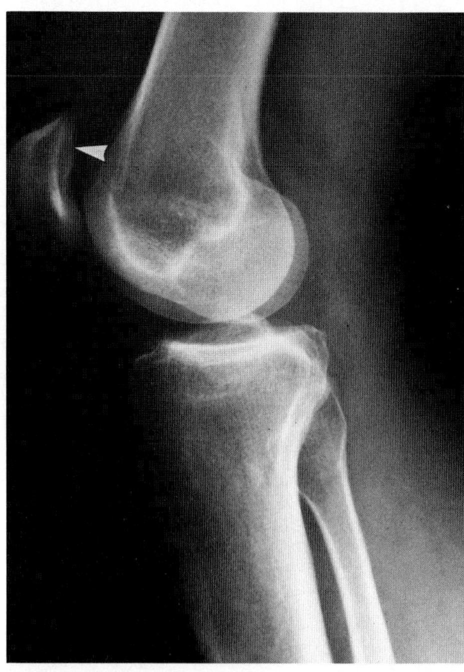

Fig. 6-27 Lateral view of the knee with an effusion and subtle lucency due to patellar fracture (arrowhead).

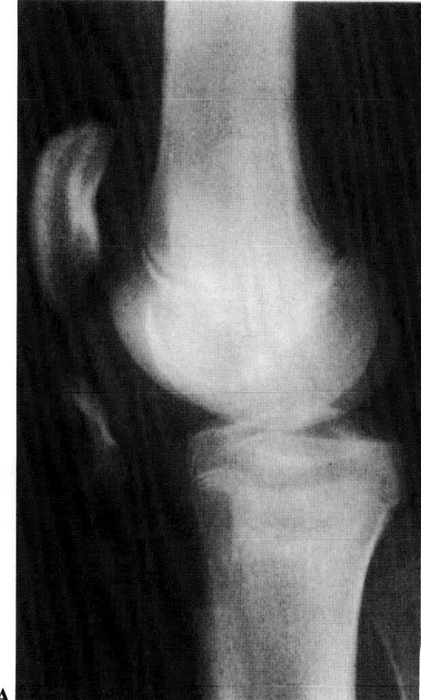

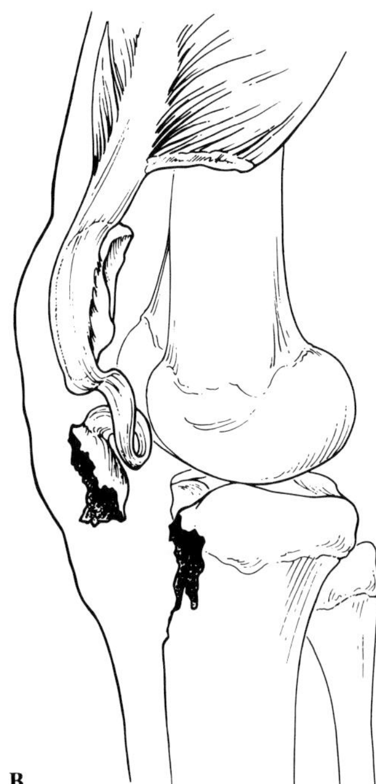

Fig. 6-28 (**A**) Lateral radiograph and (**B**) illustration of anterior tibial tuberosity avulsion. The avulsed fragment is rotated so that the irregular fracture surface lies anteriorly. *Source:* Reprinted with permission from Tehranzadeh J, The spectrum of avulsion and avulsion-like injuries of the musculoskeletal system in *RadioGraphics* (1987;7:945–974), Copyright © 1987, Radiological Society of North America.

associated with recurrent lateral subluxation, dislocation, chondromalacia, and avulsion of the patellar ligament (Figs. 6-24 and 6-28).[68,78,91,110] A low-riding patella or patella infra may be seen with dysplasias or in the athlete after trauma with avulsion of the quadriceps tendon (Fig. 6-29).[78,110]

More subtle changes such as an effusion or subtle lucent lines in the patellar surface may also be seen on the lateral view (Fig. 6-27). Subtle calcification or ossification at the upper or lower poles may also be evident with chronic stress syndrome. These changes may be due to ossification or calcification in necrotic tendon or patellar fragmentation.[106]

The AP view is less useful in evaluating fractures, but it can be of value in measurement of the Q angle radiographically or in detecting subtle displacement of the patella medially or laterally. The axial patellar view, however, is much more useful in this regard. The axial view clearly demonstrates the relationship of the articular surface of the patella with that of the femoral condyles (Fig. 6-30). Numerous techniques for axial patellar imaging have been developed. The Merchant view, taken with the knees flexed and the tube angled 45° toward the feet, is most common, but it is also common to obtain axial images in 30°, 45°, and 60° of flexion. This allows evaluation of articular contact in multiple degrees of flexion.[78]

The axial view is of great value in providing significant measurement information[68,77,94–96,100] with regard to the trochlea, patella, and patellofemoral congruence. The sulcus angle (Fig 6-30A) is defined as the angle formed by the highest point on the medial and lateral femoral condyles and the lowest point in the intercondylar sulcus. The normal sulcus angle is 141° to 142°.[63,68] An increase in the sulcus angle above this value predisposes the patient to subluxation. A second useful angle is the lateral patellofemoral angle, which is defined by two lines. The first is a line joining the summits of the femoral condyles, and the second is a line through the articular surface of the lateral patellar facet (Fig. 6-30B). The lateral

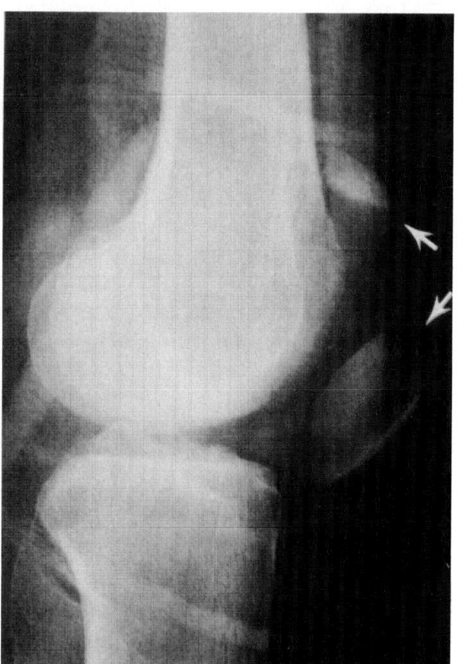

Fig. 6-29 Patella infra due to proximal pole avulsion (upper arrow). The patella (lower arrow) is pulled distally. *Source:* Reprinted with permission from Tehranzadeh J, The spectrum of avulsion and avulsion-like injuries of the musculoskeletal system in *RadioGraphics* (1987;7:945–974), Copyright © 1987, Radiological Society of North America.

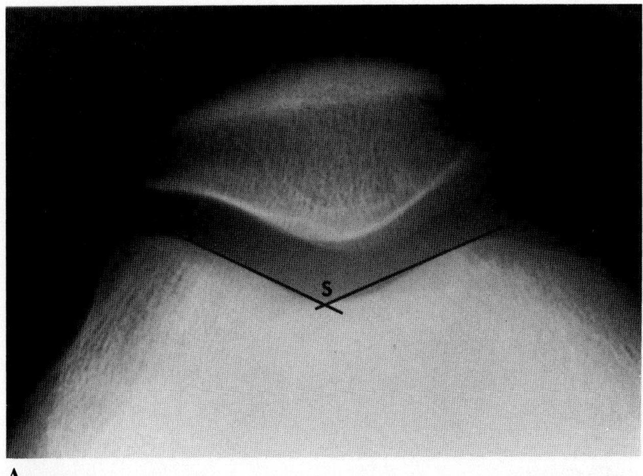

A

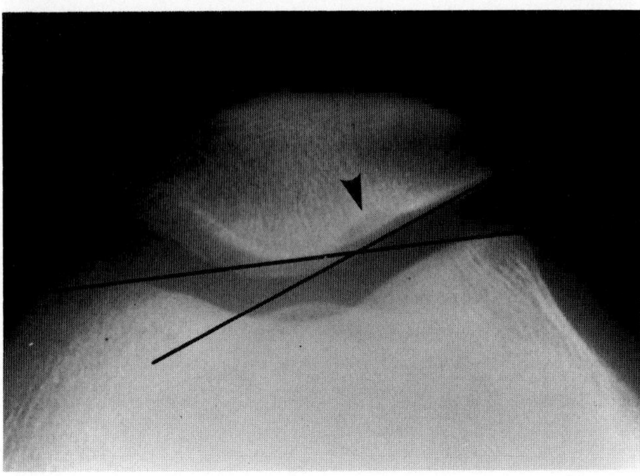

B

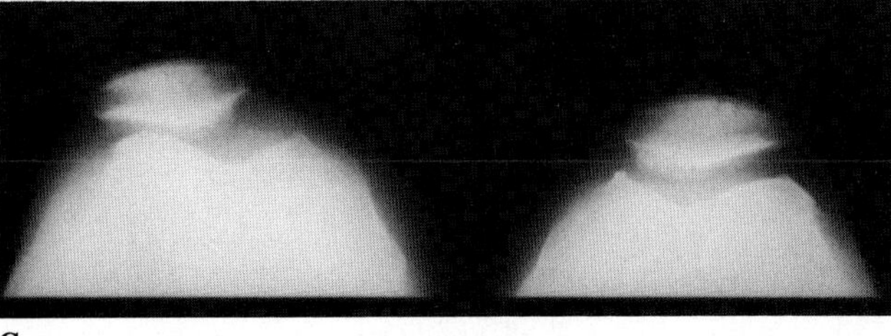

C

Fig. 6-30 (**A**) Normal axial view of the patella. Note the symmetric joint space. The sulcus angle (S) is less than 142°. (**B**) Patella with early chondromalacia (arrowhead). Note the normal lateral patellofemoral angle (opens laterally). (**C**) Axial views of the knees demonstrating a subluxed patella on the left.

patellofemoral angle is open laterally in 97% of normal knees and parallel in 80%, and it opens medially in 20% of knees with subluxing patella. Other patellar measurements may also be useful but can be complex if not routinely used.[68] Axial radiographs of the patella also are useful for visualizing osteochondral fractures, which frequently are noted along the lateral femoral condyle in patients with recurrent patellar dislocation (Fig. 6-31).[68,81,97,101] In addition, calcification or heterotopic ossification in the medial patellar retinaculum from previous dislocation and tearing of the structure may be evident on axial views.

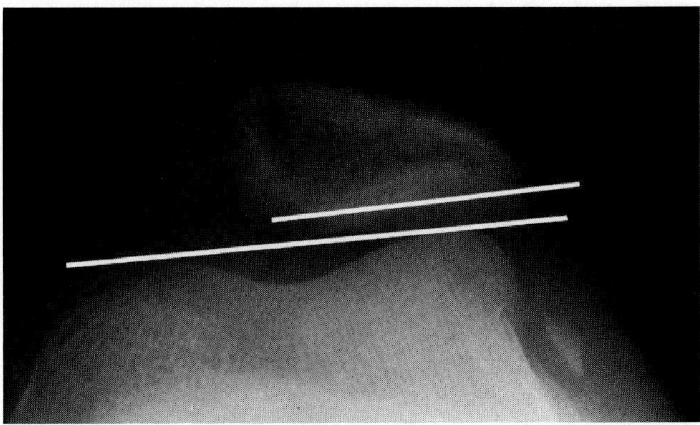

Fig. 6-31 Axial patellar view with a subluxed patella (note the lateral angle) and an avulsion fracture of the femoral condyle.

Table 6-1 MR Features of Chondromalacia

Stage	*Pathologic Change*	*MR Features*
I	Palpable softening of articular cartilage	Normal
II	Surface intact but blistered	Focal signal intensity abnormality
III	Surface erosion with no bone exposure	Irregularity or local thinning
IV	Cartilage erosion with bone exposure	Bone uncovered with significant area of cartilage loss

Sources: Berquist TH, *Imaging of Orthopedic Trauma*, ed 2, 1991, Raven Press; Hayes CW, Sawyer RW and Conway WF, *Radiology* (1990;176: 479–483), Radiological Society of North America.

New imaging techniques may also be useful, particularly in subtle patellofemoral disorders where evaluation of articular cartilage, soft tissues, and patellofemoral relationships in multiple degrees of flexion and extension may be necessary.[68,89,98,105,109,111] The study of osseous change is most easily accomplished with new ultrafast CT techniques.[109] MRI may be better suited for evaluation of subtle changes in the articular cartilage, in which case fast-scan gradient-echo techniques should be employed.[68] MR images correlate well with commonly used classification systems for chondromalacia (Table 6-1).[85,107] Lesions that are stage II or greater are detected easily with gradient-echo or T2-weighted spin-echo sequences.[68,85] T1-Weighted sequences may also be useful (Fig. 6-32) in more advanced cases.[85] Sagittal MR images are ideally suited for evaluating early inflammatory changes in the quadriceps and patellar tendons.[68,69] Sonography is useful on occasion, but MRI is preferred for soft tissue disorders of the knee.[68,80]

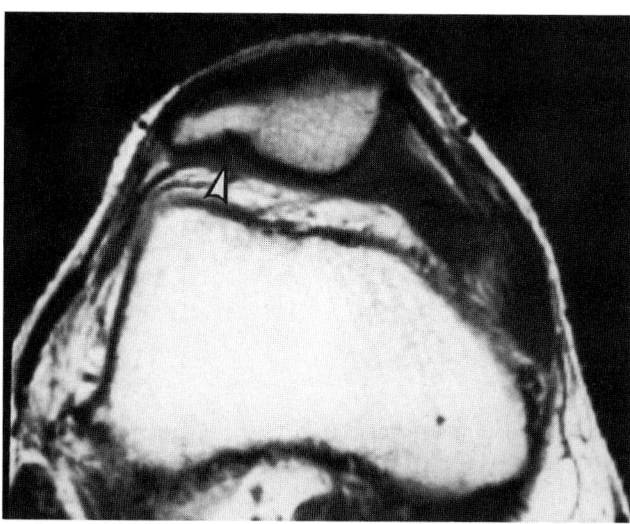

Fig. 6-32 Axial (SE 500/20) MR image demonstrating advanced chondromalacia with underlying bone irregularity (stage IV, arrowhead).

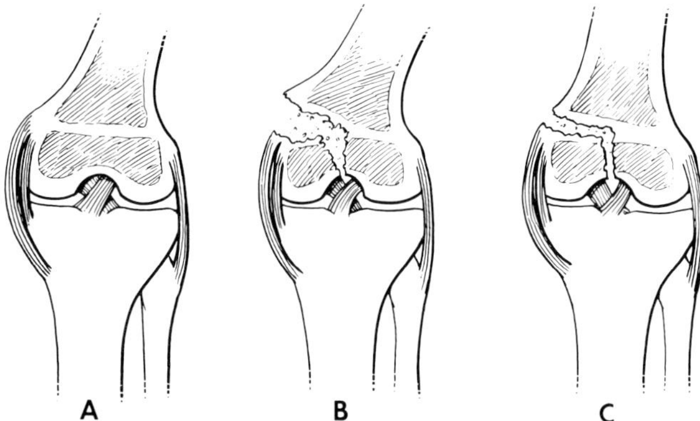

Fig. 6-33 Illustration of distal femur anatomy (**A**) and mechanism of physeal fracture of the distal femur (**B** and **C**). The proximal tibial physis receives more support from the collateral ligaments and is rarely fractured.

FRACTURES

Major fractures are infrequently associated with sports injuries. More subtle fractures, however, such as physeal fractures, stress fractures, or osteochondral fractures, are fairly common. Associated ligament injuries are frequently present and, because of newer imaging techniques, are more easily appreciated. Awareness of the fracture and soft tissue injury patterns and mechanisms of injury is important for complete imaging evaluation.

Physeal Fractures

Growth plate fractures of the distal femur and proximal tibia occur most frequently in adolescent athletes.[145] Injuries in boys outnumber those in girls by approximately 5 to 1.[138,149] The distal epiphysis of the femur is among the most common sites of injury; fractures here are usually associated with twisting injuries, which are most commonly seen in football players.[132,150,153] Fractures of the proximal tibial epiphysis are rare except for tuberosity fractures; the latter are discussed separately. The higher incidence of fractures in the distal femur compared to fractures in the proximal tibia (which are rare) is at least partially due to the anatomic configuration of the capsule and supporting ligaments of the knee. The MCL and LCL attach distal to the femoral growth plate, making it more susceptible to injury (Fig. 6-33). The distal attachment of these ligaments is located below the proximal tibial growth plate, affording it more protection.[115,116,149,153] Because rotary or valgus forces are common in football, basketball, and other sports that result in knee injury, it is not unusual to see separation of the medial distal femoral growth plate in a Salter-Harris II or III configuration (Figs. 6-33 and 6-34).

Fractures of the tuberosity frequently involve the growth plate and may extend through the growth plate, causing posterior displacement of the metaphysis. The injury is most commonly seen with high jumping, handball, track, and basketball and may be due to direct or indirect trauma (Fig. 6-35).[134,138,149] Fracture is caused by violent extension or forced quadriceps contraction with the knee in slight flexion. The injury has been classified in several fashions, including that of Watson and Jones.[134,150] Type I fractures involve the tuberosity alone. Type II fractures involve the tuberosity and proximal tibial epiphysis but do not involve the articular surface (Fig. 6-36). Type III fractures include the injuries described in type II together with involvement of the articular surface of the tibia (Fig. 6-37).[134,145,150]

When the fracture extends through the growth plate such that posterior displacement of the metaphysis occurs, the likelihood of posterior neurovascular injury is high (Fig. 6-36).[134,138,149]

Identification of physeal fractures is not difficult when there is displacement. AP and lateral views are usually sufficient for diagnosis of distal femoral, proximal tibial (Fig. 6-38), or tuberosity fractures.[116,133] In cases of subtle injury, fluoroscopically controlled stress views may be useful (Fig. 6-34C). AP and lateral tomograms or CT scans may be useful on occasion but are rarely indicated. It is not unusual to detect subtle growth plate injuries with MRI when the athlete is referred for a suspected soft tissue injury or a meniscal injury of the knee (Fig. 6-39).

Osteochondral Fractures

Osteochondral fractures involving the joint surface may occur from direct trauma or indirect injury, specifically shearing or rotary injuries. This section also includes discussion of avulsion and flake fractures, although these may not involve the articular surface. Osteochondritis dissecans is trauma

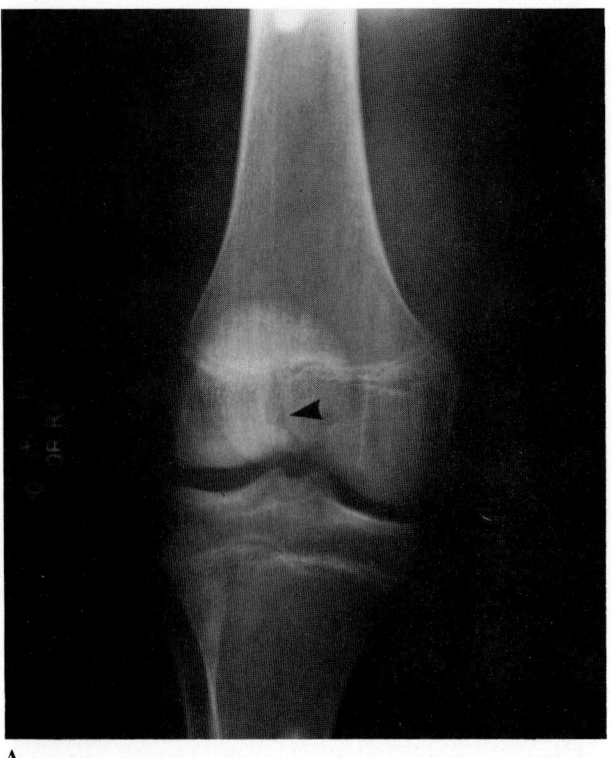

A

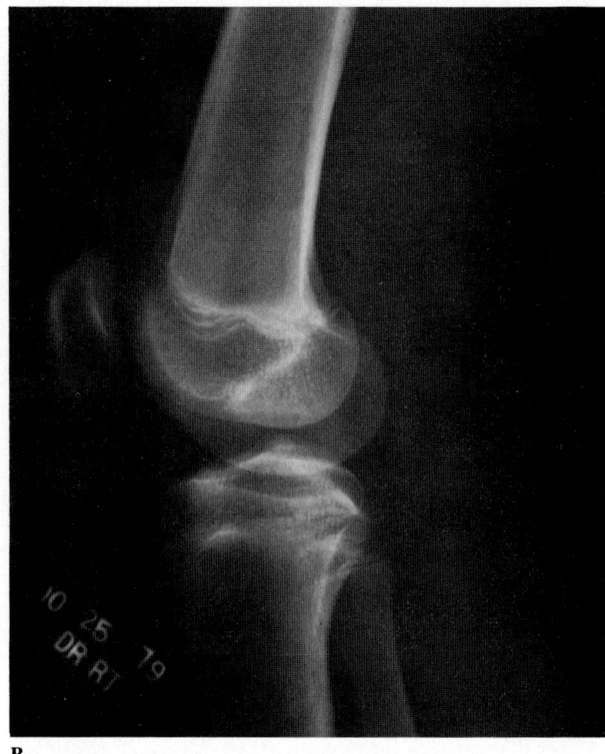

B

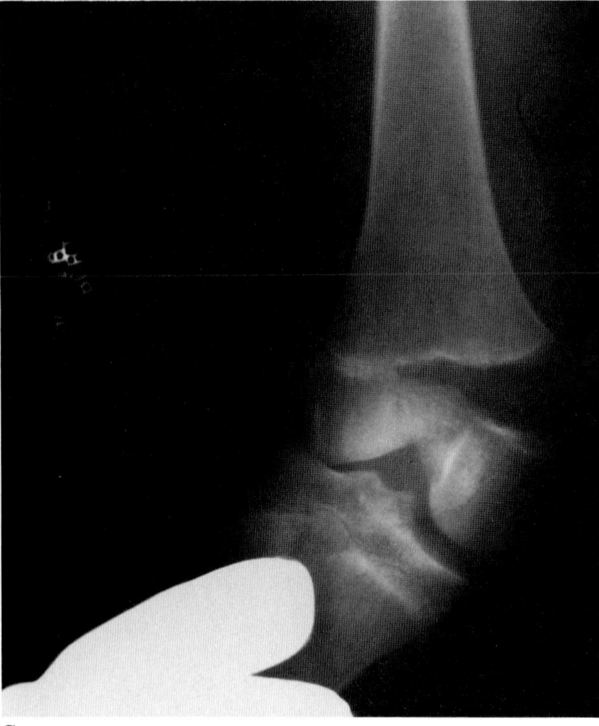

C

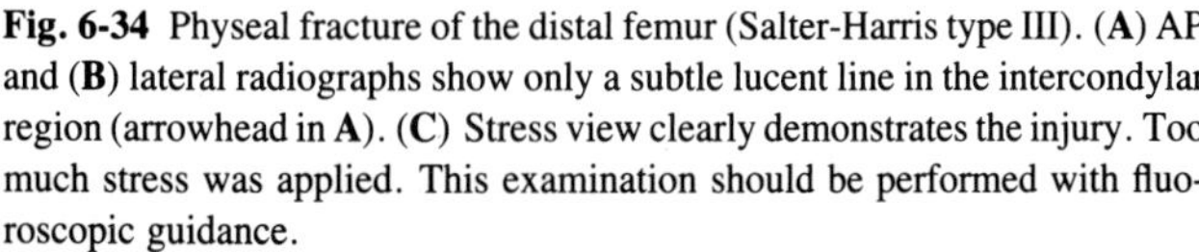

Fig. 6-34 Physeal fracture of the distal femur (Salter-Harris type III). (**A**) AP and (**B**) lateral radiographs show only a subtle lucent line in the intercondylar region (arrowhead in **A**). (**C**) Stress view clearly demonstrates the injury. Too much stress was applied. This examination should be performed with fluoroscopic guidance.

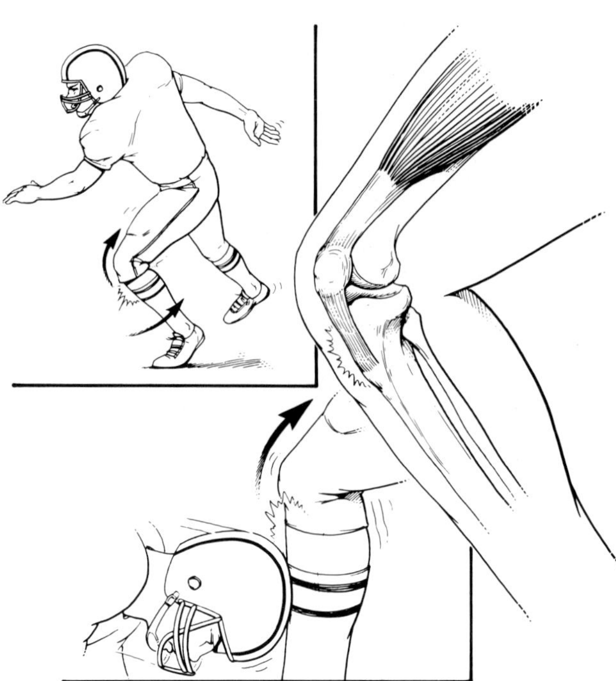

Fig. 6-35 Illustration of mechanism of tibial tuberosity fracture.

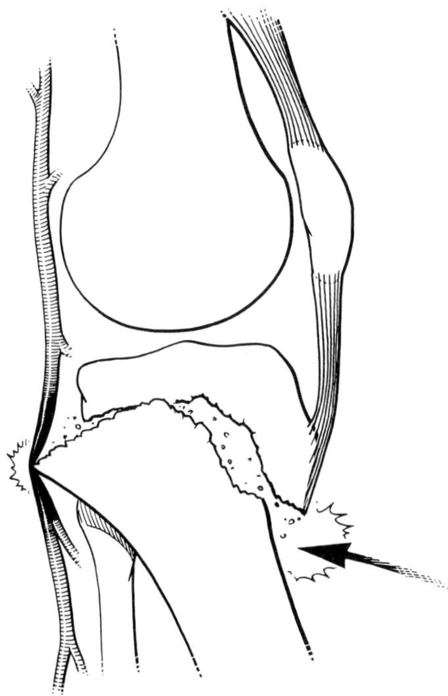

Fig. 6-36 Illustration of tibial tuberosity fractures with displaced distal fragment and neurovascular injury (type II). Arrow indicates direction of force application.

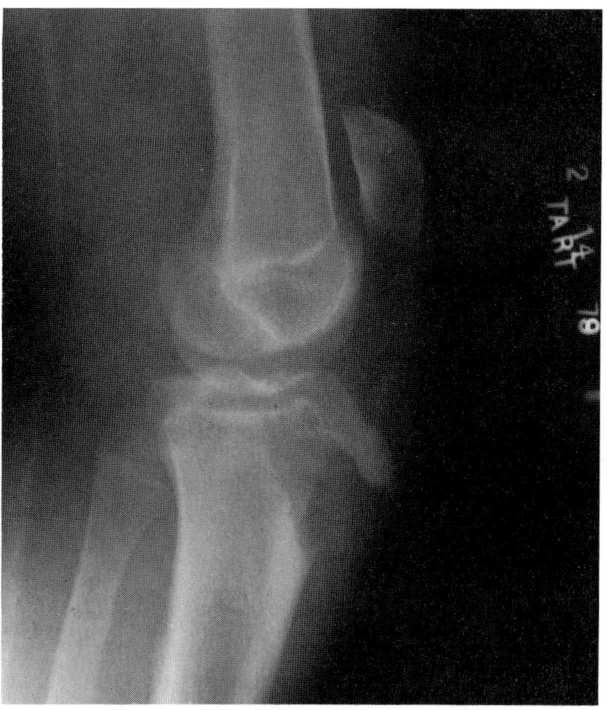

Fig. 6-37 Fracture of the tibial tuberosity extending into the anterior articular surface (type III) in an adolescent athlete.

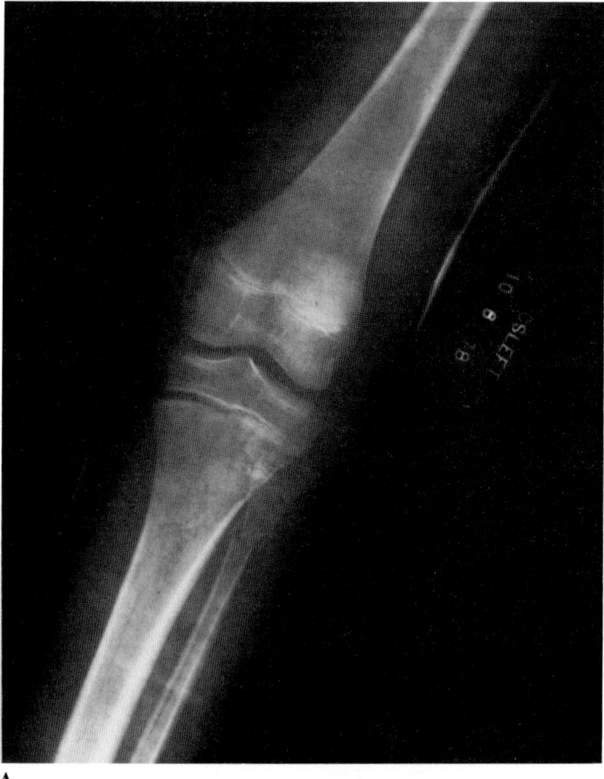

A

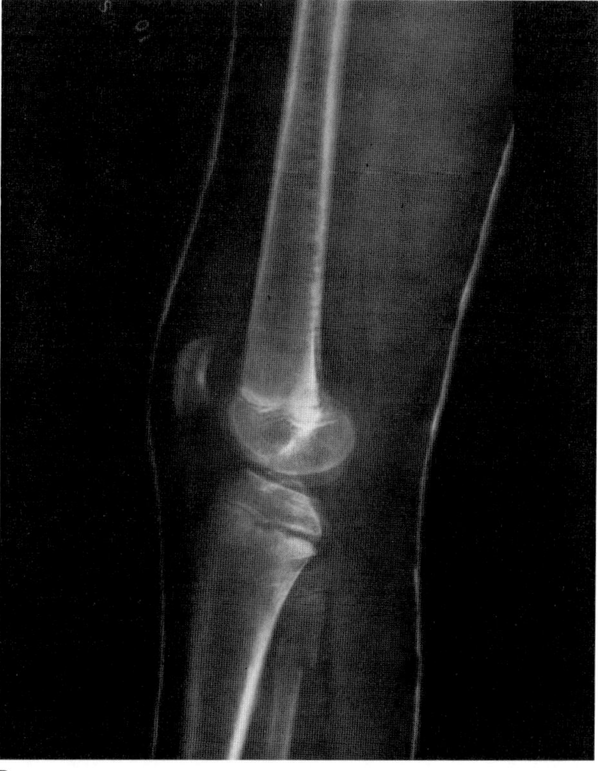

B

Fig. 6-38 (**A**) AP and (**B**) lateral casted views of the knee in a football player with a rotary valgus injury resulting in fracture of the proximal tibial physis and upper fibula.

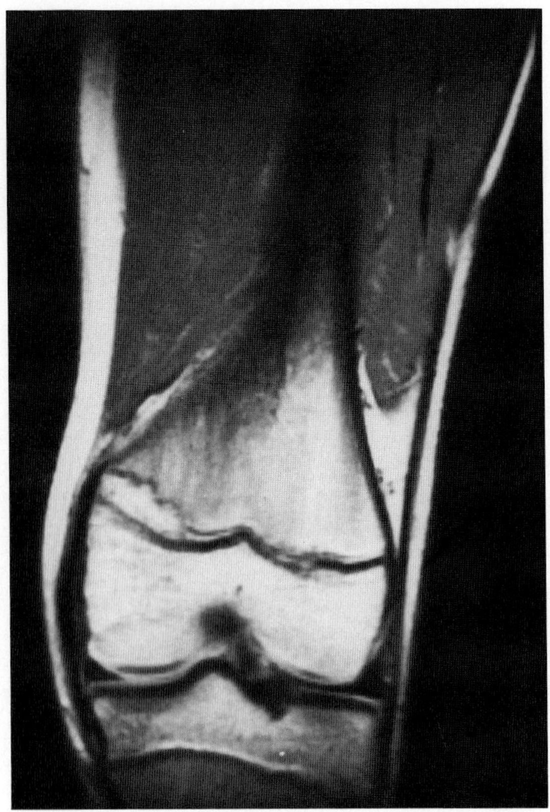

Fig. 6-39 Coronal (SE 2000/30) MR image demonstrating a subtle (radiograph negative) medial femoral growth plate fracture. The MCL and meniscus are normal.

related and also is discussed here.[116,129] Figure 6-40 illustrates several mechanisms of osteochondral fracture. Location of the osteochondral fracture depends upon the position of the knee (flexion, extension, weight bearing, etc) and whether trauma was direct or indirect.[115,130,133,136,142]

Osteochondritis dissecans most frequently occurs along the lateral aspect of the medial femoral condyle near the intercondylar notch. A lesion may also be detected in the lateral condyle and along the posterior surface of the patella.[129,141]

Avulsion fractures may be subtle and difficult to detect radiographically. Detection of these fractures should lead one to search for associated ligament and meniscal injuries.[120,122,125,144] Included in this group of fractures are the Segond fractures,[120,125] flake fractures,[132] fractures of the interchondylar tibial eminence,[116,149] and meniscal avulsions.[144] Tibial tuberosity fractures are also essentially avulsion injuries and were discussed above.

The Segond fracture is a small, flakelike avulsion fracture from the lateral aspect of the proximal tibia below the level of the tibial plateau. The mechanism of injury is typically internal rotation with varus stress.[125] Associated tears of the ACL and the menisci are common, being reported in more than 70% of cases.[120,125] Fractures that may mimic the Segond fracture include avulsion of the iliotibial band, which may cause an avulsion of Gerdy's tubercle. This fracture is usually more inferior and anterior than the Segond fracture. Avulsion fractures of the fibular head by the biceps femoris or LCL may also be confusing, but these fractures are typically more inferior and posterior than the Segond fracture. The Segond fracture

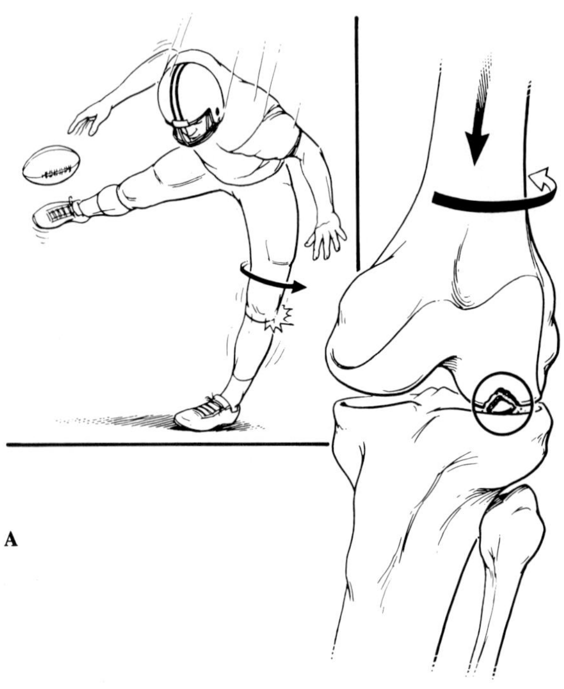

A

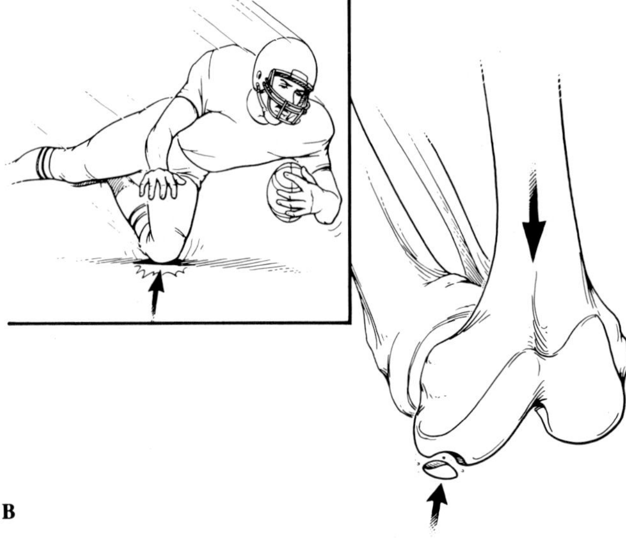

B

Fig. 6-40 Osteochondral fractures of the knee: mechanisms of injury. (**A**) Lateral femoral condyle fracture due to rotation with weight bearing. (**B**) Osteochondral fracture due to direct trauma during a fall with the knee flexed.

may be associated with dislocation of the proximal tibiofibular articulation.[117,118]

Avulsion of the posterior attachment of the medial meniscus usually results in a small, flakelike bone fragment posteriorly, which is seen near the tibial spines on the AP view (Fig. 6-41).

Fractures of the tibial spines may be subtle and minimally displaced (type I). Type II fractures are displaced anteriorly, and type III fractures are completely displaced and rotated (Fig. 6-42). Radiographic evaluation is important because the first two types may be treated conservatively (Fig. 6-43). Displaced and rotated fragments, however, may require internal fixation.

Imaging of osteochondral fractures generally requires both oblique and notch views in addition to AP and lateral views. Certain fractures, such as displaced tibial spine fractures (Fig. 6-44), may be evaluated with AP and lateral views. Notch views (Fig. 6-45) and oblique views, however, are especially useful for identification of subtle fractures, Segond fractures, and other avulsion fractures of the upper tibia and fibula. Because of the subtlety of some of these fractures as well as the frequency of associated meniscal and ligament injuries, MRI is frequently performed as a second technique to evaluate these injuries more completely. MRI is particularly useful for the evaluation of osteochondritis dissecans and undisplaced osteochondral fractures to assess the integrity of the overlying articular cartilage and the position of the fragments (Fig. 6-46). Figure 6-47 demonstrates the Berndt and Harty classification for osteochondral lesions. MRI has been shown to correlate well with the arthroscopic appearance of these osteochondral fractures.[141] Although routine films are still indicated, MRI is the technique of choice for evaluating acute soft tissue and subtle osteochondral injuries about the knee.[116,119,141]

Supracondylar Fractures of the Femur

By definition, a supracondylar fracture of the femur involves the distal 9 cm of the femur as measured from the articular surface of the femoral condyles.[116] These fractures are usually due to high-velocity trauma and, therefore, are not common except in high-velocity sports such as skiing, snowmobiling, motorcycling, and auto racing. Associated local injuries are common. These may include fractures of the ipsilateral tibial plateau or ligaments of the knee.[116,140,148]

The appearance of the fracture radiographically is important in determining the mechanism of fixation (Fig. 6-48). Seinsheimer[148] described these fractures and recognized four categories of injury. Type I fractures are nondisplaced and have less than 2 mm of separation of the fragments. Type II fracture involves the distal metaphysis but does not extend into the intercondylar notch of the femur. The type III fracture involves the intercondylar notch, and with type IV more comminution of the femoral condyles is usually present.

Detection and staging of supracondylar fractures is usually accomplished with routine AP and lateral views of the knee. Because of the mechanism of injury and frequency of associated injuries, further imaging of the knee such as MRI to evaluate the ligaments and routine radiographs of the ipsilateral extremity may be required.[116]

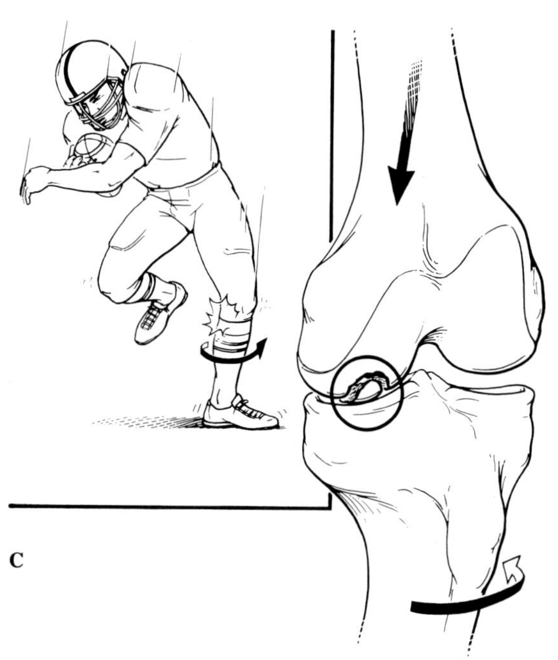

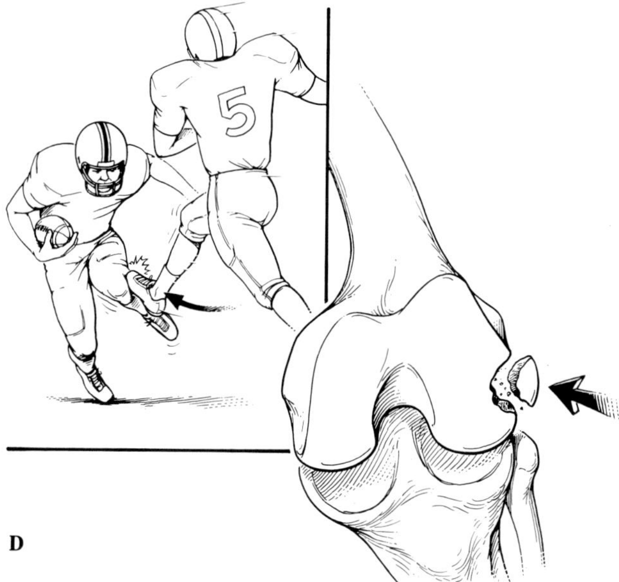

Fig. 6-40 contd (**C**) Shearing fracture of the medial femoral condyle. (**D**) Osteochondral fracture due to direct trauma.

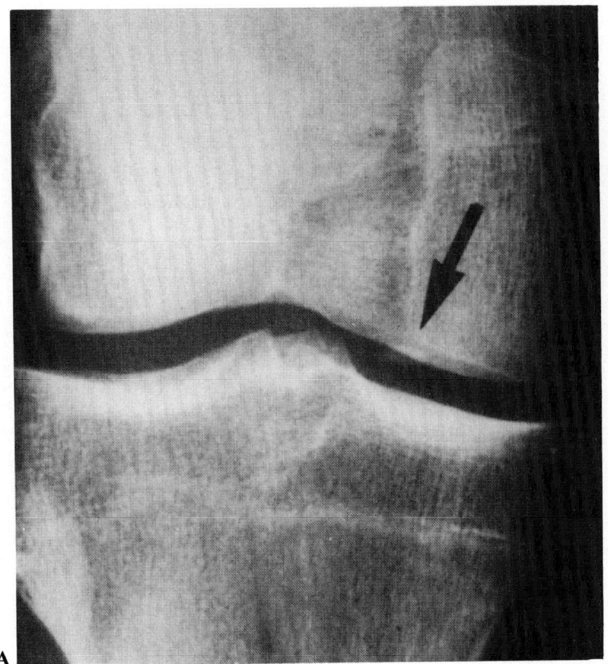

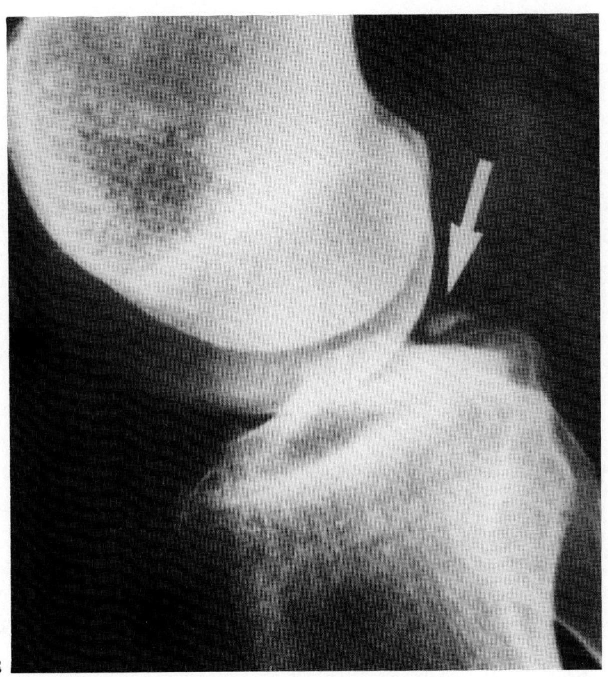

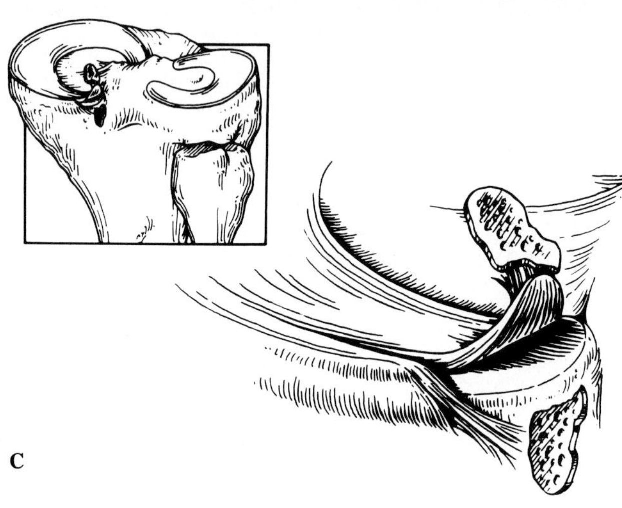

Fig. 6-41 Avulsion of the posteromedial meniscal attachment. (**A**) Routine AP and (**B**) lateral radiographs demonstrate a small posteromedial osseous fragment (arrows). (**C**) Illustration of the site of avulsion of the posterior medial meniscus and the bone fragment avulsed with the meniscal tibial ligament. *Source:* Reprinted with permission from Richmond J and Sarno RC, Post traumatic intracapsular bone fragments: association with meniscal tears in *American Journal of Roentgenology* (1988;150:159–160), Copyright © 1988, American Roentgen Ray Society.

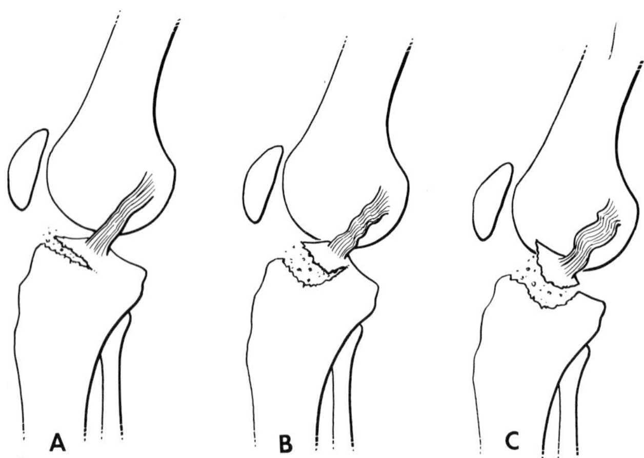

Fig. 6-42 Illustration of tibial spine fracture classification. (**A**) Type I: minimal displacement. (**B**) Type II: anterior displacement. (**C**) Type III: complete displacement.

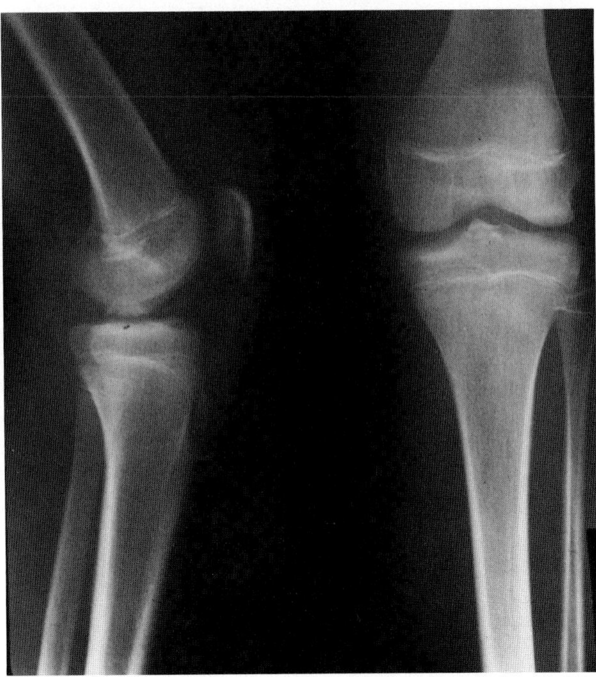

Fig. 6-43 AP and lateral views of the knee demonstrating an undisplaced tibial spine fracture.

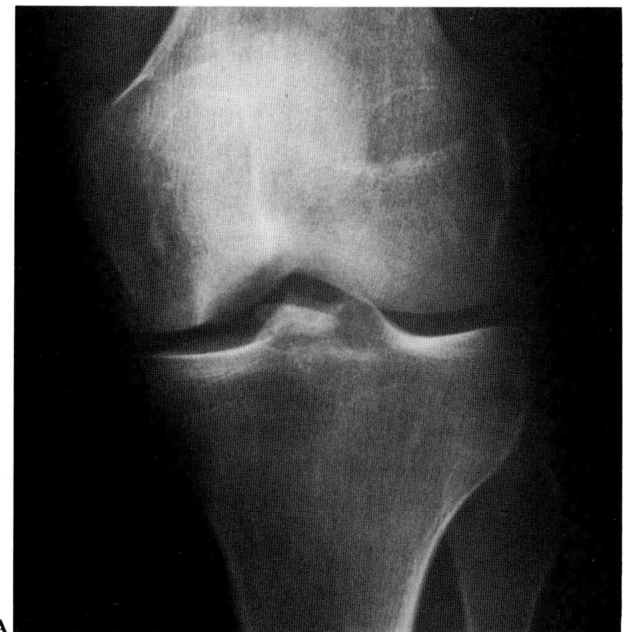

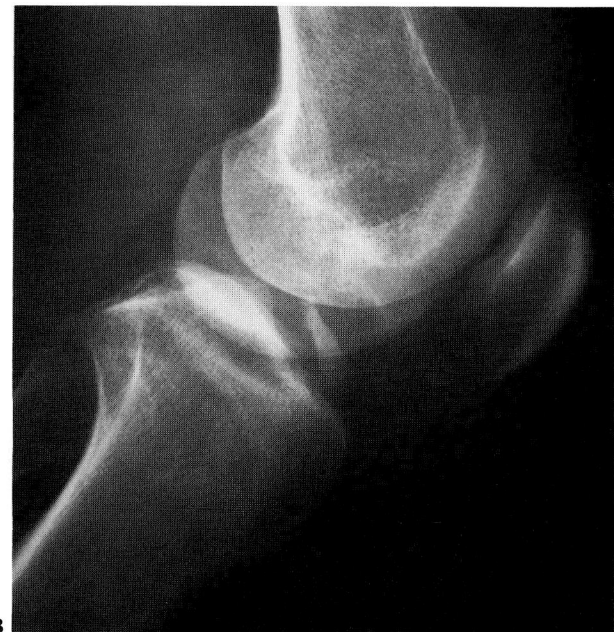

Fig. 6-44 (**A**) AP and (**B**) lateral views of the knee demonstrating a displaced osteochondral fracture from the medial femoral condyle.

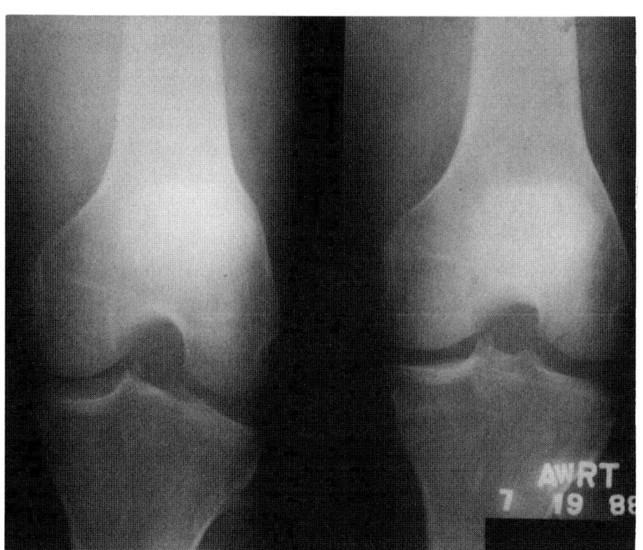

Fig. 6-45 Notch view demonstrating a subtle tibial spine fracture.

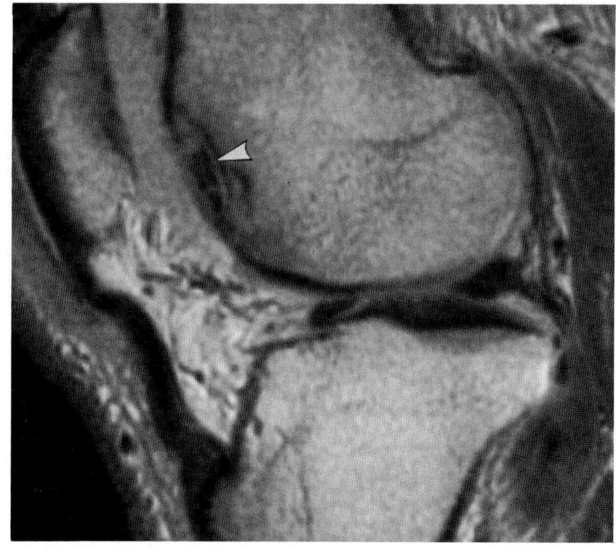

Fig. 6-46 Sagittal (SE 2000/20) MR image demonstrating an undisplaced osteochondral fracture (arrowhead) and a large effusion.

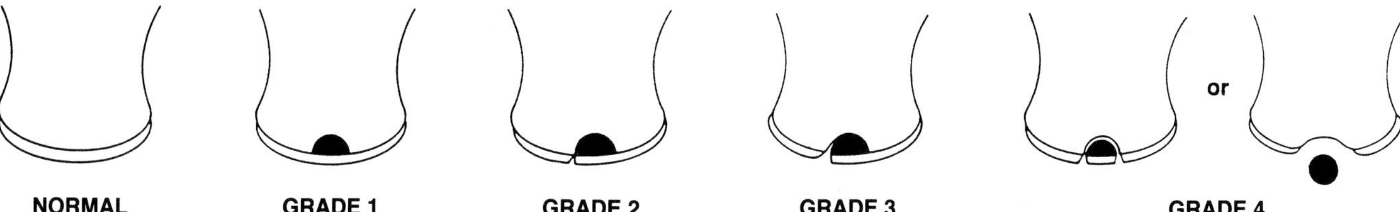

Fig. 6-47 Illustration of Berndt and Harty classification of osteochondral lesions. In grade 1, the subchondral lesion (black) is covered with intact articular cartilage. Grade 2 has a slight cartilage defect with no displacement. Grade 3 has a cleft between the fragment and bone (linear area of high signal on T2-weighted MR images). In grade 4 the fragment separated but not displaced. *Source:* Reprinted with permission from Nelson DW, DiPaola J, Colville M, and Schmidgall J, Osteochondritis dissecans of the talus and knee: prospective comparison of MR and arthroscopic classification in *Computer Assisted Tomography* (1990;14:804–808), Copyright © 1990, Raven Press.

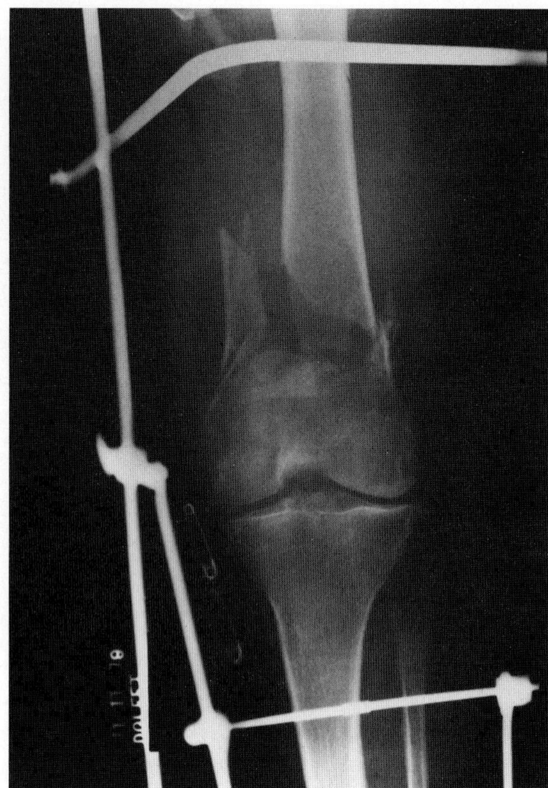

Fig. 6-48 AP view of a comminuted supracondylar fracture in traction.

Tibial Plateau Fractures

Fractures of the tibial plateaus most commonly involve the lateral plateau and are associated with valgus injuries during sports.[116,135,137] Associated ligament injuries and peroneal nerve palsy have been reported.[113,114,116,117,120,126] Peroneal nerve palsy may be present in approximately 5% of patients.[117] Injuries of the menisci and ligaments are more frequent. Up to 30% of patients may have associated ligamentous injury, most frequently of the MCL.[152] Shelton et al[149] reported MCL tears in association with all plateau fractures and an associated proximal fibular fracture. Failure to diagnose or properly treat soft tissue injury can result in instability. Up to 20% of patients have been noted to have unstable injuries due to residual ligament insufficiency.[152]

Classification and radiographic evaluation of plateau fractures is useful in selection of treatment and detection of associated soft tissue injury.[127,131] Hohl[127] classified fractures of the lateral plateau with minimal displacement as type I, those with local compression as type II, those with compression and splitting of the fracture fragment as type III, those with total depression of the condyle as type IV, and those with involvement of both condyles as type V. The main factor affecting the type of fracture is the point of impact, which in turn determines the size of the fragment (Fig. 6-49).[147] The extent of depression of the plateau depends upon the extent of trauma, the age of the patient, and the degree of knee flexion. Most fractures are produced by the femoral condyle being driven like a wedge into the underlying tibial plateau.[116,146] Therefore, lateral plateau fractures usually result from combined valgus and axial compression forces. Radiographic evaluation of plateau fractures is important in determining therapy. Therefore, it is important to evaluate the articular surface, degree of depression or separation of the fragments, and extent of soft tissue injury.[139] The osseous trauma can usually be evaluated with routine films, but CT or conventional tomography may be useful to define better the position of the fragments and the degree of articular involvement (Fig. 6-50).[116,121,143] MRI is best suited to evaluate soft tissue changes but can also be used to evaluate the position of bony fragments. Appreciation of the full extent of the injury may require both techniques before any decisions regarding therapy are made (Fig. 6-51).[116,128,151]

Combined ipsilateral fractures of the femur and tibia are unusual in athletes except in the case of extremely high-velocity injury.[123,124]

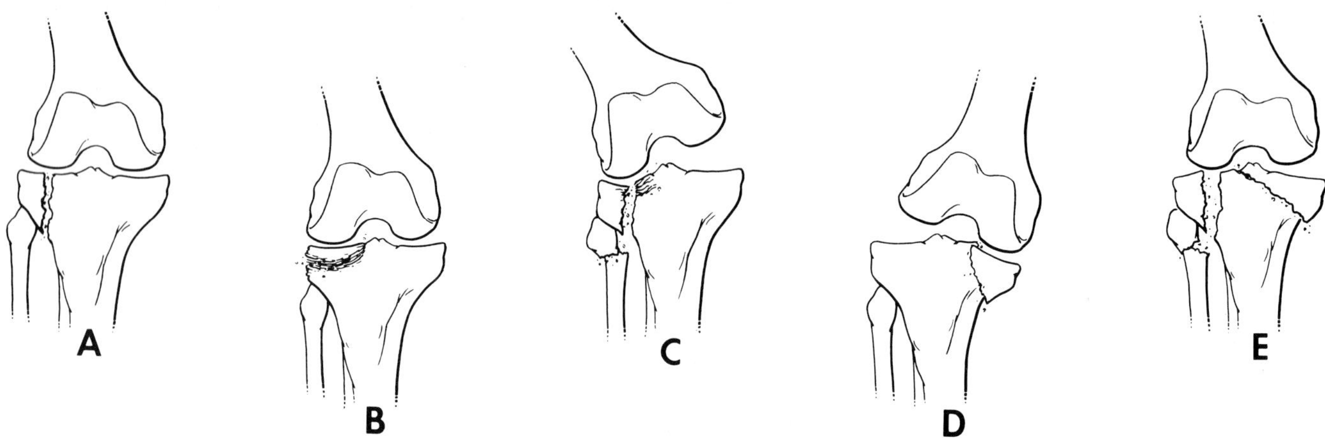

Fig. 6-49 Illustration of tibial plateau fractures (after Hohl[127]). (**A**) Type I: lateral plateau fracture with minimal displacement. (**B**) Type II: local compression. (**C**) Type III: compression and splitting of fragment. (**D**) Type IV: depression of condyle. (**E**) Type V: both condyles fractured.

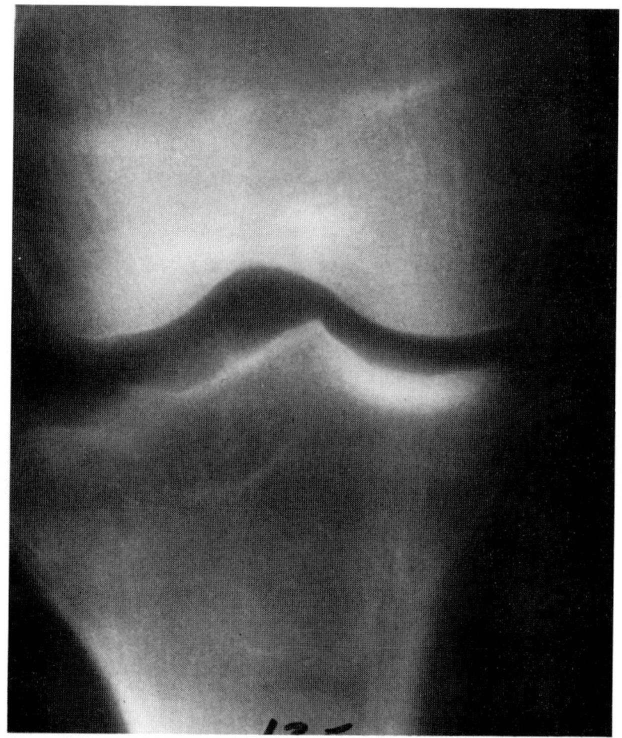

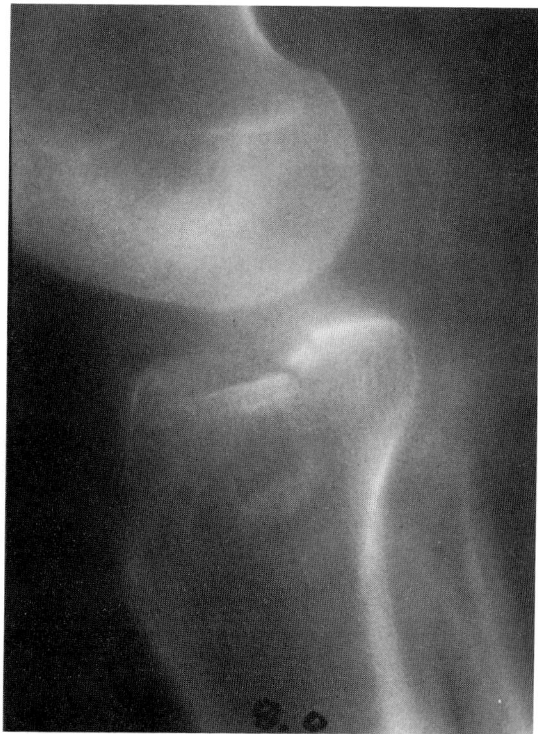

Fig. 6-50 (**A**) AP and (**B**) lateral tomograms demonstrating the degree of depression of a tibial plateau fracture.

LIGAMENT, MENISCUS, AND SOFT TISSUE INJURIES

Knee injuries account for up to one-third of all sports-related injuries.[190,210] Most are related to acute or chronic soft tissue injuries and overuse syndromes (Table 6-2).[190,204,209,217,232,243]

Attempts to prevent knee injuries have increased in recent years. Improved training, physical therapy, and preventive measures are important. Bracing has been used in football players in hopes of reducing major ligament injury. To date, however, there is no consensus as to whether this technique is useful. Some reports demonstrate an increase in injuries with prophylactic knee bracing.[160,189,245]

History and physical findings may be adequate for treatment planning in certain situations. Nevertheless, imaging plays a vital role in clearly defining the nature and extent of injuries. This information is essential to ensure institution of optimal therapy programs.[223,237,238,241]

Ligament Injuries

Ligament injuries may occur by direct trauma but most frequently result from indirect mechanisms.[155,164,230] Early diagnosis of these injuries is essential. The prognosis varies depending on the extent of the initial injury, the mode of treatment, the type of athletic activity, and whether reinjury occurs. The natural history of ligament injuries, the techniques for diagnosis, and the classification of these injuries must be thoroughly understood by the treating physician and those involved in diagnostic imaging.[164,165,194,198]

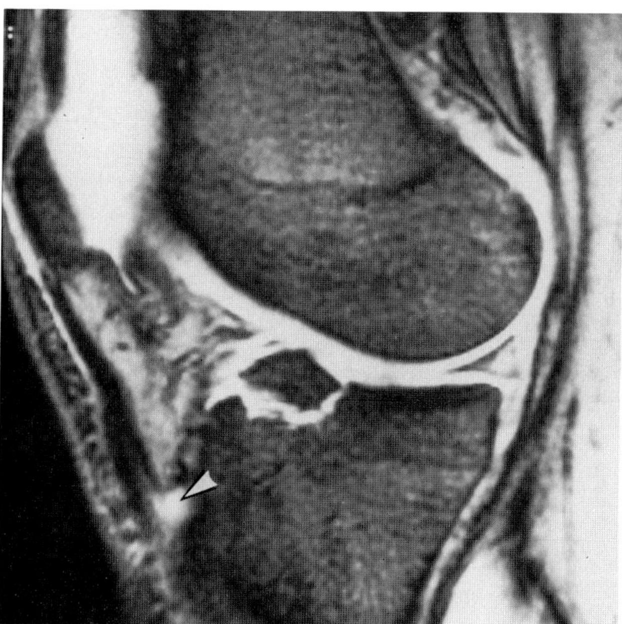

Fig. 6-51 Sagittal MPGR image demonstrating a tibial plateau fracture and partial avulsion of the patellar tendon (arrowhead). There is a large effusion.

Table 6-2 Soft Tissue Injuries of the Knee in Athletes

Articular
- Meniscal tears
- ACL tear
- PCL tear
- MCL tear
- Plicae

Periarticular
- LCL tear
- Muscle tears
- Patellar bursitis
- Patellar ligament tears
- Pes anserinus bursitis
- Iliotibial band syndrome
- Popliteal tendinitis
- Popliteal cyst

Sources: Baylis WJ and Rzonca EC, *Clinics in Pediatric Medicine & Surgery* (1988;5:571–589), WB Saunders; Berquist TH, *Imaging of Orthopedic Trauma*, ed 2, 1991, Raven Press; Mattalino AJ, Deese JM and Campbell ED, *Clinics in Sports Medicine* (1989;8:461–475), WB Saunders; Patel D, *American Journal of Sports Medicine* (1978;6:217–225), American Orthopaedic Society for Sports Medicine.

The ligaments and capsule form the passive restraints of the knee.[183,230] Injury to these structures may result in several types of instability. Medial injury may affect the MCL and the secondary restraints, which include the middle third of the medial capsule, the posterior oblique ligament, and the cruciate ligaments.[172,200,230,254] Lateral restraints are the LCL, the middle third of the lateral capsule, the popliteus and biceps femoris, and the cruciate ligaments.[158,159] The anterior restraints include the ACL with secondary support from the iliotibial band, capsule, MCL, and LCL.[157,181,254] Finally, posterior stability is provided by the PCL, posterolateral capsule, popliteus, and both collateral ligaments (Figs. 6-3 and 6-4).[172,200,221,222,230,254]

The medial ligaments are most commonly injured. Injury is generally the result of running, cutting, or abrupt deceleration leading to valgus stress. Direct trauma to the lateral aspect of the knee when the foot is planted can result in a similar stress. The extent of injury to the MCL depends upon the force and the strength of the secondary restraints (medial capsule, posterior oblique ligament, and cruciate ligaments).[201,212,254] LCL injuries are unusual. When they do occur they are a result of varus stress with the knee flexed and the tibia internally rotated.[202,207,212] Associated rupture of the ACL is common in this setting.[212,254]

Rupture of the cruciate ligaments frequently occurs with other knee injuries.[203,230,237] Isolated cruciate injuries are more controversial. Internal tibial rotation leads to ACL injury, and hyperextension forces can lead to disruption of either the ACL or the PCL.[157,170,171,173,176,181,222,237] PCL injuries have also been reported with a posteriorly directed force to the upper tibia with the knee in the flexed position.[159,203,212]

It is essential for radiologists to understand the clinical data and physical findings recorded by orthopaedists. The terms used are useful in planning the examination and ensuring that all potentially injured structures are thoroughly imaged.[164] Therefore, the most common terms and tests used to evaluate knee injuries are reviewed below.

Diagnosis of acute ligament injuries may be difficult. Intact secondary restraints may mask injury to the collateral ligaments and ACL.[254] Combined injury to the MCL and ACL is common.[230]

Patients with ACL tears frequently present with a history of an acute pop during the injury. This finding is reported by 90% of patients.[198] Hemarthrosis, swelling, and inability to bear weight are reported in more than 75% of patients.[222,230] The combination of a pop at the time of injury, gross swelling, and inability to bear weight or to continue activity is about 85% accurate for clinical diagnosis of acute ACL tear.[182,230] Patients with MCL injuries are more frequently able to bear weight after acute injury.[212]

Clinical Tests

Physical examination of the acutely injured knee may be difficult as a result of pain and swelling. Also, the degree of involvement of the secondary restraints influences the usual physical findings. For example, if the secondary restraints are intact, a low-grade injury to the primary restraint (ACL, MCL, PCL, or LCL) may be overlooked. Accuracy is increased with anesthesia.[176,222,230]

It is important for imagers to understand the implications of the clinical tests in planning the imaging examination. These tests are basically designed to evaluate instability.[212] Both the injured and the uninvolved knee are examined.[212,230]

The valgus stress test is performed with the knee flexed approximately 30° to evaluate the MCL. Joint laxity is graded from I to IV on the basis of the amount of medial joint opening. Grade I indicates 5 mm or less; grade II, 6 to 10 mm; grade III, 11 to 15 mm; and grade IV, greater than 15 mm.[212,230] The knee is also stressed in the extended position. Medial opening in the extended position suggests posterior capsule and/or PCL disruption.[212]

Varus stress is also applied in both flexed and extended positions. When the knee is extended the LCL is stressed, so that lateral joint line opening indicates injury to this structure.[198,212,217,221,230]

AP instability (drawer sign) is evaluated with the knee flexed 60° to 90°. The drawer test is performed with the evaluator's hands below the patient's knee so that stress can be applied in an anterior and posterior direction through the upper tibia. Increased anterior mobility indicates an ACL tear. Posterior laxity suggests PCL injury.[212,230] The same grading system described above is used. A positive anterior drawer sign may be noted in up to 90% of patients with ACL tears.[230] The posterior drawer sign is evident in 50% to 67% of PCL injuries.[159,203,212,230]

Table 6-3 Ligament Instability of the Knee

Type	*Major Structures Injured*	*Physical Findings*
Single plane medial instability	MCL, PCL	Opening of medial joint with valgus stress
Single plane lateral instability	LCL, PCL, ACL	Opening of lateral joint with varus stress
Anteromedial instability	MCL, ACL, medial meniscal tear	Medial laxity with medial tibial displacement with anterior drawer test
Anterolateral instability	LCL, cruciate ligament, ACL, posterior horn, lateral meniscus	Anterior and lateral subluxation of tibia on femur
Posterolateral instability	Cruciate ligament, LCL, popliteus muscle, gastrocnemius muscle, biceps femoris, lateral capsular ligament, ± PCL	Increased external rotation of tibia
Posteromedial instability	Superficial MCL, ACL, posterior oblique ligament, medial capsule	Increased posteromedial tibial subluxation

The Lachman test performed with the knee flexed 20° to 30° is more reliable than the anterior drawer sign. This test is positive in 85% of patients without anesthesia. The examiner's upper hand supports the patient's distal femur while the other hand attempts to draw the tibia forward. Anterior movement of the tibia without a firm end point is a positive Lachman test.[212,230]

Rotary instability is evaluated with the knee flexed 60° and the foot initially internally rotated to tighten the lateral structures of the knee. The foot is then externally rotated to evaluate the medial structures. Forward and backward stress is applied to evaluate the medial and lateral structures.

These physical findings may be used to describe several types of instability. Instability may be single plane (AP, medial, or lateral), rotary (anteromedial, anterolateral, posteromedial, or posterolateral), or combined.[201–203,230] Table 6-3 summarizes the types of instability and structures injured. Single-plane instability indicates that the axis of rotation has been lost because of a PCL tear. With rotary instability the PCL is intact, providing an axis for rotation.[201,230]

Imaging of Ligament Injuries

Routine radiography remains a valuable screening technique for bone trauma and also provides valuable information regarding soft tissue injury.[164,209,227,253]

AP, lateral, notch, and patellar views allow effusions and subtle osteochondral fractures to be identified.[164,209] Effusions are common, especially with ACL injuries. This finding (Fig. 6-27) may be noted on the lateral view in more than 70% of patients.[252] Soft tissue swelling or irregularity of the medial fat planes can be seen on the AP view in patients with MCL injuries. Notch and patellar views are useful for evaluating osteochondral fractures associated with cruciate ligament avulsions.[209,227] Avulsions of the ACL occur near the tibial spine. PCL avulsions affect the posterior tibia and are most easily identified on the lateral view. Avulsion of the lateral upper tibia (Segond fracture) is often associated with ACL disruption.[227]

Stress views have not been used as commonly since the introduction of MRI. Nevertheless, varus, valgus, and AP stress views are useful in confirming instability (see Fig. 6-11).[164,230]

Arthrography with routine film techniques or combined with CT has been useful for detection of certain soft tissue injuries.[187,246] Except for meniscal injury, however, MRI is far more sensitive and specific for evaluating ligament injuries.[165,173,233,234]

Complete evaluation of the capsule, MCL, LCL, and cruciate ligaments in the knee has been difficult with conventional arthrography and arthrotomography.[164] Multiplanar MRI provides significant improvement in the ability to assess these structures.[165,168,247] The anatomy of the ligaments of the knee was discussed in the initial section of this chapter, but some review is necessary in discussing the technical aspects for evaluating these structures. The ACL, because of its oblique course (Fig. 6-52), can be more difficult to identify.[165,219,226,228,233]

The ACL, through its oblique course, is intraarticular but extrasynovial.[172,200] Typically the anatomic appearance on MR images varies, with the ACL having multiple fibers seen as linear areas of low signal intensity compared to the thicker and more uniform low signal intensity of the PCL (Fig. 6-53).

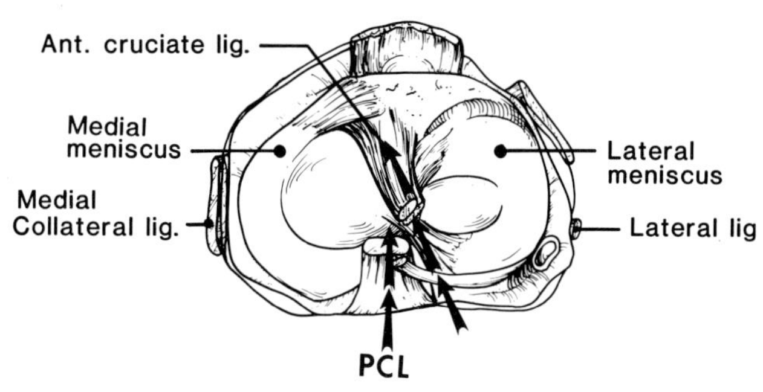

Fig. 6-52 Axial illustration of the knee demonstrating the courses of the anterior cruciate ligament (ACL) and posterior cruciate ligament (PCL).

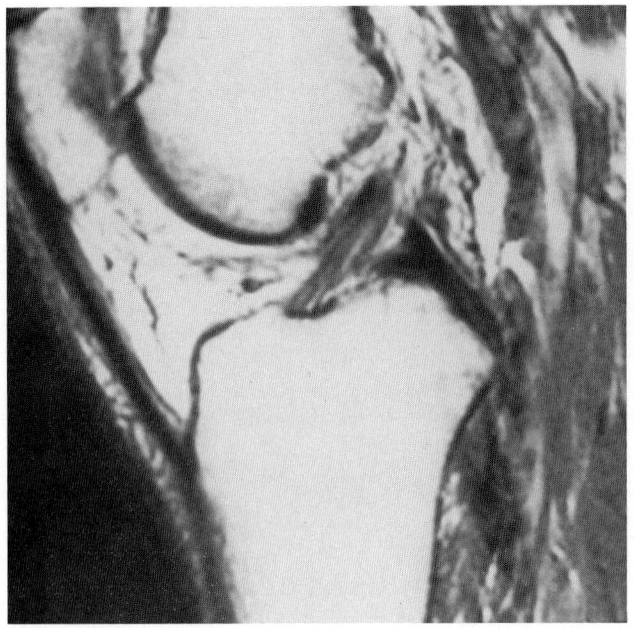

A

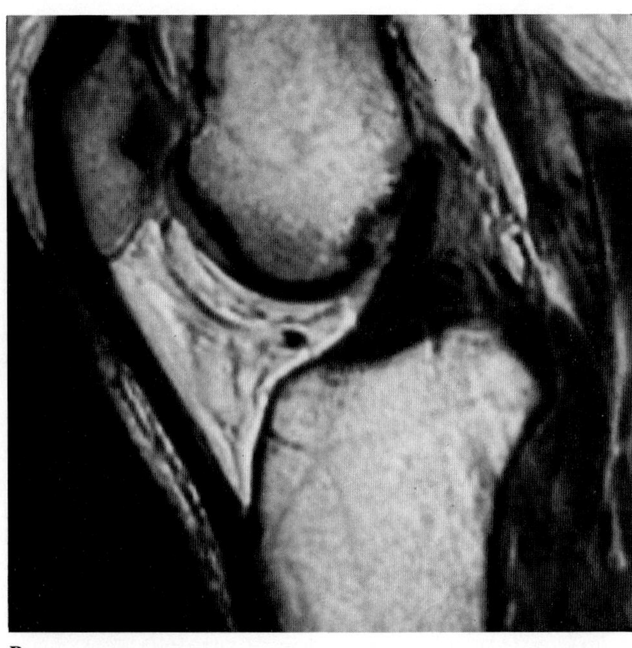

B

Fig. 6-53 Normal ACL appearance on sagittal MR images. (**A**) Normal ACL with thin, low-intensity bands. (**B**) Normal but thicker appearing ACL. Note the straight oblique (anteroinferior to posterosuperior) course.

Although oblique, sagittal, or externally rotated (20° to 30°) true sagittal images are optimal, the ACL should also be studied in other image planes. Tears in the ACL occur with internal rotation of the femur on the tibia with the knee extended. Up to 70% of patients have other intraarticular injuries, most often of the posteromedial meniscus.[165,230] The PCL is thicker and has a midline sagittal course; therefore, it is not difficult to visualize on MR sagittal images (Fig. 6-54).[161,165,184,191]

Technique for routine examination of the knee was described above and is generally adequate for evaluation of the cruciate ligaments, MCL, and LCL. In certain cases the ACL may be incompletely seen; in these cases repeat oblique images can be obtained easily. One should strive to demonstrate both cruciate ligaments completely on a single slice to assess abnormalities more easily (Fig. 6-55).

MR findings with disruption of either the ACL or the PCL are similar. The appearance or signal intensity will, of course, vary with the age of the lesion. We prefer T2-weighted images for assessment of the cruciate ligaments because the high signal intensity seen with acute lesions provides excellent contrast compared to the normally low-signal (black) ligaments (Fig. 6-56).[165] Mink et al[219,220] found T2-weighted sequences to be more sensitive and accurate than T1-weighted sequences. Sensitivity was 85%, specificity 95%, and accuracy 94% with T1-weighted sequences compared to 100%, 91%, and 97%, respectively, with T2-weighted sequences. We prefer the double echo (SE 2000/60,20) technique because increasing signal intensity on the second echo (SE 2000/60) confirms the acute nature of the injury (Fig. 6-56). Acute tears are seen as areas of high signal intensity in the ligaments, usually at either the tibial or the femoral attachments. Disruption at the femoral attachment is more common (Fig. 6-57).[214,220] With complete tears, the

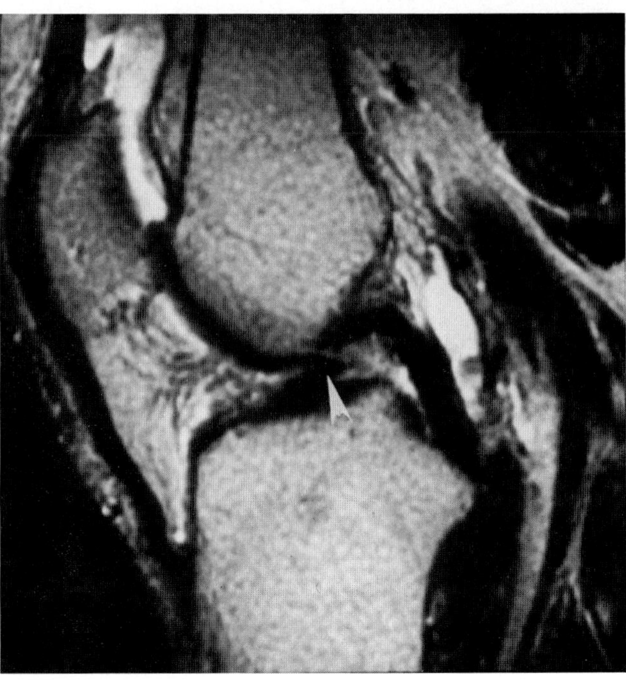

Fig. 6-54 Sagittal (SE 2000/60) MR image demonstrating the normal appearance of the PCL. There is an effusion with a tear (flat segment, arrowhead) in the ACL.

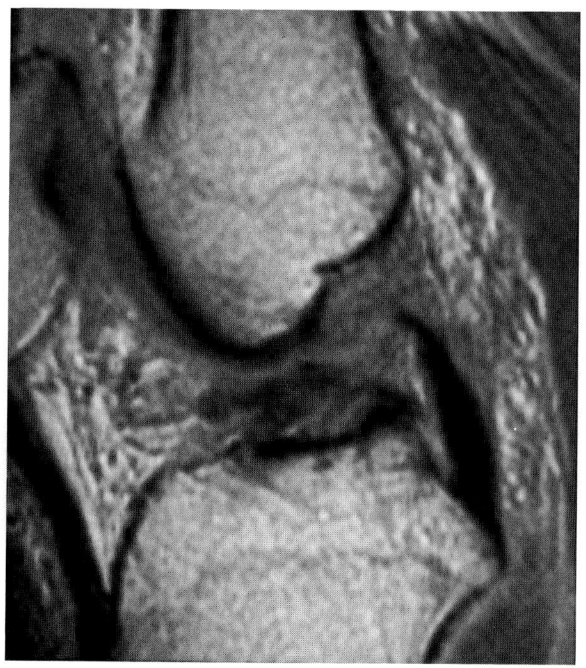

Fig. 6-55 Sagittal MR image demonstrating tears in both cruciate ligaments.

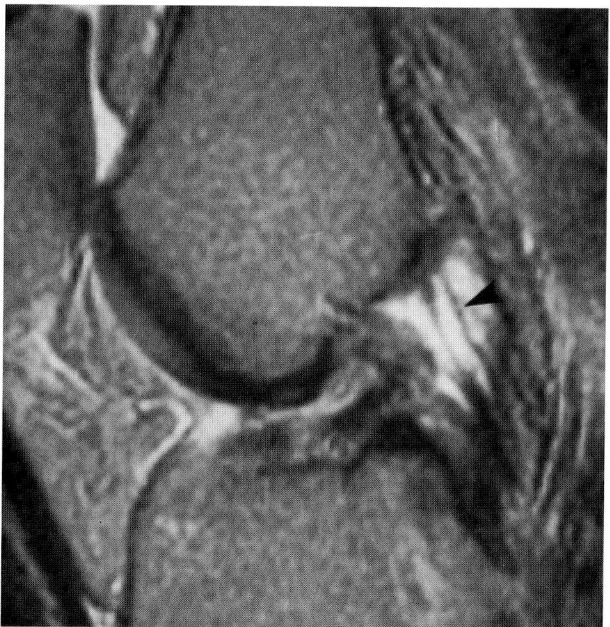

Fig. 6-56 Sagittal (SE 2000/60) MR image demonstrating an area of high signal intensity (arrowhead) due to a tear of the ACL at the femoral attachment. Note that there is no visible normal ligament on this section.

signal intensity extends throughout the width of the tendon, and there is usually separation of the tendon ends at the site of the tear with laxity or loss of the normal straight appearance of the ACL (Figs. 6-53 through 6-56). Chronic tears are seen as areas of intermediate signal intensity, typically with tendon thickening and associated ligament laxity (Fig. 6-58). The MR findings in PCL tears are similar to those in ACL tears except that the course of the ligament is not as useful. The PCL typically has a more curved appearance with convexity of its upper surface (Figs. 6-54 and 6-58). Changes in the configuration of the PCL are useful as a secondary sign of ACL disruption. An acute angle in the upper portion of the PCL forming a question mark configuration suggests a positive drawer sign due to ACL tear.[165,219,220,228,233]

Early and recent arthrographic studies of these ligaments indicate an accuracy of 91% for evaluation of the PCL but only 50% for the ACL with conventional arthrography or CT arthrography. Accuracy of detecting ACL injury may be increased by using stressed cross-table lateral techniques.[164] MRI is more accurate than arthrographic techniques. With the criteria described above, Mink et al[219,220] found that MRI correlated with arthroscopy in 95% of cases. Data obtained in practice at the Mayo Clinic have demonstrated an accuracy of 95%, specificity of 98%, positive predictive value of 88%, and negative predictive value of 96%.[165]

Evaluation of the MCL and LCL is generally easily accomplished with routine MR examination. In some cases, however, additional axial and coronal sections may be necessary to define subtle lesions more clearly. The MCL is typically divided into superficial and deep bands.[172,200] The superficial portion of the ligament typically arises from the medial femoral condyle and passes distally to insert approximately 5 cm below the joint line. Superficial fibers are separated from the deep fibers by a bursa, which may be inflamed and

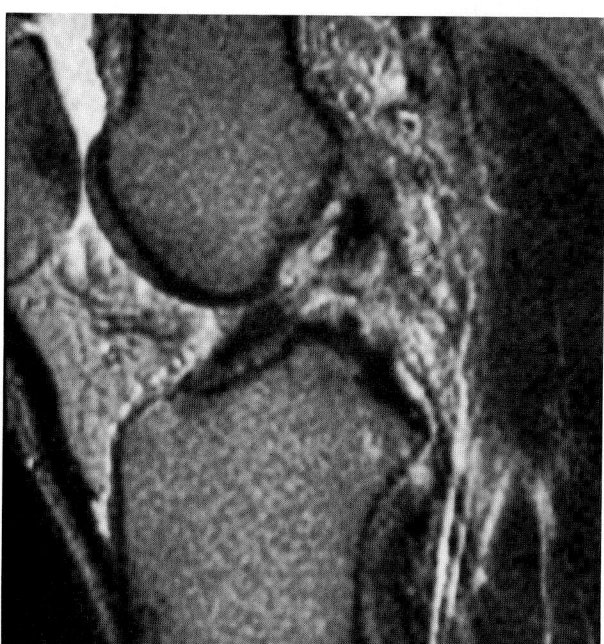

Fig. 6-57 Sagittal (SE 2000/60) MR image demonstrating an area of high signal intensity in the middle ACL due to an acute tear. Note the effusion in the suprapatellar bursa.

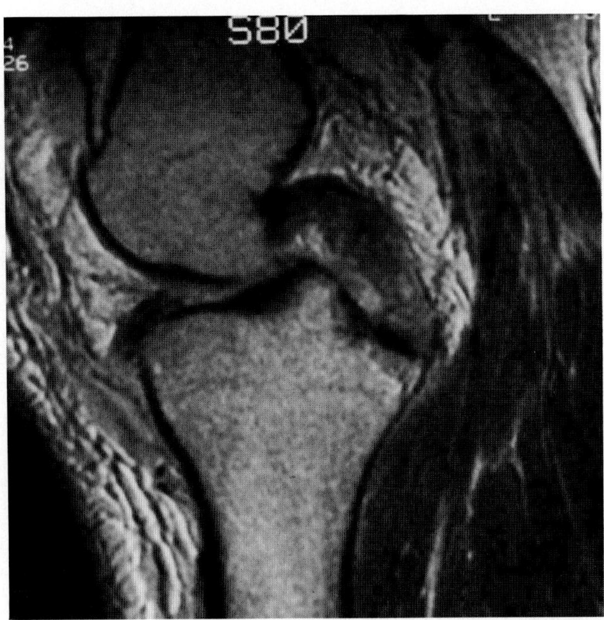

Fig. 6-58 Sagittal (SE 2000/60) MR image demonstrating thickening and slight increased signal intensity due to chronic injury to the PCL.

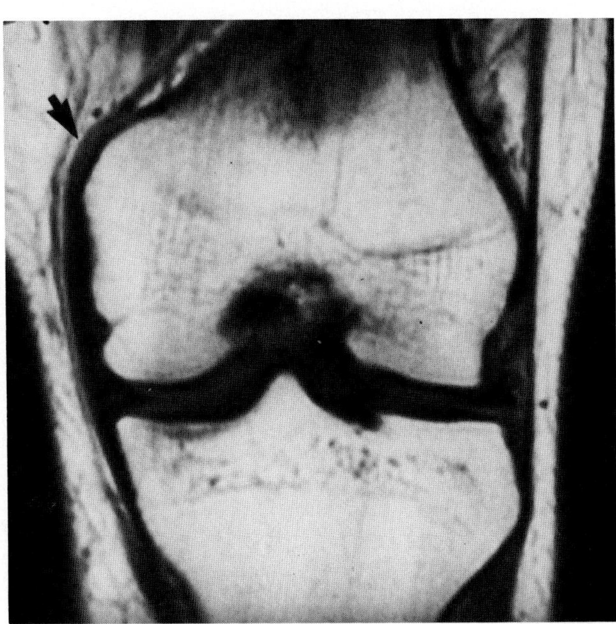

Fig. 6-59 Coronal (SE 2000/20) MR image demonstrating a first-degree sprain (arrow) at the femoral attachment of the MCL.

enlarged and should not be confused with a tear in the MCL (Fig. 6-59). The deep ligament is firmly attached to the capsule and midportion of the medial meniscus and attaches to the femur and tibia closer to the joint. The MCL is a stabilizer that resists external rotation and anterior forces and is more often injured than its lateral counterpart. Tears of the ACL are frequently noted in association with MCL tears (30%; Fig. 6-60).[165,213,219]

The LCL (Fig. 6-3) originates from the lateral epicondyle above the popliteus tendon and courses posteriorly and inferiorly to join the biceps femoris tendon; together, these insert on the fibular head. These structures, along with the iliotibial band, fabellofibular ligament, and arcuate ligament, provide the lateral support for the knee.[172,200] The LCL is not immediately associated with the capsule and is much less frequently injured than the MCL. When the ligament is disrupted, it is not uncommon to identify associated tears in the PCL.[230]

Acute incomplete tears result in areas of increased signal intensity in the soft tissues and within the normally dark appearing ligaments. When an incomplete tear is present, the joint space is normal and the course of the ligament unchanged. Care should be taken not to misinterpret the MCL bursa or the fat between its superficial and deep fibers as an incomplete injury. Complete tears in either ligament are identified by increased signal intensity at the site of the tear with

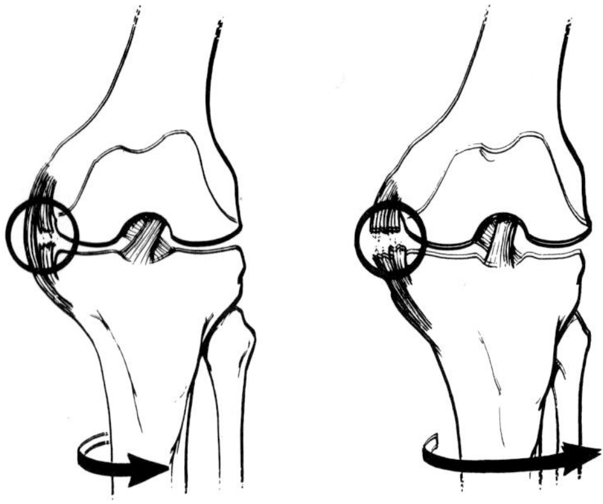

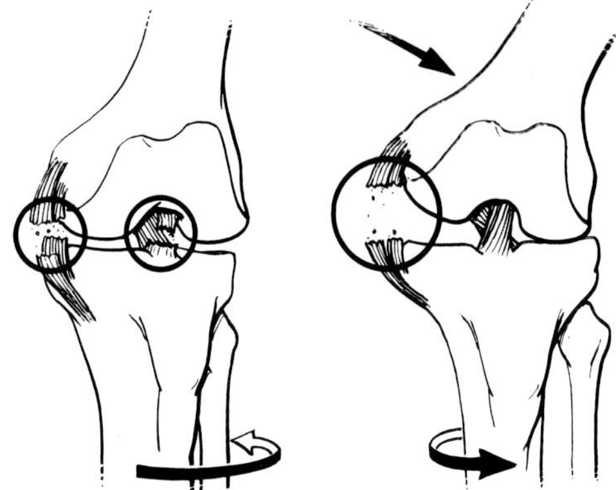

Fig. 6-60 Illustration of mechanism of injury to the MCL progressing to ACL tear (far right). Arrows indicate direction of force application.

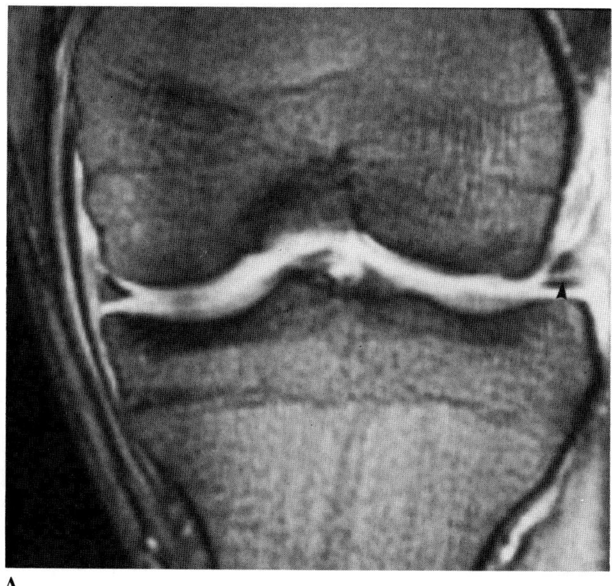

Fig. 6-61 (**A**) Normal and (**B**) partially torn MCL seen on coronal gradient-echo images. Note the lateral meniscal tear (arrowhead in **A**).

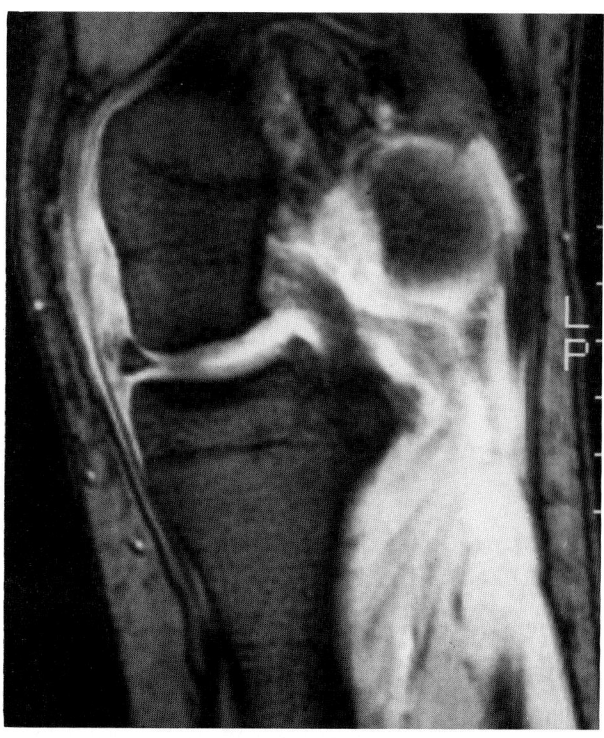

lack of continuity of the ligament and typically retraction of the torn ends (Figs. 6-61 and 6-62). Secondary findings, such as joint space widening, are not unusual.[165,219,220]

Meniscal Injury

The meniscus serves important functions in the knee related to shock absorption, stability, and distribution of synovial fluid for cartilage nutrition.[212,230] Certain anatomic features also deserve reemphasis.

The normal medial meniscus is C shaped (Figs. 6-2 and 6-4B). The transverse length is greater posteriorly (average, 14 mm) than anteriorly (average, 6 mm).[165,172,230] The meniscus is firmly attached to the capsule and deep portion of the MCL. This reduces mobility and results in an increased incidence of tears compared with the lateral meniscus.[230] Anteriorly, the medial meniscus is attached to the tibia anterior to the ACL attachment. Posteriorly, the medial meniscus attaches to the tibia midway between the lateral meniscus and the PCL attachment (Fig. 6-52).

The lateral meniscus is smaller, more circular, and more equal in width (Figs. 6-2 and 6-4B) than the medial meniscus. The anterior two-thirds of the meniscus is attached to the coronary ligament. Posteriorly the popliteus tendon with its synovial sheath passes through the joint capsule (Fig. 6-3). This results in incomplete attachment of the meniscus posteriorly. In some cases the popliteus muscle may partially attach to the lateral meniscus posteriorly.[172,200] The lateral wall of the tendon is attached to the joint capsule in most cases. Therefore, contrast medium or fluid on MRI will not completely surround the tendon.[165] The meniscus maintains superior and inferior attachments except where the tendon enters the joint inferiorly and exits superiorly (Fig. 6-3). Failure to visualize these attachments or the appearance of changes in the

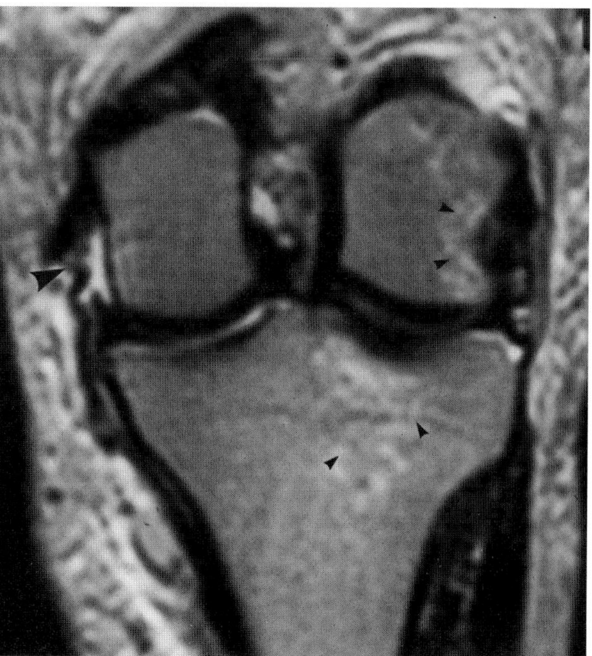

Fig. 6-62 Coronal (SE 2000/60) MR image showing valgus injury with MCL tear (large arrowhead) and impaction bone bruises laterally (small arrowheads).

normal configuration of the tunnel may be associated with meniscal tears (Fig. 6-3).[172,200,219,220]

Clinical Evaluation

Meniscal tears have been classified on the basis of appearance, mechanism of injury, and location.[164,212,219,220] Acute traumatic injuries usually occur in young athletes, leading to bucket-handle or peripheral tears.[164,208,212]

Partial or peripheral tears may go undetected after acute injury. Continued trauma leads to progressive tearing and degeneration. Patients will complain of locking in this setting or with displaced bucket-handle tears.[164,198,243] Laxity may be related to progressive degeneration and associated ligament injury.[212]

Meniscal symptoms are generally related to capsular inflammation or mechanical interference with joint motion. Associated soft tissue injury can easily mask meniscal injury in the acute setting.[212,230]

Historically, the athlete usually describes a catch or snapping sound when cutting or changing direction.[229,230] Joint effusion develops more slowly (6 to 12 hours) than with acute ligament injury.

Physical examination reveals joint line tenderness due to capsular and synovial inflammation. Pain may be produced during squatting with the feet internally and externally rotated. In the former, pressure is placed on the medial compartment, and a lateral meniscal tear may be displaced into the joint. When the feet are externally rotated, pressure is distributed to the lateral compartment, and tension is placed on the medial meniscus. Pain will often be described in the region of the meniscal injury.[212]

Clinical diagnosis of meniscal tear varies with the experience of the examiner. Accuracy is even more unpredictable in women.[212] The frequency of associated ligament and capsular injury has led to the common use of imaging to confirm clinical findings before arthroscopic evaluation is considered.

Imaging of Meniscal Injuries

Routine radiography is rarely useful in the primary diagnosis of meniscal injury. Osteochondral injury can occur at the point of bony attachment, however. The avulsed fragment can be identified in the posteromedial joint space (Fig. 6-41).

Arthrography has largely been replaced by MRI but is 90% to 95% accurate in detecting meniscal tears (Fig. 6-63).[164,179,187,209] Single- or double-contrast techniques may be used. The joint is usually entered laterally, and 6 to 10 mL of contrast agent or 4 to 6 mL of iodinated contrast agent plus 10 to 20 mL of air is injected. Normally, no contrast agent or air should enter the meniscus. Medially the meniscus is firmly attached to the capsule. The lateral meniscus is more difficult to evaluate because of the popliteus tendon, which passes through the posterolateral meniscus peripherally. Thus accuracy may be reduced in this area. Disadvantages of arthrography are its invasiveness and reduced ability to evaluate ligament and soft tissue injury compared to MRI.[164,252] Advantages include the ability to aspirate the knee in the presence of significant effusion and joint access for injection of anesthetic or steroid.[165]

CT is rarely used for meniscal injury in our practice. Accuracy approaches that of arthrography, however.[216,224] MRI has essentially replaced arthrography for imaging of knee injuries.

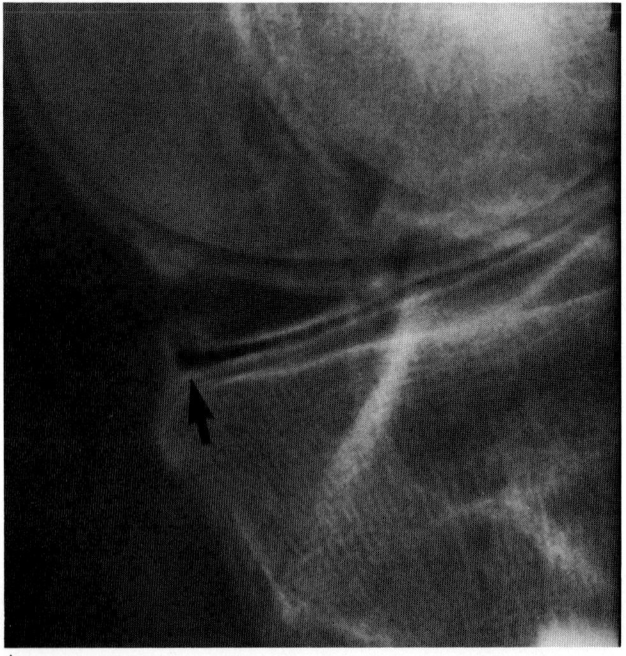

A

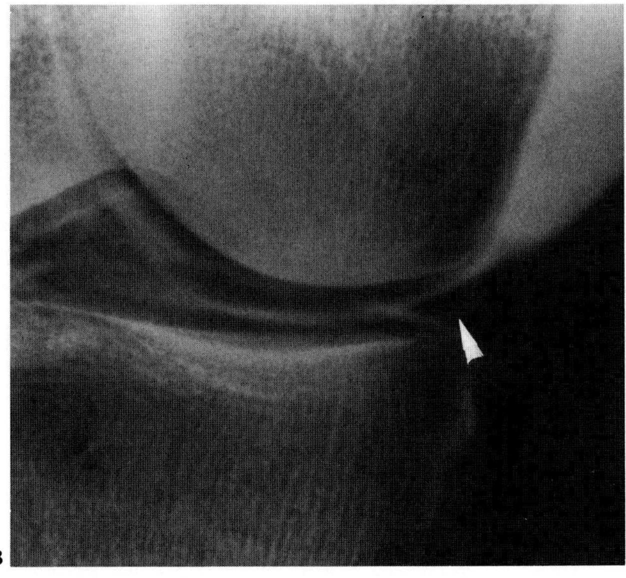

B

Fig. 6-63 (**A**) Normal double-contrast view of the posteromedial meniscus demonstrating a normal inferior recess (arrow). (**B**) Oblique tear in the anteromedial meniscus (arrow).

MR examination techniques vary depending on the software and preferences of the examiner.[165,196] Throughput and ease of lesion detection are both important. We prefer T2-weighted spin-echo or gradient-echo sequences. The high signal intensity of the lesions compared to the normal low signal intensity (black) of the menisci allows defects to be more easily appreciated.[165] Some clinicians prefer T1-weighted sequences or three-dimensional gradient-echo sequences.[211,219,220,244]

The appearance of normal menisci and meniscal tears has been well documented in the MRI literature (Fig. 6-64).[218] Increased signal intensity has been noted on T1- and T2-weighted sequences and on gradient-echo sequences.[165,173,177,184,208] These changes can be seen with mucoid degeneration as well as meniscal tears.

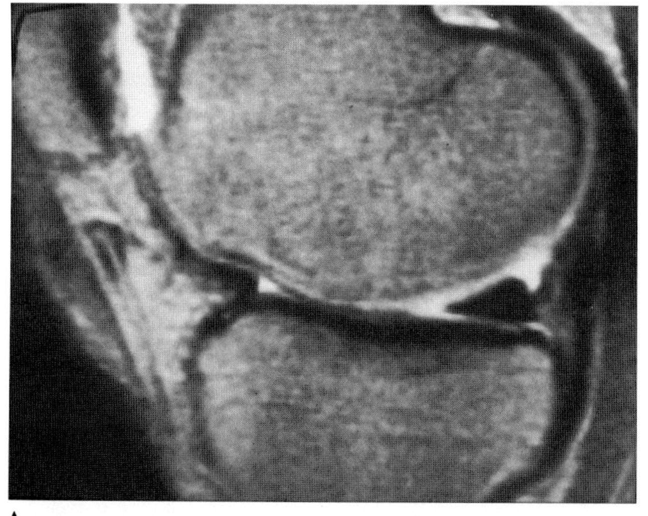

A

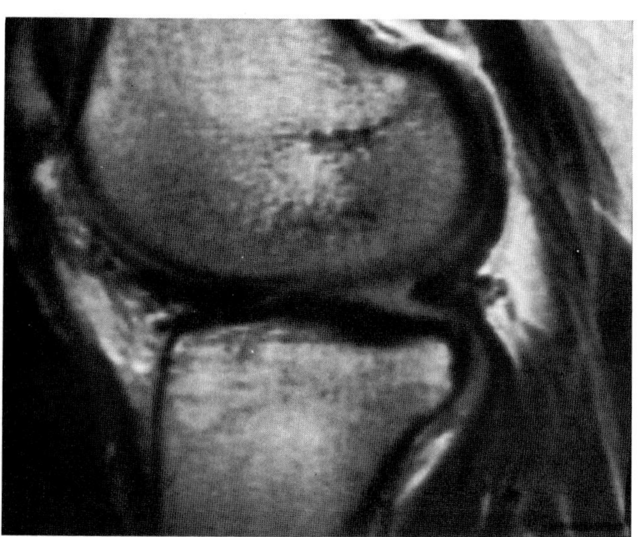

B

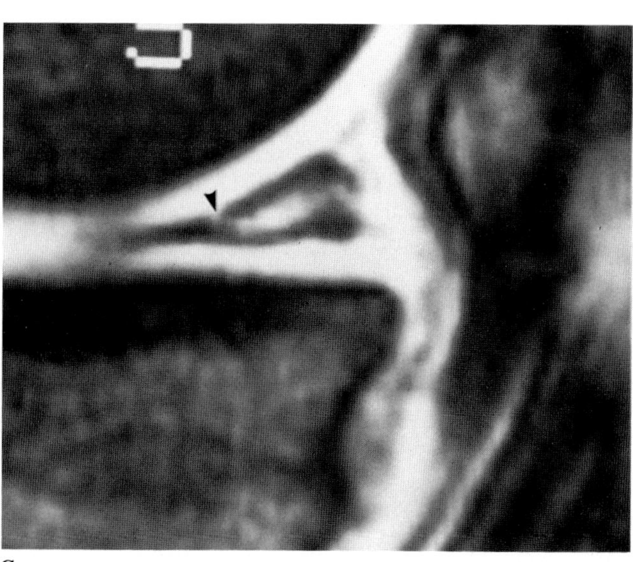

C

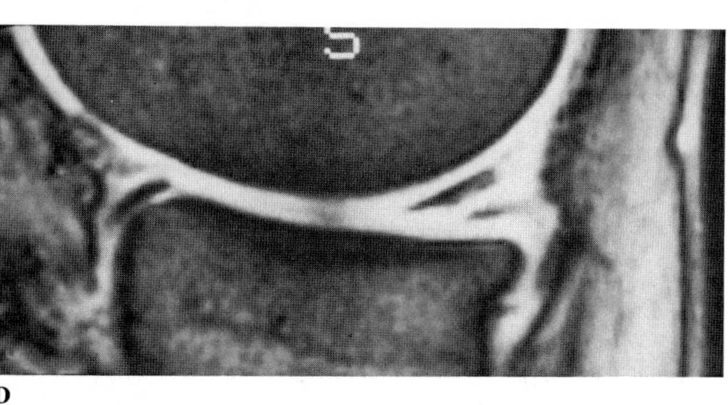

D

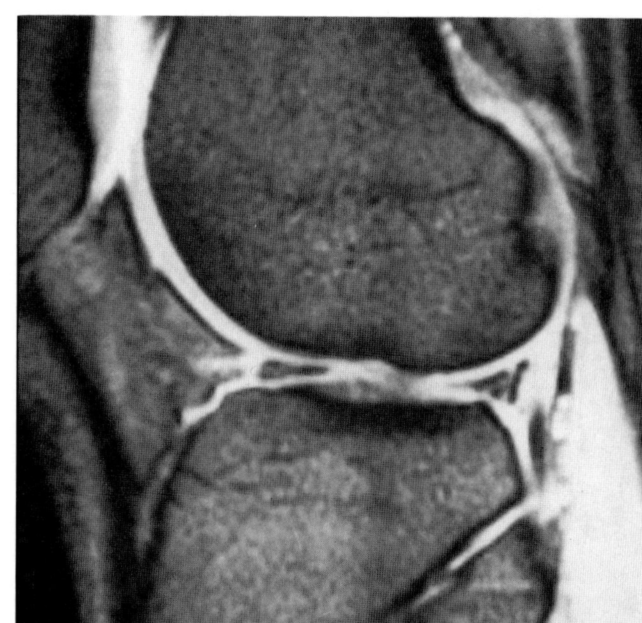

E

Fig. 6-64 Meniscal features on MR images. (**A**) SE 2000/60 image of a normal posteromedial meniscus. (**B**) SE 2000/20 image demonstrating blunting of the inner margin due to a radial tear. (**C**) Gradient-echo image demonstrating a grade 3A tear that communicates with the superior articular surface (arrowhead). (**D**) Gradient-echo image demonstrating a grade 3B lesion with irregularity of the inferior articular surface. (**E**) Gradient-echo image of a complex posterior horn tear (grade 4 lesion).

Grading systems for meniscal tears have been described by Stoller,[244] Crues,[173] and Mink[219,220] and their colleagues on the basis of pathologic findings in cadaver specimens (Fig. 6-64). A grade 1 meniscal lesion is globular in nature and does not communicate with the articular surface (Fig. 6-61). Histologically this stage correlates with early mucoid degeneration. It is believed that these changes are not symptomatic but represent a response to mechanical stress and loading, which result in increased production of mucoid polysaccharide ground substance.[173,244]

Grade 2 signal intensity is linear in nature and remains within the substance of the meniscus. Once again there is no evidence of communication with the articular surface of the meniscus. Histologically, these changes are characterized by more extensive bands of mucoid degeneration. Most investigators hold that stage 2 changes represent progression of stage 1 and that stage 2 lesions are precursors to complete tears.[173,178,219,244]

With grade 3 tears there is increased signal intensity within the meniscus that extends to the articular surface (Fig. 6-64, C and D). Mink et al[219,220] have further divided grade 3 lesions into two subcategories. Grade 3A signal intensity is a linear intermeniscal signal that abuts the articular margin (Fig. 6-64C). Grade 3B is a more irregular area of signal intensity that abuts the articular margin (Fig. 6-64D). Grade 3B lesions are most often associated with more extensive degenerative changes in the adjacent areas of the meniscus associated with the tear.

Grade 4 menisci are distorted (Fig. 6-64E) and show the changes described for grade 3 lesions.

The MR appearances of different types of meniscal tears are similar to those described for arthrography. Vertical tears are usually traumatic compared with horizontal tears, which are more often degenerative. Degenerative fraying of the surface of the meniscus may also be evident on MR images and is demonstrated as areas of irregular increased signal intensity on the meniscal surface compared to the normal dark or low intensity of the body of the meniscus. Radial tears may be somewhat difficult to diagnose but are typically seen as areas of increased signal in the inner margin of the menisci. Bucket-handle tears are vertical tears with displacement of the inner fragment for variable distances (Fig. 6-65).

When bucket-handle tears are identified, one must search carefully to be certain that the entire displaced fragment is identified.[242,243] Loose bodies or fragments of menisci in the intercondylar regions are not uncommon.[165,243] These lesions may be so subtle that reduction in the size of the meniscus may be the only finding (Fig. 6-65D). Parrot beak tears (Fig. 6-65A) are horizontal tears with vertical or radial components at the meniscal margin. These lesions are most common at the junction of the body and posterior horn of the lateral meniscus.[219,244] Peripheral tears or separations in the menis-

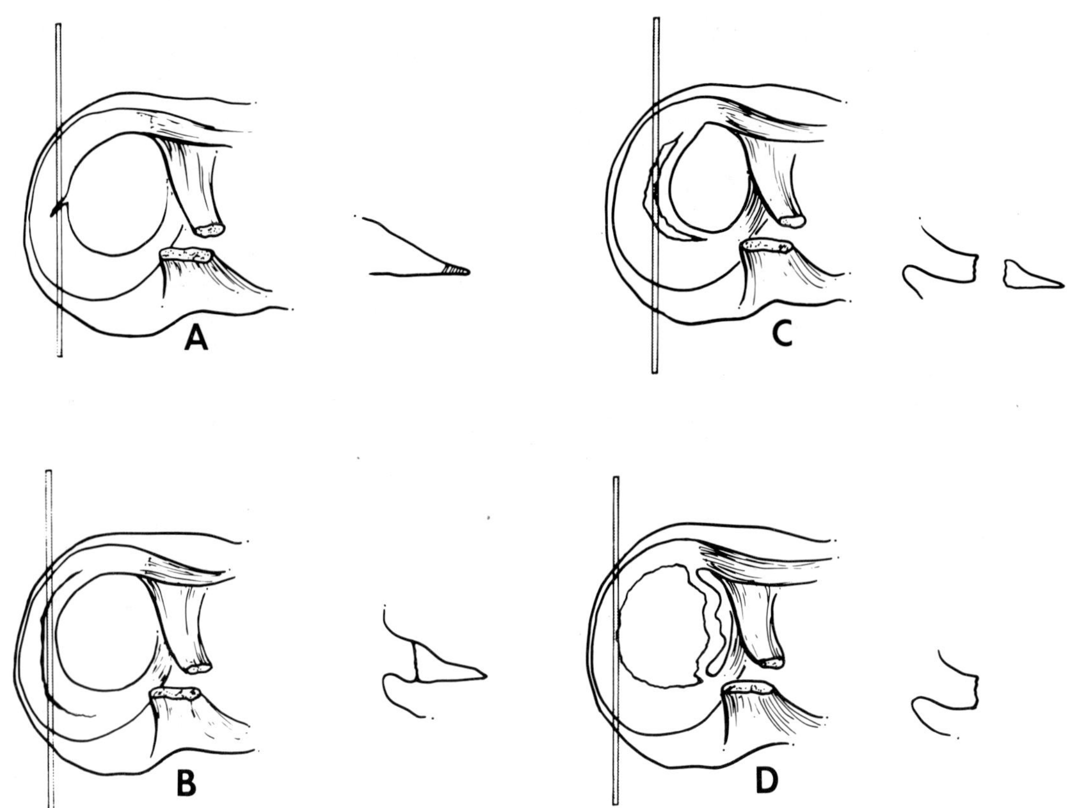

Fig. 6-65 Illustrations of meniscal tears. (**A**) Radial (parrot beak). (**B**) Vertical. (**C**) Bucket-handle. (**D**) Bucket-handle with medial fragment displaced into the intercondylar region.

cus can also be identified. These are usually easily diagnosed with arthrography but can be subtle on MR images because of vascular tissue and the synoviomeniscal junction along the margins of the meniscus.[165,199,248,249] It is important to define clearly the location (medial, lateral, inner margin, or peripheral) and type of tear when possible. Grade 1 and 2 lesions will not be identified arthroscopically. Many peripheral lesions are stable and can heal with conservative therapy, so that arthroscopy may be avoided. The vascular tissue along the periphery of the menisci allows healing to occur.[251]

Several reports in the MRI literature have described the accuracy of this modality in identification of meniscal tears.[165,234] Sensitivity of MRI in detecting meniscal tears seen at arthroscopy ranges from 75% to 100%. Reicher et al,[234] by means of meniscal grading systems, reported a specificity of 92% and a sensitivity of 89% for detection of meniscal lesions with MRI compared to arthroscopy. This same group found that the negative prediction value of MRI approached 100%. Review of data gathered at the Mayo Clinic demonstrated a sensitivity of 99%, specificity of 90%, accuracy of 90%, positive prediction value of 96%, and negative prediction value of 98% for the medial meniscus.[165] MRI of the lateral meniscus showed 97% sensitivity, 97% specificity, and 91% accuracy.[165]

One could consider arthrography an equally effective tool in evaluating isolated meniscal lesions (accuracy, 91% for the medial meniscus and 81% for the lateral meniscus), although it is clearly not as valuable in evaluating the other structures in the knee.[164,187,235,236] Even in this setting, however, there are two situations in which MRI is clearly superior and a more effective technique. These are children with knee pain and patients with acute trauma and hemarthrosis.

MRI is also of value in studying patients who have had either partial or complete meniscectomy or arthroscopic repairs of the meniscus. Patients who have been treated in this manner are generally referred to exclude residual fragments, remnants of a tear that was not completely resected, or new tears. Interpretation of MR images after surgery for meniscal tears should not be approached differently than for MRI performed on nonoperated knees. Signal intensity changes noted within the menisci are similar, and unless communication with the articular surface is identified a tear should not be suggested.[180,205,239]

Meniscal Cysts

MRI is also of value in detecting other pathology that may mimic meniscal tears, such as meniscal cysts. Meniscal cysts have been reported in up to 1% of patients undergoing meniscectomy. Most cysts are located in the lateral meniscus, but they may occur along the margin of either meniscus (Fig. 6-66).[165,219] Patients typically present with localized tenderness and occasionally swelling along the joint line. Similar presentations can be noted in patients with periarticular ganglion cysts. Ganglion cysts may or may not have a clearly defined connection with the joint. They may also occur along the periarticular tendon sheaths and tibiofibular joint.[165,219] Popliteal cysts are typically located posteromedially near the medial head of the gastrocnemius.[164,165] Distinction among these conditions is important because operative management of meniscal cysts is more commonly required. Popliteal and ganglion cysts, however, if persistently symptomatic, may also require resection. Medial cysts, although less common, frequently tend to be asymptomatic, even though they may be larger than cysts in the lateral meniscus.[169,219]

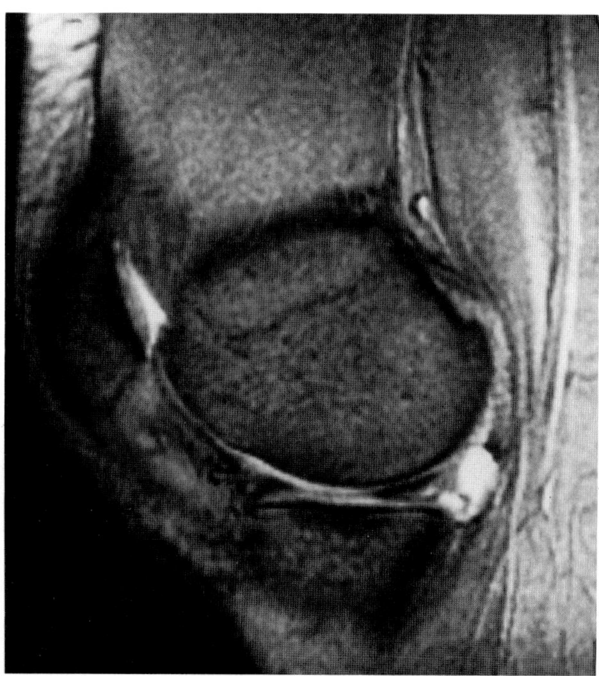

Fig. 6-66 Sagittal gradient-echo image demonstrating a meniscal cyst posteriorly.

The etiology of meniscal cysts is controversial. Various theories have been proposed, including chronic infection, hemorrhage, and mucoid degeneration. Because the fluid is similar to synovial fluid, it is hypothesized that a tear in the meniscus may lead to fluid accumulation within the meniscal tear itself, leading to cyst formation. It is likely that the etiology is multifactoral, but most investigators exclude hemorrhage and infection as causes.[165,219]

MR features of meniscal cysts and ganglia are easily appreciated on T2-weighted and gradient-echo sequences (Fig. 6-66). Both are well-marginated, high-intensity lesions. Meniscal cysts tend to be within or at the margin of the meniscus, and ganglion cysts may extend from the capsule or be located in the periarticular soft tissues.[165,219] Sonography has also been used for evaluation of meniscal cysts.[175]

Discoid Menisci

Discoid menisci are uncommon, being reported in 1.5% to 15.5% of lateral menisci.[165,193,219] Discoid medial menisci are rare. Both the etiology and the classification of discoid menisci are controversial. Hall[193] has described an arthrographic classification that is preferred at the Mayo Clinic.

Discoid menisci are typically broad and disc shaped. This configuration and the extension into the joint make this meniscus more susceptible to tearing. Type 1 discoid menisci are thick, slablike menisci with parallel superior and inferior surfaces. Type 2 are more slablike with a thin central portion. Type 3 discoid menisci are only slightly larger than normal menisci. Type 4 are asymmetric with the anterior horn extending farther into the joint than the posterior horn. Type 5 is between normal and slablike, and type 6 is any of the above with an associated tear.[193]

Clinically patients with a discoid meniscus present with symptoms of snapping and occasionally pain because these menisci are more prone to tear. Although there is no large series of MR findings in discoid menisci, Hartzman et al[197] did report a series describing MR findings. The transverse diameter of the normal meniscus is approximately 10 to 11 mm, and therefore the increased transverse diameter of a discoid meniscus can result in typical findings on both coronal and sagittal MR images. For example, on sagittal 5-mm slices, only two slices should demonstrate the meniscus. Visualization of the meniscus in more than three slices is indicative of a discoid meniscus. Coronal and radial images of the meniscus are perhaps more useful in that the true extension into the joint can be better demonstrated.[193,197,240]

Arthroscopy

Arthroscopy plays a valuable role in diagnosis and treatment of knee injuries. The complementary role of imaging and arthroscopy makes it essential for imagers to understand the place of each technique in evaluating knee injuries.

Arthroscopy allows early diagnosis, treatment, and prognostic information that is particularly useful in athletes.[229] Clinical diagnosis of knee injuries is 70% accurate. Arthroscopy is 84% to 97% accurate for evaluation of the cruciate ligaments, menisci, capsule, and synovium when performed by an experienced examiner.[229,230]

Arthroscopic evaluation with a probe allows the extent of cruciate injury to be assessed more completely. This is useful in determining whether surgical repair will be possible. At the same time meniscal injuries can be studied carefully and partial arthroscopic menisectomy performed. Athletes may return to activity in 2 weeks after partial menisectomy.[212,229,230] Arthroscopy is also useful for evaluating osteochondral fractures and patellofemoral disorders.

Arthroscopy traditionally has blind areas that are difficult to evaluate. These include the posterior horn of the medial meniscus and the retropatellar fat pad.[230]

In the acute setting, imaging, specifically MRI, is useful in defining the type of injury and assisting the orthopaedic surgeon in determining whether arthroscopy or other surgical intervention is indicated. For example, a minor MCL injury with no meniscal tear or a partial peripheral tear is likely to be treated conservatively. Demonstration of a cruciate injury or central meniscal tear may require arthroscopic assessment with partial menisectomy.[229,230]

MISCELLANEOUS INJURIES

There are numerous other conditions that may require imaging to confirm the diagnosis or to exclude more significant injury. Many of these are chronic overuse syndromes. Iliotibial band syndrome, patellofemoral stress syndrome, and patellar or quadriceps tendinitis account for more than 75% of injuries in runners.[225] Other conditions, such as bursitis and plicae, may require imaging and diagnostic or therapeutic injection (Table 6-4).[154,162,204,232,250]

Plicae

The significance of synovial plicae was not fully recognized before the advent of arthroscopy.[195,229] Plicae are embryonic synovial remnants that may be present in an asymptomatic knee. During fetal development there are thin membranes that divide the knee into medial, lateral, and suprapatellar compartments.[172,200] During development these membranes involute, resulting in a single cavity in the knee. When the membrane or a portion of it persists into adult life, it is termed a plica. These remnants are reported in up to 20% of the population.[165,195] These plicae (Fig. 6-67) are classified as suprapatellar, mediopatellar, and infrapatellar on the basis of the location of the original fetal membrane.[156,195]

The suprapatellar plica is the remnant that separated the suprapatellar bursa from the medial and lateral compartments (Fig. 6-67). Several forms have been observed, including a transverse septum with a small central communication, or medial and/or lateral remnants (Fig. 6-67). The medial suprapatellar plica is the most common. On sagittal MR or CT images this can be seen as a fold of soft tissue extending through the suprapatellar bursa above the patella. The mediopatellar plica begins above the patella medially and progresses distally to insert on the synovium above the infrapatellar fat pad (Fig. 6-67).[195] The infrapatellar plica is detected most

Table 6-4 Common Chronic Knee Injuries[162,190,215,225,231]

Condition or Syndrome	*Symptomatic Location*
Plicae syndrome	Medial
Iliotibial band syndrome	Lateral
Patellofemoral arthralgia	Anterior
Anserine bursitis	Medial
Medial retinaculitis	Medial
Popliteal tenosynovitis	Posterolateral
Patellar tendinitis	Anterior
Quadriceps tendinitis	Anterior
Snapping semitendinosus tendon	Medial

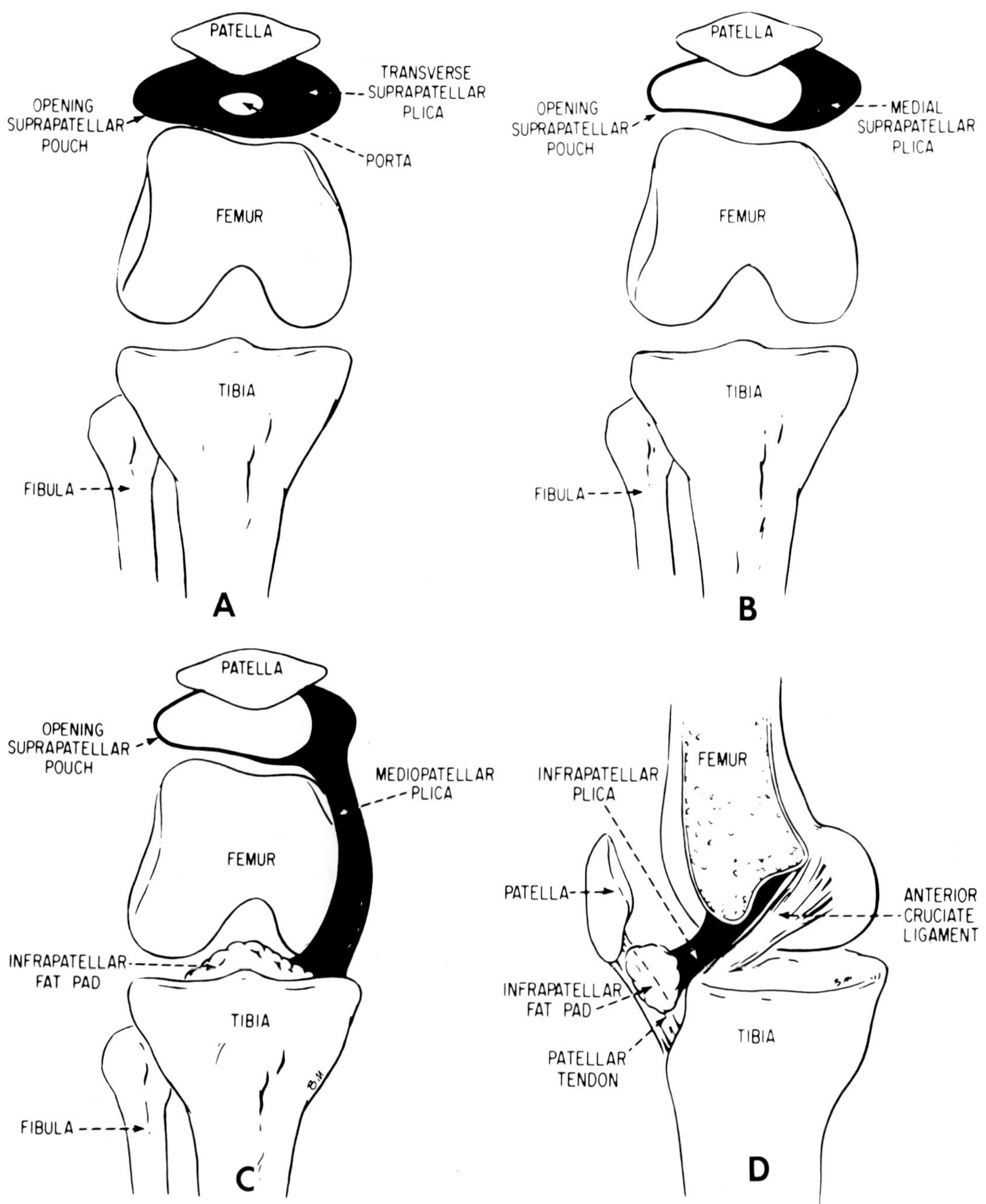

Fig. 6-67 Illustration of plicae of the knee. (**A**) Transverse suprapatellar plica with porta, anterior view. (**B**) Medial suprapatellar plica, anterior view. (**C**) Mediopatellar plica. (**D**) Infrapatellar plica. *Source:* Reprinted with permission from *Journal of Bone and Joint Surgery* (1980;62A:221–225), Copyright © 1980, Journal of Bone and Joint Surgery.

frequently. This plica follows a course along the upper margin of the ACL. It is rarely symptomatic.[165,195]

With chronic inflammation these membranes can become thickened and cause clicking or snapping as they pass over the femoral condyles. When left untreated, synovitis and cartilage damage can occur.[195,229,230] The exact etiology is unclear, but trauma and other associated conditions such as osteoarthritis, loose bodies, and the like may be evident. Most patients (90%) present with tenderness above the joint near the superior pole of the patella. A snap can be demonstrated in 71% of patients. Symptoms are generally due to thickening of the mediopatellar plica, but the suprapatellar plica has been implicated in patellar tracking abnormalities. Arthroscopic or open synovectomy may be necessary to relieve symptoms.[195,230]

When patients present with symptoms suggesting plica syndrome (snapping or peripatellar pain), either MRI or CT arthrography is most useful.[165,230] T2-Weighted sagittal MR images are adequate for identification of the suprapatellar and infrapatellar plicae. Axial T1-weighted or T2-weighted

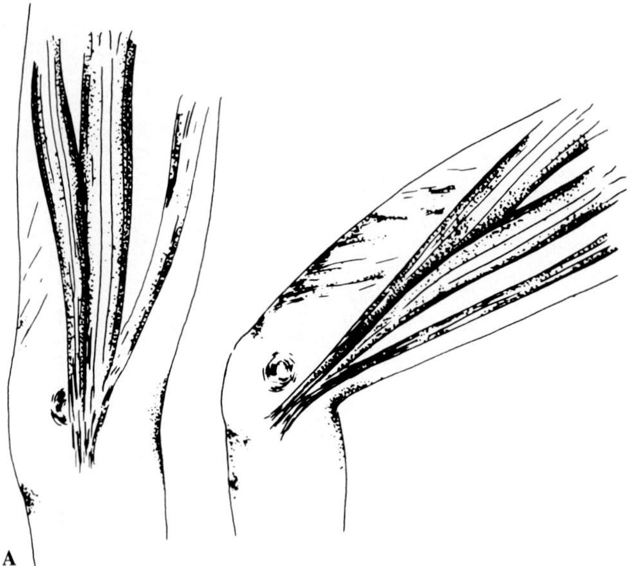

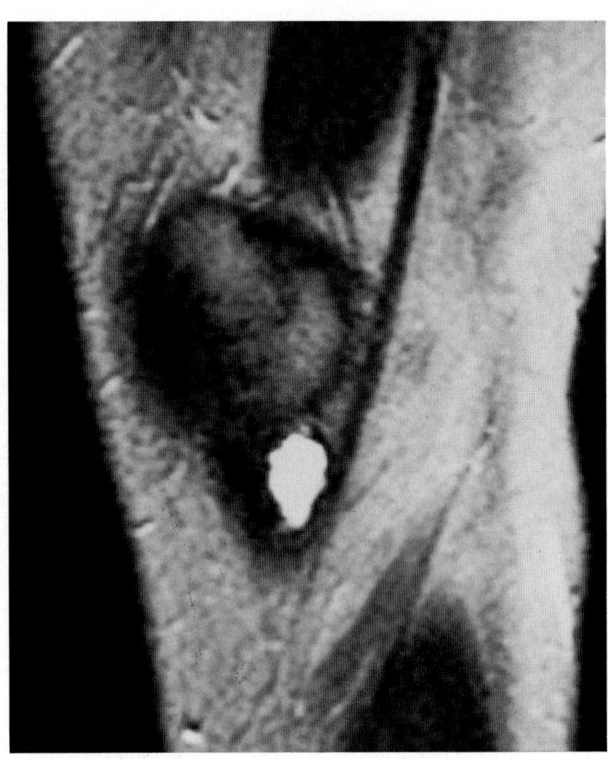

Fig. 6-68 (**A**) Illustration of friction of the iliotibial band over the femoral condyle. *Source:* Reprinted with permission from *Skeletal Radiology* (1987;16:57–59), Copyright © 1987, Springer-Verlag. (**B**) Sagittal MR image demonstrating an enlarged bursa that caused snapping of the adjacent tendon with flexion and extension.

images, however, are indicated to identify mediopatellar plicae. In the presence of an effusion a T2-weighted sequence or gradient-echo sequence is preferred. The low-signal plica is more easily seen against the high-signal synovial fluid.[165]

Iliotibial Band Syndrome

Iliotibial band syndrome is an overuse syndrome commonly seen in long distance runners.[165,217,232] Often, there is a history of recent increase in distance or hill running. The pain tends to intensify in the middle of the program and is bilateral in 20% of runners.[225]

The pain is caused by chronic inflammation or bursitis due to friction of the iliotibial band over the lateral femoral condyle (Fig. 6-68).[225,232] Physical examination reveals pain and point tenderness laterally. There may be crepitus with flexion and extension.[192,204,225]

Diagnosis may be established with clinical history and physical examination. Other lateral injuries and popliteal tendinitis may be difficult to differentiate clinically. In this setting MRI is best suited to confirm the diagnosis and exclude other injuries.[165] T2-Weighted images in the axial and sagittal planes (SE 2000/60,20; 3- to 5-mm sections, skip 1.5 mm) are usually adequate. Fast-scan or gradient-echo images in the sagittal plane can be performed with cine technique to demonstrate motion of the iliotibial band. Ultrasonography may also be useful in this setting but is less effective in excluding other disorders.[165]

Bursitis

There are numerous bursae about the knee (Table 6-5). Some communicate with the knee joint, but others are extraar-

Table 6-5 Bursae About the Knee[165,172,200]

Knee Region	*Anatomic Location*
Anterior	
Prepatellar	Between patella and skin
Retropatellar	Between patellar ligament and upper tibia
Pretibial	Between tibial tuberosity and skin
Suprapatellar*	Between quadriceps and femur (communicates with joint)
Lateral	
Gastrocnemius	Between lateral gastrocnemius and capsule
Fibular	Between LCL and biceps tendon
Fibulopopliteal	Between LCL and popliteus tendon
Popliteal*	Between popliteus tendon and lateral femoral condyle (communicates with joint)
Medial	
Gastrocnemius*	Between medial head of gastrocnemius and capsule (often communicates with joint)
Pes anserine	Between MCL and gracilis, sartorius, and semitendinosus tendons

*Communicating bursae.

Source: Reprinted from *Magnetic Resonance Imaging of the Musculoskeletal System* by TH Berquist, 1990, Raven Press, © Mayo Foundation.

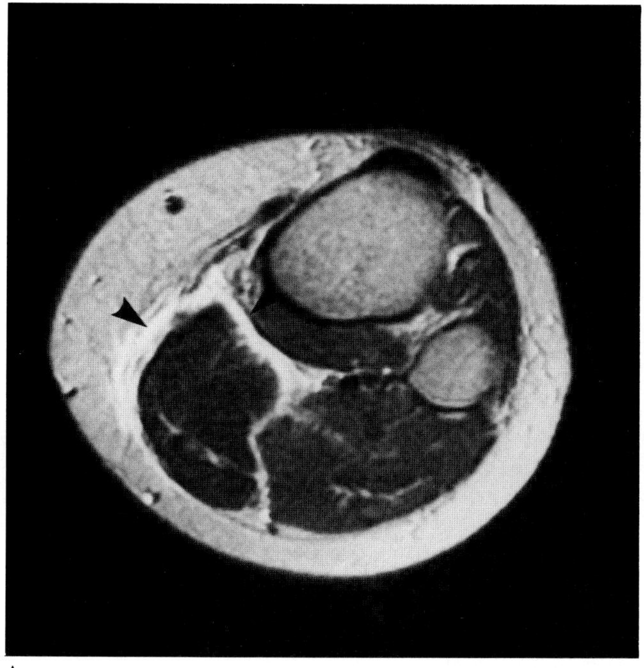

A

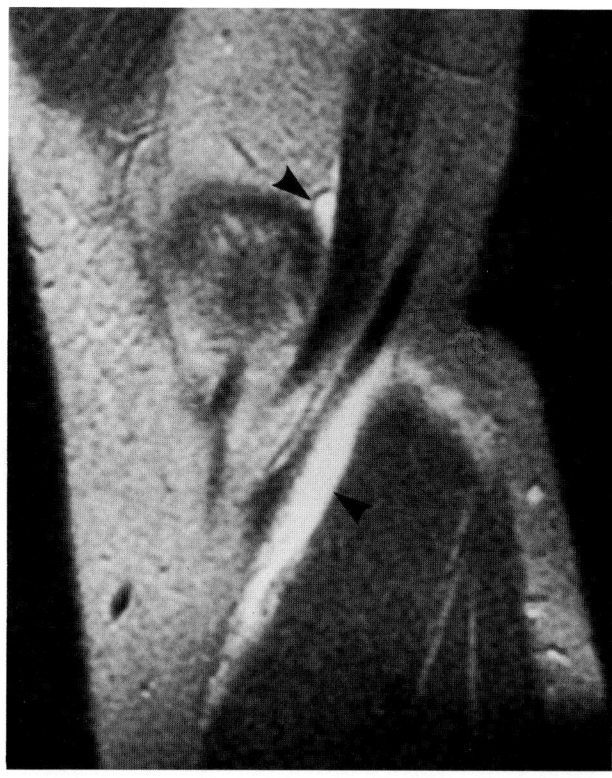

B

Fig. 6-69 (**A**) Axial and (**B**) sagittal MR images of the knee demonstrating pes anserine bursitis (arrowheads).

ticular and become inflamed with overuse syndromes.[167] Direct trauma can also lead to acute inflammation and/or hemorrhage in the bursae of the knee.[167] In the acute setting vasodilation leads to transudate formation, which may continue to evolve into an exudate with leukocytosis. In the chronic setting, thickening, fibrosis, and calcification may occur in and about the bursa.[167,217]

Pes anserine bursitis leads to medial knee pain (Fig. 6-69). The bursa lies between the pes anserinus (gracilis, semitendinosus, and sartorius) and the upper tibial metaphysis. Inflammation occurs with contusion or running.[162,186] Pain, swelling, and tenderness occur over the upper medial tibia. Differential diagnosis includes stress fractures, meniscal tears, and neoplasms.[167,208,217]

MRI and ultrasonography can be used to confirm the diagnosis. Because of the differential diagnostic possibilities, MRI is preferred. Axial and sagittal T2-weighted or T2* gradient-echo sequences are usually adequate for diagnosis of pes anserine bursitis (Fig. 6-69).[165] Other conditions that may cause medial knee pain may require additional imaging planes if the diagnosis is not obvious on axial and sagittal images.[165]

Tendinitis

Inflammation of the tendons about the knee can occur in the quadriceps, patellar, popliteal, and pes anserine tendons. A snapping semitendinosus tendon is a related condition due to inflammation of the tendon, which snaps over the posterior tibia (Fig. 6-69) with internal rotation of the tibia.[215,231]

Patellar and quadriceps tendinitis is usually associated with overuse of the extensor mechanism. Patellar tendinitis (jumper's knee) is usually noted in basketball players or other athletes for whom recurrent jumping is required.[166,167] Pain is noted over the inferior patellar pole. With quadriceps tendinitis, pain is elicited over the upper pole of the patella. Either ultrasonography or MRI may be required to differentiate tendinitis from partial or complete tears.[163,164,174]

Popliteal tendinitis causes posterolateral knee pain, primarily in runners.[254] Differential considerations include lateral meniscal tears, biceps femoris tendinitis, iliotibial band syndrome, and, rarely, soft tissue disorders. MRI is preferred to define the nature of the symptoms.[165,188] Sonography is also useful for evaluation of superficial tendons, however.[185,206]

REFERENCES

Introduction

1. Backx FJG, Erich WBM, Kemper ABA, Verbeek ALM. Sports injuries in school-aged children. *Am J Sports Med.* 1989;17:234–240.

2. Baylis WJ, Rzonca EC. Common sports injuries to the knee. *Clin Podiatr Med Surg.* 1988;5:571–589.

3. Gibson T, Davies JE, Crane J, Henry AN. Knee pain in sports people—a prospective study. *Br J Sports Med.* 1987;21:115–117.

4. Halpern B, Thompson N, Curl WW, Andrews JR, Hunter SC, Boring JR. High school football injuries: identifying the risk factors. *Am J Sports Med.* 1987;15:113–117.

5. Keene JS. Diagnosis of undetected knee injuries. *Postgrad Med.* 1989;85:153–161.

6. Kvist M, Kujala UM, Heinonen OJ, et al. Sports-related injuries in children. *Int J Sports Med.* 1989;10:81–86.

7. Lorentzon R, Wedren H, Pietila T. Incidence, nature and causes of ice hockey injuries. *Am J Sports Med.* 1988;16:392–396.

8. Micheli LJ. Lower extremity overuse injuries. *Acta Med Scand.* 1986;711:171–177.

9. Nicholas JA, Rosenthall PP, Gleim GW. A historical perspective of injuries in professional football. *JAMA.* 1988;260:939–944.

10. Paty JG. Diagnosis and treatment of musculoskeletal running injuries. *Semin Arthritis Rheum.* 1988;18:48–60.

11. Pritchett JW. A claims-made study of knee injuries due to football in high school athletes. *J Pediatr Orthop.* 1988;8:551–553.

12. Sherry E, Asquith J. Nordic (cross-country) skiing injuries in Australia. *Med J Aust.* 1987;146:245–246.

13. Taunton JE, Clements DB, Smart GW, McNicol KL. Non-surgical management of overuse injuries in runners. *Can J Sports Sci.* 1987;12:11–18.

14. Thompson RR. A study of the type and cost of football injuries. *Minn Med.* 1986;69:656–658.

Anatomy

15. Arnoczky S. Anatomy of the anterior cruciate ligament. *Clin Orthop.* 1983;172:19–25.

16. Bartel DL, Marshall JL, Schieck RA, Wang JB. Surgical repositioning of the medial collateral ligament. *J Bone Joint Surg Am.* 1977; 59:107–116.

17. Berquist TH. *Imaging of Orthopedic Trauma.* 2nd ed. New York: Raven; 1991.

18. Brantigan OC, Voshell AF. The mechanics of the ligaments and menisci of the knee joint. *J Bone Joint Surg Am.* 1941;23:44–66.

19. Butler DL, Noyes FR, Grood ES. Ligamentous restraints to anterior-posterior drawer in the human knee. *J Bone Joint Surg Am.* 1980;62:259–270.

20. Clemente CD. *Gray's Anatomy.* 13th ed. Philadelphia: Lea & Febiger; 1985.

21. Frankel VH. Biomechanics of the knee. *Orthop Clin North Am.* 1971;2:175–191.

22. Fukubayashi T, Kurosawa H. The contact area and pressure distribution pattern of the knee. *Acta Orthop Scand.* 1980;51:871–879.

23. Hollinshead HW. *Anatomy for Surgeons.* New York: Harper & Row; 1982;3.

24. Hughston J, Andrews J, Cross M, Arnaldo M. Classification of knee ligament instabilities. Part II: the lateral compartment. *J Bone Joint Surg Am.* 1976;58:173–179.

25. Hughston J, Andrews J, Cross M, Moshia A. Classification of knee ligament instabilities. Part I: the medial compartment and cruciate ligaments. *J Bone Joint Surg Am.* 1976;58:159–172.

26. Pope M, Johnson R, Brown D. The role of musculature in injuries to the medial collateral ligament. *J Bone Joint Surg Am.* 1979;61:398–402.

27. Rand JA, Berquist TH. The knee. In: Berquist TH, ed. *Imaging of Orthopedic Trauma.* 2nd ed. New York: Raven; 1991:333–432.

28. Shaw J, Murray D. The longitudinal axis of the knee and the role of the cruciate ligaments in controlling transverse rotation. *J Bone Joint Surg Am.* 1976;56:1603–1609.

29. Wiberg G. Roentgenographic and anatomic studies of the femoropatellar joint, with special references to chondromalacia patellae. *Acta Orthop Scand.* 1941;12:319–410.

Imaging of the Knee

30. Aisen AM, McDune WJ, MacGuire A, et al. Sonographic evaluation of cartilage of the knee. *Radiology.* 1984;153:781–784.

31. Apple JS, Martinez S, Allen NB, Caldwell DS, Rice JR. Occult fractures of the knee: tomographic evaluation. *Radiology.* 1983;148: 383–387.

32. Berquist TH. *Imaging of Orthopedic Trauma.* 2nd ed. New York: Raven; 1991.

33. Berquist TH. *Magnetic Resonance Imaging of the Musculoskeletal System.* 2nd ed. New York: Raven; 1990.

34. Bodne D, Quinn SF, Murry WT, et al. Magnetic resonance images of chronic patellar tendinitis. *Skeletal Radiol.* 1988;17:24–28.

35. Carlson JW, Gyori M, Kaufman L. A technique for MR imaging of the knee under large flexing angles. *Magn Resonance Imag.* 1990;8:407–410.

36. Chandnani VP, Ho C, Chu P, Trudell D, Resnick D. Knee hyaline cartilage evaluated with MR imaging: a cadaveric study involving multiple imaging sequences and intra-articular injection of gadolinium and saline. *Radiology.* 1991;178:557–561.

37. Crues JV, Mink J, Levy TL, Lotysch M, Stoller DM. Meniscal tears of the knee: accuracy of MR imaging. *Radiology.* 1987;164:445–448.

38. Daffner RH, Tabas JH. Trauma oblique radiographs of the knee. *J Bone Joint Surg Am.* 1987;69:568–572.

39. DeFlaviis L, Scaglione P, Nessi R, Albisetti W. Ultrasound in degenerative meniscal disease of the knee. *Skeletal Radiol.* 1990;19: 441–445.

40. Dumas JM, Edde DJ. Meniscal abnormalities: prospective correlation of double-contrast arthrography and arthroscopy. *Radiology.* 1986;160:453–456.

41. Eqund N. The axial view of the patellofemoral joint. *Acta Radiol Diagn.* 1986;27:101–104.

42. Farley TE, Howell SM, Love KF, Wolfe RD, Neumann CH. Meniscal tears: MR and arthrographic findings after arthroscopic repair. *Radiology.* 1991;180:517–522.

43. Fisher SP, Fox JM, DelPizzow W, Friedman MJ, Snyder SJ, Ferkel RD. Accuracy of diagnosis from magnetic resonance imaging of the knee. *J Bone Joint Surg Am.* 1991;73:2–10.

44. Fornage BD, Rifkin MD, Touche DH, Segal PM. Sonography of the patellar tendon: preliminary observations. *AJR.* 1984;143:179–182.

45. Hall FH. Radiographic diagnosis and accuracy in knee joint effusions. *Radiology.* 1975;115:49–54.

46. Hayes CW, Sawyer RW, Conway WF. Patellar cartilage lesions: in vitro detection and staging with MR imaging and pathologic correlation. *Radiology.* 1990;176:479–483.

47. Holmblad EC. Posteroanterior X-ray of the knee in flexion. *JAMA.* 1937;109:1196–1197.

48. Jensen DB, Johansen TP, Berg-Nielsen A, Henriksen O. Magnetic resonance imaging of sequelae after tibial plateau fractures. *Skeletal Radiol.* 1990;19:127–129.

49. Käebo P, Swärd L, Karlsson J, Peterson L. Ultrasonography in the detection of partial patellar ligament ruptures (jumpers knee). *Skeletal Radiol.* 1991;20:285–289.

50. Malghein J, Maldague B. Patellofemoral joint: 30° axial radiograph with lateral rotation of the leg. *Radiology.* 1989;170:566–567.

51. Passariello R, Trecco F, DePaulis F, Bonanni G, Masciocchi C, Zobel BB. Computed tomography of the knee joint: technique of study and normal anatomy. *J Comput Assisted Tomogr.* 1983;7:1035–1042.

52. Rafii M, Firooznia H, Golimbu C, Bonamo J. Computed tomography of tibial plateau fractures. *AJR.* 1984;142:1181–1186.

53. Rand JA. The role of arthroscopy in the management of knee injuries in athletes. *Mayo Clin Proc.* 1984;59:77–82.

54. Rijke AM, Tegtmeyer CJ, Weiland DJ, McCue FC III. Stress examination of the cruciate ligaments. A radiologic Lachman's test. *Radiology.* 1987;165:867–869.

55. Rosenberg TD, Paulos LE, Porter RD, Coward DB, Scott SM. The 45° posteroanterior flexion weight-bearing radiograph of the knee. *J Bone Joint Surg Am.* 1988;70:1479–1482.

56. Schwimmer M, Edelstein G, Heiken JP, Gilula LA. Synovial cysts of the knee: CT evaluation. *Radiology.* 1985;154:175–177.

57. Settegast H. Typische Roentgenobilder von normalen Menschen. *Lehmanns Med Atl.* 1921;5:211.

58. Shellock FG, Foot KF, Deutsch AL, Mark JH. Patellofemoral joint: evaluation during active flexion with ultrafast spoiled GRASS MR imaging. *Radiology.* 1991;180:581–585.

59. Shellock FG, Mink JH, Deutsch AL. Patellar tracking abnormalities: clinical experience with kinematic MR imaging in 130 patients. *Radiology.* 1989;172:799–804.

60. Stanford W, Phelan J, Kathol MH, et al. Patellofemoral joint motion: evaluation by ultrafast computed tomography. *Skeletal Radiol.* 1988; 17:487–492.

61. Surger AM, Naimork A, Felson D, Shapiro JH. Comparison of overhead and cross-table lateral views for detection of knee joint effusions. *AJR.* 1985;144:973–975.

62. Tallroth K, Lundholm TS. Stress radiographs in evaluation of degenerative femorotibial joint disease. *Skeletal Radiol.* 1987;12:617–620.

Patellar Disorders

63. Aglietti P, Insall JN, Cerulli G. Patellar pain and incongruence. I. Measurements of incongruence. *Clin Orthop.* 1983;176:217–224.

64. Aleman O. Chondromalacia post-traumatica patellae. *Acta Chir Scand.* 1928;63:149–190.

65. Andrews JR. Overuse syndromes of the lower extremity. *Clin Sports Med.* 1983;2:137–148.

66. Bassett FH II. Acute dislocation of the patella, osteochondral fractures, and injuries of the extensor mechanism of the knee. *Instr Course Lect.* 1976;25:40–49.

67. Bentley G. Chondromalacia patellae. *J Bone Joint Surg Am.* 1970;52:221–232.

68. Berquist TH. *Imaging of Orthopedic Trauma.* 2nd ed. New York: Raven; 1991.

69. Bodne D, Quinn SF, Murry WT, et al. Magnetic resonance images of chronic patellar tendinitis. *Skeletal Radiol.* 1988;17:24–28.

70. Boring TN, O'Donoghue DH. Acute patellar dislocation: results of immediate surgical repair. *Clin Orthop.* 1978;136:182–185.

71. Bourne MH, Hazel WA, Scott SG, Sim FH. Anterior knee pain. *Mayo Clin Proc.* 1988;63:482–491.

72. Brattstrom H. Shape of intercondylar groove normally and in dislocation of the patella. *Acta Orthop Scand.* 1964;68(suppl):134–148.

73. Cofield RH, Bryan RS. Acute dislocation of the patella: results of conservative treatment. *J Trauma.* 1977;17:526–530.

74. Crosby EB, Insall J. Recurrent dislocation of the patella. *J Bone Joint Surg Am.* 1976;58:9–13.

75. DeHaven KE, Dolan WA, Mayer PJ. Chondromalacia patellae in athletes: clinical presentation and conservative management. *Am J Sports Med.* 1979;7:5–11.

76. Delgado-Martins H. A study of the position of the patella using computerized tomography. *J Bone Joint Surg Br.* 1976;61:443–444.

77. Eqund N. The axial view of the patellofemoral joint. *Acta Radiol Diagn.* 1986;27:101–104.

78. Ficat RP, Hungerford DS. *Disorders of the Patellofemoral Joint.* Baltimore: Williams & Wilkins; 1977.

79. Ficat RP, Philippe J, Hungerford DS. Chondromalacia patellae: a system of classification. *Clin Orthop.* 1979;144:55–62.

80. Fornage BD, Rifkin MD, Touche DH, Segal PM. Sonography of the patellar tendon: preliminary observations. *AJR.* 1984;143:179–182.

81. Freiberger RH, Kozier LM. Fracture of the medial margin of the patella: a finding diagnostic of lateral dislocation. *Radiology.* 1967; 88:902–904.

82. Fulkerson JP, Shea KP. Disorders of patellofemoral alignment. *J Bone Joint Surg Am.* 1990;72:1424–1429.

83. Goodfellow JW, Hungerford DS, Woods C. Patellofemoral joint mechanics and pathology. II. Chondromalacia patellae. *J Bone Joint Surg Br.* 1976;58:291–299.

84. Goodfellow JW, Hungerford DS, Zindel M. Patellofemoral mechanics and pathology: I. Functional anatomy of the patellofemoral joint. *J Bone Joint Surg Br.* 1976;58:287–290.

85. Hayes CW, Sawyer RW, Conway WF. Patellar cartilage: in vitro detection and staging with MR imaging and pathologic correlation. *Radiology.* 1990;176:479–483.

86. Horns JW. The diagnosis of chondromalacia by double contrast arthrography of the knee. *J Bone Joint Surg Am.* 1977;59:119–120.

87. Hughston JC. Subluxation of the patella. *J Bone Joint Surg Am.* 1968;50:1003–1026.

88. Hungerford DS, Barry M. Biomechanics of the patellofemoral joint. *Clin Orthop.* 1979;144:9–15.

89. Inoue M, Shino K, Hirose H, Horibi S, Ono K. Subluxation of the patella: computed tomography of patellofemoral congruence. *J Bone Joint Surg Am.* 1988;70:1331–1337.

90. Insall JN, Aglietti P, Tria AJ. Patellar pain and incongruence. II. Clinical application. *Clin Orthop.* 1983;176:225–232.

91. Insall JN, Falvo KA, Wise DN. Chondromalacia patellae. *J Bone Joint Surg Am.* 1976;58:1–8.

92. Jackson RW. Etiology of chondromalacia patellae. *Instr Course Lect.* 1976;25:36–40.

93. Larson RL, Cabaud HE, Slocum DB, James SL, Keenan T, Hutchinson T. The patellar compression syndrome: surgical treatment by lateral release. *Clin Orthop.* 1978;134:158–167.

94. Laurin CA, Dussault R, Levesque HP. The tangential X-ray investigation of the patellofemoral joint: X-ray technique, diagnostic criteria, and interpretation. *Clin Orthop.* 1979;144:16–26.

95. Laurin CA, Levesque HP, Dussault R, Labille H, Peides JP. The abnormal lateral patellofemoral angle. *J Bone Joint Surg Am.* 1978;60:55–60.

96. Leach RE. Malalignment syndrome of the patella. *Instr Course Lect.* 1976;25:49–54.

97. Malghem J, Maldegue B. Patellofemoral joint: 30° axial radiograph with lateral rotation of the leg. *Radiology.* 1989;170:566–567.

98. Martinez S, Koroliken M, Fondren FB, Hedlund LW, Goldner JL. Diagnosis of patellofemoral malalignment by computed tomography. *J Comput Assisted Tomogr.* 1983;7:1050–1053.

99. Mattalino AJ, Deese JM, Campbell ED. Office evaluation and treatment of lower extremity injuries in the runner. *Clin Sports Med.* 1989; 8:461–475.

100. McDougall A, Brown D. Radiological sign of recurrent dislocation of the patella. *J Bone Joint Surg Br.* 1968;50:841–843.

101. Merchant AC, Mercer RL, Jacobsen RM, Cool CR. Roentgenographic analysis of patellofemoral congruence. *J Bone Joint Surg Am.* 1974;56:1391–1396.

102. Outerbridge RE. The etiology of chondromalacia patellae. *J Bone Joint Surg Br.* 1961;43:752–757.

103. Outerbridge RE. Further studies on the etiology of chondromalacia patellae. *J Bone Joint Surg Br.* 1964;46:179–190.

104. Outerbridge RE, Dunlop JAY. The problem of chondromalacia patellae. *Clin Orthop.* 1975;110:177–197.

105. Perrild C, Hejgaard N, Rosenklint A. Chondromalacia patellae: a radiographic study of the patellofemoral joint. *Acta Orthop Scand.* 1982;53:131–134.

106. Schmidt DR, Henry JH. Stress injuries of the adolescent extensor mechanism. *Clin Sports Med.* 1989;8:343–355.

107. Shellock FG, Mink JH, Deutsch AL, Fox JM. Patellar tracking abnormalities: clinical experience with kinematic MR imaging in 130 patients. *Radiology.* 1989;172:799–804.

108. Sikorski JM. The importance of femoral rotation in chondromalacia patellae as shown by serial radiography. *J Bone Joint Surg Br*. 1979; 61:435–442.

109. Stanford W, Phelan J, Kathol MH, et al. Patellofemoral joint motion: evaluation by ultrafast computed tomography. *Skeletal Radiol*. 1988; 17:487–492.

110. Tehranzadeh J. The spectrum of avulsion and avulsion-like injuries of the musculoskeletal system. *RadioGraphics*. 1987;7:945–974.

111. Thyn CJB, Hiller B. Arthrography and the medial compartment of the patellofemoral joint. *Skeletal Radiol*. 1984;11:183–190.

112. Wiberg G. Roentgenographic and anatomic studies of the femoropatellar joint, with special reference to chondromalacia patellae. *Acta Orthop Scand*. 1941;12:319–410.

Fractures

113. Apley AG. Fractures of the tibial plateau. *Orthop Clin North Am*. 1979;10:61–74.

114. Bakalim G, Wilppula F. Fractures of the tibial condyles. *Acta Orthop Scand*. 1973;44:311–322.

115. Baylis WJ, Rzonca EC. Common sports injuries to the knee. *Clin Podiatr Med Surg*. 1988;5:571–589.

116. Berquist TH. *Imaging of Orthopedic Trauma*. 2nd ed. New York: Raven; 1991.

117. Burri C, Bartzke G, Coldewey J, Muggler E. Fractures of the tibial plateau. *Clin Orthop*. 1979;138:84–93.

118. Clews AG. Dislocation of the upper end of the fibula. *Can Med Assoc J*. 1968;98:169–170.

119. DeSmet AA, Fisher DR, Graf BK, Lange RH. Osteochondritis dissecans of the knee: value of MR imaging in determining lesion stabilization and presence of articular cartilage defects. *AJR*. 1990;155:549–553.

120. Dietz GW, Wilcox DM, Montgomey JB. Second tibial condyle fracture: lateral capsular ligament avulsion. *Radiology*. 1986;159:467–469.

121. Elstrom J, Pankovich AM, Sassoon H, Rodriguez J. The use of tomography in assessment of fractures of the tibial plateau. *J Bone Joint Surg Am*. 1976;58:551–555.

122. Fairclough JA, Johnson SR. Ski injuries, the significance of flake fractures. *Injury*. 1988;19:79–80.

123. Fraser RD, Hunter GA, Waddel JP. Ipsilateral fracture of the femur and tibia. *J Bone Joint Surg Br*. 1978;60:510–515.

124. Gillquist J, Rieger A, Sjodahl R, Bylund P. Multiple fractures of a single leg. *Acta Chir Scand*. 1973;139:167–172.

125. Goldman AB, Pavlov H, Rubenstein D. The segond fracture of the proximal tibia: a small avulsion fracture that reflects ligamentous damage. *AJR*. 1988;151:1163–1167.

126. Gottfries A, Hagert CG, Sorensen SE. T and Y fractures of the tibial condyles. *Injury*. 1971;3:56–63.

127. Hohl M. Tibial condylar fractures: long-term follow-up. *Tex Med*. 1974;70:46–54.

128. Jensen DB, Johansen TP, Berg-Nielsen A, Henriksen O. Magnetic resonance imaging in evaluation of the sequelae of tibial plateau fractures. *Skeletal Radiol*. 1990;19:127–129.

129. Kaye JJ, Nance EP. Pain in the athlete's knee. *Clin Sports Med*. 1987;6:873–888.

130. Kennedy JC, Grainger RW, McGraw RW. Osteochondral fractures of the femoral condyle. *J Bone Joint Surg Br*. 1966;48:436–440.

131. Lansinger O, Bergman B, Korner L, Andersson GBJ. Tibial condylar fractures: a twenty year follow-up. *J Bone Joint Surg Am*. 1986;68:13–18.

132. Larson RL. Epiphyseal injuries in the adolescent athlete. *Orthop Clin North Am*. 1973;4:839–851.

133. Lee J, Weissman B, Nikpoor N, Aliabodi P, Sosman JL. Lipohemarthrosis of the knee: a review of recent experiences. *Radiology*. 1989;173:189–191.

134. Maar DC, Kerneck CB, Pierce RO. Simultaneous bilateral tibial tubercle avulsion fracture. *Orthopedics*. 1988;11:1599–1601.

135. Manco LG, Schneider R, Pavlov H. Insufficiency fractures of the tibial plateau. *AJR*. 1983;140:1211–1215.

136. Mathewson MH, Dandy DJ. Osteochondral fractures of the lateral femoral condyle. A result of indirect violence to the knee. *J Bone Joint Surg Br*. 1978;60:199–202.

137. McConkey JB, Meeuwisse W. Tibial plateau fractures in alpine skiing. *Am J Sports Med*. 1988;16:159–164.

138. Mirbey J, Besarcenot J, Chambers RT, Durey A, Vichard P. Avulsion fractures of the tibial tuberosity in the adolescent athlete. *Am J Sports Med*. 1988;16:336–340.

139. Moore TM, Harvey JP. Roentgenographic measurement of tibial plateau depression due to fracture. *J Bone Joint Surg Am*. 1974;56:155–160.

140. Neer CS, Grantham A, Sheldon ML. Supracondylar fracture of the adult femur. A study of one hundred and ten cases. *J Bone Joint Surg Am*. 1967;49:591–613.

141. Nelson DW, DiPaola J, Colville M, Schmidgall J. Osteochondritis dissecans of the talus and knee: prospective comparison of MR and arthroscopic classification. *J Comput Assisted Tomogr*. 1990;14:804–808.

142. O'Donoghue DM. Chondral and osteochondral fractures. *J Trauma*. 1966;6:469–481.

143. Rafii M, Firooznic H, Golimbo C, Bonaino J. Computed tomography of tibial plateau fractures. *AJR*. 1984;142:1181–1186.

144. Richmond J, Sarno RC. Post traumatic intracapsular bone fragments: association with meniscal tears. *AJR*. 1988;150:159–160.

145. Roberts JM. Fractures and dislocations of the knee. In: Rockwood CA, Wilkins KE, King RE, eds. *Fractures in Children*. Philadelphia: Lippincott; 1984;3:891–982.

146. Schatzker J, McBroom R, Bruce D. The tibial plateau fracture. The Toronto experience: 1968–1975. *Clin Orthop*. 1979;138:94–104.

147. Schulak DJ, Gunn DR. Fractures of the tibial plateau. A review of the literature. *Clin Orthop*. 1975;109:167–177.

148. Seinsheimer F. Fractures of the distal femur. *Clin Orthop*. 1980; 153:169–180.

149. Shelton ML, Neer CS, Grantham SA. Occult knee ligament ruptures associated with fractures. *J Trauma*. 1971;11:853–856.

150. Steiner ME, Grana WA. The young athlete's knee: recent advances. *Clin Sports Med*. 1988;7:527–546.

151. Vellet AD, Marks PH, Fowler PJ, Munro TG. Occult post-traumatic osteochondral lesions of the knee: prevalence, classification, and short term sequelae evaluation by MR imaging. *Radiology*. 1991;178:271–276.

152. Wilppula E, Bakalim G. Ligamentous tear concomitant with tibial condylar fracture. *Acta Orthop Scand*. 1972;43:292–300.

153. Wong JC, Gregg JR. Knee, ankle and foot problems in the preadolescent and adolescent athlete. *Clin Podiatr Med Surg*. 1986;3:731–745.

Ligament, Meniscus, and Soft Tissue Injuries and Miscellaneous Injuries

154. Andrews JR. Overuse syndromes in the lower extremities. *Clin Sports Med*. 1983;2:137–148.

155. Andrish JT. Ligamentous injuries of the knee. *Primary Care*. 1984;11:77–88.

156. Apple JS, Martinez S, Hardaker WT, Daffner RH, Gehweiler TA. Synovial plicae of the knee. *Skeletal Radiol*. 1982;7:251–254.

157. Arnold JA, Coher TP, Heaton LM, Park JB, Harris WD. Natural history of anterior cruciate tears. *Am J Sports Med*. 1979;7:305–313.

158. Baker CL, Norwood LA, Hughston JC. Acute combined posterior cruciate and posterolateral instability of the knee. *Am J Sports Med*. 1984;12:204–208.

159. Baker CL, Norwood LA, Hughston JC. Acute posterolateral rotary instability of the knee. *J Bone Joint Surg Am*. 1983;65:614–618.

160. Balkfors B. Course of knee-ligament injuries. *Acta Orthop Scand.* 1982;198:1–9.

161. Bassett LW, Grover JS, Seeger LL. Magnetic resonance imaging of knee trauma. *Skeletal Radiol.* 1990;19:401–405.

162. Baylis WJ, Rzonca EC. Common sports injuries of the knee. *Clin Podiatr Med Surg.* 1988;5:571–589.

163. Berlin RC, Levinsohn EM, Chrisman H. The wrinkled patellar tendon: an indication of abnormality in the extensor mechanism of the knee. *Skeletal Radiol.* 1991;20:181–185.

164. Berquist TH. *Imaging of Orthopedic Trauma.* 2nd ed. New York: Raven; 1991.

165. Berquist TH. *Magnetic Resonance Imaging of the Musculoskeletal System.* New York: Raven, 1990.

166. Bodne D, Quinn SF, Murry WT. Magnetic resonance images of chronic patellar tendinitis. *Skeletal Radiol.* 1988;17:24–28.

167. Boland AL. Soft tissue injuries of the knee. In: Nicholas JA, Hershman EB, eds. *The Lower Extremity and Spine in Sports Medicine.* St Louis, MO: Mosby; 1986:983–1012.

168. Brunner MC, Floover SP, Evancho AM, Allman FL, Apple DF, Fayman WA. MRI of the athletic knee. Findings in asymptomatic professional basketball and collegiate football players. *Invest Radiol.* 1989; 24:72–75.

169. Burk DL, Dalinka MK, Kanal E. Meniscal and ganglion cysts of the knee. *AJR.* 1988;150:331–336.

170. Cabaud HE, Slocum DB. The diagnosis of chronic anterolateral rotary instability of the knee. *Am J Sports Med.* 1977;5:99–104.

171. Clancy WG, Ray M, Zoltan DJ. Acute tears of the anterior cruciate ligament: surgical vs conservative treatment. *J Bone Joint Surg Am.* 1988;70:1483–1488.

172. Clemente CD. *Gray's Anatomy.* 13th ed. Philadelphia: Lea & Febiger; 1985.

173. Crues JV III, Mink J, Levy TL, Lotysch M, Stoller DW. Meniscal tears of the knee: accuracy of MR imaging. *Radiology.* 1987;164:445–448.

174. Daffner RH, Riemer BL, Lupetin AR, Dash N. Magnetic resonance imaging in acute tendon rupture. *Skeletal Radiol.* 1986;15:619–621.

175. Deflaviis L, Scaglione P, Nessi R, Albisetti W. Ultrasound in degenerative cystic meniscal disease of the knee. *Skeletal Radiol.* 1990;19:441–445.

176. DeHaven KE. Arthroscopy in the diagnosis and management of anterior cruciate deficient knee. *Am J Sports Med.* 1977;5:99–104.

177. Deutsch AL, Mink JH, Fox JM, et al. Peripheral meniscal tears: MR findings after conservative treatment or arthroscopic repair. *Radiology.* 1990;176:485–488.

178. Dillon EH, Pope CF, Kokl P, Lynch K. The clinical significance of stage 2 meniscal abnormalities on magnetic resonance knee images. *Magn Resonance Imag.* 1990;8:411–415.

179. Dumas J, Edde DJ. Meniscal abnormalities: prospective correlation of double-contrast arthrography and arthroscopy. *Radiology.* 1986; 160:453–456.

180. Farley TE, Howell SM, Love KF, Wolfe RD, Neumann CH. Meniscal tears: MR and arthrographic findings after arthroscopic repair. *Radiology.* 1991;180:517–522.

181. Feagin JA. The syndrome of the torn anterior cruciate ligament. *Orthop Clin North Am.* 1979;10:81–90.

182. Feagin JA, Abbott HG, Rokous JR. The isolated tear of the anterior cruciate ligament. *J Bone Joint Surg Am.* 1972;54:1340–1341.

183. Fetto JF, Marshall JL. The natural history and diagnosis of anterior cruciate ligament insufficiency. *Clin Orthop.* 1980;147:29–38.

184. Fischer SP, Fox JM, DelPizzo W, Friedman MJ, Snyder SJ, Ferkel RD. Accuracy of diagnosis from magnetic resonance imaging of the knee. *J Bone Joint Surg Am.* 1991;73:2–16.

185. Fornage BD, Rifkin MD, Touche DH, Segal PM. Sonography of the patellar tendon: preliminary observations. *AJR.* 1984;143:179–182.

186. Fornasier VL, Czitrom AA, Evans JA, Hastings DE. Case report 398. *Skeletal Radiol.* 1987;16:57–59.

187. Freiberger RH, Pavlov H. Knee arthrography. *Radiology.* 1988; 166:489–492.

188. Gallimore GW Jr, Harms SS. Knee injuries: high resolution MR imaging. *Radiology.* 1986;160:457–461.

189. Garrick JG, Regua RK. Prophylactic knee bracing. *Am J Sports Med.* 1987;15:118–123.

190. Gibson T, Davies JE, Crane J, Henry AN. Knee pain in sports people—a prospective study. *Br J Sports Med.* 1987;12:115–117.

191. Glaskow JL, Katz R, Schneider M, Scott WN. Double-blind assessment of the value of magnetic resonance imaging in the diagnosis of anterior cruciate and meniscal lesions. *J Bone Joint Surg Am.* 1989;71:113–119.

192. Grody JF, O'Connor KJ, Bender J. Iliotibial band syndrome. *J Am Podiatr Med Assoc.* 1986;7:558–561.

193. Hall FJ. Arthrography of the discoid lateral meniscus. *AJR.* 1977; 128:993–1002.

194. Halperin N, Hendel D, Fisher S, Agasi M, Copeliovitch L. Anterior cruciate insufficiency syndrome. *Clin Orthop.* 1983;179:179–184.

195. Hardaker WT, Sipple TL, Bassett FH III. Diagnosis and treatment of plicae syndrome of the knee. *J Bone Joint Surg Am.* 1980;62:221–225.

196. Harms SE, Flamig DP, Fisher CF, Febner JM. 3D MR Imaging of the knee using surface coils. *J Comput Assisted Tomogr.* 1986;10:773–777.

197. Hartzman S, Reicher MA, Bassett LW, Duckwiler GR, Mandelbaum B, Gold RH. MR Imaging of the knee. Part II: chronic disorders. *Radiology.* 1987;162:553–557.

198. Henning CE, Lynch MA, Glick KR. Physical examination of the knee. In: Nicholas JA, Hershman EB, eds. *The Lower Extremity and Spine in Sports Medicine.* St Louis, MO: Mosby; 1986:715–800.

199. Herman LJ, Beltran J. Pitfalls in MR imaging of the knee. *Radiology.* 1988;167:775–781.

200. Hollinshead WH. *Anatomy for Surgeons.* 3rd ed. New York: Harper & Row; 1982;3.

201. Hughston JC, Andrews JR, Cross MJ, Arnaldo M. Classification of knee ligament instabilities. Part I: the medial compartment and cruciate ligaments. *J Bone Joint Surg Am.* 1976;58:159–172.

202. Hughston JC, Andrews JR, Cross MJ, Arnaldo M. Classification of knee ligament instabilities. Part II: the lateral compartment. *J Bone Joint Surg Am.* 1976;58:173–179.

203. Hughston JC, Bowden JA, Andrew JR, Norwood A. Acute tears of the posterior cruciate ligament. *J Bone Joint Surg Am.* 1980;62:438–450.

204. Jones DC, James SL. Overuse injuries of the lower extremities. *Clin Sports Med.* 1987;6:273–290.

205. Jorgensen U, Sonne-Holm S, Sauridsen F, Rosenklint A. Long-term follow-up of menisectomy in athletes. *J Bone Joint Surg Br.* 1987;69:80–83.

206. Kälebo P, Sward L, Karlsson J, Peterson L. Ultrasonography in detection of patellar ligament ruptures (jumper's knee). *Skeletal Radiol.* 1991;20:285–289.

207. Kanniss P. Nonoperative treatment of grade II and III sprains of the lateral ligament compartment of the knee. *Am J Sports Med.* 1989;17:83–88.

208. Kaplan PA, Nelson NL, Garvin KL, Brow DE. MR of the knee: the significance of high signal in the meniscus that does not clearly extend to the surface. *AJR.* 1991;156:333–336.

209. Kaye JE, Nance EP. Pain in the athlete's knee. *Clin Sports Med.* 1987;6:873–883.

210. Kujala UM, Österman K. Knee injuries in athletes. *Sports Med.* 1986;3:447–460.

211. Kursunoglu-Brahme S, Schwaighefer B, Gundry C, Ho C, Resnick D. Jogging causes acute changes in the knee joint: an MR study in normal volunteers. *AJR.* 1990;154:1233–1235.

212. Larson RL, Jones DC. Dislocation and ligamentous injuries of the knee. In: Rockwood CA, Green DP, eds. *Fractures in Adults.* 2nd ed. Philadelphia: Lippincott; 1984;2:1480–1592.

213. Lee JK, Yao L. Tibial collateral ligament bursa: MR imaging. *Radiology.* 1991;178:855–857.

214. Lee JK, Yao L, Phelps CT, Wirth CR, Czajka J, Lozman J. Anterior cruciate ligament tears: MR imaging compared with arthroscopic and clinical tests. *Radiology.* 1988;166:861–864.

215. Lyu S, Wu J. Snapping syndrome caused by the semitendinosus tendon. *J Bone Joint Surg Am.* 1989;71:303–305.

216. Manco LG, Kavanaugh JH, Fay JJ, Bilfield BS. Meniscus tears of the knee: prospective evaluation with CT. *Radiology.* 1986;159:147–151.

217. Mattalino AJ, Deese JM, Campbell ED. Office evaluation and treatment of lower extremity injuries in the runner. *Clin Sports Med.* 1989; 8:461–475.

218. Middleton WD, Lawson TL. *Anatomy and MRI of the Joints: A Multiplanar Atlas.* New York: Raven; 1989.

219. Mink JH, Levy T, Crues JV III. Tears of the anterior cruciate ligament and menisci of the knee. MR imaging evaluation. *Radiology.* 1988;167:769–774.

220. Mink JH, Reicher MA, Crues JV III. *Magnetic Resonance Imaging of the Knee.* New York: Raven; 1987.

221. Noyes FR, Grood ES, Torzilla PA. The definitions for motion and position of the knee and injuries of the ligaments. *J Bone Joint Surg Am.* 1989;71:465–472.

222. Noyes FR, Mooar PA, Matthews DS, Butler DL. The symptomatic anterior cruciate deficient knee. Part I: the long-term functional disability in athletically active individuals. *J Bone Joint Surg Am.* 1983;65:154–162.

223. O'Donoghue DH. An analysis of the end results of major injuries of the knee. *J Bone Joint Surg Am.* 1955;37:1–13.

224. Passarello R, Trecco F, dePaules F, Mascrocchi G, Zobel BB. Meniscal lesions of the knee joint—CT diagnosis. *Radiology.* 1985;57:29–34.

225. Patel D. Arthroscopy of the plicae–synovial folds and their significance. *Am J Sports Med.* 1978;6:217–225.

226. Paty JG. Diagnosis and treatment of musculoskeletal running injuries. *Semin Arthritis Rheum.* 1988;18:48–60.

227. Pavlov H. The radiographic diagnosis of the anterior cruciate ligament deficient knee. *Clin Orthop.* 1983;172:57–64.

228. Polly DW, Callaghan JJ, Sites RA, McCabe JM, McMahon K, Savory CG. The accuracy of selective magnetic resonance imaging compared with findings of arthroscopy of the knee. *J Bone Joint Surg Am.* 1988; 70:192–198.

229. Rand JA. The role of arthroscopy in the management of knee injuries in athletes. *Mayo Clin Proc.* 1984;59:77–82.

230. Rand JA, Berquist TH. The knee. In: Berquist TH, ed. *Imaging of Orthopedic Trauma.* 2nd ed. New York: Raven; 1991:333–432.

231. Ray MJ, Clancy WG, Lemon RA. Semimembranosus tendinitis: an overlooked cause of medial knee pain. *Am J Sports Med.* 1988;16:347–351.

232. Renne JW. Iliotibial band fraction syndrome. *J Bone Joint Surg Am.* 1975;57:1110–1111.

233. Reicher MA, Hartzman S, Bassett LW, Mandelbaum B, Duckwiler G, Gold RH. MR Imaging of the knee. Part I: traumatic disorders. *Radiology.* 1987;162:547–551.

234. Reicher MA, Hartzman S, Duckwiler GR, Bassett LW, Anderson LJ, Gold RH. Meniscal injuries: detection using MR imaging. *Radiology.* 1986;159:753–757.

235. Renstrom P. Swedish research in sports traumatology. *Clin Orthop.* 1984;191:144–158.

236. Salazar JE, Dake RA, Winer-Murain HT. Locking and unlocking the knee: arthrographic demonstration. *AJR.* 1986;146:575–576.

237. Sandberg R, Balkfors B. Partial rupture of the anterior cruciate ligament: natural course. *Clin Orthop.* 1987;220:176–178.

238. Scott SG. Current concepts in the rehabilitation of injured athletes. *Mayo Clin Proc.* 1984;59:83–90.

239. Shellock FG, Mink JH. Knees of trained long-distance runners: MR imaging before and after competition. *Radiology.* 1991;179:635–637.

240. Silverman JM, Mink JH, Deutsch AL. Discoid menisci of the knee. MR imaging appearance. *Radiology.* 1989;173:351–354.

241. Simonet WT, Sim FH. Current concepts in the treatment of ligament instability of the knee. *Mayo Clin Proc.* 1984;59:67–76.

242. Singson RD, Feldman F, Staron R, Kierman H. MR Imaging of displaced buckle-handle tear of the medial meniscus. *AJR.* 1991; 156:121–124.

243. Steiner ME, Grana WA. The young athlete's knee: recent advances. *Clin Sports Med.* 1988;7:527–546.

244. Stoller DW, Martin C, Crues JV III, Kaplan L, Mink JH. Meniscal tears: pathologic correlation with MR imaging. *Radiology.* 1987;163: 731–735.

245. Tietz CC, Hermanson BK, Kronmal RA, Diebs PH. Evaluation of the use of braces to prevent injury to the knee in collegiate football players. *J Bone Joint Surg Am.* 1987;69:2–8.

246. Trecco F, dePaulis F, Bonanni G, et al. The use of computerized tomography in the study of the cruciate ligaments of the knee. *Ital J Orthop Trauma.* 1984;10:109–120.

247. Turner DA, Prodromos CC, Petasnick JP, Clark JW. Acute injury of the ligaments of the knee: magnetic resonance evaluation. *Radiology.* 1985;154:717–722.

248. Vahey TN, Bennett HT, Arrington LE, Shelbourene KD, Ng J. MR Imaging of the knee: pseudotear of the lateral meniscus caused by the meniscofemoral ligament. *AJR.* 1990;154:1237–1239.

249. Watonabe AT, Carter BC, Teitelbaum GP, Bradley WG. Common pitfalls in magnetic resonance imaging of the knee. *J Bone Joint Surg Am.* 1989;71:857–862.

250. Webb LY, Toby EB. Bilateral rupture of the patellar tendon in an otherwise healthy male patient following minor trauma. *J Trauma.* 1986;26:1045–1048.

251. Weiss CB, Lindberg M, Hamberg P, DeHaven KE, Gillquist J. Nonoperative treatment of meniscal tears. *J Bone Joint Surg Am.* 1989; 71:811–822.

252. Wolfe RD, Dieden JD. Cruciate ligament injury: diagnostic difficulty in the presence of meniscal injury. *Radiology.* 1985;157:19–21.

253. Wood GW, Stanley RF, Tullos HS. Lateral capsular sign: X-ray clue to a significant knee instability. *Am J Sports Med.* 1979;7:27–33.

254. Zarins B, Boyle J. Knee ligament injuries. In: Nichols JA, Hershman EB. *The Lower Extremity and Spine in Sports Medicine.* St Louis, MO: Mosby; 1986:929–982.

Chapter 7

Tibia, Fibula, and Calf

The type and incidence of bone or soft tissue injury varies with gender, age, and activity.[14,25,29,30] Older individuals (mean age, 57 ± 6 years) tend to engage more frequently in walking or racquet sports, whereas younger patients (mean age, 30 ± 8 years) tend to be involved in more vigorous activity such as running, fitness class, and field sports.[25] Marti et al[21] reviewed data on 4358 joggers and noted injuries in 45.8%. Fourteen percent of patients required medical treatment. Injuries to the calf and Achilles tendon occurred most frequently.

In organized or varsity sports up to 75% of injuries involve the lower extremity. The knee and ankle are most frequently injured. Injury to the calf, tibia, and fibula occurs in 6% to 10% of varsity athletes.[2,12,15] Fractures are most commonly noted in contact sports such as football or high-velocity sports such as cycling, skiing, and horse racing.[14,22–25]

ANATOMY

A brief review of certain anatomic features of the tibia, fibula, and key adjacent soft tissue structures is important in understanding sports injuries and selecting the proper imaging techniques.

The tibia has three borders (anterior, medial, and interosseous) and three surfaces (medial, posterior, and lateral). The anteromedial surface is subcutaneous. The slender fibula has interosseous, anterior, posterior, medial, and lateral borders. The two osseous structures are joined by the tibiofibular joint proximally and by the interosseous membrane and the tibiofibular syndesmosis distally.[3,17,20] The muscle attachments are illustrated in Figure 7-1. The distribution of tracer uptake on radionuclide studies can be correlated with these origins and insertions in certain syndromes, so that it is important to be familiar with tibial and fibular muscle attachments.[17,20] A more complete review of muscle anatomy and compartments is included in the section on soft tissue injury, below.

Major vessels and nerves of the calf arise from parent structures in the popliteal space (Fig. 7-2). Major popliteal arterial branches include the anterior tibial, posterior tibial, and peroneal arteries. The origin of the anterior tibial artery is at the level of the popliteus muscle. Accompanied by the anterior tibial vein, it passes laterally and forward between the lower border of the popliteus and the upper border of the tibialis posterior to pass above the upper margin of the interosseous membrane and enter the anterior aspect of the leg.[17,20]

The posterior tibial artery (accompanied by the vein) continues inferiorly deep to the soleus and then penetrates the deep transverse fascia of the leg. It continues medially downward in a fascial canal with the tibialis posterior and flexor digitorum longus. Most of the posterior tibial artery branches supply the muscles of the posterior compartment.[17]

The peroneal artery branches approximately 1 inch below the origin of the posterior tibial artery. Beneath the soleus, it is accompanied by two veins. The peroneal artery passes obliquely downward and laterally across the upper posterior

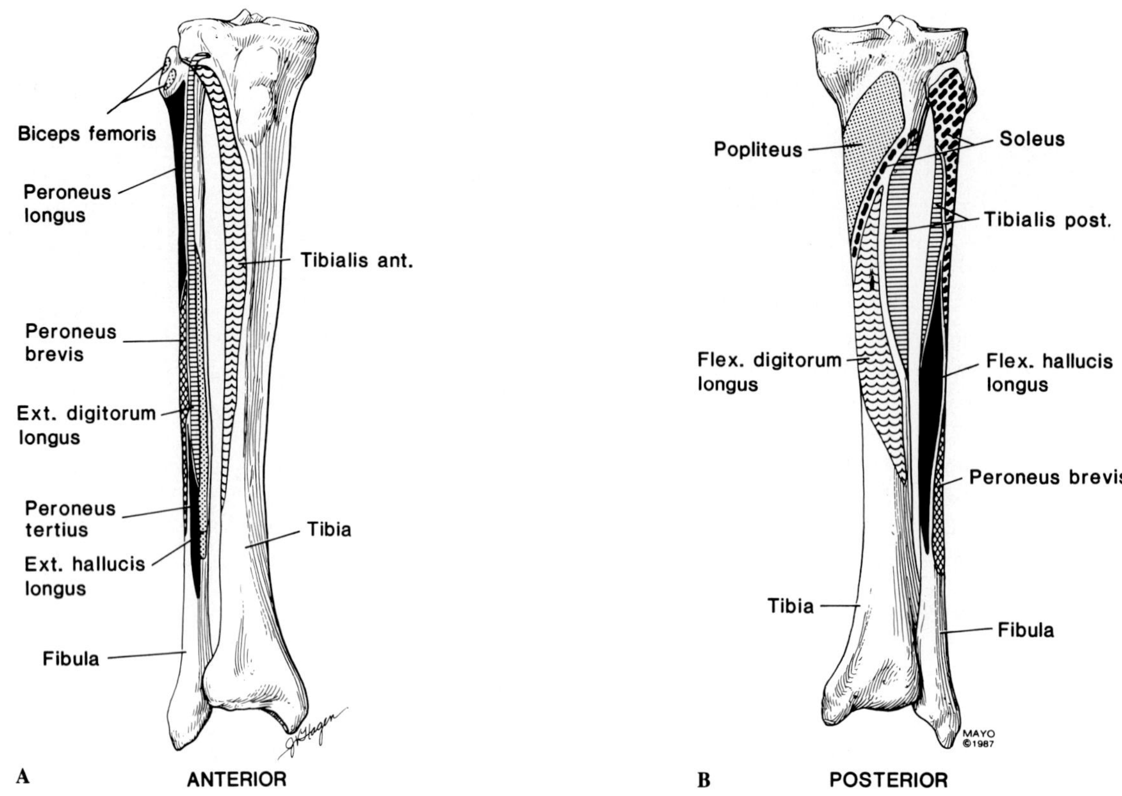

Fig. 7-1 (**A**) Anterior and (**B**) posterior illustrations of the tibia and fibula with muscle attachments. *Source:* Reprinted from *Magnetic Resonance Imaging of the Musculoskeletal System* by TH Berquist, 1990, Raven Press, © Mayo Foundation.

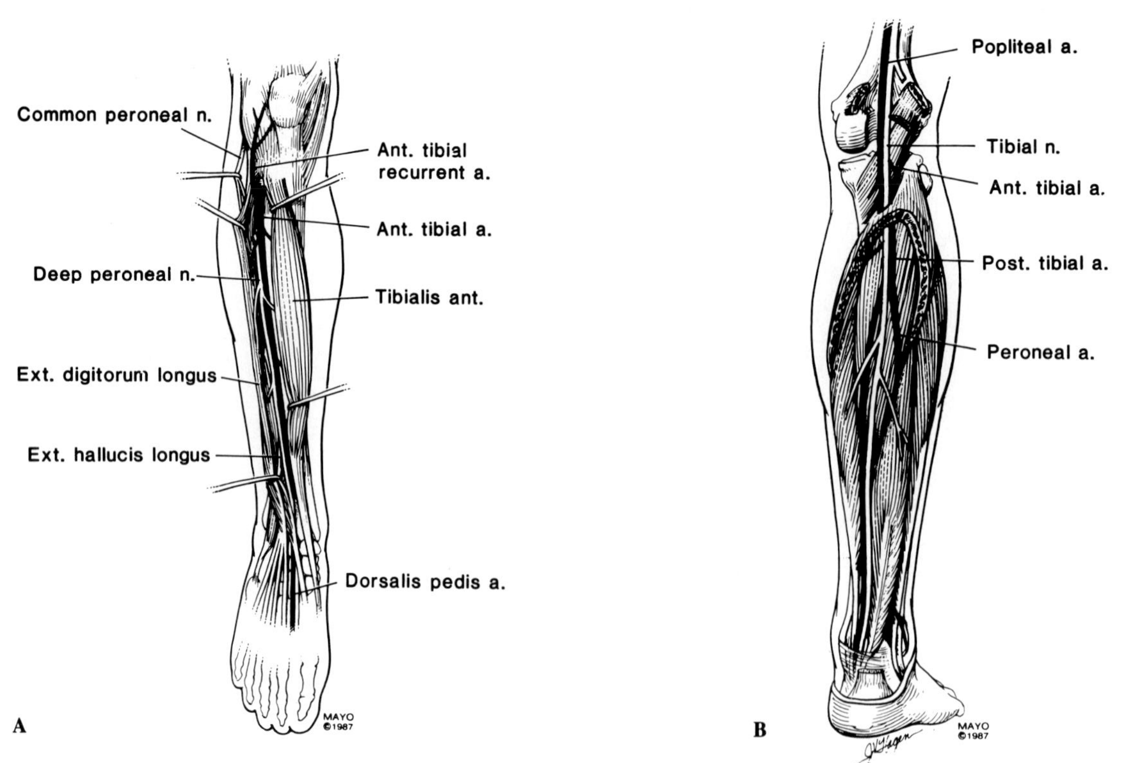

Fig. 7-2 (**A**) Anterior and (**B**) posterior illustrations of neurovascular structures in the calf. *Source:* Reprinted from *Magnetic Resonance Imaging of the Musculoskeletal System* by TH Berquist, 1990, Raven Press, © Mayo Foundation.

surface of the tibialis muscle and enters a canal formed by the fibula anterolaterally, the tibialis posterior anteromedially, and the flexor hallucis longus from behind. As it passes downward, some of its branches pass through the interosseous membrane to supply the anterior muscle group.[17,20]

Three blood supply systems nourish the tibia: the nutrient artery, the periosteal system, and the epiphyseal-metaphyseal system. The major blood supply to the tibial shaft is the nutrient artery, which arises close to the upper end of the posterior tibial artery at the junction of the upper and middle thirds of the shaft. It enters the tibia posteriorly and has a rather long oblique intracortical course. When it reaches the intramedullary space, it divides into ascending and descending branches, which form a dense network of vessels. These vessels supply approximately two-thirds of the cortex of the tibial shaft.[17,20]

The periosteal vessels originate from the anterior tibial artery or vessels of the interosseous membrane. These vessels run transversely to the long axis of the tibia. Abundant anastomoses exist between these transverse branches and with adjacent muscle arteries.[17]

The fibula is similarly supplied by the nutrient artery, periosteal system, and epiphyseal-metaphyseal system. The nutrient artery typically originates from the proximal peroneal artery.[17,20]

Major nerves in the leg include the tibial and peroneal nerves (Fig. 7-2). The tibal nerve courses through the popliteal fossa lying lateral to the popliteal vessels. It then passes behind them to their medial side as the popliteal vessels enter beneath the soleus muscle. The nerve continues downward with the posterior tibial vessels on the tibialis posterior muscle, and then on the posterior aspect of the tibia, before entering the neurovascular compartment of the flexor retinaculum.[17,20]

The common peroneal nerve is located subcutaneously just behind the head of the fibula, where it is extremely vulnerable to injury (Fig. 7-2). It courses laterally and forward around the neck of the fibula deep to the peroneus longus. At this level, it divides into the superficial and deep peroneal nerves. The superficial peroneal nerve runs downward, paralleling the fibula, and supplies the peroneus longus and brevis. The deep peroneal nerve continues forward to penetrate the anterior intermuscular septum to reach the anterior compartment. It courses inferiorly with the tibial vessels.[3,17]

FRACTURES

Tibial and fibular shaft fractures are the most common long bone fractures.[20] Fractures may result from a fall, a direct blow in contact sports, rotation with the foot in a fixed position, or high-velocity forces.[4,5,20,24] Fractures may involve the tibia or fibula alone (Fig. 7-3), but more frequently both structures are involved (Fig. 7-4).[5,20] Fractures are commonly oblique or spiral (Fig. 7-4) and most frequently involve the middle or lower thirds. It is not unusual for the ankle or knee to be injured in association with shaft fractures.[4,38] Stress fractures and microfractures are discussed completely in Chapter 12.

Imaging of tibial and fibular fractures should provide the necessary anatomic information about osseous and, when indicated, soft tissue injury (Fig. 7-5). Routine radiographs should include anteroposterior and lateral views. The knee and ankle must be included to avoid overlooking associated knee and ankle injuries (Fig. 7-6).[8,20,38]

Additional studies such as conventional tomography or computed tomography (CT) may be useful for subtle injuries and to evaluate the position of fragments after spiral fractures.[13] Magnetic resonance imaging (MRI) may be indicated when soft tissue injury or soft tissue interposition between fracture fragments is suspected.[3,18] Assessment of suspected knee injury can also be accomplished with MRI. Up to 22% of patients with tibial fractures have associated ligament injuries of the knee.[38]

SOFT TISSUE INJURIES

Soft tissue injuries and overuse syndromes are common in the calf.[6,7,19] Injuries may be related to intrinsic and extrinsic factors. Intrinsic factors include the individual's biomechanics of running, such as overpronation of the foot. Extrinsic factors include terrain, the type of surface used when running or participating in other field or court sports, and footwear.[21]

Epidemiologic studies have categorized injuries into three grades. Grade 1 injuries do not restrict training programs despite symptoms. Grade 2 injuries are sufficiently significant to cause modification or reduction in training. Grade 3 injuries interrupt training.[9] Medical assistance is most commonly sought in the last case. Many soft tissue injuries are diagnosed by history and physical examination. MRI, however, has provided a new and useful method for categorizing and clarifying the extent of many injuries.[3,11] Therefore, an understanding of soft tissue injuries and common syndromes is essential to optimize the imaging approach to their evaluation.

Muscle and Tendon Injuries

Injuries to muscle-tendon units may occur with direct trauma (contusion or hematoma) or overstretching leading to partial or complete disruption. The latter are referred to as strains and have been graded from minor (first degree) to partial (~50% of fibers torn, second degree) to complete (third degree).[1,3,12]

Muscle tears can involve any of the muscles of the leg. Marti et al[21] noted an incidence of muscle tears of 10.8% in runners. Tears in the gastrocnemius and plantaris are most frequent in experience at the Mayo Clinic. Disruption of the medial gastrocnemius (tennis leg) is most frequent.[1] Patients

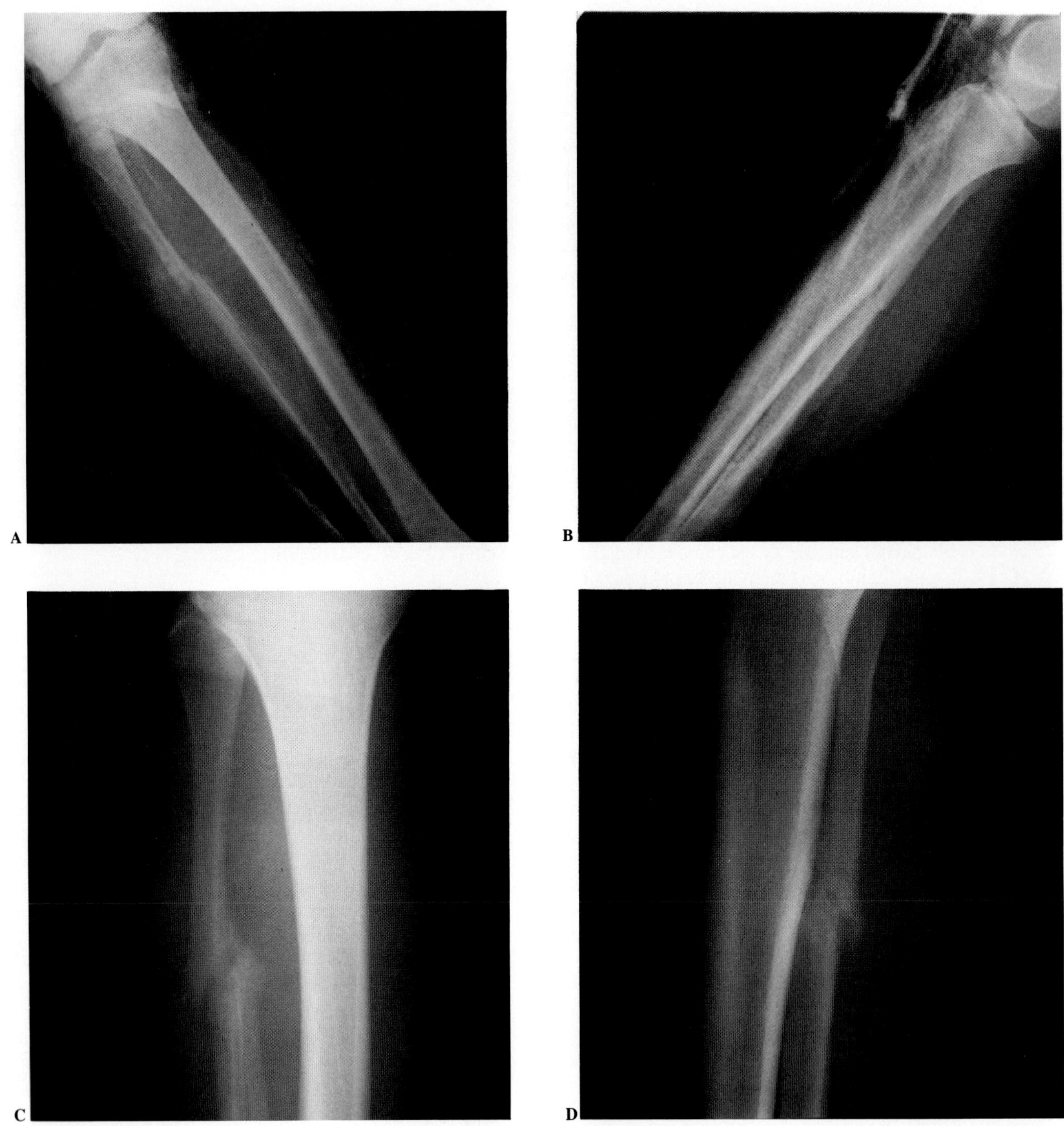

Fig. 7-3 (**A**) Anteroposterior (AP) and (**B**) lateral views of an isolated upper fibular fracture due to a direct blow during a football game. The fibula is a non–weight-bearing bone for all practical purposes. The athlete was playing with the leg protected in 5 weeks (**C** and **D**).

with muscle tears generally present with sudden onset of calf pain during exercise. Clinical symptoms and physical examination are generally sufficient for diagnosis,[1,12] but MRI is the technique of choice for evaluating the extent of injury. Both T1- and T2-weighted images are usually used to define the lesion. T2-Weighted images are best for lesion detection. The extent of the lesion is optimally demonstrated by imaging in two planes (Fig. 7-7).[3] Early experience suggests that infiltrative hemorrhage (Fig. 7-7) tends to heal more quickly than hematoma (Fig. 7-8).

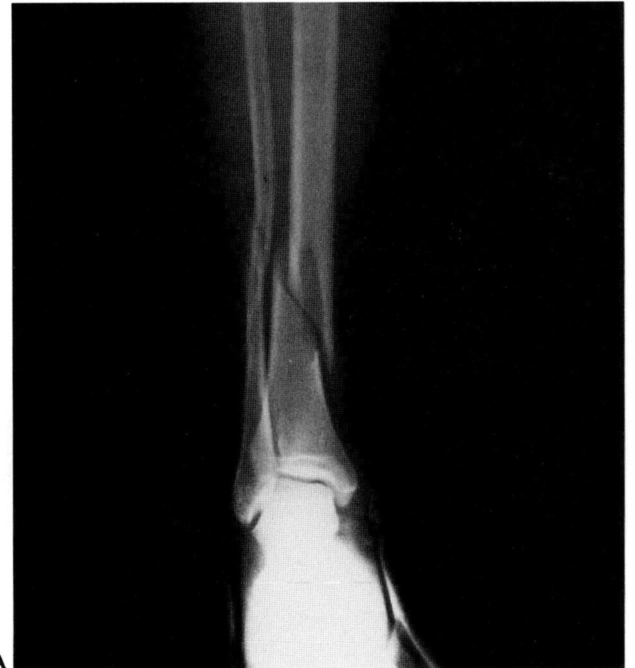
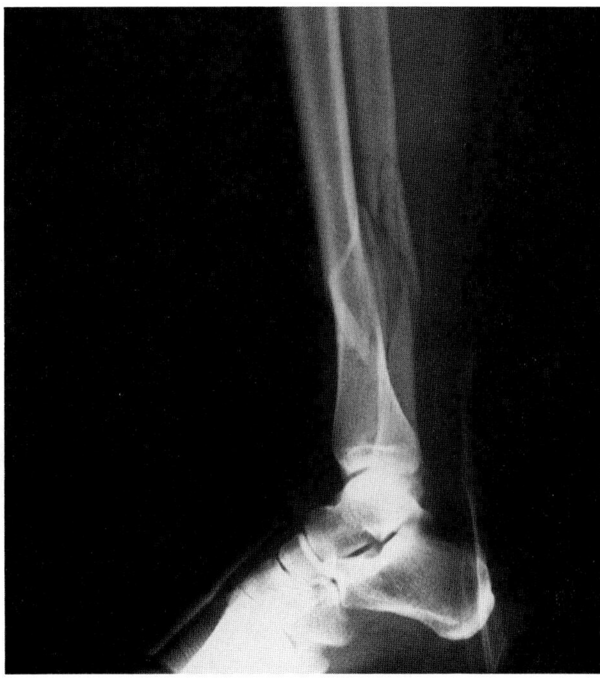

Fig. 7-4 (**A**) AP and (**B**) lateral views of typical spiral fractures of the distal tibia and fibula after a skiing accident.

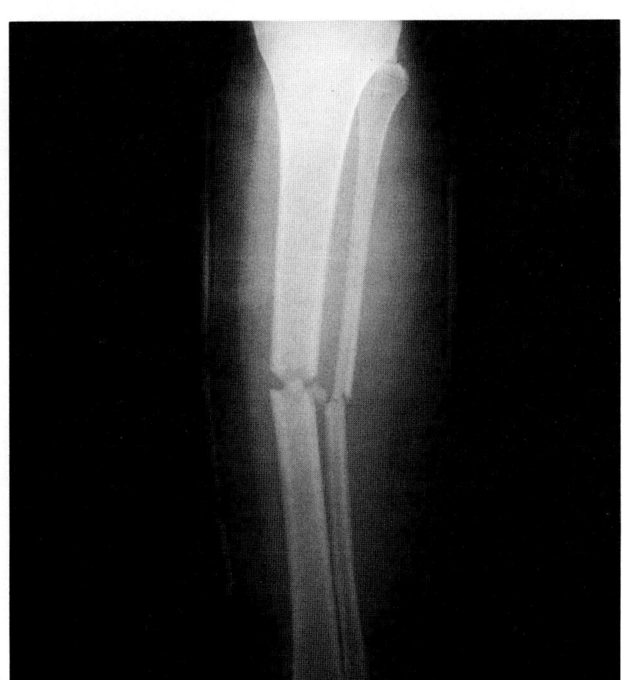
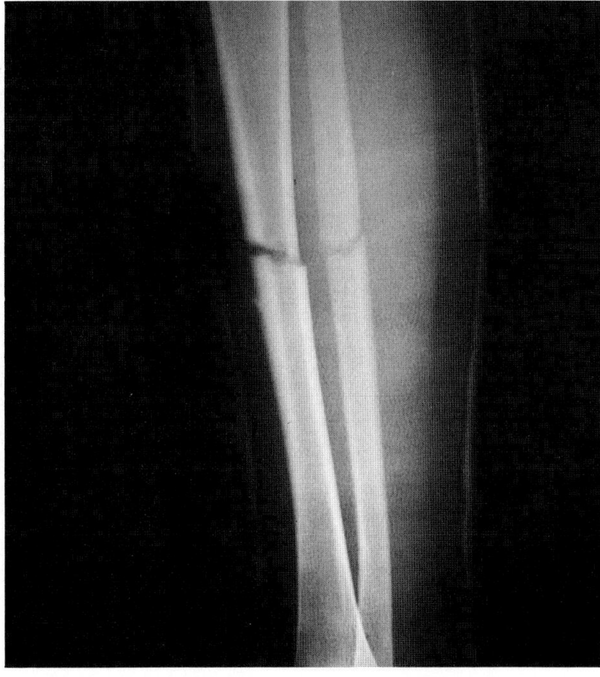

Fig. 7-5 Casted transverse midtibial and fibular fractures demonstrating medial angulation on the AP view (**A**) and normal alignment on the lateral view (**B**).

The plantaris is a small muscle with a long tendon. Therefore, MR images generally demonstrate an area of localized hemorrhage between the medial gastrocnemius and soleus (Fig. 7-9).[3]

Tendon injuries can be classified in a similar fashion, but inflammatory changes are more likely to occur than in muscle injuries. Tendon injuries (17% of runners) are common with inadequate conditioning and improper warm-up.[21] Additional

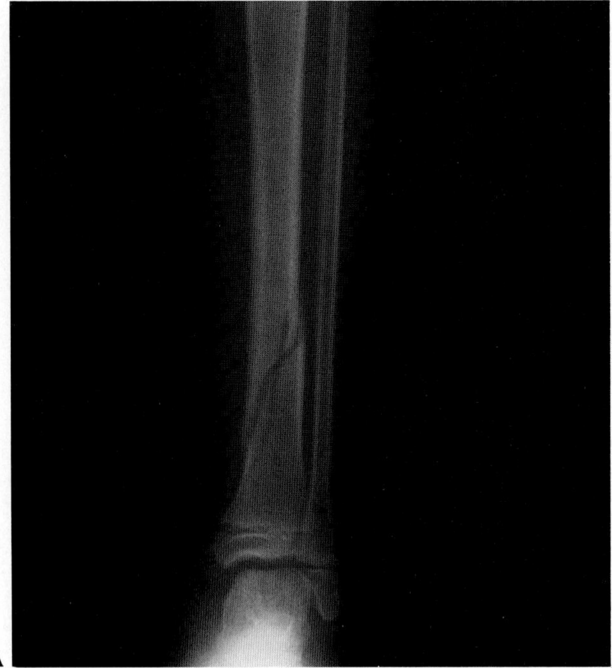
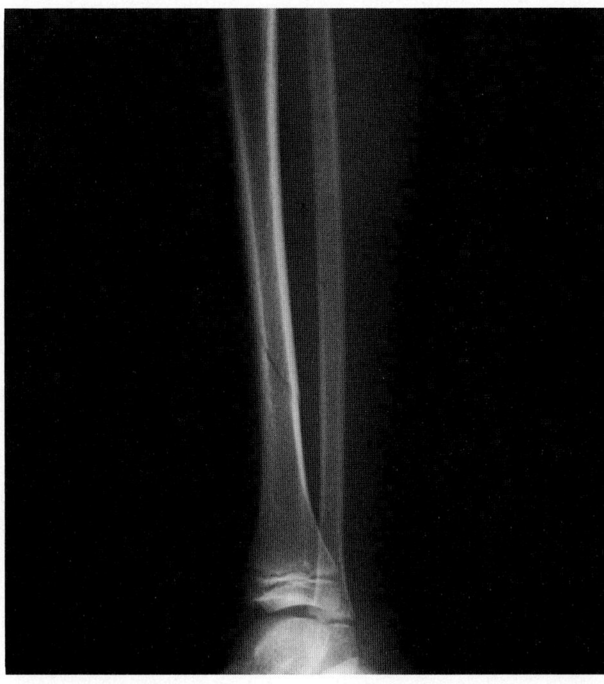

Fig. 7-6 (**A**) AP and (**B**) lateral views of a distal tibial fracture with no fibular fracture after a twisting injury during youth soccer. Note the extensive soft tissue swelling about the ankle.

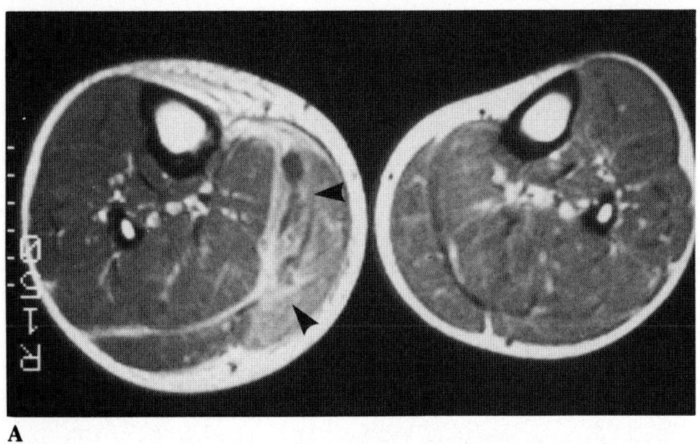
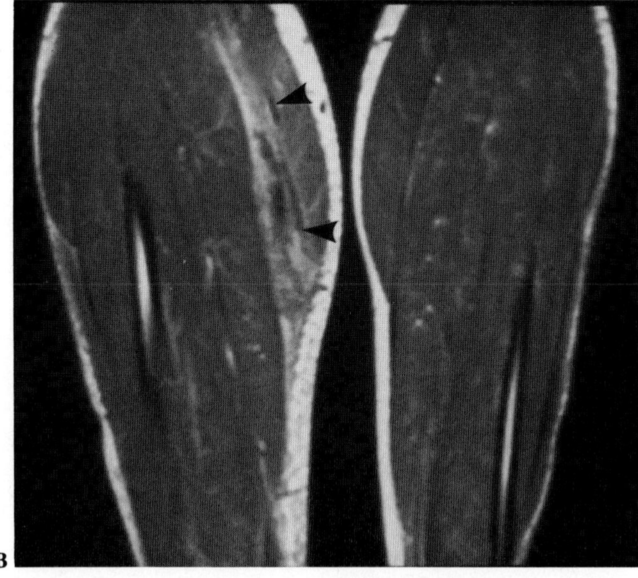

Fig. 7-7 (**A**) Axial and (**B**) coronal (SE 2000/60) T2-weighted magnetic resonance (MR) images of a grade 2 strain demonstrating hemorrhage (arrowheads) into the medial gastrocnemius. *Source:* Reprinted with permission from *Magnetic Resonance Imaging of the Musculoskeletal System* by TH Berquist, 1990, Raven Press, © Mayo Foundation.

causes of inflammation or disruption include prior injury, scarring, overstretching, cast immobilization, and prior steroid injections.[12] Table 7-1 summarizes inflammatory conditions in tendons.

MRI provides the optimal method for evaluating tendon injuries. It may be especially important when these annoying injuries do not respond to conservative therapy. The likelihood of disruption and extent of damage to the tendon can be easily identified with T2-weighted images in two planes.[3]

Shin Splints

Shin splints is a nonspecific term that has been applied to numerous painful conditions in the leg.[6] Slocum[35] defined

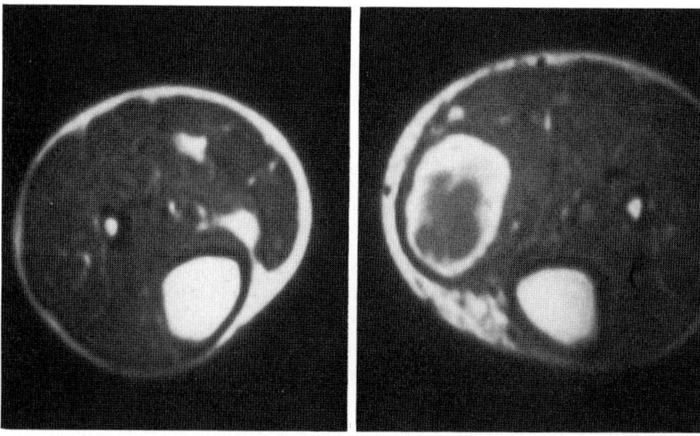

Fig. 7-8 Axial T-2 weighted MR image (SE 2000/60) demonstrating a large medial gastrocnemius hematoma acquired during a tennis match.

Table 7-1 Tendon Injuries

Injury	*Characteristics*
Tenosynovitis	Inflammation of synovial sheath and paratendon structures
Tendinitis	Inflammation of tendon due to injury or degeneration due to aging
Acute	Symptoms present < 2 weeks
Subacute	Symptoms present 2–6 weeks
Chronic	Symptoms present > 6 weeks
Tendinosis	Asymptomatic tendon degeneration; may lead to partial or complete disruption

Source: Friedman MJ in Nicholas JA and Hershman EB, *The Lower Extremity and Spine in Sports Medicine*, 1986, CV Mosby.

shin splints as a sterile inflammatory condition of muscle tendon units brought on by overexertion of the lower extremity muscles during weight bearing. The American Medical Association defines shin splints as "pain and discomfort in the leg from repetitive running on hard surfaces, with forcible use of foot flexors; diagnosis should be limited to musculotendinous inflammation excluding fracture and ischemic disorders."[27(p199)] Shin splints account for up to 18% of running injuries.[6]

Most investigators agree that *shin splints* is simply a descriptive term for exertional shin pain and not a diagnostic term.[12,26,27] More specific conditions that have been considered more loosely shin splints should be defined and used for more accurate clinical diagnosis. These include medial tibial stress syndrome, soleus syndrome, compartment syndrome, and posterior tibial tendinitis.[6,8,12,16,27]

Medial Tibial Stress Syndrome

Mubarak et al[28] describe medial tibial stress syndrome as exercise-induced pain along the distal posteromedial tibial border. Pain typically occurs during workouts in runners and is relieved by rest. Pain may return several hours later with minimal activity such as walking. In the chronic phase, this dull aching discomfort usually persists while the patient is performing ordinary daily activities.[19] Physical examination typically reveals a 3- to 6-cm area of tenderness along the

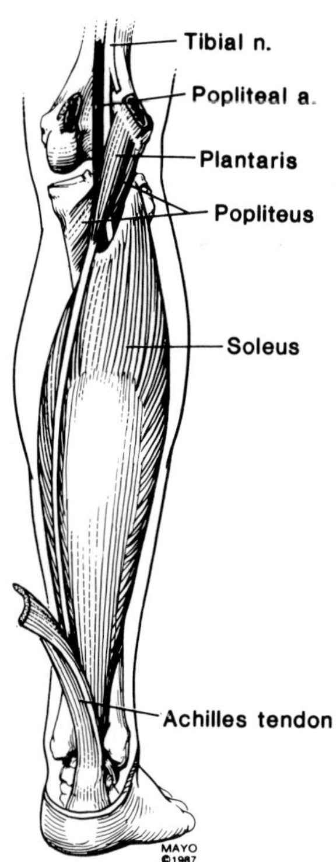

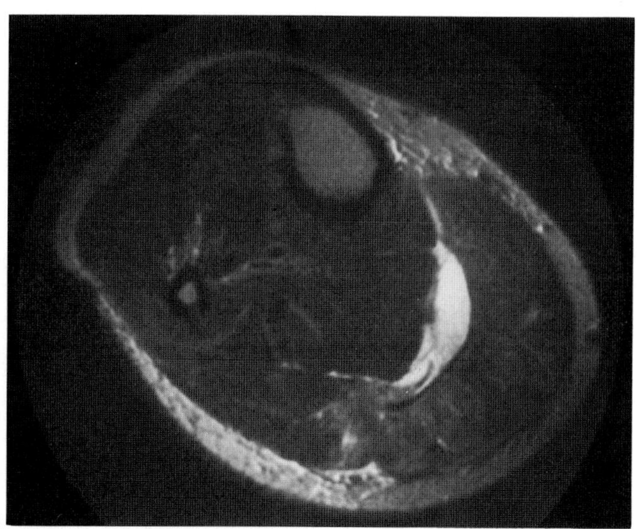

Fig. 7-9 (**A**) Illustration of the plantaris and its long tendon, which passes between the soleus and gastrocnemius. (**B**) Axial T2-weighted MR image (SE 2000/60) demonstrating a fluid collection due to plantaris tear.

distal medial tibia. Pain may be increased by plantar flexion of the foot or by inverting the foot against resistance.[12,19]

Detmer[9] classified medial tibial stress syndrome because of its importance for diagnosis, management, and prognosis. The classification was applied to chronic medial tibial stress syndrome in patients who had pain in the above-described location that reappeared after one or more periods of rest that would normally be sufficient to relieve symptoms.[9] Three basic categories were defined on the basis of the primary site of anatomic involvement. With type I the primary problem is the bone or osseous structure of the tibia (Fig. 7-10). Type II involves the periosteal-fascial junction (Fig. 7-11), and Type III involves the deep muscles posterior to the tibia (Fig. 7-10).

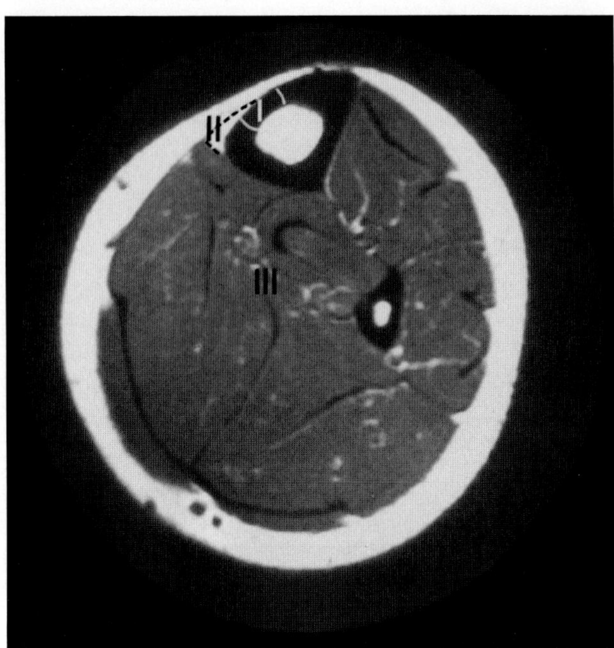

Fig. 7-10 Axial T1-weighted MR image (SE 500/20) of the calf demonstrating the sites of involvement of medial tibial stress.[9] I, Stress or microfracture of the medial tibia; II, periosteal-fascial inflammation (dotted lines); III, inflammation of deep muscles posterior to the tibia.

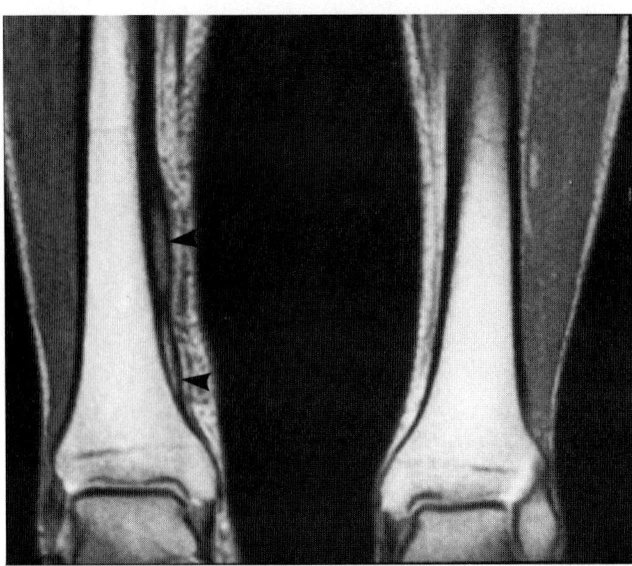

Fig. 7-11 Coronal MR image of the tibias demonstrating periosteal thickening medially (arrowheads) due to type II medial tibial stress syndrome.

Physical examination in type I injuries reveals definite bone pain, which may be more discrete in the presence of a stress fracture. Patients with periosteal or fascial inflammation (type II) have more superficial tenderness along the medial tibia. Athletes involved in track hurdling or jumping sports such as basketball more often experience this form of medial tibial stress. Type III injuries are similar to chronic compartment syndrome, which is discussed more completely later.[9,12,31]

Soleus Syndrome

Michael and Holder[26] described the soleus syndrome on the basis of the pain pattern of medial tibial stress syndrome approximating the origin of the soleus muscle (Figs. 7-1B and 7-9A). This is controversial because other investigators hold that the pain pattern more closely follows the course of the tibialis posterior muscle.[6] In either case, soleus syndrome is similar to type III medial tibial stress syndrome.

Compartment Syndrome

There are four compartments in the leg (Fig. 7-12). The anterior compartment includes the tibialis anterior, extensor hallucis longus, and extensor digitorum muscles. The lateral

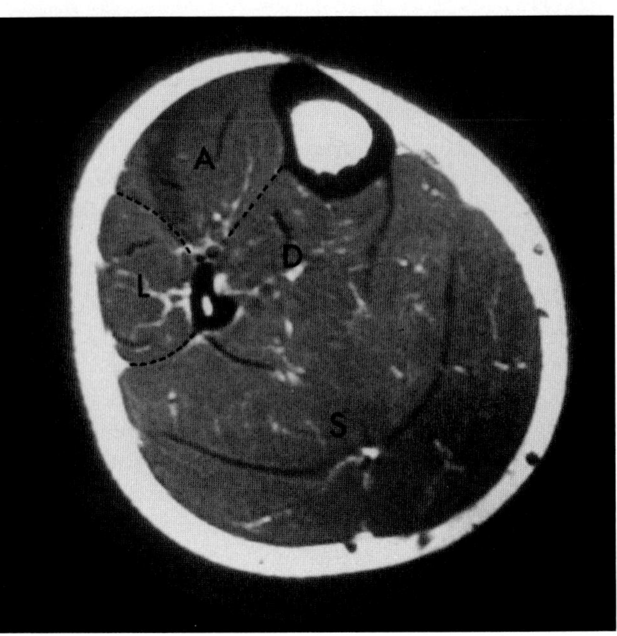

Fig. 7-12 Axial MR image demonstrating the compartments of the legs. A, Anterior: tibialis anterior, extensor hallucis longus, and extensor digitorum. L, Lateral: peroneus longus and brevis. D, Deep posterior compartment: tibialis posterior, flexor hallucis longus, and flexor digitorum. S, Superficial posterior compartment: gastrocnemius and soleus.

compartment includes the peroneus longus and brevis muscles. There are two posterior compartments: superficial and deep. The muscles of the superficial compartment are the gastrocnemius and soleus, and the deep compartment comprises the tibialis posterior, flexor hallucis longus, and flexor digitorum.[12,16,19]

Compartment syndromes are the result of muscle enlargement, hematoma, hemorrhage, or inflammation that causes increased pressure in the fascial compartment. The increased pressure leads to decreased perfusion and neurovascular compromise.[12,19]

Acute compartment syndrome has a rapid onset and usually follows fracture or blunt trauma. There is severe pain; neurovascular symptoms and muscle ischemia and necrosis can occur unless fasciotomy is performed quickly.[15,31,33,39]

Chronic or recurrent compartment syndrome more commonly involves the anterior and lateral compartments in runners and military recruits.[6,12] Muscle volume may increase up to 20% after strenuous exercise.[40] Pressures are significantly higher after exercise but decrease with rest;[6,12] normal resting pressure is less than 5 mmHg. With exercise compartment pressures may reach 50 mmHg, but normally pressures return to normal within 5 minutes of cessation of exercise. Pressures of 40 to 45 mmHg or within 30 mmHg of diastolic blood pressure are considered diagnostic. Chronic compartment syndrome is bilateral in 95% of patients.[12,33,37]

Together with pain, examination of patients with compartment syndromes may reveal changes in peripheral pulses and sensory deficits. For example, anterior compartment syndrome may present with pain and swelling anteriorly with loss of sensation (deep peroneal nerve) in the dorsal first web space of the foot. Diagnosis of compartment syndrome is confirmed most often by clinical findings and elevated compartment pressures.[12,33,37,39]

Vascular Syndromes and Injuries

Vascular injury may occur with compartment syndrome or as a result of fracture or blunt trauma.[3,12,37] Deep venous thrombosis has been reported in joggers, especially those in the 30- to 40-year age range. Sharp posterior leg pain is usually the presenting symptom. Physical examination often reveals swelling and increased calf circumference.[12]

Popliteal artery entrapment syndrome is an uncommon cause of exercise-related leg pain with associated decrease in distal pulses.[12,18] The symptoms are anomalous gastrocnemius muscles or other anatomic variations in the popliteal fossa. Injuries in men outnumber those in women, and the symptoms are bilateral in 25% of cases.[18] As with other forms of claudication, the symptoms are relieved by rest.

Imaging of Soft Tissue Injuries

Many soft tissue injuries in the leg are diagnosed on the basis of clinical findings. Therefore, imaging is usually indicated to confirm the diagnosis or to define the problem in difficult cases. The main question is usually whether soft tissue injury rather than subtle microfracture or stress fracture is present.[3,10,34]

Although routine radiographs are often normal, they are useful to exclude fractures, periosteal changes, and soft tissue ossification.[3,10] For example, tibiofibular synostosis (ossification in the interosseous membrane) may occur with repeated trauma or a single event. Routine radiography or CT would be adequate to confirm this diagnosis.[12,13]

Radionuclide bone scans (^{99m}Tc-labeled methylene diphosphorate [MPD]) are commonly used to exclude osseous injury.[3,16] Three-phase bone scans are frequently used in patients with medial tibial stress syndrome. Certain useful radionuclide uptake patterns have been defined to assist in confirming the diagnosis. Stress fractures are typically well-defined, fusiform regions of increased tracer uptake compared to the more diffuse, linear pattern described on delayed images in patients with shin splints or type II medial tibial stress syndrome (Fig. 7-13).[16,27]

Angiography and venography may be required in patients with suspected arterial or venous abnormalities.[3,32,36,37] New developments in MRI, however, have also made it possible to define these abnormalities (Fig. 7-14).[3,36,37] MRI is also an excellent technique for defining the nature of other painful conditions in the leg (Fig. 7-15). Changes in bone, soft tissue,

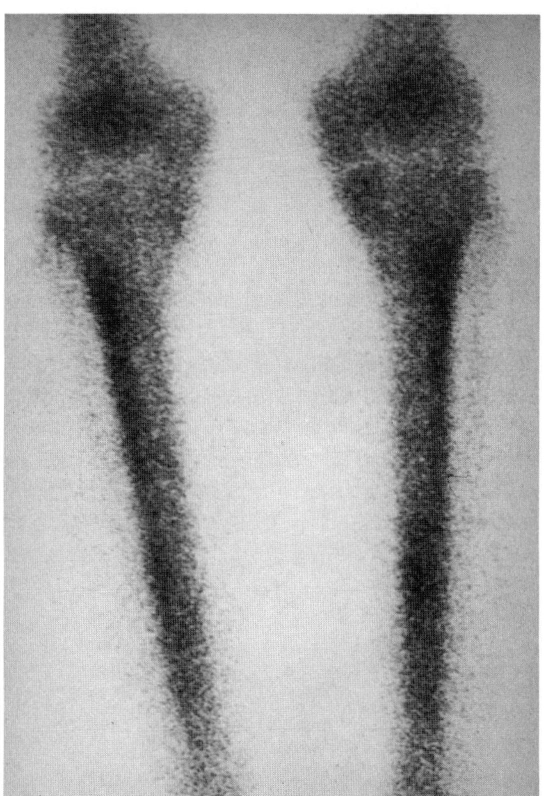

Fig. 7-13 Radionuclide bone scan demonstrating long areas of increased tracer uptake in both tibias due to shin splints.

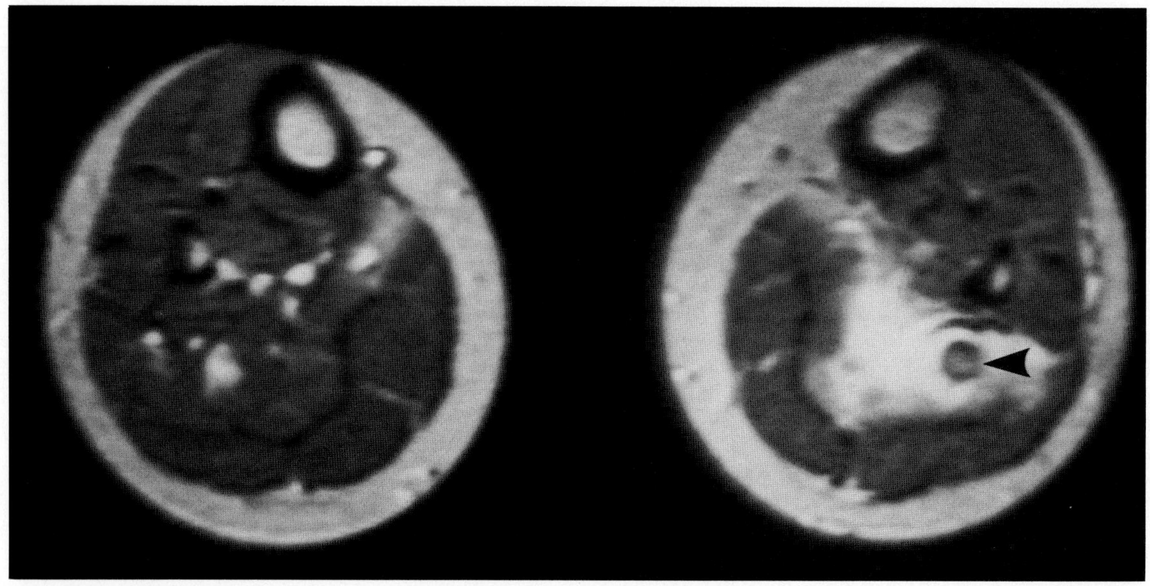

Fig. 7-14 Axial T2-weighted MR image (SE 2000/60) of the calf demonstrating increased signal intensity in the left soleus with thrombus in the vein (arrowhead).

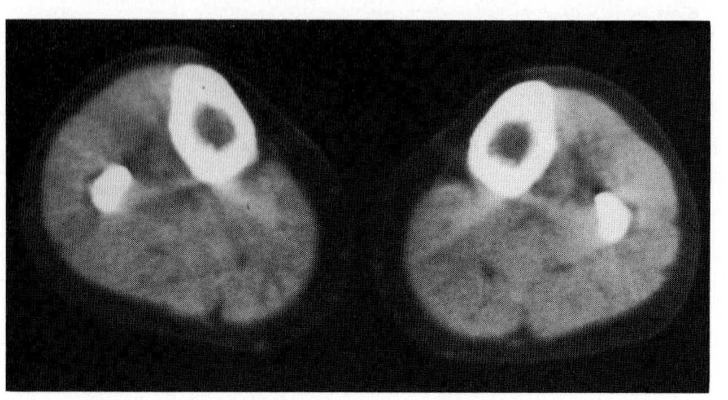

A

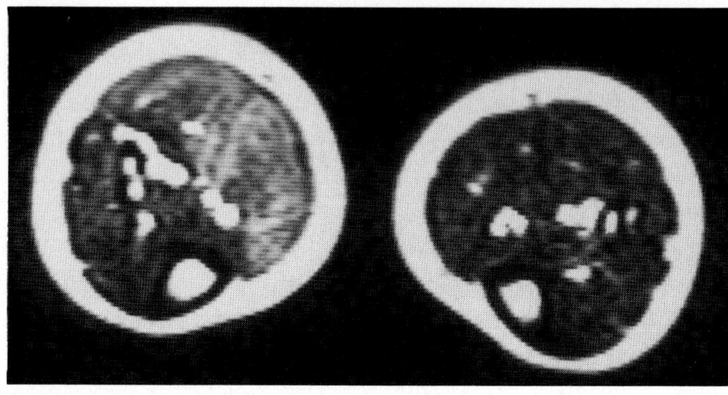

B

Fig. 7-15 Unilateral compartment syndrome that is not evident on the computed tomography image (**A**) but is obvious on the MR image (**B**).

and neurovascular structures can be defined.[3,11] Therefore, if radiographs and isotope scans do not define the nature of the injury, MRI should be considered.[3]

MR images should be performed with both T1- and T2-weighted sequences to define better subtle changes in the bone and soft tissues. Two image planes may be useful to define the extent of injury.[3] Imaging with gradient-echo techniques is most useful for evaluating vascular structures.[3,36]

REFERENCES

1. Arner O, Lindholm A. What is tennis leg? *Acta Chir Scand*. 1958;116:73–77.

2. Backx FJG, Erich WBM, Kemper ABA, Verbeek ALM. Sports injuries in school age children. *Am J Sports Med*. 1989;17:234–240.

3. Berquist TH. *Magnetic Resonance Imaging of the Musculoskeletal System*. New York: Raven; 1990.

4. Bohn WW, Durben RA. Ipsilateral fractures of the femur and tibia in children and adolescents. *J Bone Joint Surg Am*. 1991;73:429–438.

5. Boyer RS, Jaffe RB, Nixon GW, Condon VR. Trampoline fracture of the proximal tibia in children. *AJR*. 1986;146:83–85.

6. Briner WW. Shin splints. *Am Fam Physician*. 1988;37:155–160.

7. Clement DB. Tibial stress syndrome in athletes. *J Sports Med*. 1974;2:81–85.

8. Clews AG. Dislocation of the upper end of the fibula. *Can Med Assoc J*. 1968;98:169–170.

9. Detmer DE. Chronic shin splints: classification and management of medial tibial stress syndrome. *Sports Med*. 1986;3:436–446.

10. Devas MB. Stress fractures of the tibia and shin soreness. *J Bone Joint Surg Br*. 1958;40:227–239.

11. Fleckenstein JL, Conby RC, Partey RW, Peschack RM. Acute effects of exercise on MR imaging of skeletal muscle in normal volunteers. *AJR*. 1988;151:231–237.

12. Friedman MJ. Injuries to the leg in athletes. In: Nicholas JA, Hershman EB, eds. *The Lower Extremity and Spine in Sports Medicine*. St Louis, MO: Mosby; 1986;601–655.

13. Gershuni DH, Skyhar MJ, Thompson B, Resnick D, Donald G, Akeson WH. A comparison of conventional and computed tomography in the evaluation of spiral fractures of the tibia. *J Bone Joint Surg Am*. 1985;67:1388–1395.

14. Halpern AA, Nagel DA. Anterior compartment pressures in patients with tibial fractures. *J Trauma.* 1980;20:786–790.

15. Halpern B, Thomas N, Curl WW, Andrews JR, Hunter SC, Boring JR. High school football injuries: identifying the risk factors. *Am J Sports Med.* 1987;15:113–117.

16. Holder LE, Michael RH. Specific scintigraphic pattern of shin splints in the lower leg. *J Nucl Med.* 1984;25:A65–A69.

17. Hollinshead WH. *Anatomy for Surgeons.* Philadelphia: Harper & Row; 1982;3.

18. Insua JA, Young JR, Humphries AW. Popliteal artery entrapment syndrome. *Arch Surg.* 1970;101:771–775.

19. Jones DC, James SL. Overuse injuries of the lower extremity: shin splints, iliotibial band friction syndrome, and exertional compartment syndromes. *Clin Sports Med.* 1987;6:273–290.

20. Leach RE. Fractures of the tibia and fibula. In: Rockwood CA, Green DP, eds. *Fractures in Adults.* 2nd ed. Philadelphia: Lippincott; 1984;2: 1593–1663.

21. Marti B, Vader JP, Minder CE, Abelin T. On the epidemiology of running injuries. *Am J Sports Med.* 1988;16:285–294.

22. Matheson GO, MacIntyre JC, Taunton JE, Clements DB, Lloyd-Smith R. Musculoskeletal injuries associated with physical activity in older adults. *Med Sci Sports Exerc.* 1989;21:379–385.

23. Mattalino AJ, Deese M, Campbell ED. Office evaluation and treatment of lower extremity injuries in the runner. *Clin Sports Med.* 1989;8: 461–475.

24. Matter P, Ziegler WJ, Halzach P. Skiing accidents in the past 15 years. *J Sports Sci.* 1987;5:319–326.

25. Maylack FH. Epidemiology of tennis, squash, and racquetball injuries. *Clin Sports Med.* 1988;7:233–243.

26. Michael RH, Holder LE. The soleus syndrome. *Am J Sports Med.* 1985;13:87–94.

27. Moore MP. Shin splints. *Postgrad Med.* 1988;83:199–209.

28. Mubarak SJ, Gould RN, Lee FF, Schmidt DA, Hargens AR. The medial tibial stress syndrome. *Am J Sports Med.* 1982;10:201–205.

29. Paty JG. Diagnosis and treatment of musculoskeletal running injuries. *Semin Arthritis Rheum.* 1988;18:199–209.

30. Pickard MA, Tullett WM, Patel AR. Sports injuries as seen at an accident and emergency department. *Scott Med J.* 1988;33:296–297.

31. Puranen J. The medial tibial syndrome. Exercise ischemia in the medial fascial compartment of the leg. *J Bone Joint Surg Br.* 1974;56: 712–715.

32. Rappaport S, Sostman HD, Dope C, Campataro CM, Holcomb W, Gore JC. Venous clots: evaluation with MR imaging. *Radiology.* 1987; 162:527–530.

33. Reveman RS. The anterior and lateral compartment syndrome of the leg due to intensive use of muscles. *Clin Orthop.* 1975;113:69–80.

34. Rothenberger LA, Chang JI, Cable TA. Prevalence and types of injuries in aerobic dancers. *Am J Sports Med.* 1988;16:403–407.

35. Slocum DB. The shin splint syndrome. Medical aspects and differential diagnosis. *Am J Surg.* 1967;11:875–881.

36. Spritzer CE, Sussman SK, Blunder RA, Salad M, Herfkens RJ. Deep venous thrombosis evaluation with limited flip-angle, gradient refocused MR imaging: preliminary experience. *Radiology.* 1988;166:371–375.

37. Stack C. Superficial posterior compartment syndrome of the leg with deep venous compromise. *Clin Orthop.* 1987;220:233–236.

38. Templeton DC, Morder RA. Injuries to the knee associated with fractures of the tibial shaft. *J Bone Joint Surg Am.* 1989;71:1392–1394.

39. Veith RG, Matsen FA, Newell SG. The current anterior compartment syndromes. *Physician Sports Med.* 1980;8:80–88.

40. Wright S. *Applied Physiology.* 10th ed. London: Oxford University Press; 1961.

Chapter **8**

Foot and Ankle

INTRODUCTION

Fifty-five percent to 90% of sports injuries involve the lower extremity, most commonly the knee, foot, and ankle.[1,3] The majority of foot and ankle injuries are related to running, jumping, or cutting maneuvers.[3,7,8]

Acute foot and ankle injuries account for 10% of emergency department visits.[2] Overuse injuries are also common, however, and most often are not seen in an emergency setting.[4–6,9,10]

Garrick and Requa[3] reviewed more than 16,000 athletic injuries and found that foot and ankle injuries represented just over 25% of this population. In the ankle, sprains were the most common injury. Volleyball (82%) and basketball (79%) were the most frequent activities associated with ankle sprains. The fewest sprains were noted with skiing, ballet, and figure skating.[3,9] Overuse injuries in the ankle occur less frequently (27% of ankle injuries). Cycling, ice skating, ballet, and running are most commonly associated with overuse syndromes in the ankle.

Overuse syndromes in the foot account for 50% of injuries.[3,10] The highest incidence in the series reported by Garrick and Requa[3] occurred in volleyball (70%); running (59%) and tennis, racquetball, and gymnastics (~50%) had the next highest incidence rates. Sprains do occur in the foot, but they account for less than 7% of foot injuries.

Knowledge of the anatomy and clinical data are essential requirements for optimal imaging of the foot and ankle. Therefore, these aspects of foot and ankle injuries are emphasized along with specific imaging techniques.

ANATOMY

Basic osseous and soft tissue anatomy is discussed in this section. More detailed anatomic information is reviewed in the context of specific bone and soft tissue injuries in later sections of this chapter.

Osseous and Ligamentous Anatomy of the Ankle

The ankle is formed by three bones: the tibia, the fibula, and the talus (Fig. 8-1).[11–13,15,18] The tibia is the second longest bone in the skeleton. It is expanded proximally and distally. The body of the tibia (diaphysis) has three surfaces: anterior, medial, and posterior. The anterior surface ends in the medial malleolus. The medial margin is subcutaneous. The interosseous membrane attaches to the lateral margin (Fig. 8-1).[15–18]

Distally the tibia expands at the metaphysis to form the medial malleolus and the articular surface for the talus (Fig. 8-1). The inferior or articular surface is biconcave and articulates with the talar dome.[13,21] Hyaline cartilage covers the articular surface of the tibia and extends medially to the articular portion of the medial malleolus. The articular cartilage does not completely cover the posterior tibia (posterior malleolus). This is significant because, if only small segments of the posterior malleolus are fractured, the articular portion may be excluded.[17,26]

The anterior surface of the tibia is smooth except at the anteroinferior margin, where it is more irregular at the site for

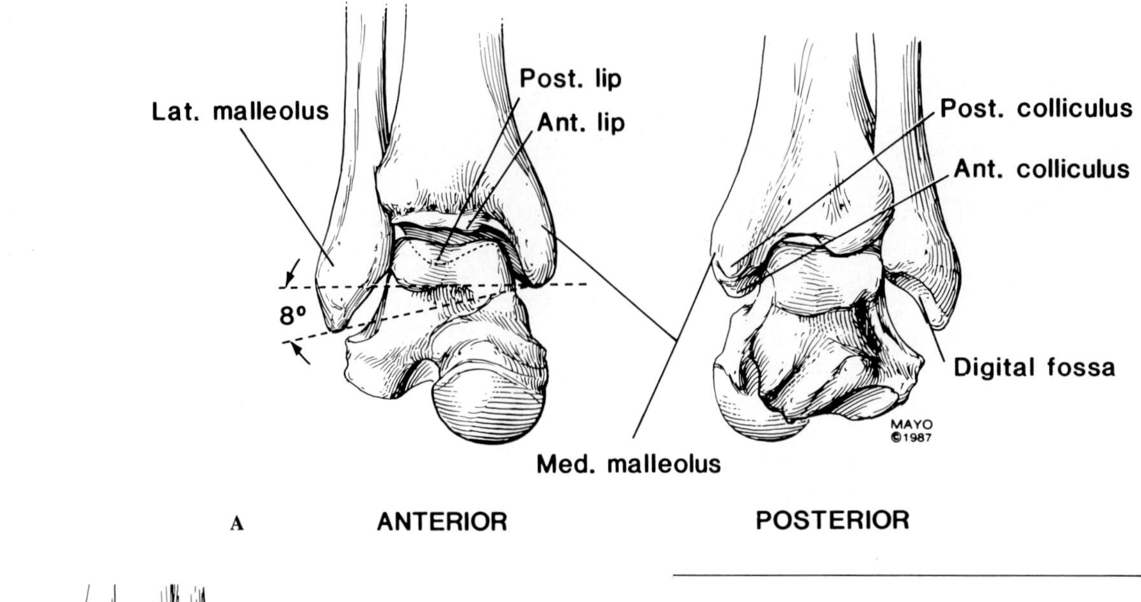

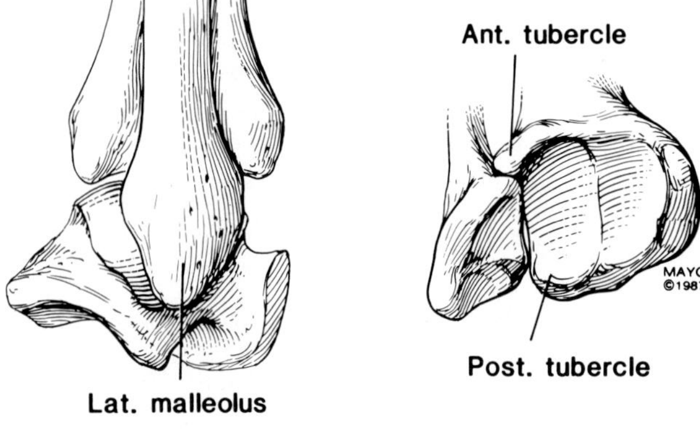

Fig. 8-1 Illustration of the bony anatomy of the ankle seen anteriorly and posteriorly (**A**) and laterally and inferiorly (**B**). *Source:* Reprinted from *Radiology of the Foot and Ankle* by TH Berquist, Raven Press, 1989, © Mayo Foundation.

attachment of the anterior ankle capsule. The posterior tibia has grooves for the flexor hallucis longus (lateral) and flexor digitorum longus and tibialis posterior tendons (medial).[11,12] The lateral surface articulates with the fibula. This articular surface is bounded anteriorly and posteriorly by ridges for insertion of the anterior and posterior distal tibiofibular ligaments (Figs. 8-1 and 8-2).[15,18] The strong medial extension (medial malleolus) articulates with the talus and forms the medial portion of the ankle mortise.

The fibula is thin and flat and does not have a direct weight-bearing surface (Fig. 8-1). The lateral malleolus is the expanded distal portion of the fibula. The fibula is irregular along its medial margin at the point of attachment for the interosseous ligament. Hyaline cartilage covers the articular surface on the inferomedial aspect. There are irregular areas anteriorly and posteriorly for insertions of the tibiofibular ligament. The fibula (lateral malleolus) is more posterior than

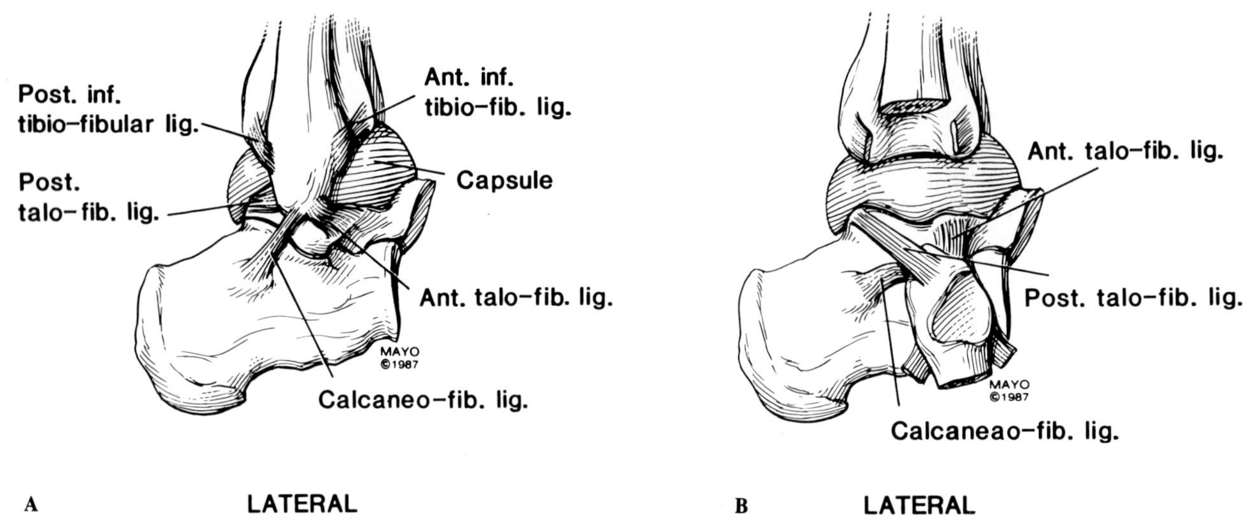

Fig. 8-2 Illustration of the ligaments of the ankle. (**A**) Lateral ligaments, (**B**) lateral ligaments with fibula displaced.

the medial malleolus, and its distal extent is below the level of the medial malleolar tip.[15,18,21] Thus an angle of about 8° is formed by a line drawn from the tips of the malleoli (Fig. 8-1A).[12,18,19] The posterior position of the lateral malleolus results in an angle of 20° between the malleoli in the axial plane. For this reason the mortise view of the ankle is taken with the foot internally rotated approximately 20°.[17,27]

The hyaline cartilage trochlear surface of the talus is usually 2 to 3 mm wider anteriorly than posteriorly. It articulates with the weight-bearing surface of the tibia and the medial and lateral malleoli. Thus the ankle mortise is formed by the tibial and fibular components of the ankle, which roofs the talus (Fig. 8-1).[20,21] The tibial portion of the mortise is termed the plafond.[13] Forces on the talus that result in position changes of this structure in the mortise are responsible for many osseous and/or ligamentous ankle injuries.[21,23]

The supporting structures of the ankle include the joint capsule, medial and lateral ligaments, and interosseous ligament (Fig. 8-2). In addition 13 tendons cross the ankle, and there are four retinacula.[13] Four ligaments support the distal tibia and fibula.[15,18] The interosseous ligament, with its oblique fibers, joins the tibia and fibula at a level just above the joint. The interosseous ligament is the thickened distal portion of the interosseous membrane. The tibial and fibular attachments of this ligament form a triangular configuration that is weakened at its base by the syndesmotic recess. This recess is an extension of the joint into the tibiofibular space. The distal anterior and posterior tibiofibular ligaments join the tibia and fibula just proximal to the tibiotalar joint (Fig. 8-2). The anterior ligament is weaker than the posterior. This explains the increased incidence of avulsion fractures posteriorly compared to ligament disruptions.[21,22] The transverse ligament is the fourth ligament of the syndesmotic group. This ligament lies anterior to the posterior tibiofibular ligament and extends from the lateral malleolus to the posterior articular margin of the tibia just lateral to the medial malleolus. The ligament actually forms part of the posterior articulation with the talus (Fig. 8-2E).[15,18]

The deltoid ligament provides medial stability.[12,22,23] This ligament is a strong, triangular-shaped group of fibers with its apex at the medial malleolus. The ligament fans out as it progresses inferiorly and divides into superficial and deep fibers.[15] The superficial fibers insert in the navicular tuberosity. Progressing posteriorly, the remaining superficial fibers insert in the sustentaculum tali and the talus. The deep fibers attach to the medial surface of the talus (Fig. 8-2).[15,19,22,23] The deltoid ligament prevents excessive abduction and eversion of the ankle and subtalar joints. In addition, eversion, pronation, and anterior displacement of the talus are restricted.[13]

There are three ligaments laterally. The anterior talofibular ligament is the weakest and most frequently injured.[26] It passes anteriorly from the fibula to insert anterior to the lateral talar articular facet.[15,18] This ligament restrains anterior talar motion.[18] The posterior talofibular ligament is much stronger

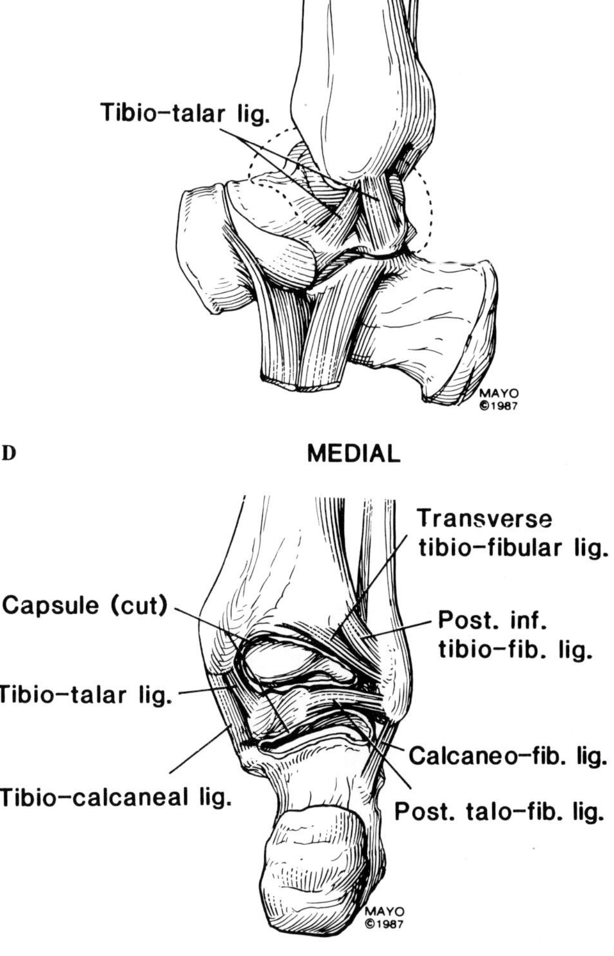

Fig. 8-2 contd **(C)** medial ligaments, **(D)** medial ligaments with superficial fibers retracted inferiorly, **(E)** posterior view of ligaments. *Source:* Reprinted from *Radiology of the Foot and Ankle* by TH Berquist, Raven Press, 1989, © Mayo Foundation.

and courses transversely from the posterior aspect of the lateral malleolus to the posterior talar tubercle. This ligament prevents posterior talar motion (Fig. 8-2). The calcaneofibular ligament (Fig. 8-2) is the longest of the three ligaments and takes a nearly vertical course from the lateral malleolus to the lateral surface of the calcaneus. The calcaneofibular ligament prevents excessive inversion.[18] The peroneal tendons are just superficial to the calcaneofibular ligament.

The synovium-lined capsule of the ankle is attached to the acetabular margins of the tibia, fibula, and talus. The anterior and posterior portions of the capsule are thin and provide much less support than the ligaments described above (Fig. 8-2).[11,26]

Foot Anatomy

For purposes of discussion, the foot can be divided into three segments: the hindfoot (talus and calcaneus), midfoot (remaining five tarsal bones), and forefoot (metatarsals and phalanges).[13,26] Three longitudinal columns have also been described. The medial column consists of the calcaneus, talus, navicular, medial and intermediate cuneiforms, and first and second metatarsals and phalanges. The middle column consists of the lateral cuneiform and the third metatarsal and phalanx. The lateral column is made up of the hindfoot (talus and calcaneus) and the fourth and fifth metatarsals with their phalanges. All articulations are synovial joints supported by strong plantar and weaker dorsal ligaments.[13,18]

Hindfoot

The hindfoot includes the talus and calcaneus.[19,33] The talus is the second largest of the tarsal bones and articulates with the tibia, medial and lateral malleoli, and calcaneus inferiorly (Fig. 8-3). The talar head articulates with the navicular.[15,18]

Superiorly the trochlea articulates with the tibia and malleoli (Fig. 8-1). It is covered with hyaline cartilage and makes up the upper portion of the body of the talus.[13] There are three articular facets on the inferior surface of the talus (Fig. 8-1).[11,15,18] The anterior and posterior facets articulate with similarly named calcaneal facets. The middle facet is just posterior to the anterior calcaneal articular facet. The middle facet articulates with the sustentaculum tali.[15] The talar sulcus lies between the middle and anterior facets. This structure with its calcaneal counterpart forms the tarsal sinus, which contains the interosseous talocalcaneal ligament. The head of the talus articulates with the navicular. The talonavicular joint is at a 20° angle medial to the midpoint of the talar dome (Fig. 8-3). The talocalcaneal relationship is also important. On the lateral radiograph of a normal foot the talus and calcaneus form an angle of 40° (Fig. 8-3B). On the anteroposterior (AP) view this angle is normally 35° (Fig. 8-3A). These values vary by as much as 20°. The angles are generally smaller in the immature foot. The talus articulates with 75% of the navicular in pronation and 100% of the navicular in supination. The normal talonavicular axis extends into the shaft of the first metatarsal (Fig. 8-3). During pronation this axis is medial, and during supination lateral, to the first metatarsal head.[13,26,30]

Several osseous growths have been described on the talus. These are usually of no clinical significance. A normal ridge is

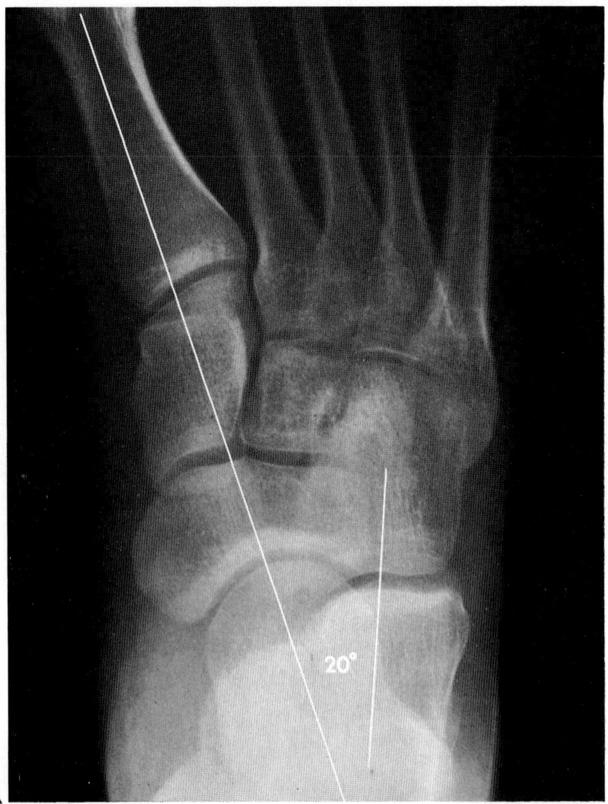

A

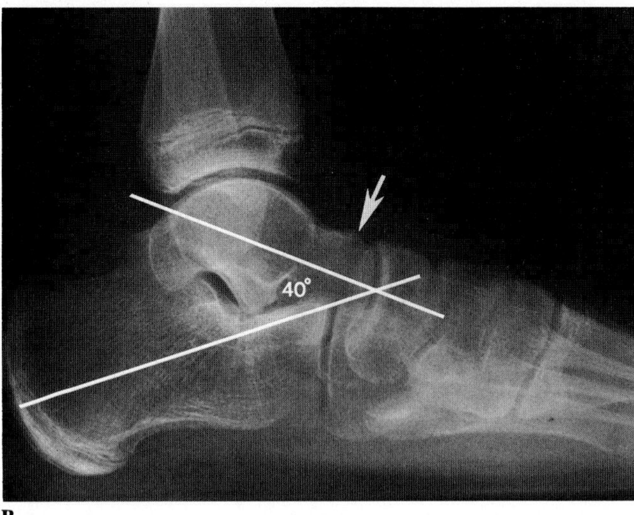

B

Fig. 8-3 (**A**) Anteroposterior (AP) and (**B**) lateral views of the foot showing the normal osseous relationships. Note the normal talar ridge (arrow in **B**).

present distal to the trochlear surface on the dorsolateral aspect of the talus.[29] This can be seen on the lateral view of the ankle and should not be confused with pathology. This ridge is the site of attachment of the dorsal talonavicular ligament and anterior tibiotalar joint capsule. Therefore, hypertrophy can occur in patients engaged in activities that require extremes of plantar flexion (football, ballet dancing, and the like; Fig. 8-3B).[29] The posterior aspect of the talus contains an oblique groove for the flexor hallucis longus tendon.[15]

The calcaneus, which is the largest tarsal bone, contains three superior articular facets.[15] The middle, most medial facet is on the sustentaculum tali. The calcaneal sulcus lies between the middle and anterior facets and forms the floor of the tarsal canal. This canal has an oblique course and measures 10 to 15 mm in height, 3 to 5 mm in width, and 15 to 20 mm in length.[29] The distal or plantar surface of the calcaneus contains two grooves. The lateral groove is for the peroneus longus tendon. More medially, the flexor hallucis longus runs in the groove beneath the sustentaculum tali.[12,18]

The posterior aspect of the calcaneus forms the prominence of the heel.[17] It contains irregular areas superiorly for insertion of the Achilles tendon (superior tuberosity). There are similar areas medially for the attachments of the plantar aponeurosi, flexor digitorum brevis and abductor hallucis, and laterally for the abductor digiti minimi muscle attachments. The calcaneus articulates with the cuboid anteriorly (Fig. 8-3).

There are two ligaments that directly support the talocalcaneal joint. These are the interosseous talocalcaneal ligament, which is located in the sinus tarsi, and the smaller lateral talocalcaneal ligament.[15,18] In addition, the ligaments of the ankle and adjacent tendons provide stabilization. The latter include the peroneal tendons, flexor hallucis longus, flexor digitorum longus, and tibialis posterior tendons.[18]

The posterior talocalcaneal joint has a synovial cavity of its own, being separated from the anterior talocalcaneal articulation by the interosseous ligament. The posterior subtalar joint communicates with the ankle in 10% of patients.[13] The anterior joint may communicate with the talonavicular joint (talocalcaneonavicular joint).[11,15,18]

Midfoot

The remaining tarsal bones make up the midfoot. These include the cuboid, the navicular, and three cuneiforms.[15,18]

The cuboid articulates with the calcaneus proximally and with the fourth and fifth metatarsals distally (Fig. 8-3). Dorsally the cuboid is roughened at the points of ligament attachment. On the plantar surface the cuboid contains a groove for the peroneus longus tendon. The medial cuboid surface contains a facet for articulation with the lateral cuneiform.[11,15,18]

The navicular is on the medial side of the foot anterior to the talus. It articulates proximally with the talus, anteriorly with the cuneiforms, and occasionally laterally with the cuboid (Fig. 8-3).[15,18]

The spring ligament is contiguous with the deltoid ligament of the ankle (Fig. 8-2C). It extends from the calcaneus to the navicular tuberosity. The cubonavicular ligament runs dorsally from the cuboid to the navicular.[15] Proximally the bifurcate ligament originates on the anterosuperior calcaneus and sends medial fibers to the lateral navicular and lateral fibers to the cuboid.[15,18] The calcaneonavicular ligament is on the plantar aspect of the capsule.[11]

There are three cuneiform bones located distal to the navicular and medial to the cuboid (Fig. 8-3). The medial cuneiform is the largest and articulates with the navicular proximally, the intermediate cuneiform laterally, and the first and second metatarsals distally (Fig. 8-3).[15] The intermediate cuneiform is the smallest cuneiform and lies between the medial and lateral cuneiforms. It articulates with the latter bones, the navicular, and the second metatarsal.[15,18] The lateral cuneiform lies between the intermediate cuneiform and the cuboid, articulating with both. It also articulates with the navicular and the second through fourth metatarsals (Fig. 8-3).[11,15,18]

The five metatarsals articulate proximally with the tarsal bones described above (Fig. 8-3), and each, except the first (great toe), typically has three phalanges distally. The metatarsals have a similar configuration except that the first is broader from the proximal articular surface distally to its head. The fifth metatarsal has a broad base compared to the second through fourth metatarsals.

Dorsal, plantar, and interosseous ligaments support the tarsometatarsal joints and bases of the metatarsals. Distally the transverse metatarsal ligament connects the heads of the metatarsals.[15] Each of the metatarsophalangeal joints is supported by collateral and plantar ligaments. The extensor tendons replace the usual dorsal ligaments in these joints.[11,15,18]

Arches of the Foot

There are three arches in the foot: one transverse and two longitudinal. The lateral longitudinal arch is formed by the calcaneus, cuboid, and fourth and fifth metatarsals. In a patient with normal gait, this arch normally receives the weight of the body before the medial longitudinal arch.[11] The peroneus longus tendon runs through the midpoint of this arch. The medial longitudinal arch is formed by the calcaneus, talus, navicular, cuneiforms, and first through third metatarsals. The vertical height of the medial arch is greater than that of the lateral arch. The apex of the arch is more posterior, being located at the calcaneotalonavicular junction. The posterior tibial tendon inserts on the navicular and sends plantar fibers below the arch, adding additional support.[15,18,21,33]

The transverse arch is completed when the feet are adjacent, so that the two medial longitudinal arches are approximated. Thus the bases of the metatarsals and midtarsal bones form the arch with support from the peroneus longus and posterior tibial tendons.[15,29,31]

Normal Variants

There are many anatomic variants that can mimic more serious pathologic conditions.[13,28,32] These changes are most

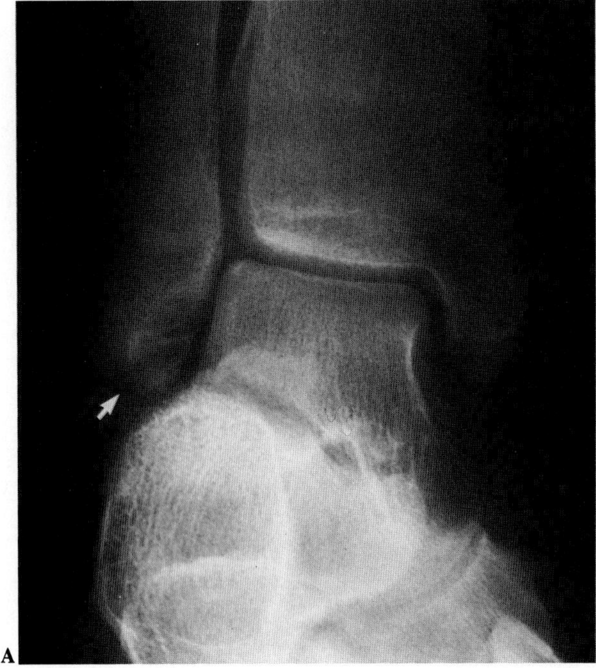

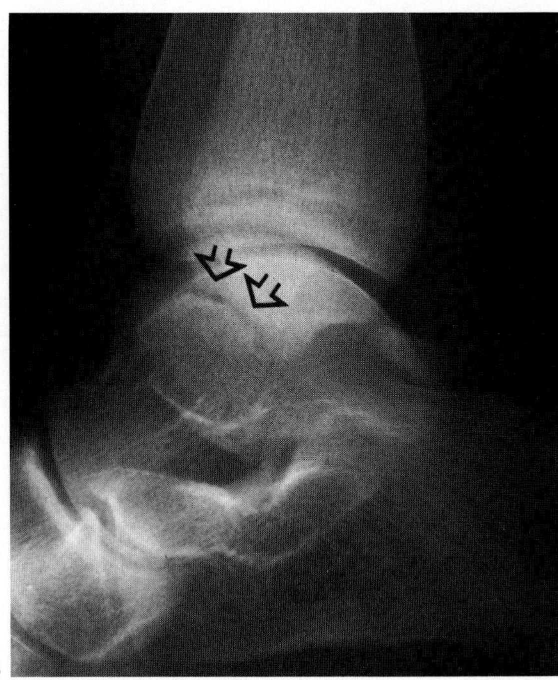

Fig. 8-4 (**A**) AP and (**B**) lateral views of the ankle showing the os subfibulare (arrows). This normal variant has a well-defined cortical margin and should not be confused with a fracture. *Source:* Reprinted from *Radiology of the Foot and Ankle* by TH Berquist, Raven Press, 1989, © Mayo Foundation.

common in the metaphyseal and epiphyseal areas adjacent to the growth plates.[13,14] Occasionally small ossification centers are evident adjacent to the growth plates, simulating fractures.[13,16,28] Ossicles are also commonly noted near the medial and lateral malleoli. These frequently cause confusion in diagnosing patients with recent injury (Fig. 8-4). They occur medially in 17% to 24% of girls and up to 47% of boys. Most are bilateral, and they are commonly seen from 6 to 12 years.[13,19] Normal variants are also common in the tarsal bones.[13,14]

The secondary ossification center of the talus is located posteriorly. It appears at 8 to 11 years of age and normally fuses at 16 to 20 years of age. This somewhat controversial ossification center is the posterior part of the talar tubercle and is located lateral to the flexor hallucis longus tendon.[13,14,28] If this center does not fuse to the talus, it is called the os trigonum tarsi and is frequently mistaken for a fracture (Fig. 8-5).[25] In forced plantar flexion the ossicle can separate, or fracture can occur in the fused center.[13,27]

Another common finding is the accessory navicular, or os tibiale externum (Fig. 8-6). This lies in the posterior tibial tendon just proximal to the medial margin of the navicular. This ossicle may affect tendon function, especially during puberty when growth is accelerated.[13,14] Resection may be required to relieve the painful symptoms. The os supranaviculare (Fig. 8-6) is located at the proximal dorsal margin of the navicular distal to the joint space. This is more distal than the os supratalare, which would be proximal to the talonavicular joint. The most frequently noted ossicles in the foot are summarized in Fig. 8-6.[13,14,28]

Soft Tissue Anatomy

The muscles of the calf are divided into anterior, posterior, and lateral compartments. Because of their action on the foot and ankle, a brief review of anatomy and function is indicated.

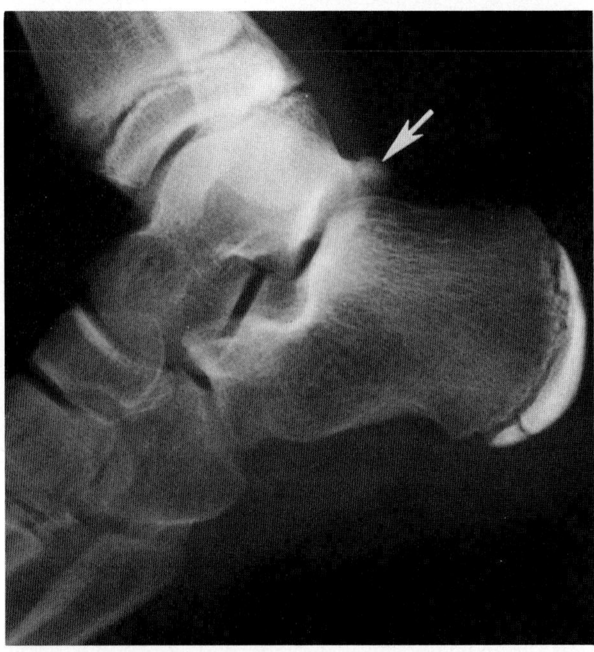

Fig. 8-5 Lateral view of the hindfoot demonstrating a normal sclerotic calcaneal apophysis. There is also normal-appearing os trigonum tarsi (arrow).

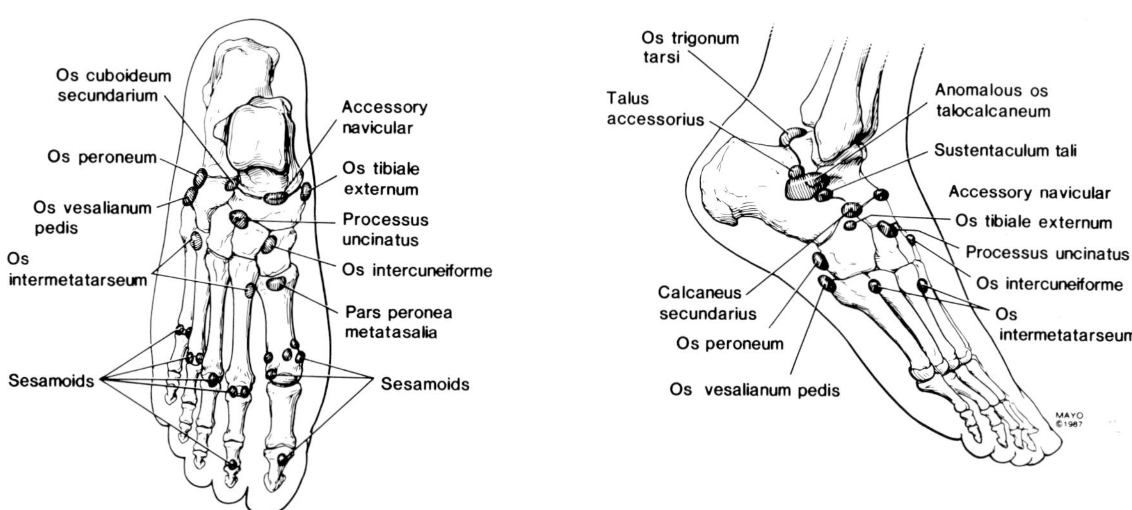

Fig. 8-6 Illustration of the accessory ossicles of the foot. *Source:* Reprinted from *Radiology of the Foot and Ankle* by TH Berquist, Raven Press, 1989, © Mayo Foundation.

The posterior compartment contains superficial and deep muscle groups divided by crural fascia (Fig. 8-7).[15,18] The gastrocnemius and soleus are the major superficial muscles. Their tendons join to form the Achilles tendon, which inserts on the posterior calcaneus. The muscles serve as plantar flexors of the foot.[11,15,18] The accessory soleus muscle may be evident in a small percentage of patients as a normal variant. When present, symptoms, especially in runners, may mimic those of a muscle tear or neoplasm. Comparison with the normal ankle and magnetic resonance imaging (MRI) demonstration of characteristic muscle tissue confirm the diagnosis.[13,16]

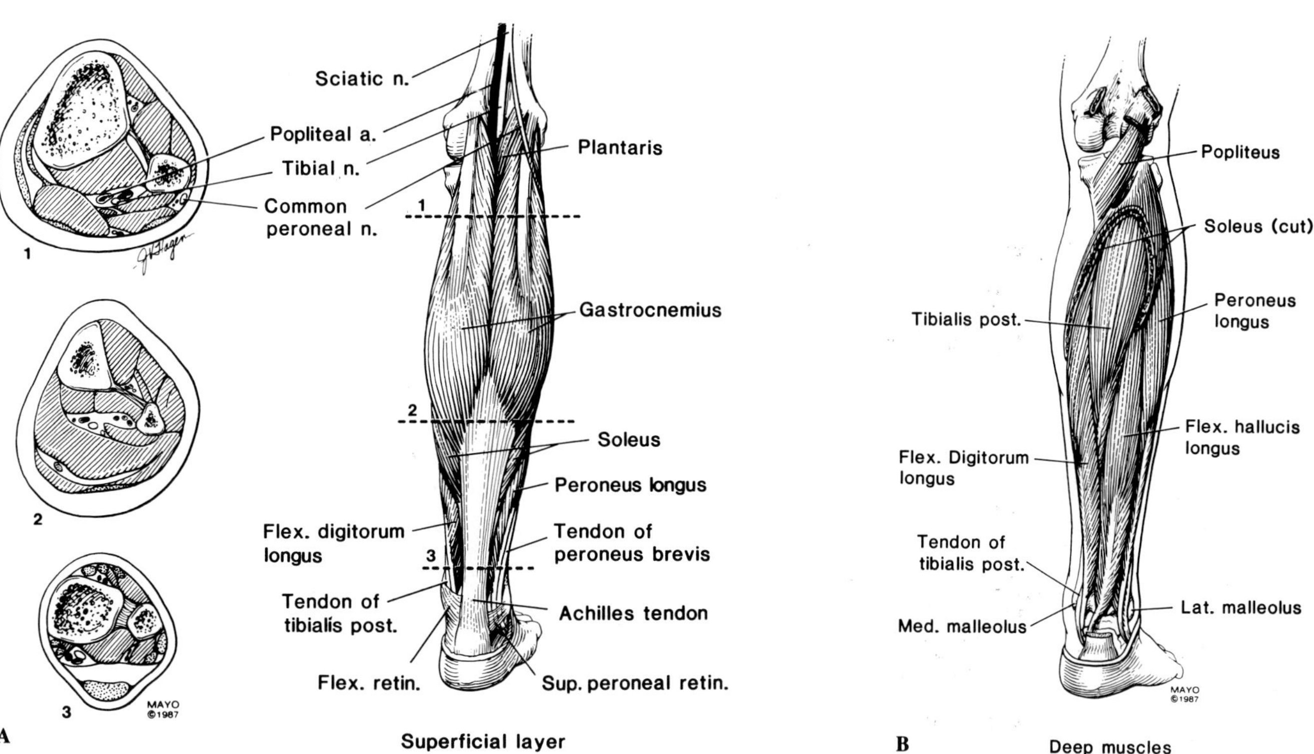

Fig. 8-7 Illustration of the posterior superficial (**A**) and deep (**B**) muscles acting on the foot and ankle. *Source:* Reprinted from *Radiology of the Foot and Ankle* by TH Berquist, Raven Press, 1989, © Mayo Foundation.

The muscles of the deep posterior compartment (popliteus, tibialis posterior, flexor hallucis longus, and flexor digitorum longus; Fig. 8-7B) also act on the foot and ankle except for the popliteus, which serves as a flexor of the knee.[15,18] The flexor hallucis longus serves as a flexor of the great toe, and the flexor digitorum longus assists in plantar flexing the foot and serves as a flexor of the lateral four toes.[15] The tibialis posterior is the deepest muscle of the posterior compartment. Its tendon passes anterior to the flexor digitorum under the flexor retinaculum to insert on the navicular and tarsal bones. This muscle aids in adduction, inversion, and plantar flexion.[15,18] Neurovascular supply to the posterior muscles is via the tibial nerve and posterior tibial artery.[15]

The peroneus longus and brevis are the muscles of the lateral compartment (Fig. 8-8). The tendons enter a common sheath above the ankle and pass posterior to the lateral malleolus and deep to the peroneal retinacula. On the lateral surface of the foot the peroneus brevis inserts on the fifth metatarsal base. The peroneus longus passes under the foot to insert on the medial cuneiform and first metatarsal base. Both muscles assist in eversion and plantar flexion of the foot.[13,15]

The anterior compartment comprises the extensor digitorum longus, peroneus tertius, extensor hallucis longus, and tibialis anterior (Fig. 8-9).[11,15] The extensor digitorum longus aids in dorsiflexion of the foot and lateral four toes. The extensor hallucis longus serves mainly for dorsiflexion of the great toe. The tibialis anterior inserts at the midfoot and aids in dorsiflexion and inversion of the foot.[13,15,31] Neurovascular supply to the anterior and lateral compartments is via the peroneal nerve and anterior tibial and peroneal arteries.[11,15,18]

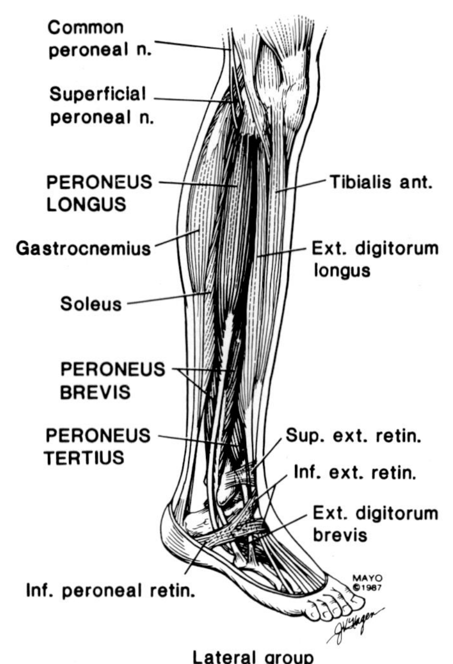

Fig. 8-8 Illustration of the lateral muscles acting on the foot and ankle. *Source:* Reprinted from *Radiology of the Foot and Ankle* by TH Berquist, Raven Press, 1989, © Mayo Foundation.

The musculature of the foot is complex. A complete discussion of origins and insertions is beyond the scope of this text. Certain functional aspects will be discussed, but the reader is referred to other texts for a more indepth discussion.[13,15,18]

The muscles of the foot are divided into four layers (Fig. 8-10).[15,18] The superficial muscles include the abductor hallucis, flexor digitorum brevis and abductor digiti minimi. The former is a weak abductor of the great toe and is supplied by the medial plantar artery and nerve.[15] The centrally located flexor digitorum brevis has the same neurovascular supply. It serves as a flexor of the lateral four toes. The abductor digiti minimi is a flexor and abductor of the fifth toe.[13,15,18]

The second layer of muscles includes the quadratus plantae, lumbrical muscles, and tendons of the flexor hallucis longus and flexor digitorum longus.[15] These muscles assist in flexion of the toes. Neurovascular supply is via both medial and lateral plantar artery and nerve branches.[15,18,24]

The third layer includes the flexor hallucis brevis, adductor hallucis, and flexor digiti minimi brevis. The flexor hallucis aids in flexion of the great toe, and the adductor hallucis serves as an adductor of the great toe. The flexor digiti minimi flexes the small toe.[15,18,24]

The fourth and deepest muscle layer includes the three plantar and four dorsal interosseous muscles. The dorsal interossei act as abductors and the plantar interossei as adductors of the foot.[15,18,33]

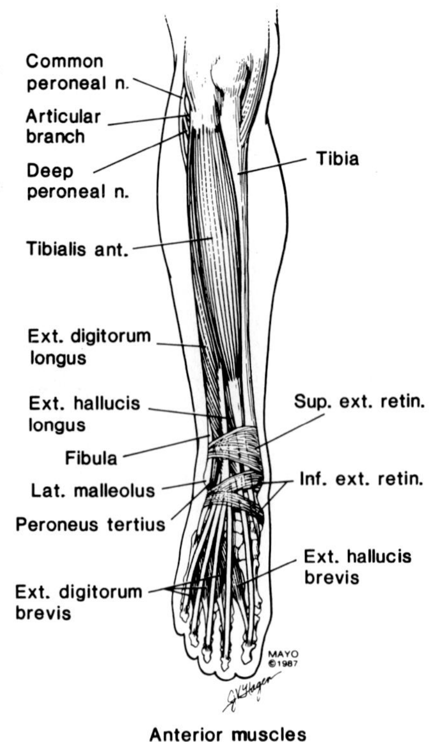

Fig. 8-9 Illustration of the anterior muscles acting on the foot and ankle. *Source:* Reprinted from *Radiology of the Foot and Ankle* by TH Berquist, Raven Press, 1989, © Mayo Foundation.

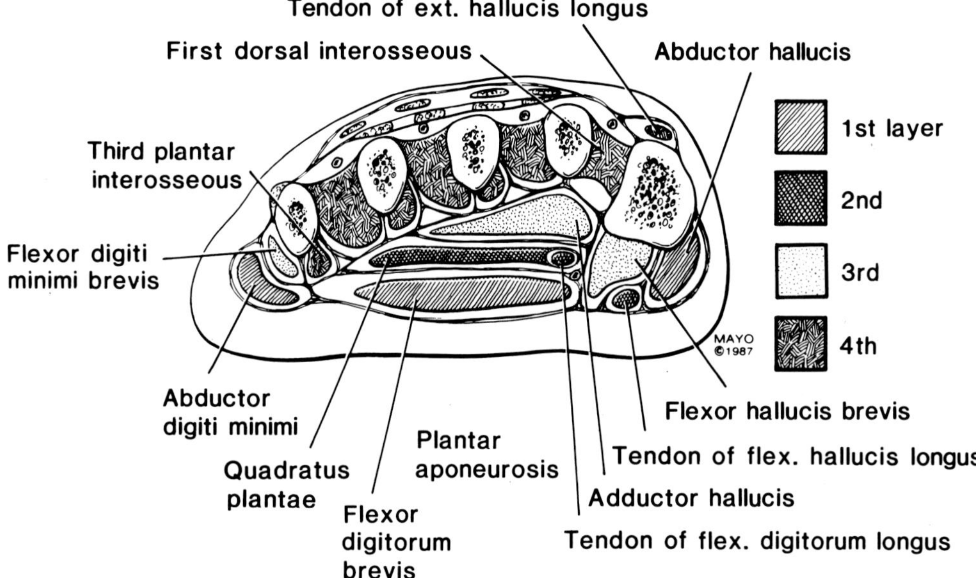

Fig. 8-10 Illustration of the muscle layers of the foot. *Source:* Reprinted from *Radiology of the Foot and Ankle* by TH Berquist, Raven Press, 1989, © Mayo Foundation.

The extensor digitorum brevis is the dorsal muscle of the foot. The muscle is a dorsiflexor of the great toe and second through fourth toes.[13,18]

Common Terms

Terms used to describe the movements in the foot and ankle are often misused (Fig. 8-11). This results in some confusion when descriptive terms such as *supination, eversion, pronation,* and the like are used. Definitions of these commonly used terms are listed below as they apply during physiologic motion of the foot and ankle.[13,19,21,31]

- *Plantar flexion*: The hinge motion at the tibiotalar joint allows the foot to plantar flex (sole of the foot is depressed). Several other motions and position changes occur with plantar flexion. During plantar flexion the gastrocnemius muscle pulls the calcaneus upward, which shifts the calcaneus into a slight varus position (posterior heel is rotated medially). The head of the talus turns in and downward during plantar flexion, which causes the foot to move inward.[13,19,31]
- *Dorsiflexion*: The hinge motion of the ankle allows the foot to be elevated or dorsiflexed (foot is lifted toward the anterior leg). The gastrocnemius muscle is relaxed, and the heel shifts into a valgus position (heel is rotated laterally). The talus turns upward and outward, so that the foot also turns outward during dorsiflexion.[13,19,31]
- *Inversion*: During inversion the sole of the foot is turned inward. In the European literature the terms *supination* and *adduction* (see below) are often used interchangeably with *inversion*.[21] The foot tends to dorsiflex slightly during inversion.
- *Eversion*: During eversion the sole of the foot is turned outward. The terms *pronation* and *abduction* have been used interchangeably with eversion.[21] The foot tends to plantar flex slightly during eversion.
- *Adduction*: By definition, *adduction* means movement of a part toward the axis or midline.[22] The term is most

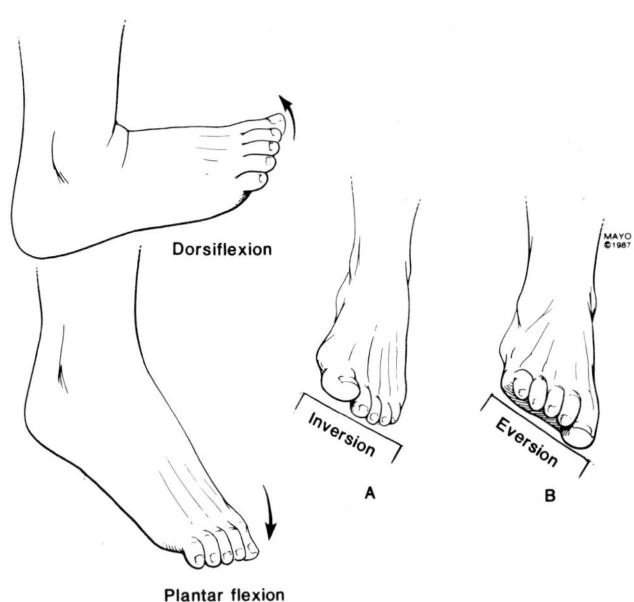

Fig. 8-11 Illustration of common positions of the foot. *Source:* Reprinted from *Radiology of the Foot and Ankle* by TH Berquist, Raven Press, 1989, © Mayo Foundation.

frequently used to describe forces acting on the foot or ankle. *Inversion* has been equated with *adduction* in the literature. The term *adduction* is preferred when describing forces applied to the foot and ankle.[13,19,21,31]

- *Abduction*: This term indicates motion of a given part away from the midline. Again, terms such as *eversion* have been used interchangeably with *abduction*; *abduction* is preferred when describing forces moving the foot or ankle outward.[13,19,21,31]
- *Supination and pronation*: Supination and pronation are commonly used for describing the rotation that occurs at the wrist.[21] Technically the foot is pronated when the sole is flat. Pronation can occur to a minimal degree with the forefoot abducted and dorsiflexed. Limited supination is possible. Typically the literature has used the terms *pronation* and *eversion,* and *supination* and *inversion,* interchangeably.[21–23] The terms *supination* and *pronation* should be reserved for the upper extremity. *Eversion* and *inversion* are less confusing when describing foot and ankle position.
- *External rotation*: This term is typically used to define outward rotation of the foot in relation to the longitudinal axis of the leg. With many athletic injuries the leg actually rotates medially with the foot fixed. Therefore, the foot then is actually rotated in an outward (external) position compared to the leg.[13,22,23]
- *Varus*: Varus indicates rotation, bending, or positioning inward or toward the midline axis. The term should be used to describe position, not motion.
- *Valgus*: Valgus is used to denote rotation, bending, or positioning away from the axis of the midline. Like *varus,* the term *valgus* denotes position.

SOFT TISSUE TRAUMA

Injuries affecting the soft tissues of the foot and ankle are common.[34,35,47,55] Cass and Morrey[47] reported an incidence of about 500 ankle sprains per year. Sprains in the foot occur less frequently.[57] Many injuries can be treated conservatively with satisfactory results. Proper imaging evaluation, however, is needed to determine the extent of injury so that chronic instability and function loss can be avoided.[40]

Ankle Ligament Injuries

The ligaments and other supporting structures of the ankle are discussed earlier in this chapter. Certain aspects of ankle anatomy bear repeating, however, to provide a complete discussion of ligamentous trauma.

The distal tibia and fibula are supported in their anatomic relationship by the distal anterior and posterior tibiofibular ligaments and the interosseous membrane (Fig. 8-12).[42,67,83] Other ligament structures maintain the ankle joint. Medially, the deltoid ligament is triangular and broadens as it extends from the medial malleolus to its talar and calcaneal insertions. The deltoid ligament is composed of an anterior and posterior superficial ligament and an intermediate deep or tibiotalar

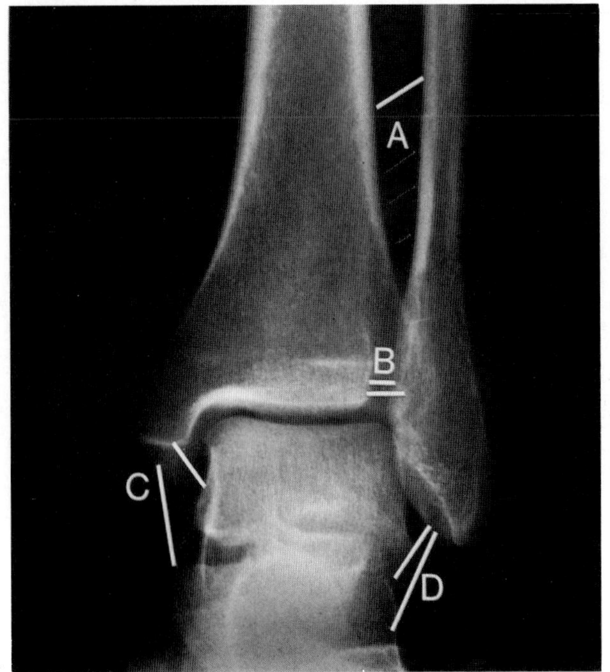

A

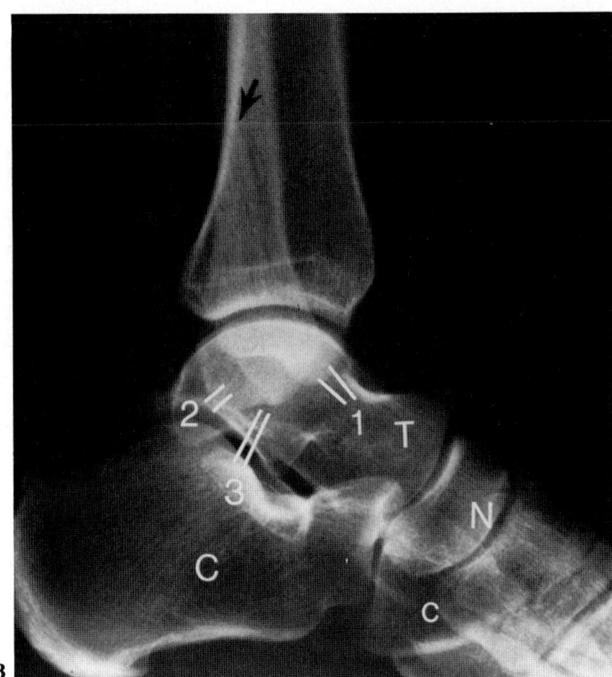

B

Fig. 8-12 (**A**) AP and (**B**) lateral radiographs of the ankle demonstrating ligamentous support. (**A**) A, interosseous membrane; B, distal tibiofibular ligament; C, deltoid ligament; D, calcaneofibular ligament. (**B**) 1–3, lateral ligament complex; C, calcaneus; c, cuboid; T, talus; N, navicular. Note the subtle fibular fracture (arrow).

ligament.[83] The latter ligament is essentially a triangular thickening with a medial capsule. There are three ligaments laterally (Fig. 8-12B). The anterior talofibular ligament extends from the anterior fibula to insert in the lateral talus just below the articular surface. With the ankle in a neutral position, this ligament is horizontally oriented and resists internal rotation. Recent studies also indicate that it is significant in resisting varus tilt, particularly with the ankle in plantar flexion. The posterior tibiofibular ligament extends from the posterior fibula to the posterior talus. The calcaneofibular ligament originates at the lateral malleolar tip and inserts on the calcaneus, restricting inversion. The calcaneofibular ligament supports both the ankle and the subtalar joints and is intimately associated with the peroneal tendon sheaths.[47,83]

Ankle sprains are most commonly due to inversion with adduction of the foot. The injury commonly occurs during sporting events or falls on uneven surfaces[45,47] (Fig. 8-13). Isolated rupture of the deltoid ligament (an eversion injury) is rare.[45] Clinically ankle sprains present with variable degrees of pain, swelling, and ecchymosis. In assessing ankle sprains it is important to classify the degree of injury so that proper treatment can be instituted and chronic instability avoided. Typically ankle sprains are divided into three grades.[42,47] Patients with grade 1 sprains present with mild stretching of the ligaments but no disruption or instability. These athletes can still ambulate and generally have mild swelling with pain and tenderness over the anterior talofibular ligament.[83] Grade 2 sprains are incomplete ligament tears. There is generally significant pain, marked swelling, and ecchymosis. Physical examination is difficult in this setting. Discomfort on palpation over the calcaneal fibular ligament is not uncommon. Grade 3 sprains are complete ligament tears. Both the anterior talofibular ligament and the calcaneofibular ligament may be involved, resulting in ankle instability.[47] The degree of swelling is variable, but there is usually tenderness over both the anterior talofibular and the calcaneofibular ligaments.[83]

Diagnosis of ligament disruption usually requires special studies. Routine ankle views (AP, lateral, and mortise) are not effective in differentiating the types of ankle sprains. Secondary signs, however, are important in determining which additional techniques may be most useful.[96] Patients with grade 1 sprains generally present with mild soft tissue swelling over the lateral malleolus. This can be identified on AP and mortise views. A bright light is frequently needed to evaluate the soft tissues. No fracture or effusion is evident on the lateral view. Grade 2 and 3 sprains have more significant swelling that can be identified clinically and on both AP and lateral radiographs. This finding has little value, however. Attempts at correlating ligament injury with the degree of swelling seen radiographically have been unsuccessful. The presence of an effusion in the joint is somewhat useful in that it generally indicates that the capsule is intact (Fig. 8-14). Effusions are best seen on the lateral view. Small avulsion fractures (grade IV sprain) can also be seen on plain films. Measuring the tibiotalar joint to differentiate second- and third-degree sprains is not usually helpful.[40,99] If the talus is shifted, however, resulting in asymmetry of the ankle mortise, a ligament injury is generally present (Fig. 8-15).

Stress views of the ankle are useful in diagnosing ligament disruption.[63,83] This technique requires adequate anesthesia of the involved joint, however, and is highly dependent upon the experience of the examiner. Comparison with the normal ankle under stress is also necessary. The ankles should be stressed in varus and valgus positions with the foot in neutral and plantar flexed positions. AP stress views (drawer sign) should also be obtained.

For best results the examination should be fluoroscopically guided to ensure proper positioning and monitoring. When performing varus and valgus stress tests, it is important to remember normal variations in ankle motion. Normal talar tilt ranges from 5° to 23°.[47,49,65,83] This problem is overcome by

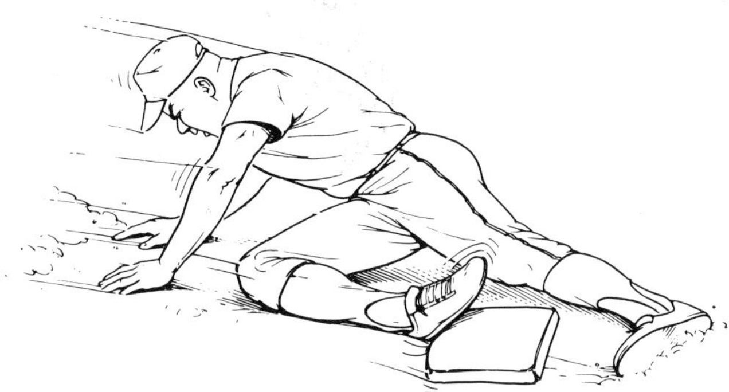

Fig. 8-13 Illustration of ankle injury during sliding into base.

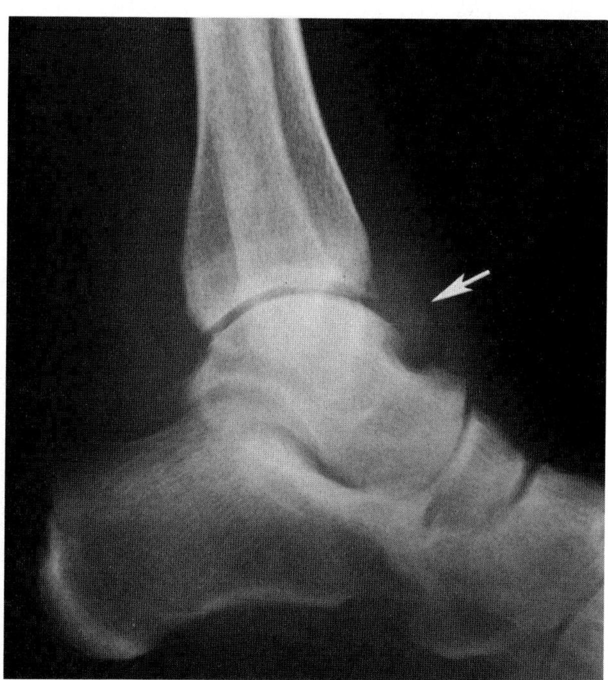

Fig. 8-14 Lateral view of the ankle demonstrating an effusion anteriorly (arrow).

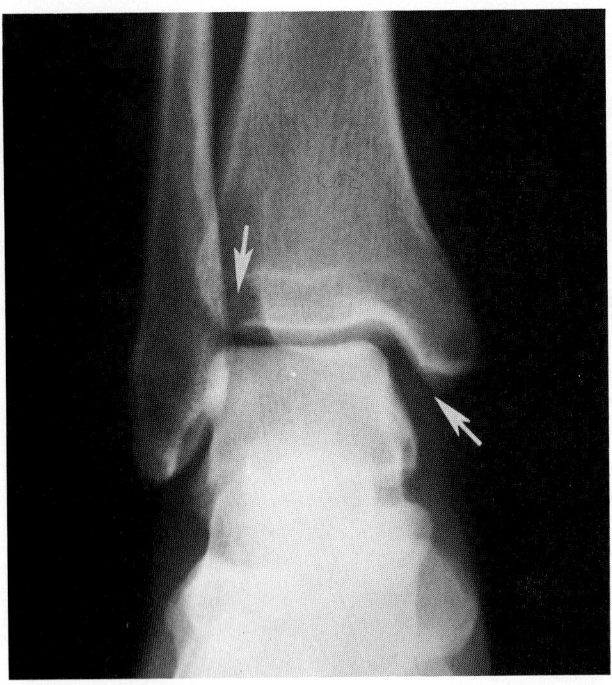

Fig. 8-15 AP view of the ankle demonstrating talar shift due to medial and distal tibiofibular ligament tears (arrows).

comparing the injured and uninjured sides. Measuring varus and valgus stress views can be accomplished by means of angle or distance measurements. With the angle technique a line is drawn along the talar dome and tibial plafond. The change in the angle with stress is measured, and both ankles are compared (Fig. 8-16). If the angle (talar tilt) of the injured ankle is about 10° greater than that of the normal side, it generally indicates that both the anterior talofibular and the calcaneofibular ligaments are torn.[47,62] These changes should be noted with the foot in both plantar flexed and neutral positions during stress. In neutral, if the angle is 6° greater than on the normal side, both ligaments are probably torn. If this only occurs in plantar flexed stress, it is likely that only the anterior talofibular ligament is torn.[62] It has been demonstrated experimentally that accuracy is best with 10° of plantar flexion and the leg internally rotated 25°.[73] The change in height from the talar dome to the plafond can also be measured. A difference of 3 mm between the normal and injured ankle indicates ligament disruption.[83] AP stress can be applied with several techniques. For consistency, we prefer the double-exposure technique with the foot plantar flexed 10°.[40,73,83] This allows the change in talar or tibial position to be measured easily on one film. A shift of greater than 2 or 3 mm between the injured and uninjured sides is considered significant.[83,103]

Stress views are less accurate compared to arthrography or tenography.[35,83,94,95] Sauser et al[94] studied 55 patients with stress views and arthrography within 72 hours of injury. They noted that stress views were accurate if talar tilt increased by 10° or more but that the test was only positive in 38% of patients with positive arthrograms.

Blanchard et al,[42] Black et al,[41] and Schweigel et al[95] reported significantly improved accuracy (approaching 96%) when stress tenography was used to evaluate the calcaneofibular ligament. The false-negative rate with conventional arthrography approaches 21%.[41,99] The ankle tenogram

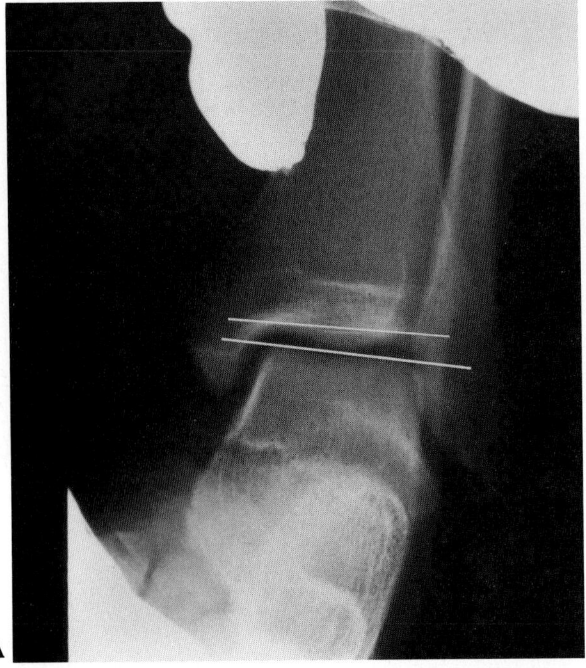

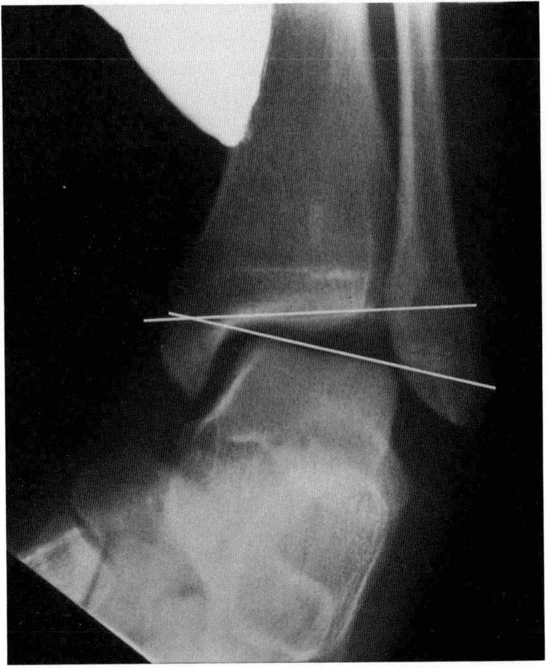

Fig. 8-16 Stress views (varus) of the normal ankle (**A**) and the injured ankle (**B**) demonstrating a lateral ligament tear.

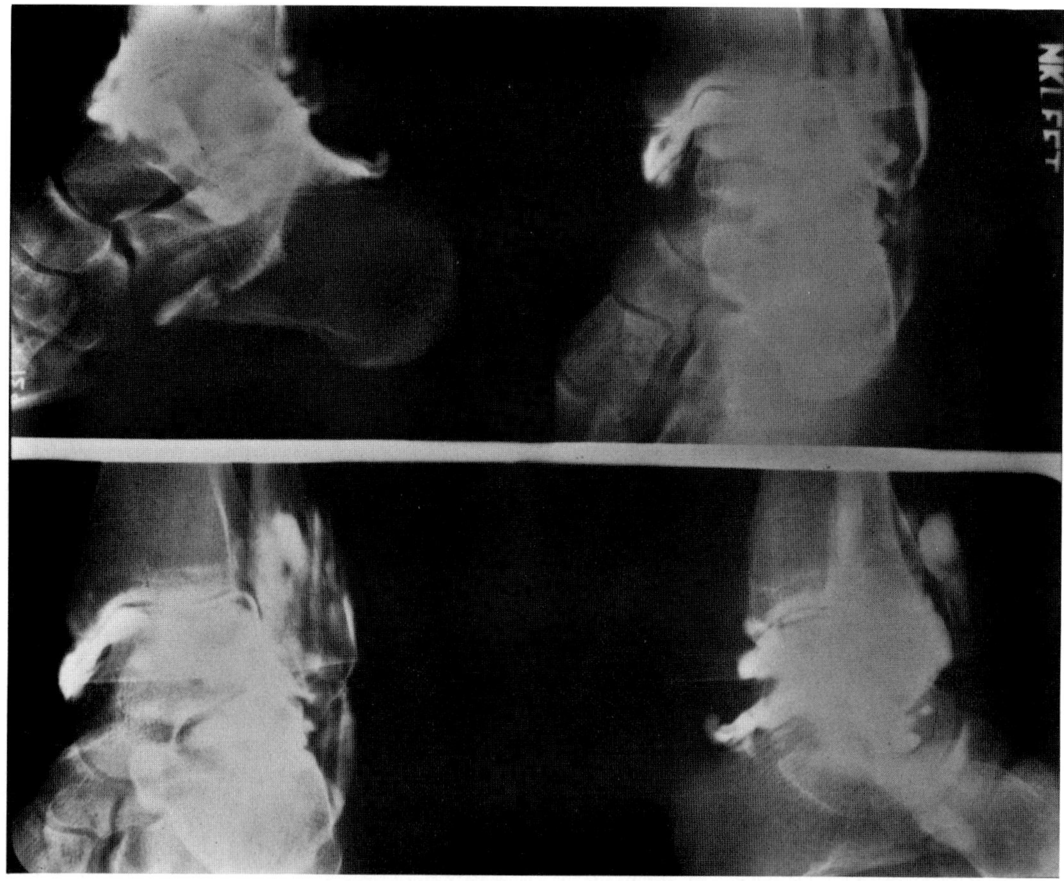

Fig. 8-17 Four views of the ankle after lateral tenography. Note that contrast medium fills the joint as a result of a lateral ligament tear.

is positive when contrast medium injected into the peroneal tendon sheath enters the joint space (Fig. 8-17). This decompresses the sheath, however, and can make it more difficult to demonstrate anterior talofibular ligament tears. This ligament and the deltoid ligaments are intimately associated with the capsule, so that ankle arthrography is more useful in demonstrating these ligament injuries (Fig. 8-18). Because stress views are most accurate after anesthetic injection, it would seem wise to combine arthrograms or tenograms with stress views to allow the most accurate assessment of the injury. Therefore, we recommend using one of these combinations in assessing ankle injury. This decision should be based on clinical findings and whether surgery or treatment modifications will be made as judged from the degree of ligament injury. Surgical intervention is a more important consideration in professional athletes or young active individuals. Generally, assessment of the calcaneofibular ligament is most crucial because conservative treatment is most often used if only the anterior talofibular ligament is torn. Therefore, a stress tenogram is the technique of choice.[41,42,56] Computed tomography (CT) and MRI are useful in evaluating the tendons around the ankle but, in our experience, are less effective in evaluating the capsule and ligaments.[39,54,77]

Ligament injuries also occur in the foot.[40] Gymnastics, long distance running, and aerobic activities are frequently

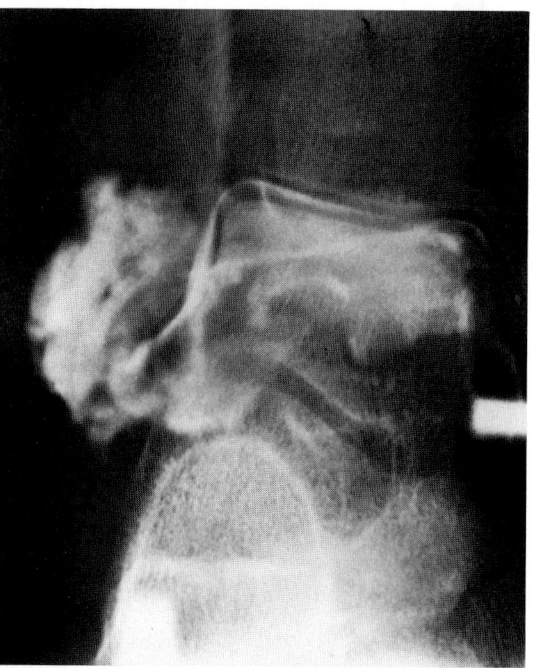

Fig. 8-18 AP view of the ankle after arthrography demonstrating extravasation of contrast medium laterally, but no filling of the peroneal tendon sheaths, due to an anterior talofibular ligament tear.

implicated.[57] Inversion injuries, which may mimic typical ankle sprains, may affect the bifurcate ligament, which extends between the calcaneus and cuboid.[57] Other midtarsal ligaments are also stressed in gymnasts and dancers (ballet). Diagnosis of these conditions may be difficult clinically.[80]

Cuboid subluxation may be particularly difficult to diagnose. The athlete typically presents with lateral midfoot pain and is unable to run, cut, or jump. Pain or point tenderness may be noted on plantar pressure over the cuboid.[80]

Sinus tarsi syndrome is commonly associated with inversion injuries of the foot and ankle sprains. The talocalcaneal interosseous ligament carries the hindfoot nerve fibers, and even minor injury may cause significant pain. On physical examination there is point tenderness over the lateral aspect of the sinus tarsi.[46,57,87]

Middle-aged joggers commonly develop subluxation of the metatarsophalangeal joint, specifically the second joint.[76] Patients present with metatarsal pain and often have claw toe deformities.[76]

Imaging of ligament injuries of the foot is difficult. Routine radiographs, CT, or conventional tomography may be useful to identify subtle associated avulsion fractures.[40] MRI is useful in specific situations.[39] Diagnostic and therapeutic injections, however, are most useful in localizing the pain and confirming the clinical diagnosis. Fluoroscopically monitored injections can be accomplished in all articulations. A mixture of bupivacaine and betamethasone (1:1 ratio) is injected after confirming needle position with a small amount of contrast medium.[40]

Tendon Injuries

Thirteen tendons cross the ankle.[67] These tendons include the peroneus brevis and longus laterally; the Achilles tendon posteriorly; the tibialis posterior, flexor digitorum longus, and flexor hallucis longus medially; and the tibialis anterior, extensor hallucis longus, extensor digitorum longus, and peroneus tertius anteriorly. All tendons are enclosed in sheaths with the exception of the Achilles tendon (Fig. 8-19). Tendon injury may occur as an isolated event, in association with a fracture, or as a result of previous fracture with degenerative joint disease. Tendons may also rupture in patients on steriod therapy (systemic or direct injection) or with chronic inflammatory diseases.[40,61,78,91]

Peroneal Tendons

The peroneal muscles assist in pronation and eversion of the foot (Fig. 8-8).[67,91] The peroneus brevis tendon is anterior to the peroneus longus as they pass posterior to the lateral malleolus (Fig. 8-19C). In about 80% of patients there is a notch (variable in size) in the fibula that accommodates a portion of the peroneus brevis. In 20% of patients this notch is shallow or

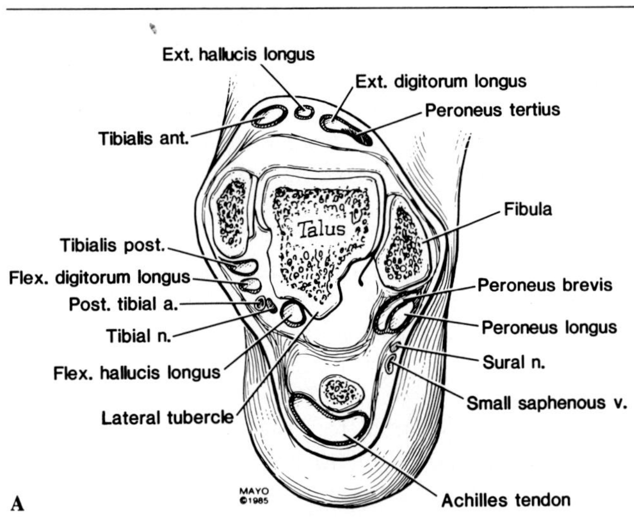

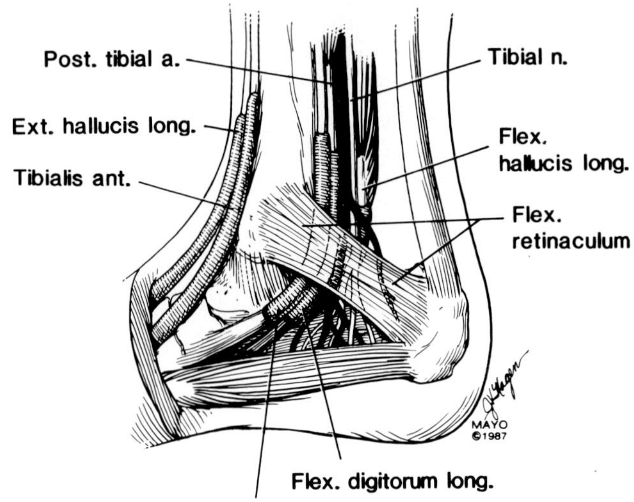

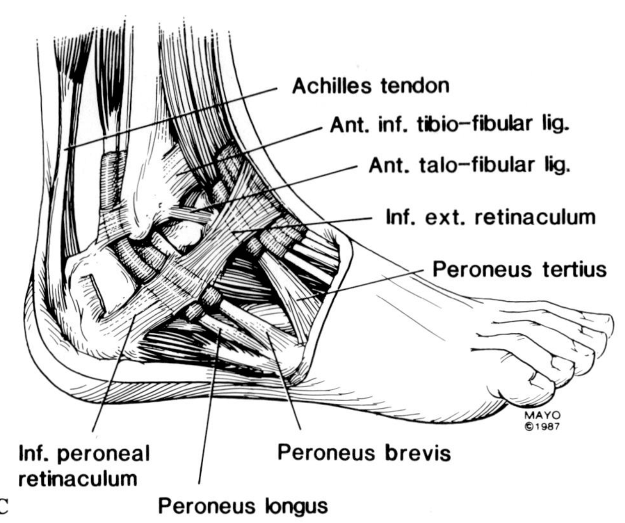

Fig. 8-19 Illustration of the tendons about the ankle seen in the axial (**A**), medial (**B**), and lateral (**C**) projections. *Source:* Reprinted from *Radiology of the Foot and Ankle* by TH Berquist, Raven Press, 1989, © Mayo Foundation.

absent, which may lead to recurrent subluxation.[67,91] The tendons also pass through the superior and inferior peroneal retinacula (Fig. 8-18). It is between these two structures that they are immediately adjacent to the calcaneofibular ligament.[67] The peroneal tendons share a common sheath to the inferior margin of the superior peroneal retinaculum. At this point the sheath of the peroneus longus separates from that of the peroneus brevis. The peroneus longus progresses inferior to the peroneal tubercle of the calcaneus to the plantar aspect of the foot, where it inserts in the base of the first metatarsal and medial cuneiform. The peroneus brevis passes inferiorly, inserting on the base of the fifth metatarsal.[40,61] Evaluation of the tendons and normal osseous sulci is easily accomplished with MRI or CT.[39,94,101]

Dislocation. Diagnosis of peroneal tendon injury first requires that the problem be considered. Many patients present with a sprained ankle or repeated giving-way, and dislocation of the peroneal tendons is not considered (Table 8-1).[34,82] The mechanism of injury is not clear, but dislocation is probably due to an inversion-dorsiflexion or abduction-dorsiflexion injury. Patients present with pain and swelling over the posterosuperior aspect of the lateral malleolus.

Swelling may make actual palpation of the tendon difficult, and pain with motion can limit the detection of subluxation on physical examination. Routine radiographs will demonstrate soft tissue swelling laterally, but the distribution is not characteristic or different from that of an inversion sprain. A characteristic longitudinal flake fracture along the distal fibular metaphysis is useful when present.[84] This is best seen on the internal oblique view.[67] Murr[85] reported this finding in 15% to 50% of peroneal tendon dislocations. Usually other imaging procedures are more useful. CT, MRI, or tenography should be considered to confirm the diagnosis. CT provides excellent bone detail and is useful in assessing the peroneal notch in the fibula.[91,92] The tendons are less well demonstrated with CT than with MRI.[39] Subtle tears or complete disruptions are more easily seen on MRI, where the tendons are normally of low signal intensity (black) compared to the high intensity seen in the tendon that has torn. These noninvasive techniques do have disadvantages. For example, if the tendons have returned to normal position or are only slightly displaced, fluoroscopic observation after tenography may be more useful in demonstrating subluxation. This may also be possible to demonstrate with new fast-scan (gradient-echo) MR techniques.[39,40]

Table 8-1 Ankle Sprains: Differential Diagnosis[47,48,52,67]

- Fractures
  - Talus
    - Neck
    - Dome
    - Lateral process
    - Posterior process
  - Calcaneus (anterior process)
  - Cuboid
  - Malleolar fractures or avulsions
  - Fifth metatarsal base
- Soft tissue injuries
  - Peroneal tendon
    - Subluxation
    - Dislocation
  - Subtalar subluxation or dislocation
  - Deltoid ligament ruptures
  - Talonavicular subluxation or dislocation

Rupture of the peroneal tendon. Rupture of the peroneal tendons is not common. The lesion may be overlooked as a cause of ankle instability, however, and therefore the true incidence is not known.[34] Patients may present acutely with an ankle sprain or have symptoms of chronic instability. Cavovarus foot and compartment syndromes have also been reported with peroneal tendon rupture.[44,51,52] When the tendons are torn, the patient will be unable effectively to evert the foot.[34,67]

Routine radiographs are usually not useful. Displacement of the os peroneum, however, may indicate peroneal rupture.[102] Tenography may demonstrate the site of the tear, but because this technique outlines the tendon and does not provide direct assessment it is less useful than MRI. Both CT and MRI have been described as useful techniques for evaluating the peroneal tendons.[38,91,101] MRI has superior soft tissue contrast and can define incomplete, complete, and chronic inflammatory changes in both the tendon and the sheath (Figs. 8-20 and 8-21). If a complete tear is present, the tendon ends can be defined as well as the absence of the tendon in its sheath in the torn region. If a partial tear has occurred there will be increased signal intensity in the tendon due to blood and fluid. These findings are most easily demonstrated on T2-weighted (SE 2000/60) or gradient-echo T2* sequences. The contrast of the blood and fluid compared to the normally low-intensity (black) tendon is most striking with these sequences. In patients with old tears the tendon will look thickened with areas of intermediate intensity (gray on the MR image), and there is often fluid in the tendon sheath. The latter is not seen in normal patients (Table 8-2).

Achilles Tendon

The Achilles tendon is the largest and strongest tendon in the foot and ankle. The tendon originates where the gastrocnemius and soleus tendons join and inserts on the posterior calcaneus. In its axial presentation the tendon thickens distally, becoming elliptical with concave anterior and convex posterior surfaces (Fig. 8-19). Approximately 2 to 6 cm above its calcaneal insertion, the fibers in the tendon cross. The posterior fibers course medial to lateral, and the anterior fibers lateral to medial, before inserting in the calcaneus. Most tendon tears occur just above this, perhaps partially because of

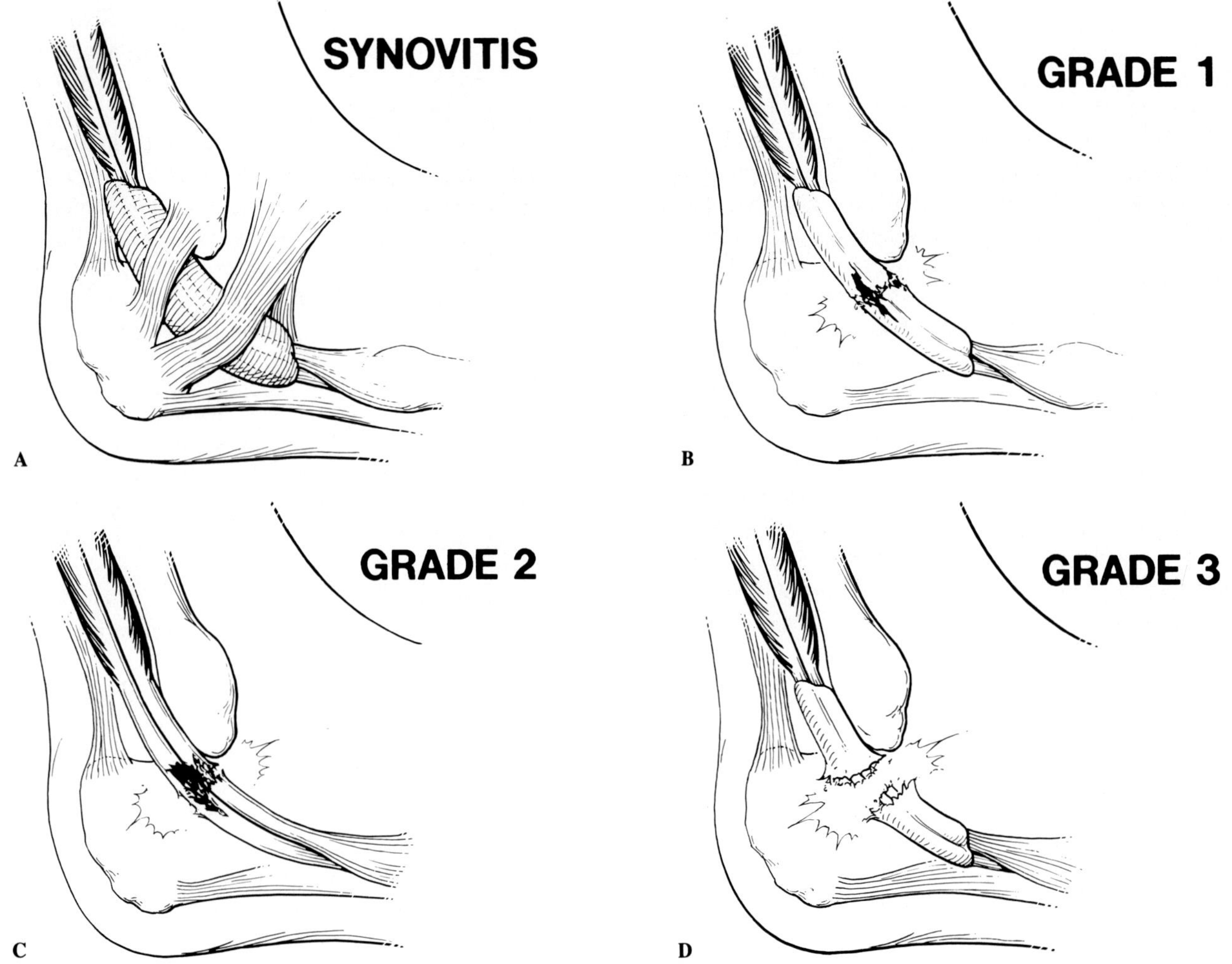

Fig. 8-20 Illustration of peroneal tendon injuries. The same features can be applied to other tendons about the ankle. (**A**) Synovitis. (**B**) Grade 1 injury, few fibers torn. (**C**) Grade 2 injury, partial tear (≤50% of fibers). (**D**) Grade 3 injury, complete tear.

the reduced blood supply in this region. The Achilles tendon does not have a true tendon sheath.[39,64,67]

Acute and chronic inflammation of the Achilles tendon is common in runners. Up to 11% of runners develop Achilles tendinitis.[97] Inflammation is usually due to errors in training (running up hills or wearing hard-soled shoes).[36] The injury is also common in racquet sports and most commonly occurs in 30- to 50-year-old men.[74]

The Achilles tendon, although strong, is commonly torn. Fifty-nine percent of ruptures are related to sports injuries.[66,77] Ruptures are usually the result of indirect trauma. The injury can occur during athletic activity at any age. It usually ocurs in strenuous activities with frequent plantar flexion during raising up on the toes or with pushing off or jumping with the knee extended. Falling or landing on the forefoot, which leads to abrupt dorsiflexion of the foot, can also lead to Achilles rupture. Certain systemic and local conditions predispose to tendon disruption. Gout, systemic lupus erythematosus, rheumatoid arthritis, hyperparathyroidism, chronic renal failure, steroids, and diabetes have all been implicated.[70,86]

Clinically, patients present with pain, local swelling, and inability to raise up on their toes on the affected side.[67] If the tendon is completely torn, a defect may be palpable on physical examination. Clinical examination is not always accurate, however. The exact nature of the injury can be misdiagnosed in more than 25% of patients.[74] This is because a gap in the tendon may not be palpable (especially in incomplete tears) and because the patient may be able to plantar flex the foot with the toe flexors. Differentiation of Achilles tears from gastrocnemius or plantaris tears may also be difficult.[40] The Thompson test may be useful. This test is performed by squeezing the gastrocnemius muscle belly. If the Achilles tendon is intact, the foot will plantar flex during the maneuver (positive response). If the tendon is torn, the foot will not respond (negative response).[40,67]

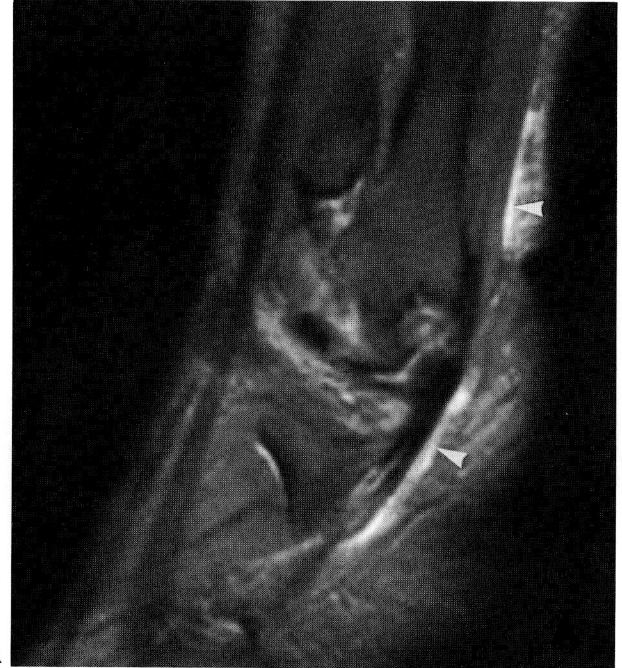

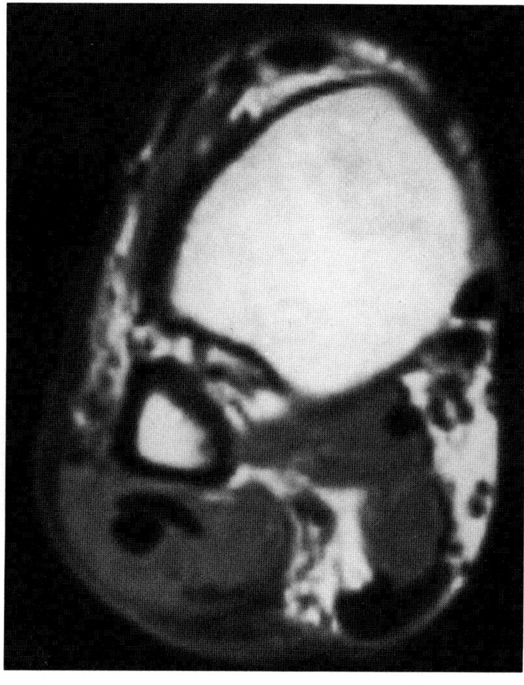

Fig. 8-21 Peroneal tendon injuries. (**A**) Sagittal (SE 2000/80) magnetic resonance (MR) image demonstrating synovitis (arrowheads) with intact tendons. (**B**) Axial (SE 500/20) MR image demonstrating extensive synovitis in a patient with subluxing peroneal tendons.

In addition to ruptures, Achilles tendinitis is one of the most common overuse syndromes. Because there is no tendon sheath, the peritenon becomes inflamed.[71,93] Inflammation is frequently related to footware (rigid sole) and a pronated heel and is seen in runners who use hilly terrain.[93]

Imaging of Achilles tendon pathology can be accomplished with several modalities. Routine radiographs are usually nonspecific. Newmark et al,[86] however, described fracture of a calcaneal osteophyte in association with Achilles tendon avulsion. Low-kilovoltage radiography and Xerox techniques may demonstrate swelling, thickening of the tendon, and irregularity of the pre-Achilles fat or Kager's triangle.[40] These findings are best seen on the lateral view. Ultrasound can also be effective in elucidating the architecture of the tendon.[43,58,72] This requires experience on the part of the examiner and interpreter. Ultrasound images can be difficult to interpret by those who do not routinely use the technique (Fig. 8-22).

Table 8-2 Ligament and Tendon Injuries: MR Features

Injury	*MR Features*
Acute complete disruption	T2-Weighted (SE 2000/60); tendon ends separated, high signal intensity between tendon ends and in sheaths; tendon ends may be thickened
Acute partial disruption	Tendon not separated; high signal for a portion of width of tendon; high signal in tendon sheath; tendon usually thickened in area of tear
Chronic disruption	Tendon thickened or separated and thickened; slightly increased intensity in area of tear; high signal in tendon sheath
Inflammation	High signal in tendon sheath; tendon may appear normal; thickened tendon or ligament with normal intensity (chronic)

CT and MRI, although more expensive than the techniques mentioned above, provide more information about the tendon and surrounding structures. MRI is particularly useful because of its superior soft tissue contrast and ability to image in the axial, sagittal, coronal, and off-axis oblique planes.[40,50,68] At the Mayo Clinic, we find MRI to be useful in detecting complete, incomplete (Fig. 8-23), and old Achilles injuries (Table 8-2) as well as in evaluating bursitis and other causes of Achilles tendon pathology.[39] The extent of involvement can be assessed accurately with MRI. In addition, patients can be followed to determine whether healing is progressing normally or whether operative intervention is necessary.[39]

Another uncommon problem may mimic an Achilles injury or soft tissue tumor. This situation is created by the presence of an accessory soleus muscle (Fig. 8-24).[90] It is not uncommon for patients with this anomaly to experience pain after exercise.[53] Either CT or MRI can easily diagnose the condition, but MRI can more easily distinguish the accessory soleus muscle from a soft tissue tumor or hematoma.

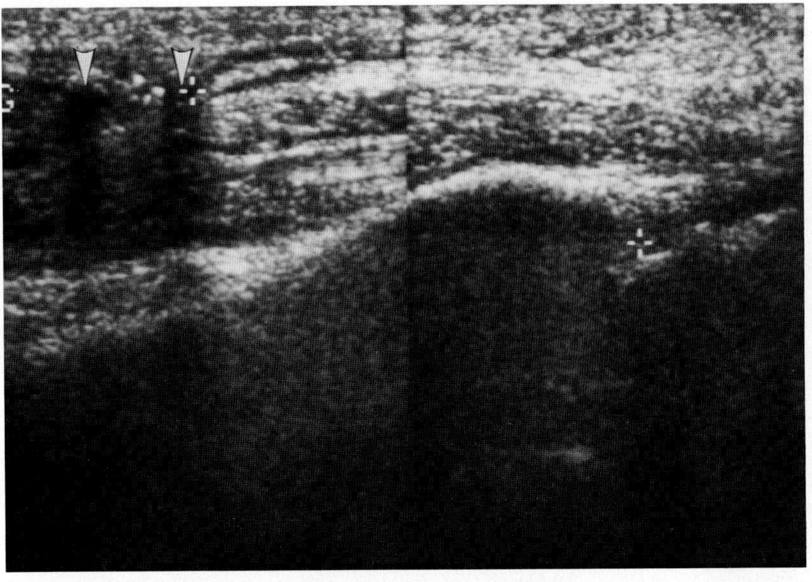
A

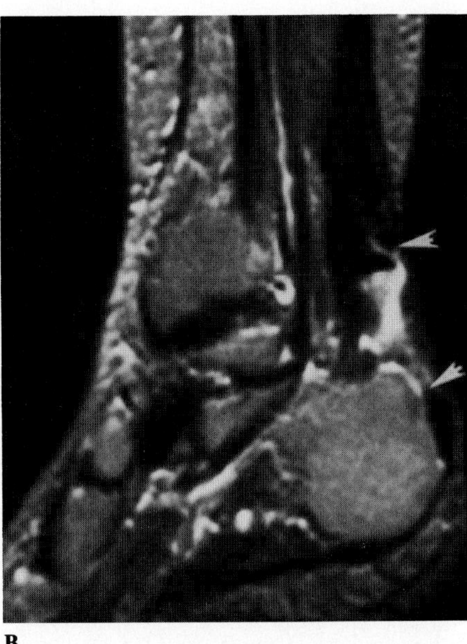
B

Fig. 8-22 (**A**) Ultrasound of the Achilles tendon in the longitudinal plane demonstrating a defect at the plus sign with calcifications proximally (arrowheads). (**B**) MR image of the same patient shows the defect (arrows) and calcifications proximally.

Medial Tendons

The posterior tibial, flexor digitorum longus, and flexor hallucis longus tendons make up the medial tendon group and are located anterior to posterior in the above order (Fig. 8-19). The posterior tibial tendon (most anterior) with its tendon sheath passes just posterior to the medial malleolus and lateral to the flexor retinaculum and broadens at its insertion in the navicular tuberosity and base of the medial cuneiform. The flexor digitorum longus takes a similar course proximally, lying between the posterior tibial tendon and the posterior tibial artery (Fig. 8-19). As it turns toward the plantar aspect of the foot, it passes superficially to the flexor hallucis longus before dividing into tendon slips that insert in the bases of the second to fifth distal phalanges. The flexor hallucis longus tendon is located more posteriorly and laterally. It passes through a fibroosseous tunnel beneath the sustentaculum tali and along the medial plantar aspect of the foot to insert in the base of the distal phalanx of the great toe.[59–61,67]

Acute rupture of the deltoid ligament is not common.[44] Similarly, the posterior tibial, flexor digitorum longus, and flexor hallucis longus tendons are rarely torn after acute trauma.[60,67,100] Dezwart and Davidson[52] have reported posterior tibial tendon rupture in association with bimalleolar fracture.

The posterior tibial tendon is the most commonly injured of the three medial tendons. Injury typically occurs during the pronation phase in running or with rapid changes in direction in basketball, soccer, football, and tennis. Patients present with pain, local tenderness, and swelling, and physical examination may reveal a nonpalpable tendon.[67] Rupture of the

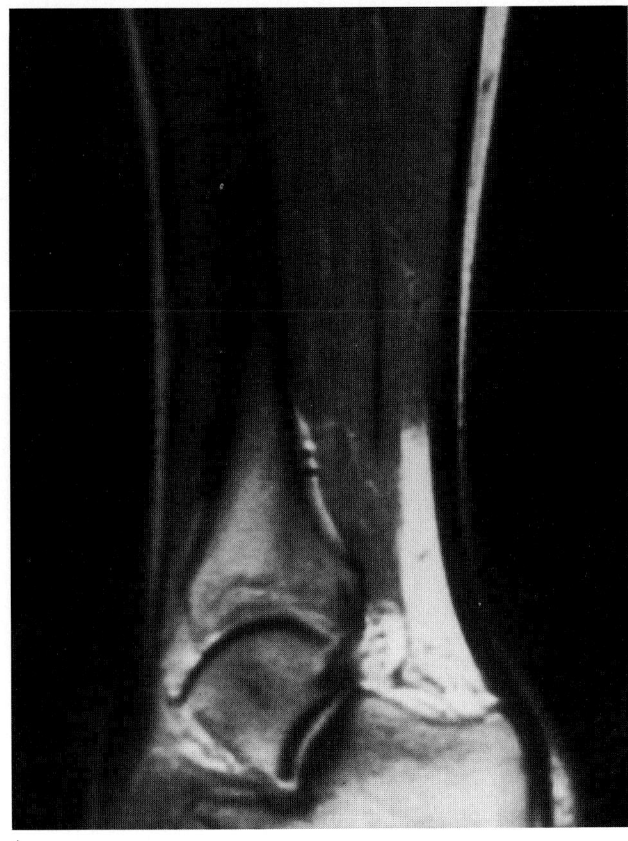
A

Fig. 8-23 Achilles tendon injuries. (**A**) Normal sagittal MR image of the Achilles tendon.

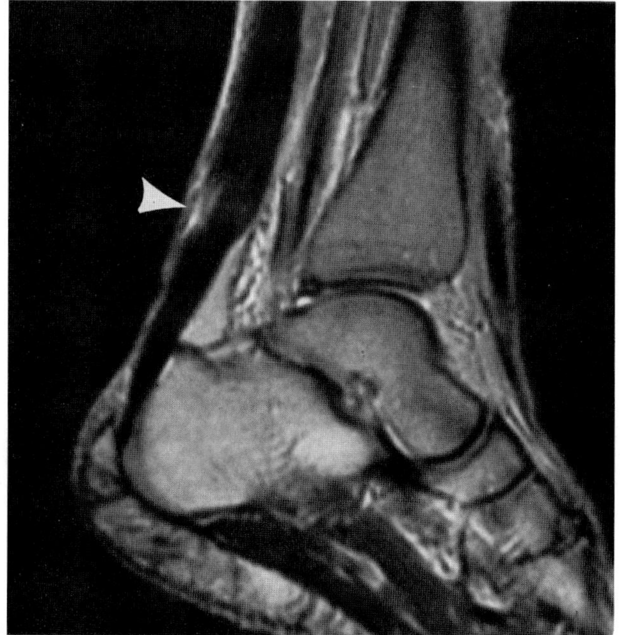

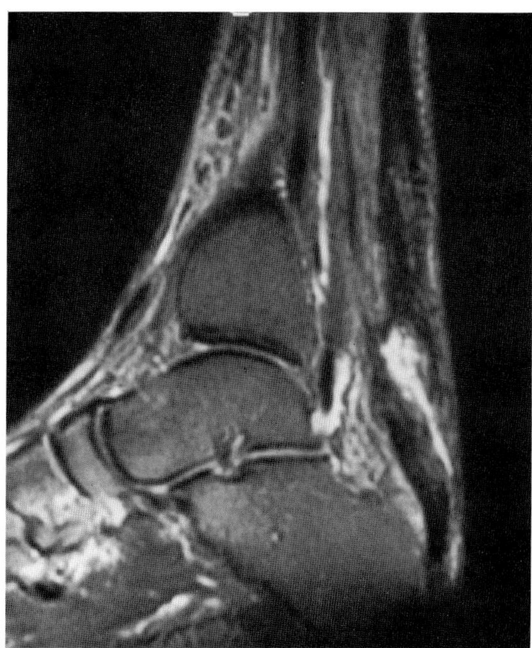

Fig. 8-23 contd (B) Sagittal T2-weighted MR image (SE 2000/60) demonstrating a low-grade (first-degree) tear (arrowhead) with associated tendon thickening. **(C)** Sagittal T2-weighted MR image (SE 2000/80) demonstrating complete disruption of the Achilles tendon.

posterior tibial tendon can lead to progressive flatfoot deformity, inability to raise up on the toes, and weakness on inversion of the foot.[59,78]

Routine radiography is usually of little value in patients with medial tendon injuries. Acute traumatic rupture of the posterior tibial tendon has been described in association with medial malleolar fractures.[52] The fracture is a mirror image of the flake fracture seen with peroneal tendon dislocation. It occurs longitudinally along the distal medial tibial metaphysis.[100] Posterior tibial tendon rupture may present with an increased talocalcaneal angle on the AP and lateral view.[59] These findings, along with soft tissue swelling, are the only plain film findings that might suggest the diagnosis. In patients with chronic disease and inflammation, the stress tenogram may show changes in the posterior tibial or adjacent tendon sheaths.[61,83] The structure of the tendon is better demonstrated with CT or MRI, however. In our experience MRI has been most useful in assessing the nature and degree of posterior tibial tendon pathology (Fig. 8-25 and Table 8-2).

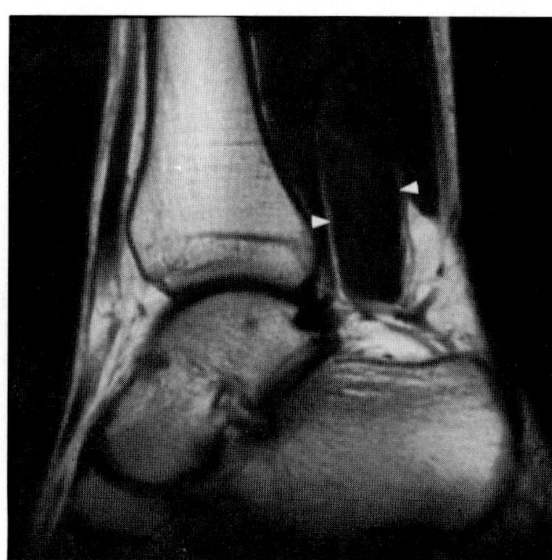

Fig. 8-24 Sagittal T1-weighted MR image (SE 500/20) demonstrating an accessory soleus muscle (arrowheads).

Rupture of the flexor digitorum and flexor hallucis longus tendons occurs less frequently but can present with similar clinical findings. Garth[60] reported rupture of the flexor hallucis longus in ballet dancers and soccer players. Patients presented with swelling, tenderness, and crepitation near the sustentaculum tali. Symptoms were increased with flexion and extension of the great toe.

Tenography of the flexor hallucis longus is tedious because of the difficulty in localizing the tendon with the needle tip. Therefore, MRI or CT is more useful.[39,40]

Anterior Tendons

Anteriorly the anterior tibial, extensor hallucis longus, and extensor digitorum longus tendons are all enclosed in tendon sheaths (Figs. 8-9 and 8-19). Acute tears are unusual, but in patients with previous fractures, degenerative arthritis, or other predisposing factors tendon rupture can occur.[61,67] Chronic inflammation or more significant involvement of the anterior tibial tendon is not uncommon in runners. Rupture of the anterior tibial tendon usually occurs as it exits the superior retinaculum. The distal segment retracts and can be palpated

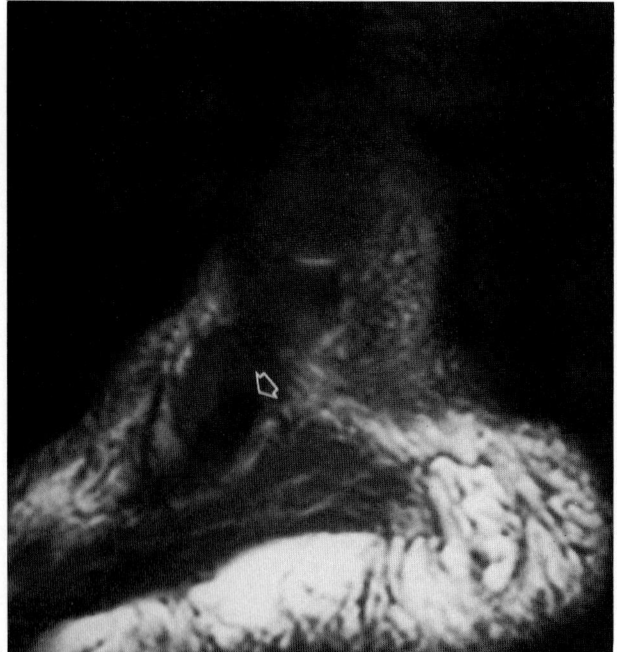

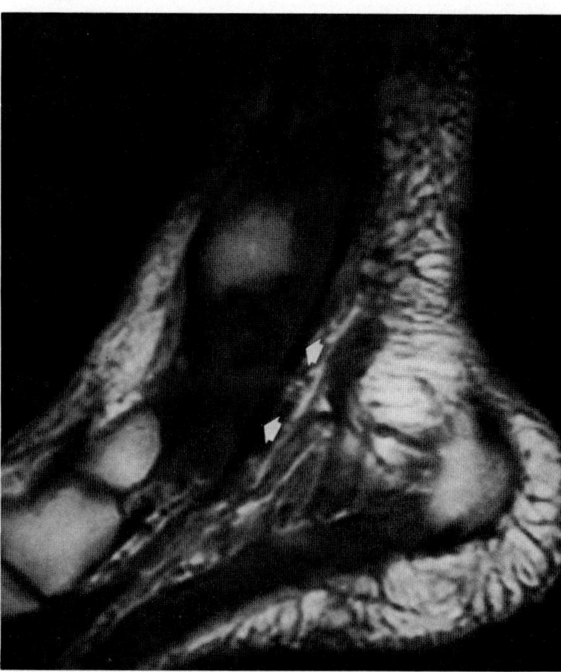

Fig. 8-25 Sagittal T1-weighted MR images (SE 500/20) demonstrating the torn end (open arrow in **A**) of the posterior tibial tendon and the adjacent flexor digitorum longus (closed arrows in **B**).

between the superior and inferior retinacula. Clinically there is pain and swelling over the ankle anteriorly. There may also be decreased dorsiflexion of the foot on physical examination.

Radiographically patients will demonstrate minimal to prominent soft tissue swelling anteriorly. This is most easily identified on the lateral and oblique views. Tenography will demonstrate abnormalities in the tendon sheaths, but more specific information can be obtained with MRI. Examinations should be performed in the axial and sagittal planes. T2-weighted sequences are generally best because the high intensity of fluid and blood provides excellent contrast with the black tendon (Fig. 8-26). Conservative treatment is adequate in older, less active patients. Surgical repair is indicated in active patients.[67]

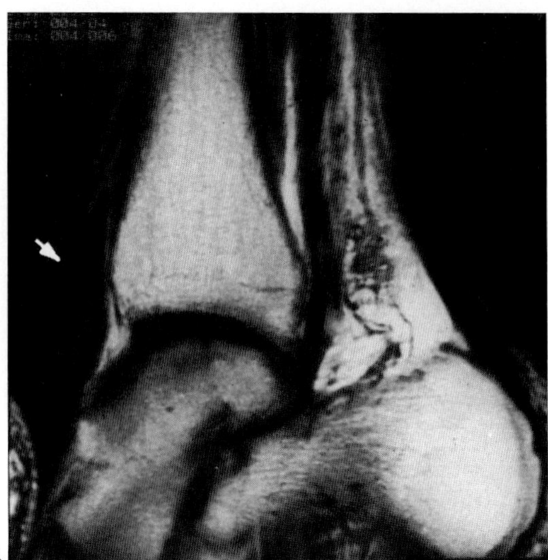

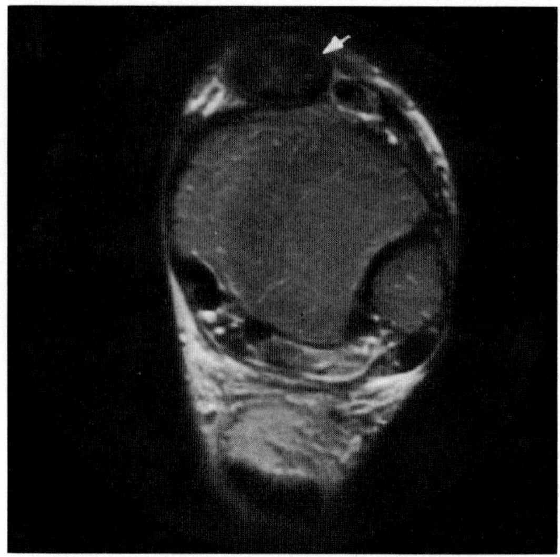

Fig. 8-26 Anterior tibial tendon injury. (**A**) Sagittal T-1 weighted MR image (SE 500/20) and (**B**) axial T2-weighted MR image (SE 2000/60) demonstrating a second-degree tear (arrows).

Table 8-3 Hindfoot Pain

Plantar
- Plantar fasciitis
- Nerve entrapment

Posterior
- Retrocalcaneal bursitis
- Achilles tendon inflammation or rupture
- Cavus foot

Lateral
- Peroneal tendinitis, subluxation, or rupture
- Nerve entrapment

Medial
- Tendinitis or rupture
- Tarsal tunnel syndrome
- Retinacular inflammation

Hindfoot Pain

Hindfoot and/or heel pain is common in athletes. For purposes of discussion, it is useful to consider four different areas (Table 8-3): plantar, posterior, lateral, and medial.[37,40]

Plantar Pain

The most common problem resulting in plantar pain is fasciitis.[75,104] The condition is noted in 7% of runners. In the acute phase there is more focal pain at the medial calcaneal attachment, but with prolonged symptoms the pain and area of tenderness on physical examination become more diffuse. The condition is more common with cavus foot or excessive pronation.[40,80]

Routine radiography may demonstrate distortion of soft tissue planes or periostitis (Fig. 8-27). These changes are most easily appreciated on the lateral view. Although radionuclide scans may be useful, MRI is most effective for differentiation of inflammation from ruptures of the plantar fascia (Fig. 8-28).[38,39]

Medial calcaneal nerve entrapment may also lead to plantar pain. The condition is most often noted in runners, and some investigators postulate the syndrome is caused by inflammation of the nerve as it passes through the abductor hallucis.[40] MRI is the most useful modality for evaluating plantar pain. Coronal and sagittal T2-weighted images (Fig. 8-28) are most effective.

Posterior Pain

Posterior heel pain may be related to Achilles tendon injury or inflammation or bursitis.[36,69] The first two were discussed previously. Retrocalcaneal bursitis is an inflammation of the bursa located between the Achilles and posterosuperior calcaneus (Fig. 8-29).[40] Patients with increased calcaneal inclination (Fowler-Phillip angle) or cavus foot are more likely to be affected.

Routine radiographs may demonstrate changes in the pre-Achilles fat. MRI will demonstrate a high-signal fluid collection on T2-weighted images. In some cases injections, performed fluoroscopically, are useful for confirming the diagnosis and treating the condition.[40]

Lateral Pain

Lateral heel pain occurs infrequently. Peroneal tendon injury, described above, and sural nerve entrapment should be considered in this setting. Nerve entrapment may be caused by tendon sheath ganglia or avulsion fractures that cause entrapment of the nerve, which runs posterior to the peroneal tendons.[40] MRI in the axial and sagittal planes is most useful for imaging this region.

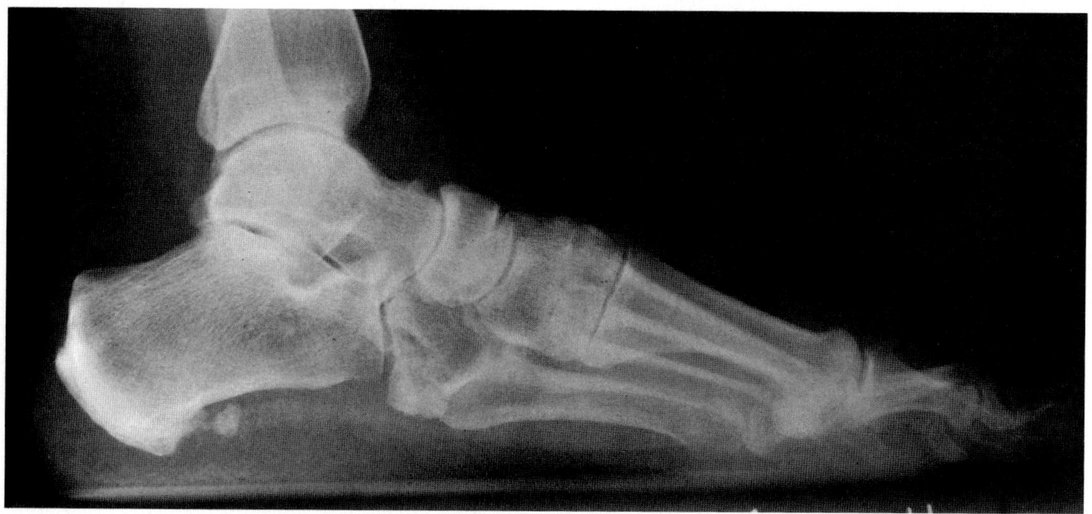

Fig. 8-27 Lateral radiograph demonstrating plantar spur avulsion in a runner.

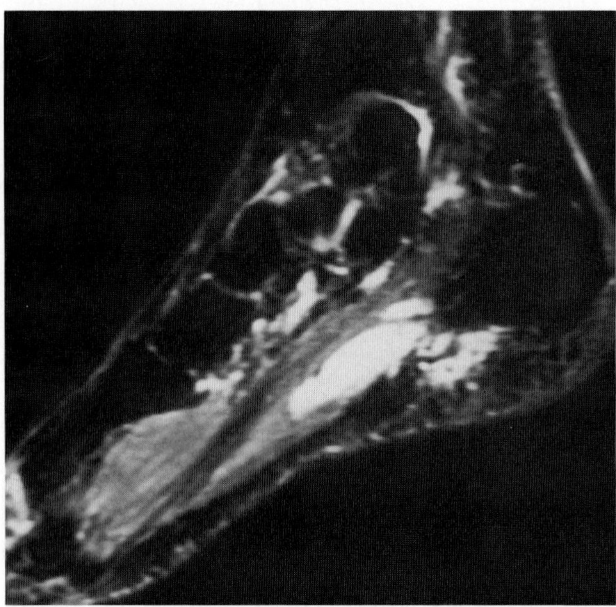

Fig. 8-28 Sagittal gradient-echo MR image demonstrating irregular increased signal intensity due to plantar fascia tear.

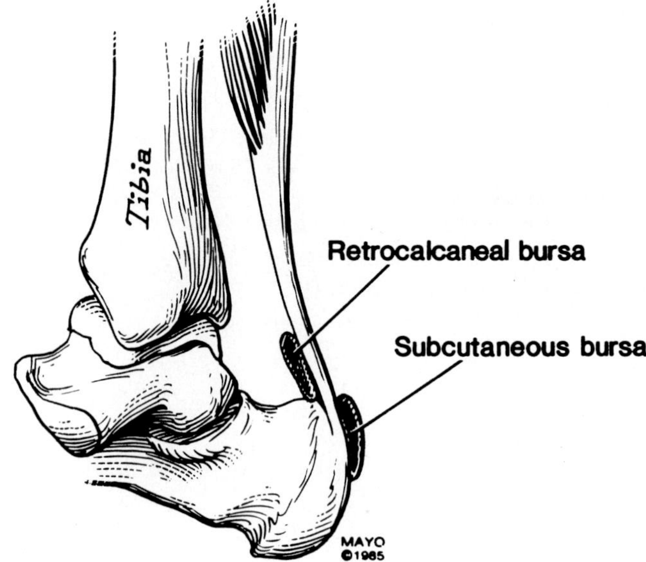

Fig. 8-29 Illustration of the retrocalcaneal bursa. *Source:* Reprinted from *Magnetic Resonance Imaging of the Musculoskeletal System* by TH Berquist, 1990, © Mayo Foundation.

Medial Pain

Medial tendon injuries were described previously. Tarsal tunnel syndrome is caused by irritation of the tibial nerve as it passes beneath the flexor retinaculum (Fig. 8-19B). Chronic trauma due to recurrent sprains and fractures or fracture-dislocations may lead to tarsal tunnel syndrome.[40,79,93]

Patients typically present with burning pain medially or heel paresthesia. Symptoms increase with weight bearing.[40] MRI is most useful for evaluation of this and other medial hindfoot syndromes. Axial and sagittal T2-weighted images are most useful in this regard.[39]

Forefoot Pain

Forefoot pain is a common problem in athletes (Table 8-4).[76] Those conditions responsible for these symptoms, excluding fractures, are reviewed below.

- *Metatarsalgia*: Metatarsal pain may be due to a long second metatarsal and a hypermobile first metatarsal.[76,81] This localized form of forefoot pain usually correlates with a metatarsal pad insert. More generalized metatarsal pain is evident in athletes with a tight Achilles tendon or anterior ankle impingement.[81] Surgical correction may be required in the latter.[40]
- *Sesamoiditis*: Sesamoid pain syndromes are common in runners.[88] The medial and lateral hallux sesamoids lie in the medial and lateral slips of the flexor hallucis brevis. Their function is to elevate the first metatarsal head to disperse impact forces, to protect the flexor hallucis tendon, and to increase the mechanical advantage of the flexor hallucis brevis tendon.[40,75] The sesamoids may become inflamed or fractured or may undergo osteonecrosis (Fig. 8-30).[40,84] Patients with simple sesamoiditis usually respond to rest and longitudinal arch support. For those who do not respond, more significant injury must be excluded.
- *Osteochondritis*: Forefoot pain in athletes may also be due to osteonecrosis of the metatarsal head. The second metatarsal head is most commonly involved (Fig. 8-31). Women are affected more frequently than men.[40,89]
- *Metatarsophalangeal subluxation and synovitis*: Synovitis and/or subluxation of the metatarsophalangeal joints result in local tenderness, swelling, and pain with passive flexion.[98] Synovitis is common in football players, especially those playing on artificial surfaces. The

Table 8-4 Forefoot Pain: Differential Diagnosis

Metatarsalgia
Sesamoiditis
Osteochondritis
Metatarsophalangeal subluxation and synovitis
Hallux rigidus
Neuromas
Turf toe
Stress fractures

Sources: Lillich JS and Baxter DE, *Foot and Ankle* (1986;7:145–151) American Orthopaedic Foot and Ankle Society Inc; Marshall P, *Clinics in Podiatric Medicine and Surgery* (1989;6:639–655) WB Saunders; Smith RW and Reischl SF, *Clinics in Sports Medicine* (1988;7:75–88) WB Saunders.

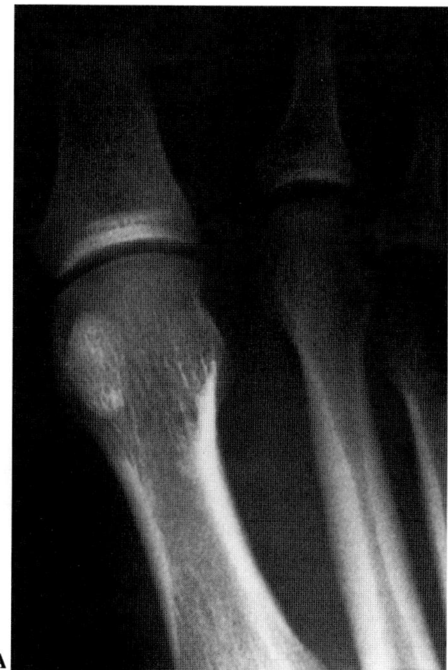

A

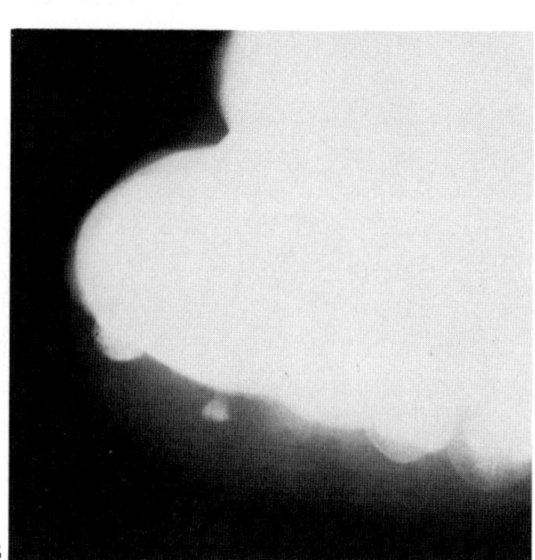

B

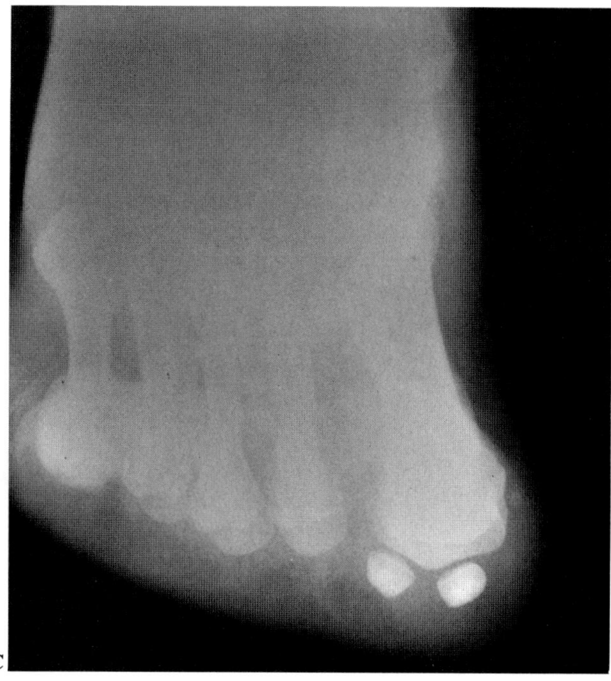

C

Fig. 8-30 Sesamoid osteonecrosis in a runner with forefoot pain. (**A**) Posteroanterior view shows an absent lateral sesamoid. (**B**) Sesamoid view shows swelling with fragmentation of the sesamoid. (**C**) Normal sesamoid view for comparison.

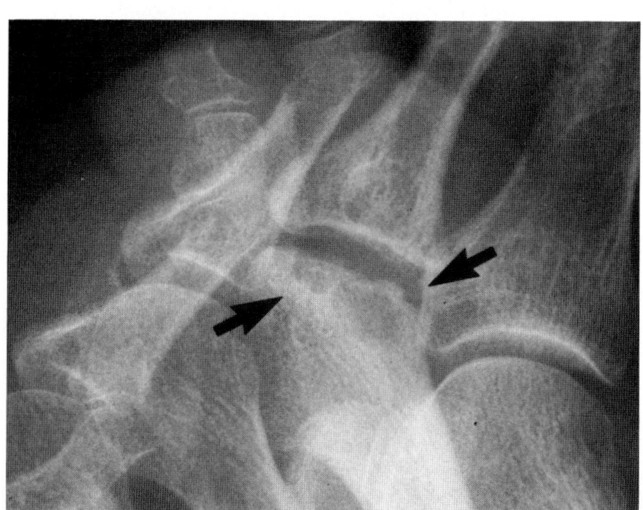

Fig. 8-31 Osteonecrosis of the second metatarsal head (arrows).

second metatarsophalangeal joint is most commonly affected; it is followed in frequency by the first and third joints. If the condition persists, hammertoe or medial or lateral translocation may develop.[98] Subluxation more often occurs in middle-aged male joggers; the second metatarsal is most commonly involved.[76] Other forefoot pain syndromes, neuromas, and stress fractures (Table 8-4) must be excluded.

- *Hallux rigidus*: Athletes frequently develop hallux rigidus, usually as a result of chronic trauma.[76] Symptoms usually occur with starting from a squatting stance, such as in football or track. Hard-soled shoes may be helpful. In certain cases surgical correction may be indicated.
- *Neuromas*: Neuromas (Morton's neuroma) are due to chronic trauma to the interdigital nerve. Symptoms are commonly noted beween the third and fourth metatarsal heads. Paresthesia and numbness in the sensory distribution of the nerve are common. On examination, pain is elicited by placing pressure on the plantar aspect of the foot while compressing the metatarsal heads.[93,98] Generally, properly fitting footwear or direct injection with anesthetic and steroid will be successful. Surgery may be required in certain cases, however. In this setting, imaging is useful before consideration and planning of surgery.[40]

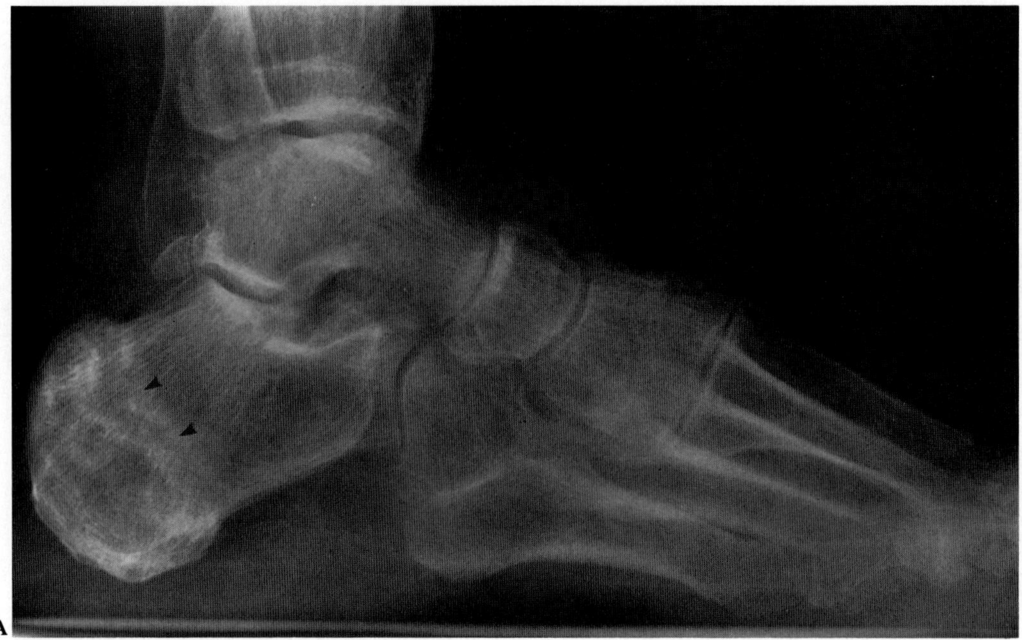

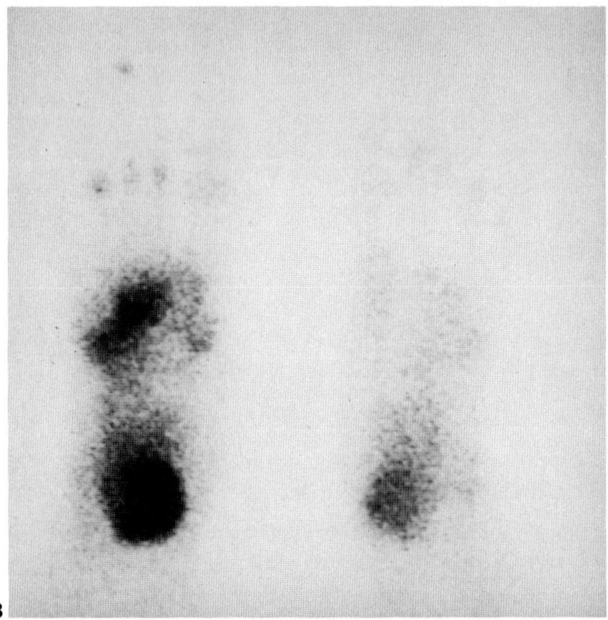

Fig. 8-32 (**A**) Cavus foot with condensation (arrowheads) in the calcaneus. (**B**) Radionuclide scan shows increased tracer uptake in this region and in the midfoot as a result of stress fractures.

Imaging of forefoot problems should begin with radiographs in the oblique and standing AP and lateral projections.[40] Normal angles, joint congruency, and phalangeal deformities provide valuable clues to injury or foot deformities such as cavus foot (Fig. 8-32) that predispose to certain pain syndromes. The position and appearance of the sesamoids should be carefully assessed. Sesamoid views (Fig. 8-30) are useful in patients with suspected abnormalities.

When routine radiographs are normal, radionuclide scans are useful to define early injuries such as stress fractures (Fig. 8-32), sesamoiditis, or early osteonecrosis. Findings on bone scan can allow more specific imaging with CT or tomography to define the lesion more effectively. Recently, MRI has become a frequent second choice after routine films. MRI can clearly define soft tissue lesions such as neuromas (Fig. 8-33) as well as osseous abnormalities.[39]

ANKLE FRACTURES

Management of foot and ankle fractures is a common problem for orthopaedic surgeons, emergency department physicians, family practice physicians, and radiologists. Imaging plays an important role in assessing the degree of bone and soft tissue injury and in following the healing process.

The detection of most fractures is not difficult. Detection of subtle fractures and evaluation of the extent of soft tissue injury, however, may be more difficult. Thus it is essential for those interpreting images to be aware of the manner in which various fractures and soft tissue injuries present so that the images can be evaluated correctly and thoroughly. Soft tissue changes may be the only clue to a subtle fracture or ligament rupture. Soft tissue swelling, obliteration of the fat planes or the pre-Achilles fat triangle, and the presence of an effusion can be useful in identifying the location of subtle fractures (Fig. 8-14).[136]

It is also important to understand the clinical significance of certain fracture patterns. Fractures may be complete (involving both cortices) or incomplete (involving one cortex). The

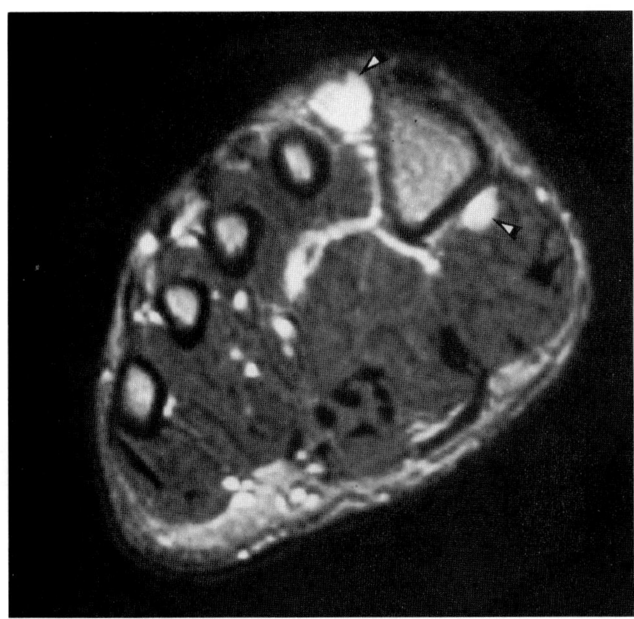

Fig. 8-33 Axial T2-weighted MR image (SE 2000/60) demonstrating multiple neuromas (arrowheads).

latter are more common in children. Avulsion fractures occur at the insertion of ligaments or tendons.

Pediatric Ankle Fractures

Ankle fractures may be simple or complex with associated ligament rupture. The latter are more common in adults. Generally, fractures in patients older than 15 to 16 years of age are classified and treated on the basis of adult criteria.

The appearance of ankle fractures in children depends upon the age (growth plate development), relationship of the ligaments to the epiphyses, and mechanism of injury.[113,114,117,120] Distal diaphyseal and metaphyseal fractures are frequently incomplete. In most cases there is a posterior cortical break with buckling (torus fracture) of the anterior cortex above the growth plate.[113] Fractures of the distal tibia and fibula frequently involve the growth plates. The distal tibia epiphysis is the second most common site for growth plate fracture.[107,113] In Rogers' series,[131] 25% of 118 physeal injuries involved the distal tibia or fibula. Physeal fractures can result in growth or articular deformity if proper diagnosis and treatment are not implemented.

There are two types of epiphyses. Pressure epiphyses are located in the ends of long bones and are subject to weight-bearing forces and forces acting on the joint. Traction epiphyses occur at sites of muscle or tendon insertions (ie, the greater and lesser trochanter). The latter are not directly associated with weight bearing.[132] The pressure epiphyses of the distal tibia and fibula contribute 45% and 40%, respectively, of the growth of the tibia and fibula. The proximal epiphyses of the tibia contribute 55%, and those of the proximal fibula contribute 60%.[132] The distal tibial and fibular epiphyses appear at age 2. The tibial epiphysis fuses by age 15 in girls and 17 in boys. The fibular epiphysis remains open longer and fuses at age 20.[113]

Histologically the growth plate is divided into four zones. Progressing distally from the metaphysis, these zones include the zone of provisional calcification, the hypertrophic cartilage zone, the proliferating zone, and the resting zone.[131,132] The cartilage cells are surrounded by longitudinally oriented collagen fibers and a chondroitin sulfate matrix. This substance is less abundant in the hypertrophic zone, which at least partially explains why this zone is the most susceptible to fracture.[131,132] The blood supply to the epiphysis and metaphysis of the long bones is separate, with the exception of the proximal radial and femoral epiphyses. Therefore, when fracture of the growth plate occurs the blood supply is generally not disrupted. This spares the proliferating zone, and normal growth can occur after healing.[107,113,114]

The same forces that cause fracture and/or ligament disruption in adults also cause fractures in children. In children the growth plates are two to five times weaker than the ligaments, so that fractures of the physes occur more commonly than ligament injuries.[107] The fracture patterns that evolve are thus related to age, the ligamentous attachments, and the type of force applied. Growth plate fractures are more common during the first year and the rapid growth phases in the early teens.[131] The growth plate fuses at different rates in boys and girls, and the method of closure in the distal tibia is important in understanding fracture patterns. Fusion of the distal tibial epiphysis begins at age 12 in girls and age 13 in boys. Fusion does not occur symmetrically. Closure of the growth plate occurs over a period of about 18 months. The process begins centrally, with the medial portion of the physes closing before the lateral portions. The medial fused portion becomes less susceptible to fracture than the lateral physis, which results in the juvenile Tillaux and triplane fracture patterns seen in patients of this age group (Fig. 8-34).[107,113,131,132] Most growth plate fractures are secondary to shearing or crushing forces that lead to opening, shifting, or compression of the physes.[107,113,114,131]

The most commonly used classification system for physeal injuries was described by Salter and Harris (Fig. 8-35).[132] This classification is useful because of its prognostic significance and easy-to-use radiographic patterns.[113,131,132] Type I fractures (Fig. 8-35) are due to separation of the epiphysis with the fracture line confined to the growth plate. The fracture usually extends through the hypertrophic zone and does not involve the epiphysis or metaphysis.[132] In Rogers' series[131] of 118 physeal fractures, 6% were type I. This type of injury may be subtle radiographically. Comparison radiographs of the uninjured ankle may be helpful. Type I injuries are uncommon in athletes and tend to occur more commonly in children younger than 5 years of age. The prognosis is generally excellent.[132]

Type II fractures (Figs. 8-35 and 8-36) are the most common (75% in Rogers' series[131]). This fracture extends through

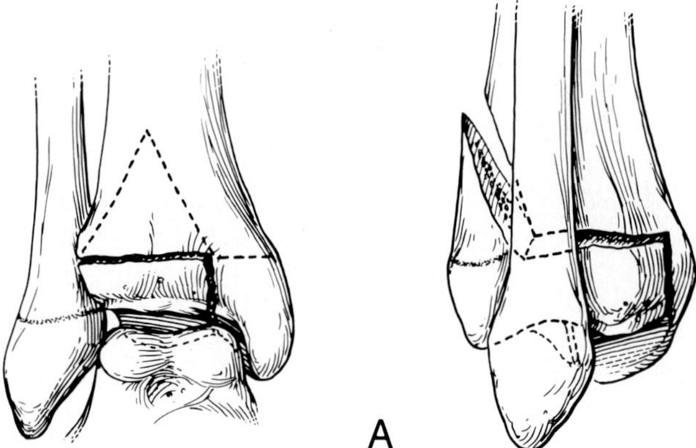

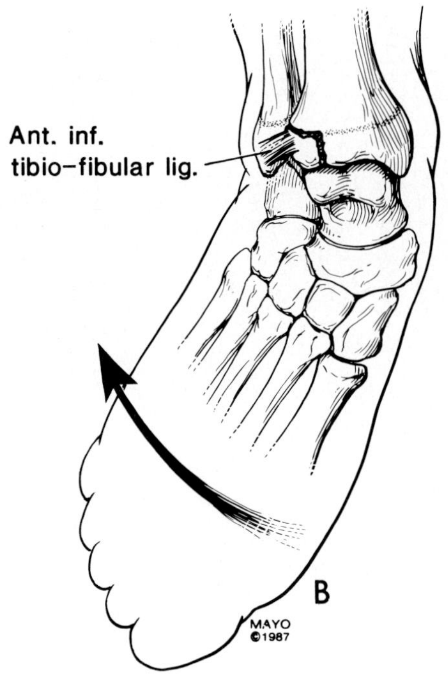

Fig. 8-34 Illustrations of triplane (**A**) and juvenile Tillaux (**B**) fractures. *Source:* Reprinted from *Radiology of the Foot and Ankle* by TH Berquist, Raven Press, 1989, © Mayo Foundation.

the growth plate for a variable distance before exiting through the metaphysis.[132] Type II fractures occur more commonly in patients older than 10 years of age. Eversion or inversion injuries with forced abduction or adduction of the foot have been implicated in this ankle fracture.[132]

Type III fractures (Figs. 8-35 and 8-37) are intraarticular, extending through the epiphysis and entering the growth plate, where they exit through the hypertrophic zone. The metaphysis is spared.[132] This injury is usually due to an intraarticular shearing force.

Type IV fractures (Fig. 8-35) extend from the articular surface of the epiphysis through the growth plate and exit through the metaphysis. Complete reduction of this fracture is essential to prevent growth disturbances. This fracture makes up 10% of Salter-Harris fractures.[132]

Type V fractures (Fig. 8-35) are the result of compression injuries that cause impaction of the growth plate. The ankle and knee are commonly involved.[132] The prognosis is guarded with type V fractures. These fractures are uncommon (1% of 118 fractures in Rogers' series[131]).

Other classifications have also been applied to growth plate fractures.[108,111,113,131] Crenshaw[111] proposed a classification similar to that of Salter and Harris that is frequently used because of its simplicity. Injuries are categorized according to forces applied: external rotation, abduction, adduction, plantar flexion, and direct trauma. The incidence and radiographic appearance of these injuries are summarized in Table 8-5. With this approach the pattern of injury can be used in fracture reduction. Fractures are reduced by gently reversing the direction of the mechanism of injury noted radiographically.[107]

External rotation injuries occur when the foot is supinated and subjected to external rotation forces. This stress leads to fracture of the posterolateral tibial physis (usually Salter-Harris II) and often a fracture of the fibula above the growth plate.[111,113,114] Abduction (eversion) injuries result in Salter-Harris I or II fractures of the anterolateral tibia. The direction of stress and talar shift usually displaces the fragment laterally. Talar forces may lead to associated fibular fractures.[111,132] Adduction forces are similar to inversion injuries, placing tension on the lateral ligament complex. This results in avul-

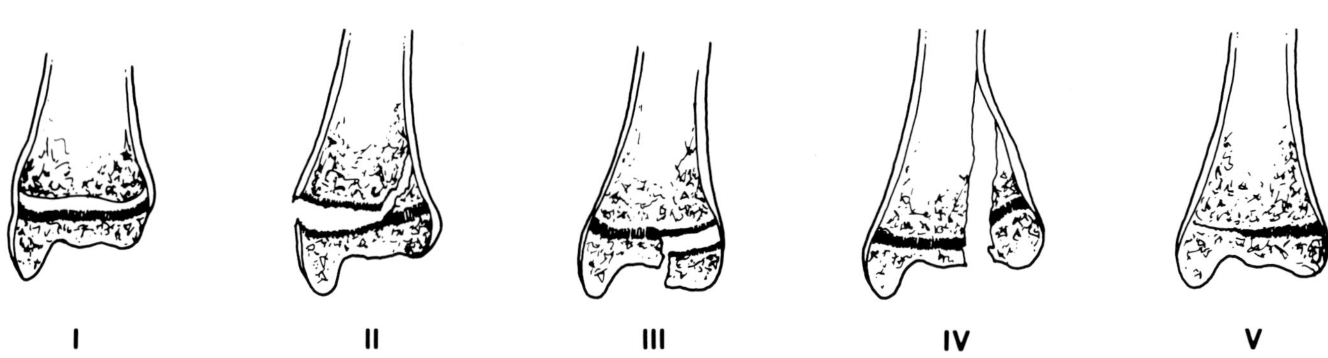

Fig. 8-35 Illustration of Salter-Harris physeal fracture classification.

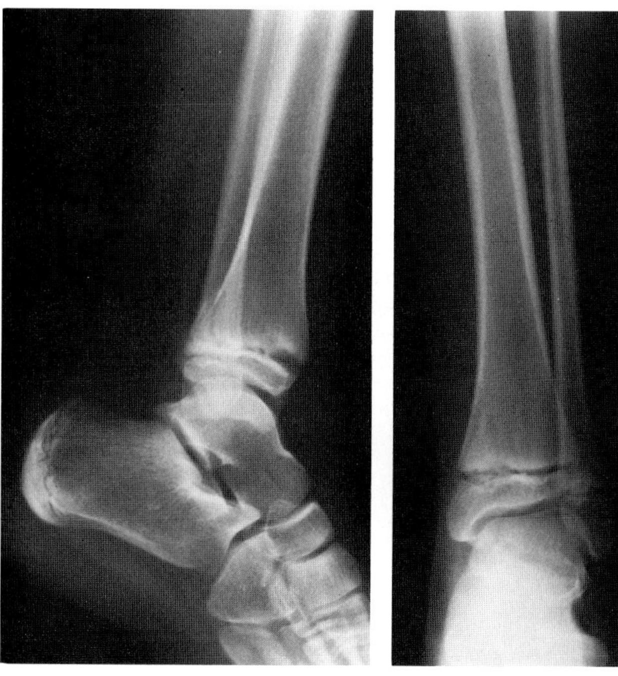

Fig. 8-36 Lateral and AP views of the ankle demonstrating a Salter-Harris II fracture of the distal tibia.

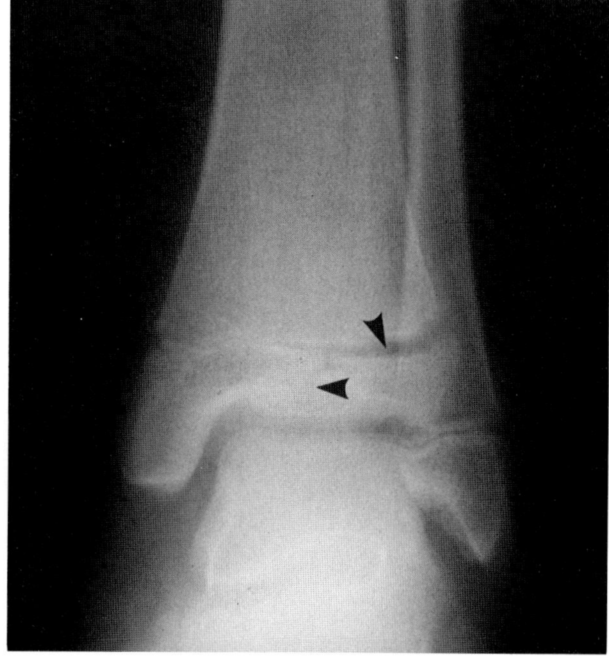

Fig. 8-37 AP view of the ankle in a baseball player who sustained a Salter-Harris III fracture (arrowheads) during a base-stealing attempt.

sion or distal fibular physeal fractures. The force, if continued, will cause impaction of the talus against the medial malleolus, leading to a Salter-Harris III or IV fracture of the medial malleolus.[113,132] Plantar flexion injuries lead to posterior epiphyseal injuries. By definition there is no external rotation force, and therefore no associated fibular fracture is evident.[111] The Crenshaw fracture patterns are most common during the 12th year, and there is a significantly higher incidence in boys.[111,132]

More recently, the Lauge-Hansen system has been combined with the Salter-Harris system.[113,114] The former is an accurate method commonly applied to adult ankle injuries and is discussed later.[121] Dias and Tachdjian[113] studied 71 patients with their combined classification system, and only 4 patients (5.6%) did not properly fit the categories. This classification, like the Lauge-Hansen system, is based on the position of the foot during the injury and the direction of the abnormal force (Fig. 8-38 and Table 8-6).

Several ankle fractures do not fit into this classification. A Salter-Harris III of the distal tibia is usually due to external rotation forces. This fracture is generally seen in the lateral portion of the tibia.[119] Triplane fractures do not fit the original Dias-Tachdjian classification (Fig. 8-34A). The injury is believed to be due to external rotation with or without associated plantar flexion.[109,123] The fracture consists of three fragments instead of the two fragments seen with most growth plate fractures. The first fragment involves the anterolateral portion of the tibial epiphysis and looks like a Salter-Harris III injury. The second fragment is the remainder of the tibial epiphysis with the metaphyseal attachment. The third fragment is the tibial metaphysis.[109,114,123,128] The fracture has a characteristic radiographic appearance. On the AP view it has the appearance of a Salter-Harris III fracture, and on the lateral view it resembles a Salter-Harris II fracture of the distal

Table 8-5 Pediatric Ankle Fractures: Crenshaw Classification

Type	*Appearance*	*Incidence (%)**
External rotation	Salter-Harris II of tibia with posterior metaphyseal fragment; associated fibular fracture common; juvenile Tillaux, triplane	39.7
Abduction	Salter-Harris I or II; anterolateral metaphyseal fragment with type II; distal fibular shaft fracture may be associated	14.2
Plantar flexion	Posterior displacement of epiphysis or metaphyseal fragment; no fibular fracture	18.6
Adduction	Avulsion of fibular tip or physeal fracture; Salter-Harris III or IV of medial malleolus	22.1

*Total <100% because approximately 5% of fractures do not fit these categories.

Sources: Crenshaw AH, *Clinical Orthopaedics and Related Research* (1965;41:98–107), JB Lippincott; Rogers LF, *Radiology* (1970;96:289–299) Radiological Society of North America. Reprinted from *Radiology of the Foot and Ankle* by TH Berquist, Raven Press, 1989, © Mayo Foundation.

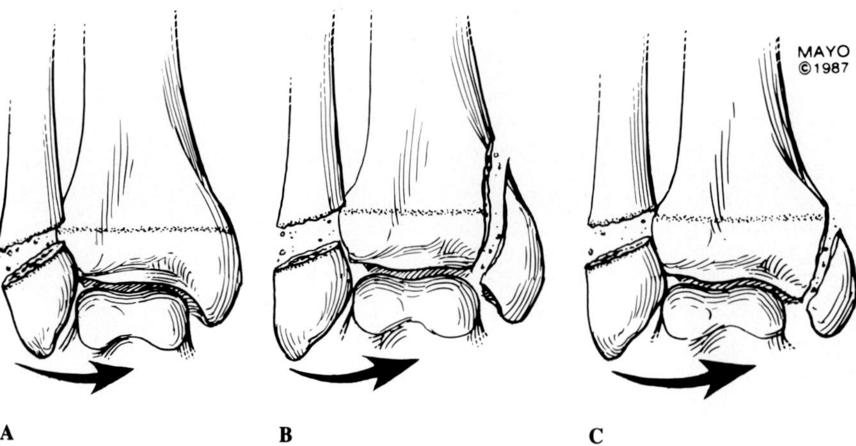

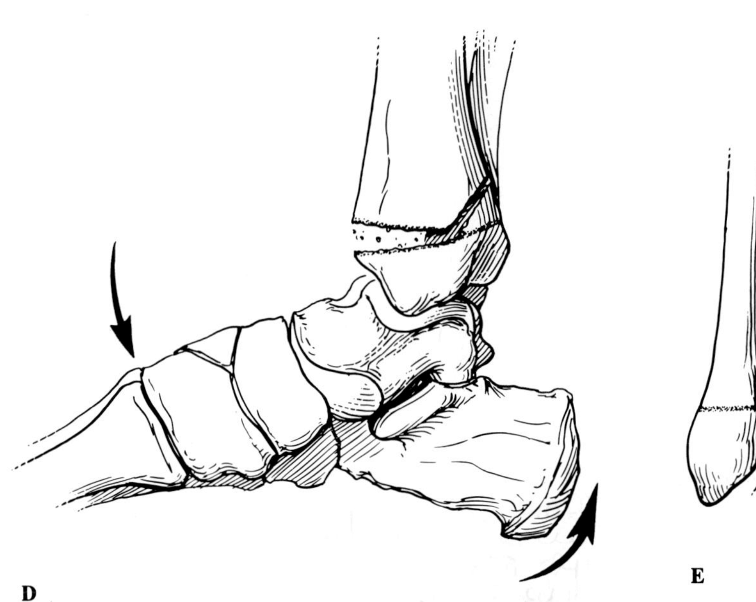

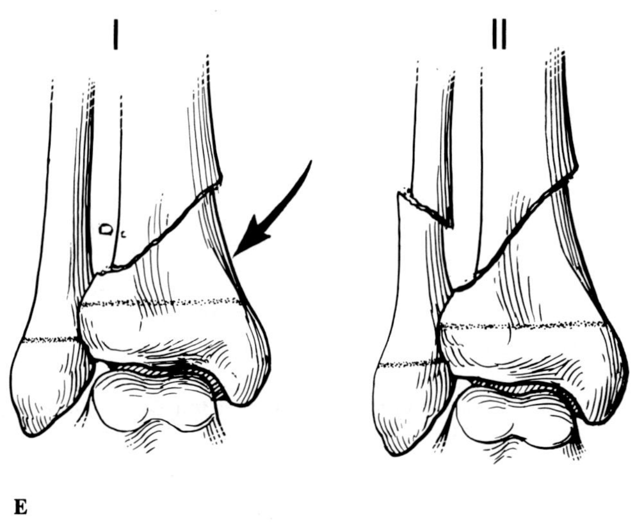

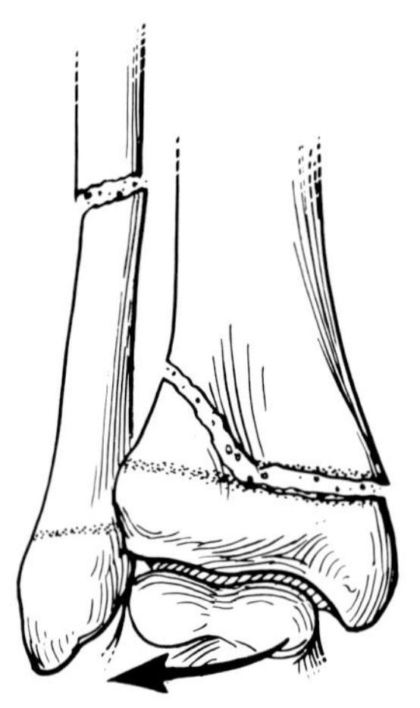

Fig. 8-38 Illustrations of the Dias-Tachdjian classification of ankle growth plate fractures. Arrows indicate direction of force application. (**A**) Inversion-supination stage I, Salter-Harris I or II of the fibula. (**B** and **C**) Inversion-supination stage II, Salter-Harris I or II of the fibula plus medial malleolar fracture. (**D**) Supination–plantar flexion, Salter-Harris I or II of the distal tibia (best seen on the lateral view). (**E**) Supination–external rotation stage I, Salter-Harris II or oblique fracture of the distal tibia; supination–external rotation stage II, stage I plus fibular fracture above the growth plate. (**F**) Pronation–eversion–external rotation, fracture of the fibula above the growth plate with Salter-Harris II of the medial tibia. *Source:* Reprinted from *Radiology of the Foot and Ankle* by TH Berquist, Raven Press, 1989, © Mayo Foundation.

tibia (Fig. 8-34A).[113] The incidence of triplane fractures is not high. Cooperman et al[110] noted an incidence of 6% in a series of 237 patients with epiphyseal fractures of the ankle. In reality the fracture behaves like a Salter-Harris IV, and since its original description many investigators hold that it is often only a two-part fracture. The medial malleolus and anteromedial portion of the epiphysis remain attached to the tibial metaphysis and form one fragment. The second fragment is the lateral portion of the epiphysis with the lateral metaphyseal attachment.[109,123] Other variations of the triplane fracture have also been described.[109]

The so-called juvenile Tillaux fracture is a Salter-Harris III fracture of the distal lateral tibia.[113] The fragment is displaced by the distal tibiofibular ligaments when the foot is externally rotated (Fig. 8-34B).

Most epiphyseal injuries can be clearly defined on the routine ankle trauma series: AP, lateral, and mortise views. In

Table 8-6 Ankle Growth Plate Fractures in Children: Dias-Tachdjian Classification

Type	*Appearance*
Inversion-supination	
Stage I	Traction on lateral ligaments leads to Salter-Harris I or II of fibula; rarely, ligament tear or avulsion fracture of fibula occurs (Fig. 8-38A)
Stage II	Greater inversion force leads to Salter-Harris III or IV of medial tibia in addition to stage I changes (Fig. 8-38, B and C)
Supination–plantar flexion	Salter-Harris I or II of distal tibia; metaphyseal fragment best seen on lateral view (Fig. 8-38D)
Supination–external rotation	
Stage I	Salter-Harris II of distal tibia with spiral component similar to supination–plantar flexion (Fig. 8-38E)
Stage II	Grade I plus spiral fibular fracture above growth plate (Fig. 8-38E)
Pronation–eversion–external rotation	Tibial and fibular physes fracture simultaneously; Salter-Harris II of tibia with fibular fracture above growth plate (5 to 6 cm) (Fig. 8-38F)

Sources: Dias LS in Rockwood CA, Wilkins KE and King RE, *Fractures in Children,* Vol 3, 1984, JB Lippincott; Dias LS and Giegerich CR, *Journal of Bone and Joint Surgery* (1983;65A:438–444). Reprinted from *Radiology of the Foot and Ankle* by TH Berquist, Raven Press, 1989, © Mayo Foundation.

most cases the entire tibia and fibula should be included on the films so that a high fibular fracture is not overlooked. Fractures of the fibular physis, the most common ankle fracture, may be very subtle.[114] Usually Salter-Harris I or, more commonly, II fractures are best seen on the mortise view. When the foot is internally rotated 15° to 20°, the fibula is viewed clear of the tibia. This fracture, however, should be suspected in any child with swelling and point tenderness over the growth plate. When no other fractures are evident (supination-inversion stage I, Table 8-6) the patient can be splinted, and a repeat study in 10 to 14 days will often demonstrate the fracture line more clearly. Slight perosteal callus may also be evident at this time. When a Salter-Harris III or IV fracture is present medially, one should assume that the growth plate or the lateral ligaments are damaged or that an avulsion fracture may be present. Salter-Harris I and II fractures of the distal tibia may also present with subtle radiographic findings. Comparison views on an approach similar to the one described above can be used to evaluate these fractures.

More complex physeal injuries, especially triplane fractures or comminuted epiphyseal fractures, can be better evaluated with CT or MRI.[109] These techniques clearly demonstrate the epiphyseal fragmentation and distal tibiofibular relationships. As is the case for adults, it is important to define the degree of articular involvement, note any articular irregularity, and clearly define the degree of separation of the fracture fragments. Displacement of more than 2 mm has significant treatment implications.[113,114]

Adult Ankle Fractures

Complete evaluation of ankle fractures in adults includes assessment of the fracture fragments and accurate description of associated ligament injuries. Evaluation of bone and soft tissue involvement is important in determining the mechanism of injury, which in turn has significant treatment implications.[105–108,118]

When evaluating ankle fractures it is common to consider the bones and ligaments a ringlike structure in the coronal plane (Fig. 8-39).[107,125] The ring is made up of the medial malleolus, tibial plafond, distal tibiofibular ligaments and syndesmosis, lateral malleolus, lateral ligaments, talus, and medial ligaments.[107,125] Breaks in the ring commonly occur at five sites either alone or in combination. Shift of the talus indicates disruption of the ring at more than one site. The five common sites of injury include the lateral malleolus, lateral ligaments, deltoid ligaments, medial malleolus, and syndesmosis.[130] Fractures of the tibial plafond occur after axial loading with various degrees of plantar flexion.[108,124,125]

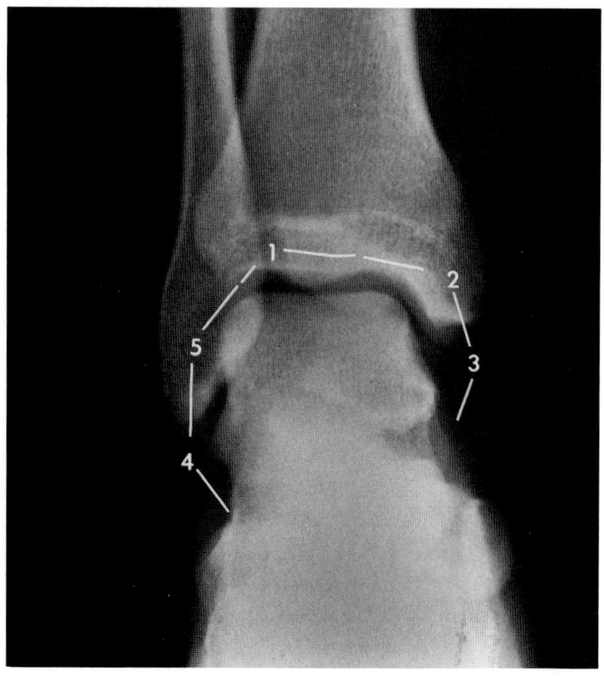

Fig. 8-39 AP radiograph of the ankle demonstrating the ring created by the bones and ligaments. 1, Distal tibiofibular ligament; 2, medial malleolus; 3, deltoid ligament; 4, lateral ligaments; 5, lateral malleolus.

Clinical Features

After ankle injury, patients generally present with various degrees of pain, swelling, and ecchymosis depending to some degree on the significance of the injury. The incidence of swelling and presence of ecchymosis is somewhat higher when fractures are present, but this is not a reliable clinical finding. With incomplete injuries and stable fractures (single break in the ring) weight bearing is usually still possible. Weight bearing is more difficult or impossible with unstable fractures.[108,124,125]

Most ankle fractures occur as a result of inversion or eversion forces (Fig. 8-40).[105,107,125] The mechanism of injury is rarely pure, however. Most often abduction, adduction, lateral rotation, or axial loading occur in addition to eversion or inversion.[107,108,137]

The value of classifications for ankle fractures is that they have a significant impact on treatment, prognosis, and establishing the mechanism of injury. Classifications must also be workable and easy to remember. With this in mind, various classifications have been developed for ankle fractures.[121,125,126,139,141] The more commonly employed classifications are those proposed by Lauge-Hansen[121] and Weber.[125] The former is accurate in predicting the mechanism of injury and extent of ligament involvement. Therefore, it is recommended to radiologists so that the description of the injury can be most accurate. The Weber classification is not as complex but is frequently used because of its value in planning appropriate therapy.[115,125]

The Lauge-Hansen classification was devised with the use of cadaver specimens. It is based on the position of the foot at the time of injury (first word) and the direction of the injuring force (second word).[105,121] With this sytem, four basic categories of injury are described. The classification considers different levels of injury in each category on the basis of the degree of the force and the length of time for which it is applied (Table 8-7).

Supination-adduction injuries (inversion; Fig. 8-41) cause traction on the lateral ligaments, resulting in either a ligament tear or an avulsion fracture of the lateral malleolus (stage I). The fracture is generally transverse and below the joint level.[105,122,125] If the force is sufficient, the talus can impact against the medial malleolus (stage II; Table 8-7). If an oblique fracture of the medial malleolus is evident but no fracture is seen in the lateral malleolus, one can assume that the lateral ligaments are disrupted (Fig. 8-42). This has to be the case if the talus is shifted (two breaks in the ring).[105]

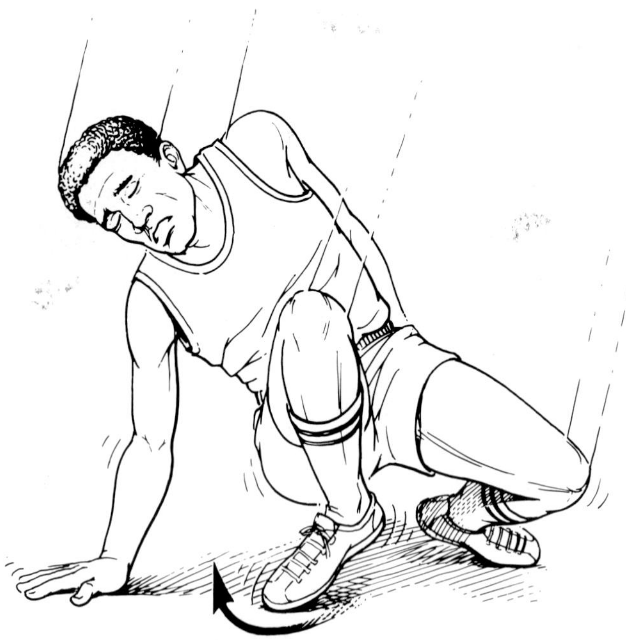

Fig. 8-40 Illustration of external rotation eversion injury in basketball.

Table 8-7 Lauge-Hansen Classification of Ankle Fractures

Type	Appearance
Pronation-abduction	
Stage I	Ruptured deltoid ligament or transverse medial malleolar fracture
Stage II	Disruption of distal tibiofibular ligaments (anterior and posterior)
Stage III	*Oblique fibular fracture at joint level (best seen on AP view)
Pronation–lateral rotation	
Stage I	Rupture of deltoid ligament or transverse medial malleolar fracture
Stage II	Disruption of anterior tibiofibular ligament and interosseous membrane
Stage III	*Fibular fracture above joint space (usually 6 cm or more above joint line)
Stage IV	Posterior tibial chip fracture or rupture of posterior tibiofibular ligament
Supination-adduction	
Stage I	Lateral ligament injury or *transverse lateral malleolar fracture below ankle joint
Stage II	Steep oblique fracture of medial malleolus
Supination–lateral rotation	
Stage I	Disruption of anterior tibiofibular ligament
Stage II	*Spiral fracture of distal fibula near joint (best seen on lateral view)
Stage III	Rupture of posterior tibiofibular ligament
Stage IV	Transverse fracture of medial malleolus

*Fibular fracture appearance is the key to determining the mechanism of injury.

Sources: Arimoto HR and Forrester DM, *American Journal of Roentgenology* (1980;135:1057–1063) American Roentgen Ray Society; Lauge-Hansen N, *Archives of Surgery* (1950;60:957–985) American Medical Society. Reprinted from *Radiology of the Foot and Ankle* by TH Berquist, Raven Press, 1989, © Mayo Foundation.

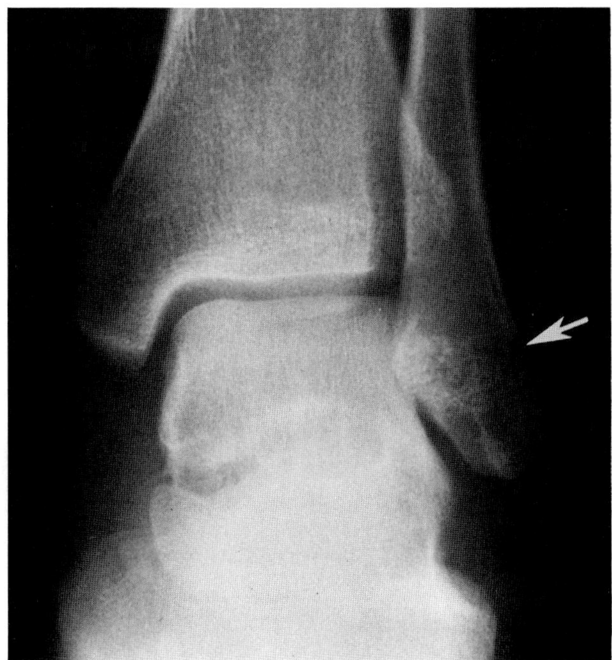

Fig. 8-41 Subtle supination-adduction stage I injury with opening of the fibular physis (arrow) in a 16-year-old baseball player.

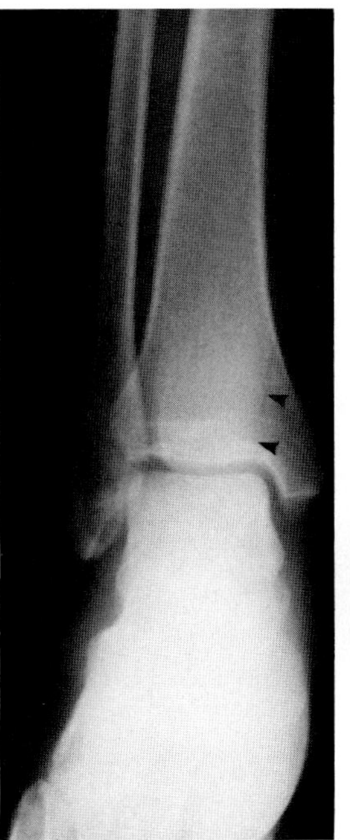

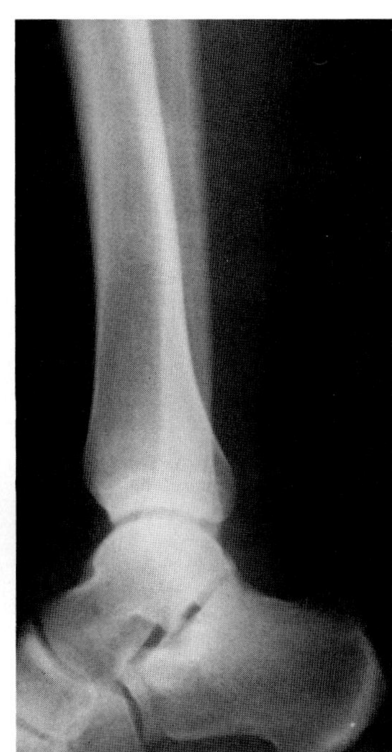

Fig. 8-42 AP and lateral views of the ankle demonstrating an oblique fracture medially (arrowheads) due to a supination-adduction injury.

Supination-adduction injuries account for 18% to 21% of ankle fractures fitting the Lauge-Hansen classification.[121,140,141]

Supination–lateral rotation injuries cause medial tension, with the talus causing posterior displacement of the lateral malleolus.[105] This causes disruption of the anterior distal tibiofibular ligament (stage I; Fig. 8-43A). As the force continues a spiral fracture of the lateral malleolus occurs at or just above the tibiotalar joint. The fracture is best seen on the lateral view (Fig. 8-43B). This stage II injury is the most common ankle fracture.[105,140,141] When the force and talar rotation continue a small posterior malleolar fracture will occur (stage III), and if the force continues an avulsion fracture of the medial malleolus or rupture of the deltoid ligament occurs (stage IV; Fig. 8-43A). Supination–lateral rotation injuries account for 55% to 58% of ankle fractures.[105]

Pronation-abduction injuries (eversion) result in abduction of the talus in the ankle mortise, placing tension on the medial structures. This leads to a transverse avulsion fracture of the medial malleolus or rupture of the deltoid ligament (stage I; Fig. 8-44). With continued force the anterior and posterior distal tibiofibular ligaments are torn, or avulsion fractures of the anterior and posterior tibial attachments occur (stage II; Fig. 8-44). With further force an oblique fibular fracture develops at or just above the tibiotalar joint.[105,121,125] This fracture is best seen on the AP view (Fig. 8-44), which differentiates it from the spiral fracture seen with supination–lateral rotation injuries. The latter is seen best on the lateral view.[105] When an oblique lateral malleolar fracture is noted on the AP view, one should assume that the tibiofibular ligaments and deltoid ligaments are ruptured even though no obvious talar shift may be noted.[105] Stress views may be needed to confirm this finding.

Pronation–lateral rotation injuries cause medial tension as the talus rotates laterally (Fig. 8-45). Initially the medial ligaments rupture, or an avulsion fracture of the medial malleolus occurs (stage I). As the force continues, the injury progresses clockwise around the ankle in the axial plane. The anterior distal tibiofibular ligament and interosseous membrane rupture (stage II); this is followed by a fibular fracture. This fracture (stage III) is typical in that it occurs well above the joint space ($\geq$5 to 6 cm), which allows differentiation of this injury from the others on the basis of the radiographic appearance (Fig. 8-45). When the force continues the posterior distal tibiofibular ligament ruptures, or a posterior tibial avulsion fracture is noted (stage IV).[105,107] Pronation injuries (abduction–lateral rotation) account for about 20% of ankle fractures.[141]

In his original series, Lauge-Hansen[121] found that 75% of injuries were either supination-adduction or supination–lateral rotation injuries. The classification is accurate for detection of fracture and ligament components of ankle injuries in 90% to 95% of cases.[105] There are exceptions, most notably fractures of the tibial plafond due to axial loading or plantar flexion injuries. The characteristic appearance of the fibular fracture and orderly progression of the injuries, however, make this classification ideal for radiologists. Accurate reporting of ankle injuries is greatly facilitated.[105,107,125,141]

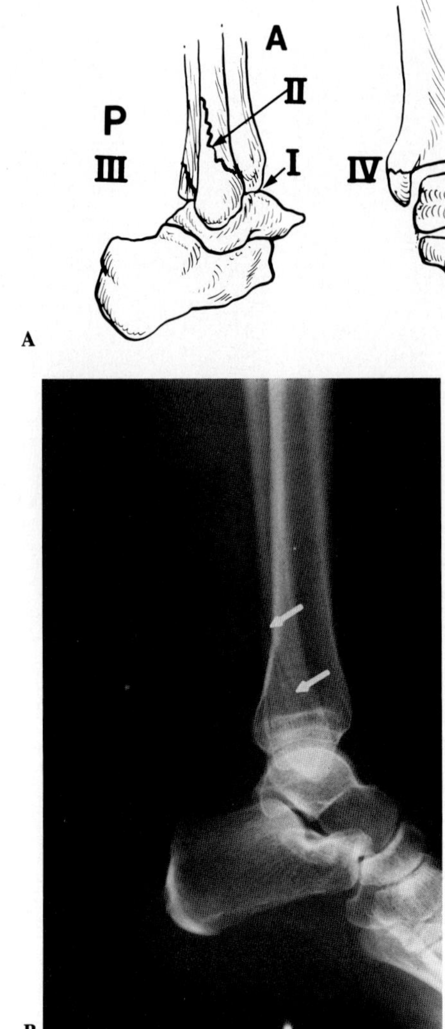

Fig. 8-43 (A) Illustration of the stages of supination–lateral rotation injuries. *Source:* Reprinted from *Radiology of the Foot and Ankle* by TH Berquist, Raven Press, 1989, © Mayo Foundation. (B) Lateral view demonstrating a stage II supination–lateral rotation injury (arrows). The AP view did not demonstrate the injury.

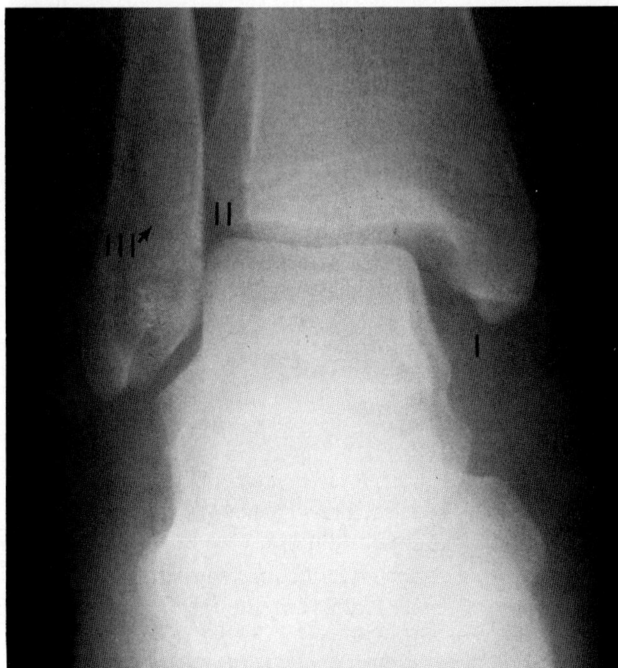

Fig. 8-44 AP view of the ankle after a pronation-abduction stage III injury. I, Rupture of the deltoid ligament; II, rupture of the distal tibiofibular ligaments; III, oblique fibular fracture (arrow).

The Weber classification is commonly used by orthopaedic surgeons.[105,125,139] This classification is much simpler because it uses the level of fibular fracture in predicting the degree of syndesmosis injury and mortise displacement.[125]

Type A injuries cause fractures below the tibiotalar joint and do not involve the syndesmosis (similar to Lauge-Hansen supination-adduction; Fig. 8-41).[125] Type B fractures occur at the joint level, producing an oblique fibular fracture (similar to Lauge-Hansen pronation-abduction) that is best seen on the AP view (Fig. 8-44).[125,139–141] Two categories of type C fractures are described. Type C1 is an oblique fibular fracture above the level of the distal tibiofibular ligaments. Type C2 lesions present with higher fibular fractures and therefore more extensive rupture of the syndesmosis (Fig. 8-45). Treatment of type A injuries can usually be accomplished closed; type B and C injuries usually require internal fixation. The Weber classification is useful for treatment purposes but is not as useful in elucidating the mechanism of injury and ligament involvement as the Lauge-Hansen system.[105,107,121,125]

Fractures of the tibial plafond do not fit neatly into either of the above classifications.[136] These injuries, although uncommon, are difficult to manage.[125,126,130,140] Fractures are due to axial loading and generally occur in association with falling from a significant height.[122,125,127] Fractures usually extend up the tibial shaft in an oblique or spiral manner (Fig. 8-46). Severe comminution with multiple articular fragments (pilon fracture) is common. Twenty percent of plafond fractures are open.[127]

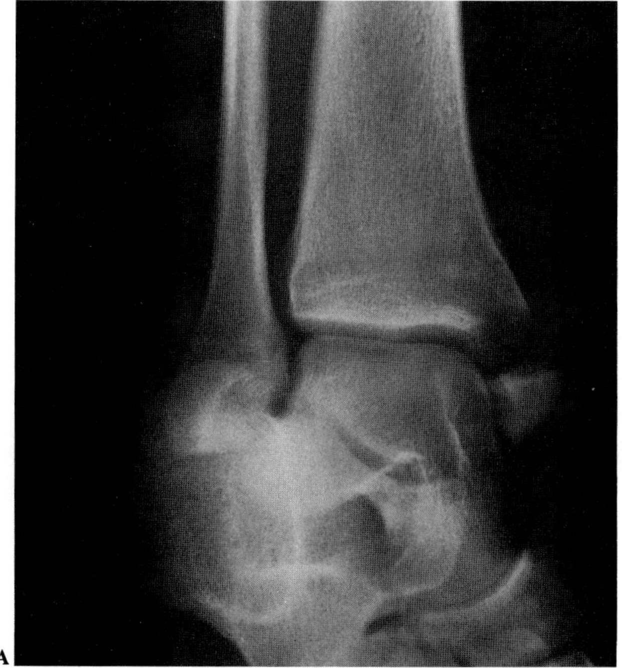

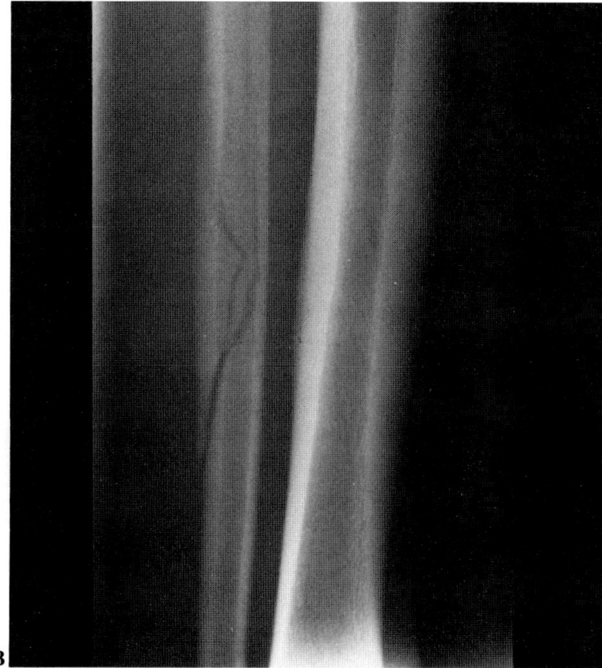

Fig. 8-45 (**A**) Mortise view of the ankle and (**B**) lateral view of the midfibula demonstrating a stage III pronation–lateral rotation injury. The entire leg should be radiographed because the fibular fracture may occur near the knee.

Radiographic Evaluation

AP, lateral, and mortise views are performed in all patients with suspected ankle fractures. At the Mayo Clinic, we also routinely obtain the external oblique view. In most cases these views provide sufficient information regarding the degree of bone and soft tissue involvement.[105,107,118,125] This is especially true in patients with fractures that fit the Lauge-Hansen classification (>95%). It is also essential to include the entire tibia and fibula when studying patients with ankle fractures. The fibular fracture, which is the key to classifying the injury, may be just below the fibular head (Fig. 8-47).[105,125] The AP view is useful in evaluating soft tissue swelling, which may lead the interpreter to a subtle fracture. The oblique fracture of the fibula (pronation-abduction stage III) is best seen on the AP view. Avulsion fractures of the tibia and fibula can also be seen on this view.[107,122,125]

The mortise view (foot internally rotated 15° to 20°) is crucial for evaluating the position of the talus and the syndesmosis. The space between the talar margin and medial malleolus and between the plafond and lateral malleolus should be equal.[107] The distance between the distal tibia and fibula should not exceed 4.5 mm.[107,125] Talar asymmetry indicates the presence of two injuries: two ligament ruptures, two fractures, or a combination of fracture and ligament rupture.[121,122,139–141]

The lateral view is most useful for detecting anterior and posterior tibial chip or avulsion fractures (Fig. 8-48). In addition, the fibular fracture seen with supination–lateral rotation stage II injuries is best seen on the lateral view (Fig. 8-43B).[105,133–135] The presence of an ankle effusion or Achilles tendon injury (obliteration of the pre-Achilles fat triangle) is also most easily noted on the lateral view.[136]

At the Mayo Clinic, we routinely obtain a 45° external oblique view in addition to the above views. This will provide

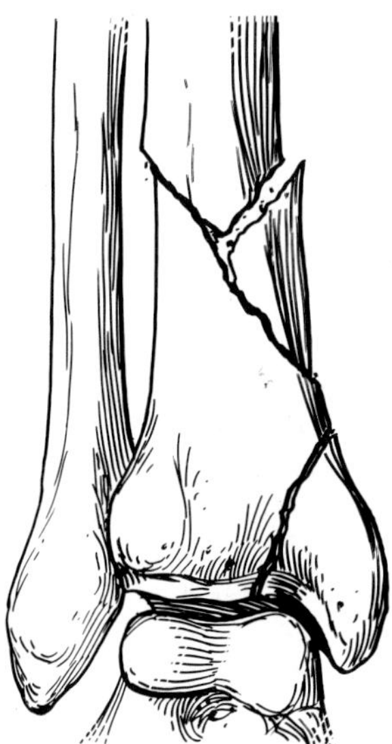

Fig. 8-46 Illustration of a tibial plafond fracture. *Source:* Reprinted from *Radiology of the Foot and Ankle* by TH Berquist, Raven Press, 1989, © Mayo Foundation.

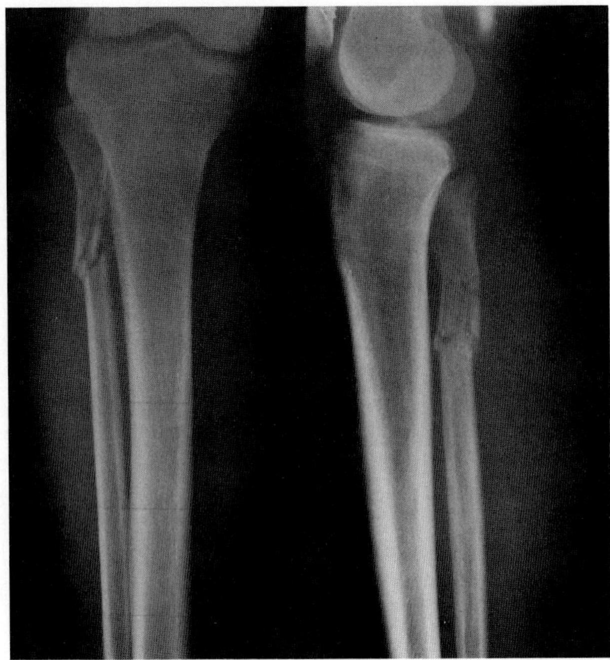

Fig. 8-47 AP and lateral views of the tibia and fibula demonstrating a high fibular fracture in association with a medial ligament and syndesmosis tear (pronation–lateral rotation stage III).

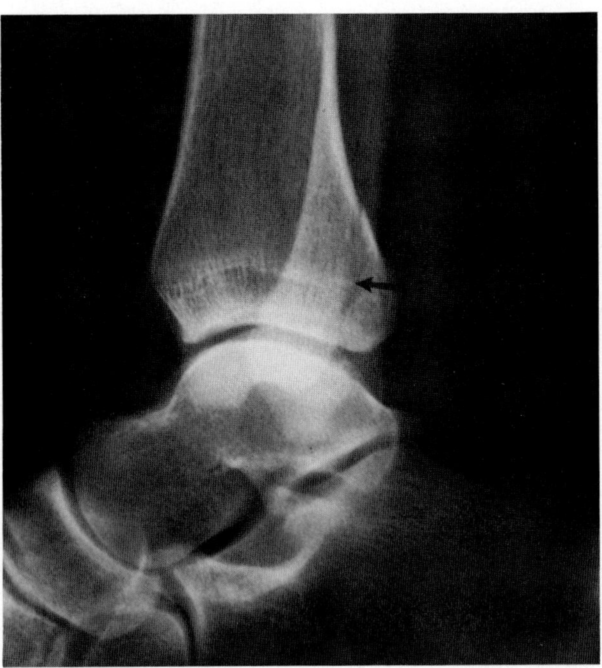

Fig. 8-48 Lateral view of the ankle demonstrating a minimally displaced posterior tibial fracture (arrow).

added information, especially when subtle posterior tibial fractures are present. Because of the frequency of associated fractures in the foot and of foot fractures that may mimic ankle injury, it may also be wise to obtain routine (AP, lateral, and oblique) views of the foot in patients presenting with ankle injury.[107]

Occasionally special studies are needed before planning conservative (closed) or operative therapy. Tomography (AP and lateral projections) is useful in evaluating the degree of articular involvement in complex plafond fractures and may also be necessary to exclude articular involvement. The position of fragments, especially articular fragments, can be better demonstrated with thin-slice (1.5- to 3.0-cm) CT. This technique offers the capability of three-dimensional reconstruction, which can be useful in planning surgical approaches for complex fractures.[107,115,125]

Complications

Complications of ankle injuries are important to the athlete and may significantly reduce the ability to compete at a varsity or professional level. Therefore, discussion of these complications is indicated. Complications may result from the initial injury or may be related to treatment (Table 8-8). Loss of reduction generally occurs with closed reduction but can occur after internal fixation as well.[125] Reduction may be difficult or impossible to maintain with closed manipulation in certain cases. For example, the fibula can become trapped behind the tibia. Also, soft tissue underposition or tendon entrapment may make it impossible to reduce fractures.[112,125] Usually routine radiographs are adequate to evaluate changes in the position of fragments. Failure to maintain reduction as a result of soft tissue interposition can be diagnosed easily with CT or MRI. If these techniques are not available, tenography can be performed.

Arthritis is the most common long-term complication, occurring in up to 30% to 40% of patients regardless of the treatment method used.[125,138] The incidence is higher with displaced plafond fractures, when the syndesmosis is poorly reduced, with chronic instability, and in older patients.[125,127] Radiographic findings of arthritis may not become obvious for 3 to 8 years. Pain symptoms may lead to operative intervention with ankle fusion or, in certain cases, ankle arthroplasty.

Table 8-8 Complications of Ankle Fractures[112,118,121,122,125,127,141]

Osteoarthritis
Chronic instability
Nonunion
Malunion
Reflex sympathetic dystrophy
Infection
Adhesive capsulitis
Tendon rupture or dislocation
Synovial chondromatosis
Tarsal tunnel syndrome
Neurovascular injury
Pes cavovarus deformity

Malunion and nonunion are uncommon when adequate reduction is obtained. Nonunion occurs most commonly after avulsion of the medial malleolus. The incidence (10% to 15%) is much higher after closed reduction compared to open reduction (0.5%).[107,125] Displaced fragments with well-defined sclerotic margins indicate obvious nonunion radiographically. Subtle cases can be detected tomographically or, more accurately, with MRI. On T2-weighted (SE 2000/60, 1.5 T) sequences there is increased signal in the fracture line with nonunion. Fibrous union will be seen as a dark area in the fracture line on both T1- and T2-weighted sequences.

Patients with internal fixation are more prone to infection. The incidence is low, however, and infections are usually superficial.[125]

Reflex sympathetic dystrophy is a syndrome of refractory pain, neurovascular changes of swelling, and vasomotor instability as well as trophic changes involving soft tissues and bone.[107,116] The etiology is unclear, but the syndrome has been attributed to trauma, infection, cervical arthritis, and the like. The severity of trauma does not correlate with the severity of the symptoms. Most investigators hold that the syndrome is due to posttraumatic reflex spasm leading to loss of vascular tone and aggressive osteoporosis.[129] Osteoporosis may have a diffuse or patchy appearance involving both medullary and cortical bone (Fig. 8-49). Prompt diagnosis can lead to more effective therapy. Isotope scans may demonstrate multiple articular changes earlier, suggesting the diagnosis and permitting treatment to be instituted earlier.

Neurovascular injury can occur during the injury or because of inadequate treatment. In the acute setting, angiography is most often employed to evaluate vascular occlusion. Doppler techniques can also be used to evaluate vascular patency.

Ossification of the syndesmosis can occur after ankle fracture.[125] Most often it is incomplete. Complete bony fusion can occur, however, usually when a syndesmosis screw has been used. These changes are usually obvious on routine radiographs. Scarring and stenosis may be purely fibrous, however, in which case CT or MRI is more useful.

TALAR FRACTURES AND DISLOCATIONS

The talus is a unique and important functional unit of the hindfoot.[150,158,181] It serves to support the body weight and to distribute forces to the foot. The talus ossifies from a single primary center, with ossification beginning in the neck. The posterior aspect ossifies last, with maturation being completed 16 to 20 years after birth.[163] Articular cartilage covers 60% of the talar surface, and there are no direct tendon or muscle attachments. Therefore, the blood supply is vulnerable.[161,164,168,172,175]

Superiorly the trochlear surface articulates with the tibia. This articular surface is wider anteriorly. Medially and laterally there are articular facets for the medial and lateral malleoli. There are bony processes posteriorly and laterally. The posterior process is divided into medial and lateral tubercles by a groove for the flexor hallucis longus tendon. This tendon in its fibrous tunnel is the closest anatomically to a tendinous attachment.[161,164,165] In up to 50% of patients the os trigonum is present as a secondary ossification center. This lies just

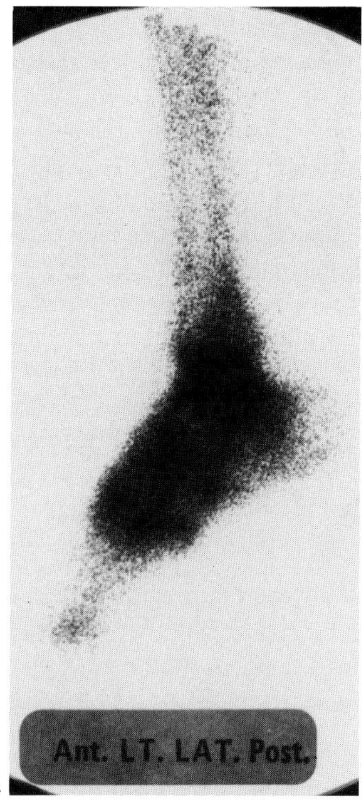

A

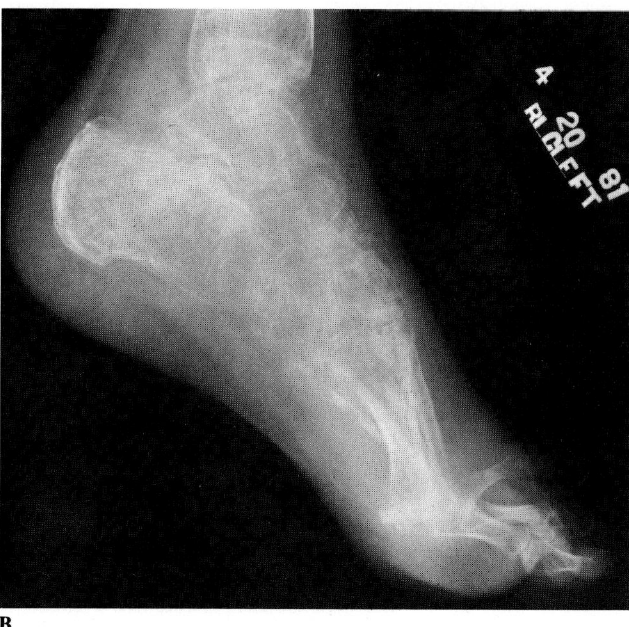

B

Fig. 8-49 (**A**) Radionuclide scan and (**B**) lateral view of the foot in a patient with reflex sympathetic dystrophy.

posterior to the lateral tubercle of the posterior process (Fig. 8-6).

Inferiorly the talus articulates with the calcaneus via the large posterior, the middle, and the anterior facets. The talus forms the roof of the tarsal tunnel between the middle and posterior facets. The talar head articulates with the navicular. Articular stability is maintained by articular capsules and ligaments.[164,169,174] Movements in the subtalar joint include eversion (lateral rotation of the hindfoot), inversion (medial rotation of hindfoot), and slight flexion and extension.[163]

The blood supply to the talus is limited by the significant articular surface area and lack of muscle and tendon insertions. The main blood supply enters the talus via the tarsal canal as a branch of the posterior tibial artery. This artery supplies the inferior neck and most of the body. Branches of the dorsalis pedis artery enter the superior aspect of the talar neck and supply the dorsal portion of the neck and the head of the talus. The peroneal artery supplies a portion of the lateral talus.[164,170]

Talar Neck Fractures

Fractures of the talar neck are uncommon in adults and rare in children. Letts and Gibeault[165] identified 12 pediatric fractures over an 18-year period. The largest series of talar fractures was reported by Coltart.[151] He noted 228 talar injuries in a total of 25,000 fractures and dislocations (0.9%); talar injuries accounted for only 6% of all foot and ankle injuries. Fractures of the talar neck are the second most common talar injury.[151,160,161] The injury usually occurs during abrupt dorsiflexion of the forefoot. This is most often associated with high-velocity sports or a significant fall.[163] Direct trauma from an object striking the top of the foot may also lead to fracture of the talar neck.[166] As usual, the mechanism of injury is rarely pure; adduction or external rotation forces are also implicated.[160,164] Talar neck fractures have also been reported with other ankle injuries involving supination, supination–lateral rotation, and, less commonly, pronation.[164]

Management of talar neck fractures and fracture-dislocations depends on accurate demonstration of the bone and soft tissue injury. The most commonly used classification system for these injuries was devised by Hawkins[160] and modified by Canale and Kelly[150] to include four categories of injury. This classification is useful in determining the prognosis of the injury, specifically in predicting the incidence of avascular necrosis.[160,166] The types of fractures and fracture-dislocations are summarized in Table 8-9.

Talar neck fractures must be undisplaced to be considered type I. These fractures enter the subtalar joint between the middle and posterior facets and may extend into the body. Type II fractures are displaced with subluxation or dislocation of the subtalar joint. The ankle joint is normal. In this setting, two and occasionally all three sources of blood supply are disrupted.[150] Type III fractures are displaced with dislocation

Table 8-9 Talar Neck Fractures and Fracture-Dislocations[149,150,160,166]

Type	*Definition*	*Incidence (%)**
I	Undisplaced vertical neck fracture	11–21
II	Displaced vertical neck fracture with subtalar subluxation or dislocation	40–42
III	Displaced vertical neck fracture with subluxation or dislocation of both tibiotalar and subtalar joints	23–47
IV	Displaced vertical fracture of talus with subtalar or tibiotalar dislocation and subluxation or dislocation of talonavicular joint	5

*Incidence >100% because of multiple series.

Source: Reprinted from *Radiology of the Foot and Ankle* by TH Berquist, Raven Press, 1989, © Mayo Foundation.

of the body from both tibiotalar and subtalar joints; all three sources of blood supply are interrupted. Type IV fractures have associated talonavicular subluxation or dislocation.[150] Twenty-four percent of type II and III injuries were open fractures in Hawkins' series.[160,168]

Radiographic Diagnosis

Routine AP, lateral, and mortise views of the ankle and AP, lateral, and oblique views of the foot are obtained in patients with suspected talar fracture. Talar neck fractures, especially undisplaced ones (Hawkins type I), can be subtle and easily overlooked on routine views (Fig. 8-50). The presence of an ankle injury should alert one to the possibility of a talar neck fracture. Too frequently the more obvious ankle injury provides too much interest for the unwary observer, and a subtle talar fracture may be overlooked. Up to 20% of patients have associated medial malleolar fractures that are often more obvious.[160] Sixteen percent of patients have fractures in other bones of the ipsilateral foot. Tomography may be needed to confirm subtle fractures or to exclude a suspected injury.[145]

Displaced talar neck fractures or fractures with dislocation are usually easily detected on routine views. Detection of subluxation may require that joint spaces and articular relationships be more carefully assessed. Stress views may be helpful. The risk of displacing a talar fracture when one is present, however, is significant, and therefore stress views are not always safe in this setting. If the tarsal relationships are not clear, CT or conventional tomography should be performed.[177]

Complications

Complications are particularly common after displaced talar neck fractures (Hawkins types II to IV).[149,160,166,167]

Avascular necrosis. Avascular necrosis usually becomes evident on routine radiographs in 6 to 8 weeks. During this

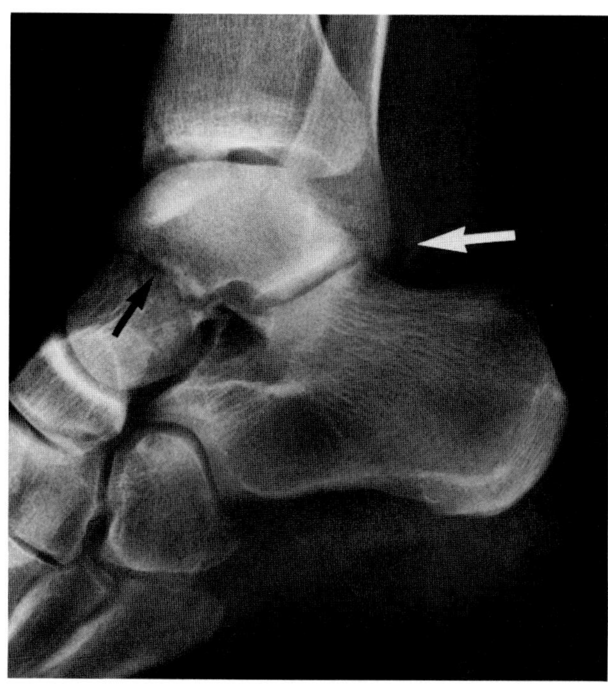

Fig. 8-50 Oblique view of the ankle demonstrating a minimally displaced talar neck fracture (black arrow) and a posterior process fracture (white arrow).

non–weight-bearing period, disuse osteoporosis develops and leads to subchondral lucency in the talar dome. This finding (Hawkins' sign) was described by Hawkins[160] and indicates an intact vascular supply. The finding is most easily identified on AP or mortise views of the ankle. Canale and Kelly[150] noted this sign in 23 patients, only one of whom developed avascular necrosis; 20 of 26 with a negative Hawkins sign developed avascular necrosis.

Although routine radiographic features are well described, changes are evident earlier with isotope scans and MRI. Technetium-99m isotope studies have been advocated to assist in determining when weight bearing should be allowed.[150] Compared to MRI, however, isotope studies do not provide the same degree of bone detail. MRI would appear to be the technique of choice in early detection and follow-up evaluation of patients with suspected avascular necrosis.[144,178]

Arthritis. Posttraumatic arthritis is common after talar neck fractures. The incidence, as expected, increases with the severity of the injury. Peterson et al[172] reported that 97% of patients in their series developed osteoarthritis. Most series show a lower incidence but indicate that degenerative changes develop in nearly two-thirds of type II and III injuries.[150,160,166] The incidence of arthritis is also higher in the subtalar joint than in the tibiotalar joint.[149,166]

Early radiographic changes may show only slight narrowing of the joint space. This may be too subtle to detect without comparison views or tomography. In certain cases, ankle or subtalar arthrography is useful for diagnosing early changes. This also allows injection of anesthetic for diagnostic purposes or a combination of steroid and anesthetic for treatment. MRI provides a new technique for assessing early changes in articular cartilage.[144]

Malunion and nonunion. Delayed healing is not uncommon after talar neck fractures (15%).[145] Delayed union is considered in fractures that have not healed by 6 months. It is not unusual for fractures to take more than 1 year to heal in adults. This is partially due to their intraarticular nature, lack of periosteum, and decreased blood supply.[161] Nonunion occurs in only about 4% of cases overall.[161,165] The incidence is higher in Hawkins type II and III fractures, however.[166]

Malunion is also more common in complex injuries (Hawkins types II to IV). Lorentzen et al[166] reported malunion in 15% of all their cases, but none of these was a Hawkins type I fracture; 28% and 18%, respectively, were Hawkins type II and III fractures. Canale and Kelly[150] noted varus deformity in 47% of type II fractures. This resulted in increased stress in the lateral subtalar joint.[150,161]

Radiographic diagnosis of malunion or nonunion can be difficult. Serial radiographs may demonstrate widening, sclerosis, and irregularity of the fracture line if nonunion has occurred.

Tomography and CT may be useful, but both have difficulty clearly distinguishing nonunion from fibrous union or early pseudarthrosis. MRI is particularly useful in this situation. T2-weighted sequences (SE 2000/60) will demonstrate high intensity (fluid) in the fracture line if nonunion is present and low intensity (black) if a fibrous union is present.[144]

Malunion is most easily demonstrated on AP and lateral radiographs, which allow measurements to be obtained and compared with those of the uninjured side. CT may be particularly useful in evaluating the degree of malunion and the resulting articular deformities of the complex subtalar joint.

Other complications. Other complications include associated fractures, infection, skin necrosis, and neurovascular damage. Ipsilateral foot and ankle fractures have been reported in 16% of patients.[145]

Talar Body, Head, and Process Fractures

Fractures of the talar body and posterior and lateral processes are uncommon in adults and rare in children.[146,147,161–163,173] Although the incidence is lower than that for talar neck fractures, complications are similar for body and neck fractures.

Most talar body fractures are due to significant falls or motor vehicle accidents that lead to axial compression of the talus between the tibial plafond and calcaneus. Fractures of the lateral process usually occur with the foot dorsiflexed and inverted.[159] The calcaneus causes shearing of the lateral process. Snepper et al[179] described six basic fracture patterns: simple compression fractures, vertical fractures in the coronal

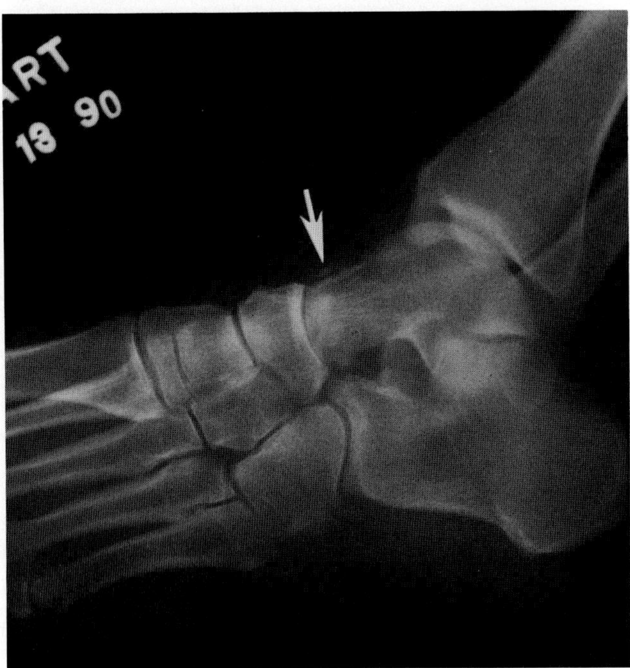

Fig. 8-51 Oblique view of the foot demonstrating a dorsal talar avulsion fracture (arrow).

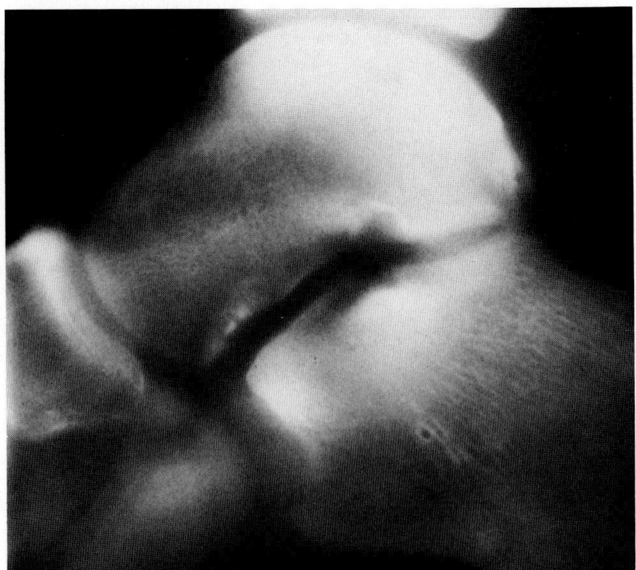

Fig. 8-52 Lateral tomogram demonstrating impaction of the anterior talar facet.

and sagittal planes, posterior tubercle fractures, lateral tubercle fractures, and comminuted crush fractures. In addition, chip or avulsion fractures may occur. These minor fractures are more common in athletes (Fig. 8-51).

AP, lateral, and mortise views of the ankle are usually adequate for diagnosis of displaced fractures. More subtle fractures (chip, avulsion, or undisplaced body fractures) require conventional tomography or CT for detection (Fig. 8-52). Views of the foot should also be obtained because multiple injuries are common.[179] Treatment planning is facilitated by CT or conventional tomography in many cases.

Talar Dome Fractures

Osteochondral fractures of the talar dome differ from other chip or avulsion fractures in that they are more difficult to detect and prognosis is potentially worse compared to a nonarticular chip fracture.[142,168] Talar dome fractures are the most common talar fracture. This injury is much more common in adults. Only 16 of 201 patients (8%) in Berndt and Harty's series[143] were younger than 16 years of age.

Many athletes present with symptoms mimicking those of ankle sprain. Talar dome fractures must be considered in this setting. The mechanism of injury and radiographic appearance of medial and lateral talar dome fractures differ significantly. Lateral fractures are due to inversion or inversion-dorsiflexion injuries (Fig. 8-53). The fracture is shallow with a flakelike fragment.[143,149] Medial lesions are deeper, not always clearly associated with trauma, and often less symptomatic.[149] Traumatic lesions are due to lateral rotation of the plantar flexed ankle.[143,156]

The most commonly used classification system for talar dome fractures was devised by Berndt and Harty.[143] Stage I lesions are compressions of the talar dome with no associated ligament ruptures and intact cartilage. These lesions are the most subtle and rarely are symptomatic. Stage II lesions are incomplete fractures with the fragment remaining partially attached. Stage III lesions are complete but not displaced fractures. Stage IV lesions are detached.[143] Stage II to IV lesions can be overlooked because of the significant ligamentous injuries that accompany them (Figs. 8-53 and 8-54).

Diagnosis

Routine AP, lateral, and mortise views of the ankle are taken in patients with suspected fracture or ligament injury. Talar dome fractures are most easily detected on mortise views (Fig. 8-53A) and occasionally on the AP view. The lateral view is rarely useful for identification of this fracture, but it should be evaluated carefully for the presence of an effusion. The presence of an effusion should lead one to search more carefully for a talar dome fracture. Stage I lesions can be especially subtle. The only finding on routine views may be a subtle change in bone density at the margin (usually lateral) of the talar dome. If an effusion is present or if clinical suspicion is high, tomography should be performed in both AP and lateral projections (Fig. 8-53B).

It is not uncommon to overlook this lesion on the initial examination. Patients are commonly treated for an ankle sprain. It is imperative to keep this lesion in mind in all athletes with ankle sprains. When a history of inversion injury, exercise-related ankle pain, clicking or catching, and persistent

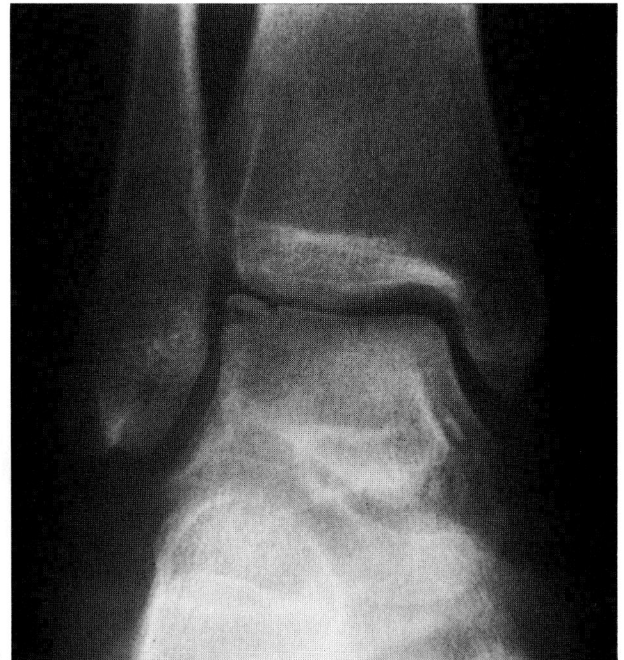

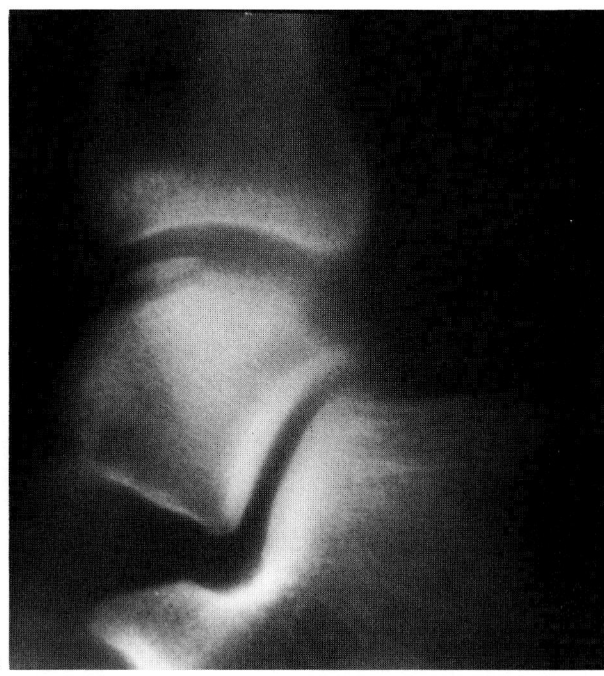

Fig. 8-53 (**A**) Mortise view and (**B**) lateral tomogram of a slightly displaced lateral talar dome fracture.

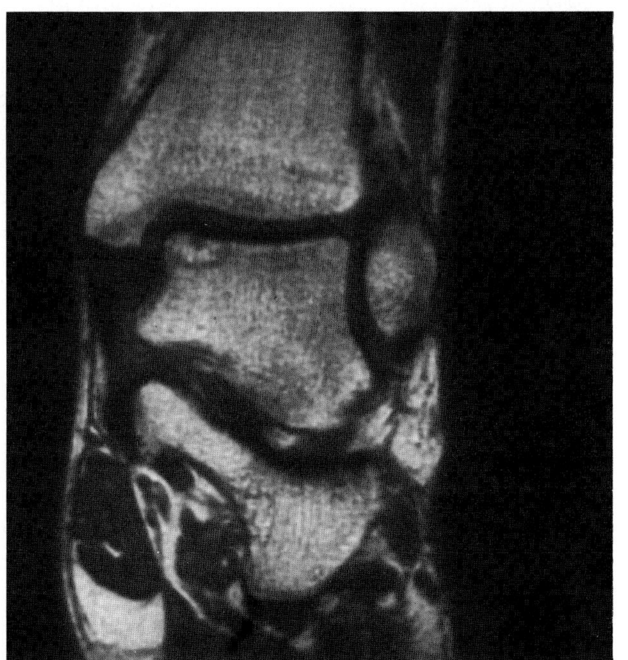

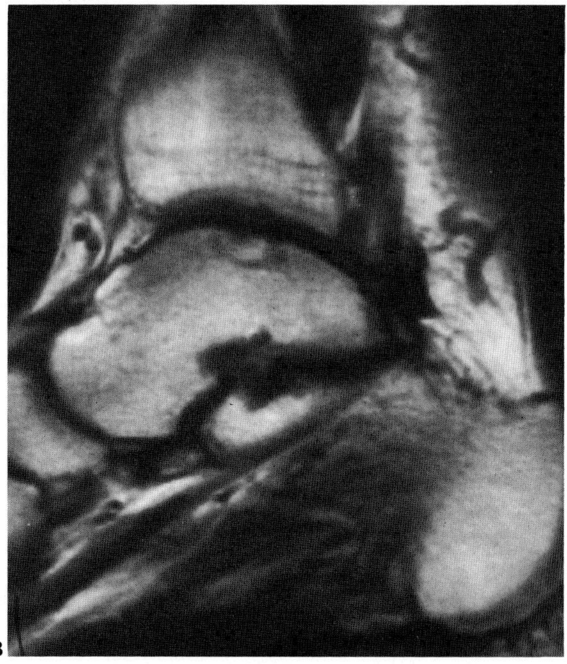

Fig. 8-54 (**A**) Coronal and (**B**) sagittal (SE 500/20) MR images of a medial talar dome fracture. Radiographs were normal.

swelling is present, one should definitely pursue the possibility of an osteochondral fracture.[171,182] If the injury is more than 48 hours old, isotope scans can be used to identify the site of injury. This is important because other fractures (Table 8-1) can also mimic ankle sprains. After isotope studies, tomography should be performed to clarify the type and significance of the lesion.[148] More than 20% of lesions are missed when tomography is not performed.[168,171]

Once the lesion is detected, it is important to determine its exact site and size. This can be done tomographically.[168] The cartilage over the lesion may be intact or interrupted. This can be determined with double-contrast arthrotomography or MRI.[144,145,153,168]

Complications

Symptoms are often more prolonged and displacement of lateral lesions more common than medial lesions. The most common complication is osteoarthritis,[149,168] which is evident in 50% of patients regardless of the treatment employed.[149] Displaced fragments lose their blood supply and are susceptible to avascular necrosis. Subchondral cyst formation has also been reported; presumably it is due to intrusion of synovial fluid through defects in the articular cartilage and subchondral bone.[145,168]

Talar and Subtalar Dislocations

The majority of eversion and inversion motion occurs at the subtalar joint. Inversion is limited by the interosseous ligament, peroneal tendons, and lateral ankle ligaments. Eversion is limited by the deltoid ligament, posterior tibial tendon, and anterior tibial tendon.[163,168]

The talus and calcaneus are connected by joint capsules and the lateral, medial, interosseous, and cervical ligaments. The talonavicular ligament provides less support than the talocalcaneal group.[155,161,163]

Pure subtalar dislocations occur with simultaneous dislocation of the talocalcaneal and talonavicular joints. Total talar dislocation occurs when the talus is dislocated from the ankle mortise in addition to the joints mentioned above.[154,161,168]

Subtalar dislocations are uncommon (1.3% to 2.0% of all dislocations).[152,168,176] Fifteen percent of all talar injuries are due to dislocation.[171] Most injuries occur during significant falls with inversion forces or with landing on the inverted ankle in sporting events (basketball and volleyball).[168,176] The injury is rare in children; DeLee and Curtis[152] reported the average age to be 33.6 years. The incidence of subtalar dislocations in men is 6 to 10 times higher than that in women.[155]

Subtalar dislocations may be medial (56%), lateral (34%), posterior (6%), or anterior (4%).[168] With medial dislocations the talus remains in the ankle mortise, and the calcaneus and navicular are dislocated medially (inversion force). Lateral dislocations occur with eversion injuries.[152] DeLee and Curtis[152] reported a higher incidence of associated fractures with lateral dislocations; articular fractures of the talus, navicular, or calcaneus occurred in 75% of patients with lateral dislocation compared to 45% with medial dislocations. Lateral dislocations are also more commonly open injuries.[152,161] Associated malleolar fractures or fractures of the fifth metatarsal base can occur with any subtalar dislocation.

Total dislocation is uncommon but potentially one of the worst hindfoot injuries.[176] Detenbeck and Kelly[154] noted only nine cases of total talar dislocation from 1959 to 1967.

Routine radiographs of the foot and ankle are usually sufficient to diagnose subtalar or total talar dislocation. In certain cases stress views may be useful. Associated fractures should be looked for carefully after reduction.[176] Tomography or occasionally CT is best for this purpose.[157,168,177,180]

CALCANEAL FRACTURES

The calcaneus is the largest tarsal bone, and because of its complex anatomy it can be difficult to image with routine radiographic techniques (Fig. 8-55). It is composed of a thin cortical shell with sparse trabecular bone, especially in adults.[190,199] The superior surface has three facets that articulate with the anterior, middle, and posterior talar facets. The middle facet is located on the sustentaculum tali and lies anterior to the sinus tarsi. There is a groove on the inferior surface of the sustentaculum for the flexor hallucis longus. The posterior facet (largest of the three) forms the posterior border of the sinus tarsi.[189,194,205]

The calcaneus is the most commonly fractured bone in the adult foot, accounting for 60% of foot fractures and 2% of all skeletal fractures.[189,192–194] Fractures occur most commonly in men. Calcaneal fractures in children are much less common (5% of all calcaneus fractures), and the patterns differ from those of adult calcaneal fractures.[188,202,206] Most calcaneal fractures in children are less extensive, and compression is less likely to occur, because of the cancellous bone.[202,206] Also, unlike fractures in adults, calcaneal fractures in children are generally extraarticular. Overall, 63% of pediatric fractures are extraarticular and 37% intraarticular. In patients younger than 7 years of age, 92% of fractures are extraarticular.[202] In adults, 70% to 75% of calcaneal fractures are intraarticular and 25% to 30% extraarticular. The adult calcaneus is more susceptible to axial loading, resulting in frequent compression and displacement of the fractured fragments.[194,199]

Most severe adult calcaneal fractures are due to falls or trauma resulting in axial loading of the calcaneus. Less severe avulsion and extraarticular fractures occur with twisting injuries or muscle pulls.[187,194] These injuries are more common in athletes.

Classification systems of calcaneal injuries have been proposed by Rowe et at[201] and Essex-Loprestie.[185] The Essex-Loprestie classification is more popular than the Rowe classification; it divides fractures into two major categories: intraarticular fractures involving the subtalar joint, and fractures not involving the subtalar joint (Table 8-10).[185,194] Types IIB and IIC are the most common intraarticular fractures.[185] To provide a more general classification that can be used for both adults and children, Schmidt and Weiner[202] have proposed a combined classification that uses both the Rowe and the Essex-Loprestie classifications (Table 8-11). A separate type six fracture has been added because of the significant soft tissue injury seen with this fracture in children.

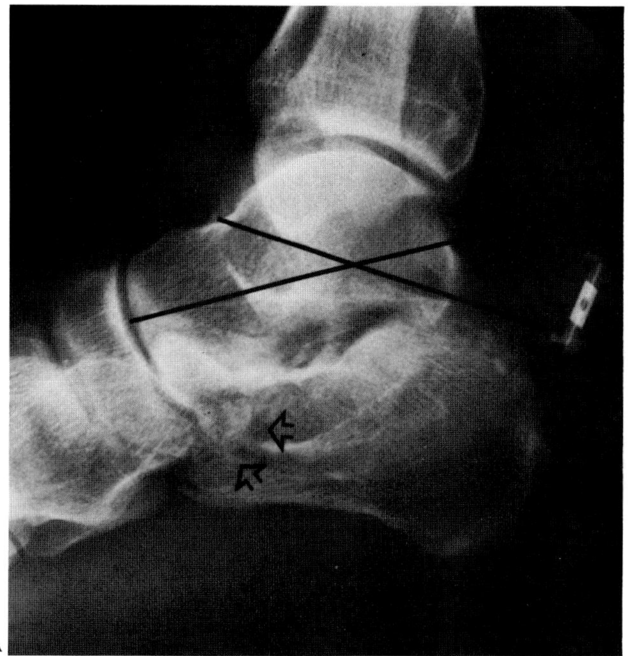

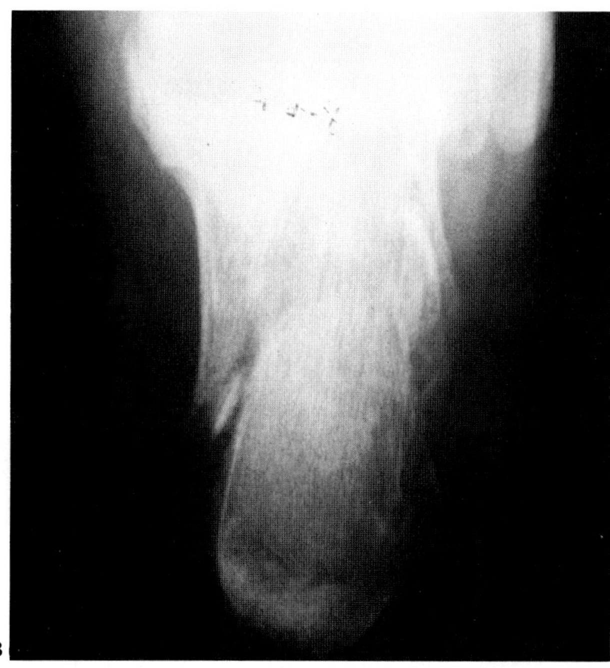

Fig. 8-55 (**A**) Lateral and (**B**) axial views of the calcaneus demonstrating a complex fracture with reduction in Böhler's angle (lines in **A**).

Type I fractures generally have a benign course and are due to avulsion or twisting injuries.[185,194,201] Types IB, IC, and ID involve articular surfaces, however, resulting in different treatment considerations. Apophyseal fractures (type IA) only occur in children. Anterior process fractures (15% of calcaneal fractures, type IC) can be particularly subtle (Fig. 8-56).[190,197] Patients often present with symptoms of an ankle sprain (Table 8-1).[197] The most common mechanism of injury is inversion with internal rotation of the foot, with the anterior process being avulsed by the bifurcate ligament.[194,197] A less common mechanism is a compression fracture (nutcracker injury) with the foot dorsiflexed during varus stress, leading to compression of the anterior process (Fig. 8-57). Other inversion fractures affecting the dorsolateral calcaneus can be confused with a sprain, an anterior process fracture, or the os peroneum (a normal variant). Norfay et al[195] noted this small flakelike fracture in 10% of patients with suspected ankle fracture.

Type 2 fractures are due to direct trauma (2A), usually with abrupt contraction of the Achilles tendon (2B) when the ankle

Table 8-10 Essex-Lopresti Classification of Calcaneal Fractures

I. No subtalar joint involvement
   A. Tuberosity fractures
      1. Beak type
      2. Medial avulsion
      3. Vertical
      4. Horizontal
   B. Calcaneocuboid joint involvement

II. Subtalar joint involvement
   A. Undisplaced
   B. Displaced
   C. Gross comminution

Sources: Essex-Loprestie P, *British Journal of Surgery* (1952;39:395–419) Surgery Society Ltd; Morrey BF, Cass JF, Johnson KA and Berquist TH (ed), *Imaging of Orthopedic Trauma* ed 2, 1991, Raven Press.

Table 8-11 Calcaneal Fractures: Classification and Incidence

Type (Schmidt and Weiner modification of Rowe and Essex-Lopresti)	*Incidence (%)*
1C (anterior process)	15
1A (tuberosity)	6
1B (sustentaculum tali)	3
1D and 1E	1
2 (A, beak, or B, Achilles avulsion)	3–4
3 (linear, extraarticular)	19
4 (linear, intraarticular)	10–24
5A (tongue type)	5
B (joint depression or comminution)	43–60

Sources: Essex-Loprestie P, *British Journal of Surgery* (1952;39:395–419), Surgery Society Ltd; Gross RH in Rockwood CA, Wilkins KE, and King RE, *Fractures in Children* Vol 3, 1984, JB Lippincott; Morrey BF, Cass JF, Johnson KA and Berquist TH (ed), *Imaging of Orthopedic Trauma* ed 2, 1991, Raven Press; Rowe CR, Sakillarides, HT and Freeman PA, *Journal of the American Medical Association* (1963;184:920–924) American Medical Association.

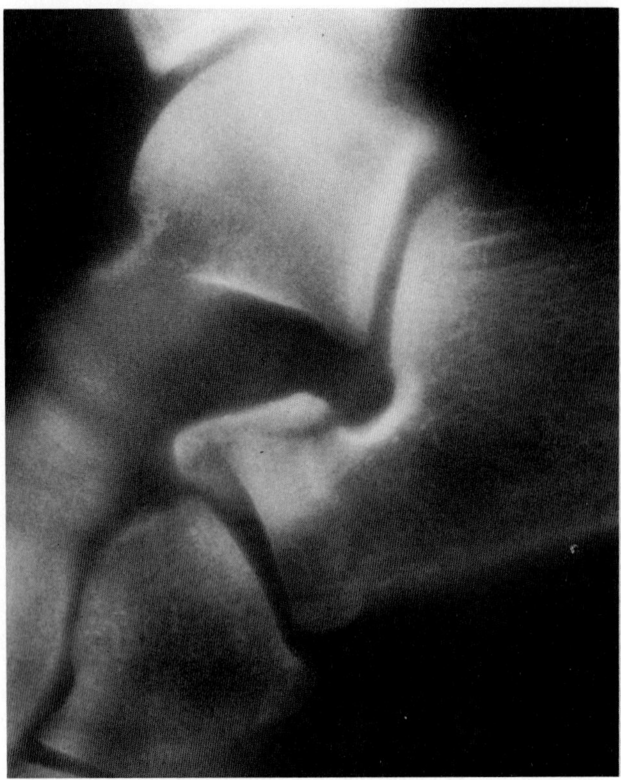

Fig. 8-56 Lateral tomogram of an anterior calcaneal process fracture.

is in a fixed position.[194] These fractures account for only about 4% of calcaneal injuries (Fig. 8-58).[201]

Type 3 to 5 injuries are usually due to axial loading. This may be a direct vertical force or a posterior force directed toward the base of the posterior facet. Generally the fracture also involves the sustentaculum tali, which is commonly

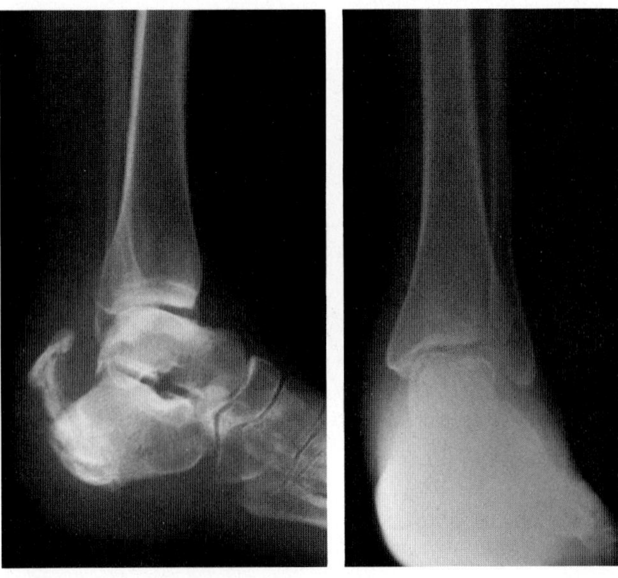

Fig. 8-58 Lateral and AP views of the ankle demonstrating marked swelling with an avulsion fracture (type 2) of the posterior calcaneus.

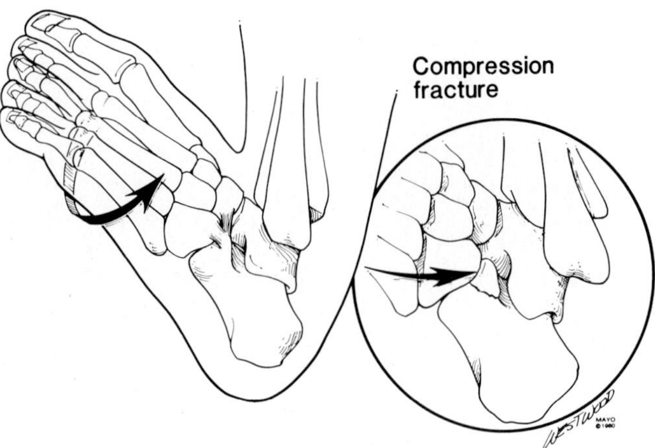

Fig. 8-57 Illustration of compression injury of the anterior calcaneal process. Arrows indicate direction of force application. *Source:* Reprinted from *Imaging of Orthopedic Trauma* ed 2 by TH Berquist, 1991, Raven Press, © Mayo Foundation.

involved because of associated sharing forces (Fig. 8-59).[187] Type 3 fractures account for about 19% of calcaneal fractures, and type 4 and 5 fractures (intraarticular) account for 70% to 75% of calcaneal fractures.[188,194,201]

Type 6 fractures involve the posterior calcaneus, tuberosity, and Achilles tendon. There is extensive posterior soft tissue injury. This injury may be seen in cyclers who catch their heel in the spokes of the wheel.

Routine radiographs in patients with suspected calcaneal fractures should include lateral, oblique, and axial views (Fig. 8-55).[184,194,198,204] Routine views are generally adequate for diagnosis of displaced fractures. Care should be taken to measure Böhler's angle and to assess the degree of articular involvement.[183] The latter problem and the need to detect more subtle injury generally mandate further studies.

Special oblique views for the subtalar joint and anterior process have been described.[186] In the acute setting, fluo-

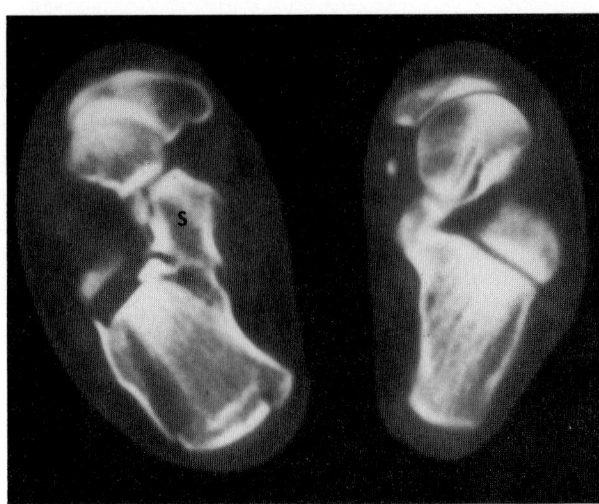

Fig. 8-59 Computed tomogram of a complex fracture of the calcaneus with involvement of the subtalar joint and sustentaculum (S).

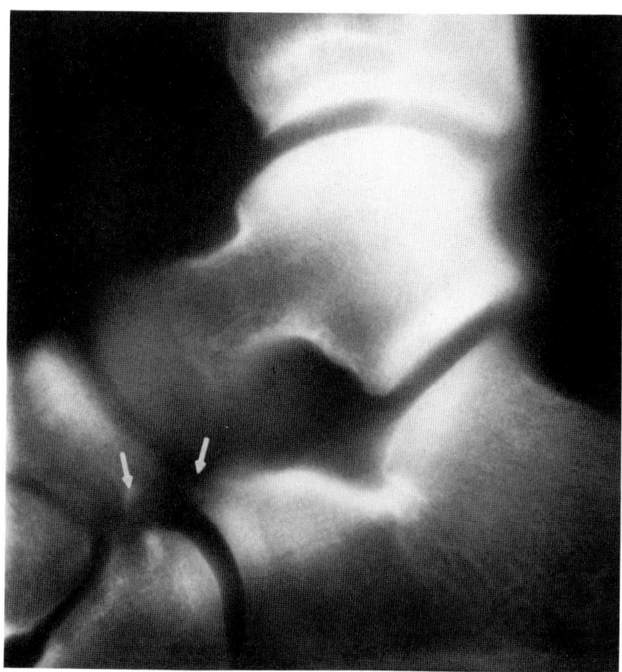

Fig. 8-60 Lateral tomogram demonstrating subtle anterior process and cuboid fractures (arrows) that could not be identified on routine views.

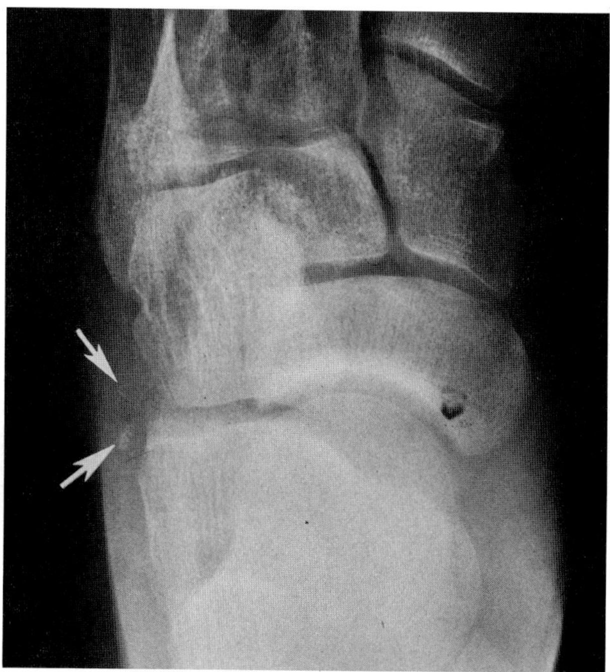

Fig. 8-61 Avulsion fractures of the calcaneocuboid articular margins (arrows) in a basketball player.

roscopically positioned spot views are most easily obtained. Conventional tomography and CT are the techniques of choice in defining more complex fractures and foot anatomy. These techniques are important not only for diagnosis but also to assist in determining the type of therapy.[187,189,194,196,200] Undisplaced type I fractures are frequently missed (Fig. 8-60). Schmidt and Weiner[202] noted that 81% of fractures overlooked radiographically in their series fell into the type I category. These fractures can be easily detected with conventional tomography (Fig. 8-60). Conventional tomograms can also be used in patients with intraarticular fractures. Generally, however, CT is preferred. CT provides advantages in defining joint alignment, detecting intraarticular fragments, and assessing the integrity of the sustentacular portion of the calcaneus. These are key factors in therapy planning.[191,196,203] Soft tissue injury can also be assessed with CT.[187,196,197] When tendon and ligament complications are suspected, however, MRI may provide better information. CT images are more easily reformatted into three-dimensional display than MR images. This needs to be decided before the examination is performed so that 1.5-mm slices can be obtained in the axial and 30° coronal planes.[203]

MIDFOOT AND FOREFOOT INJURIES

Midfoot Fractures and Fracture-Dislocations

The midfoot is made up of the lesser tarsal bones (navicular, cuboid, and three cuneiforms). There is minimal motion in the articulations of these bones, and stability is greater laterally than medially.[221] Additional plantar support is due to stronger ligaments and tendon reinforcement. The major joint (Chopart's joint) is formed by the combination of the talonavicular and the calcaneocuboid articulations.[221,226]

Injuries to the bones and midtarsal joints have been classified by Main and Jowett.[226] Their classification is based on the deforming force and resulting displacement. Five categories of injury are established: medial (30% of injuries), longitudinal (41% of injuries), lateral (17% of injuries), plantar (7% of injuries), and crush (5% of injuries).[221] When forces are applied medially, the following injuries can occur: inversion resulting in dorsal avulsion fractures of the talus (Fig. 8-51) or navicular and the lateral margins of the calcaneus or cuboid (Fig. 8-61), medial subluxation of the forefoot, and rotational dislocation of the talonavicular joint leaving the calcaneocuboid articulation intact. This is less common than subtalar dislocation.[226]

Longitudinal forces cause compression of the metatarsals; forces are transmitted to the cuneiforms, compressing the navicular between the cuneiforms and the talar head. This causes lines of force and fractures to occur parallel to the articular margins of the cuneiforms.[226]

Lateral forces are usually due to falls causing medial distraction, which may lead to avulsion fractures of the navicular or talus, and lateral impaction, which causes compression of the calcaneus and/or cuboid (Fig. 8-62). Lateral subluxation of the talonavicular joint may also occur.[221,226]

Plantar forces result in talonavicular or calcaneocuboid subluxation or dislocation with associated periarticular avul-

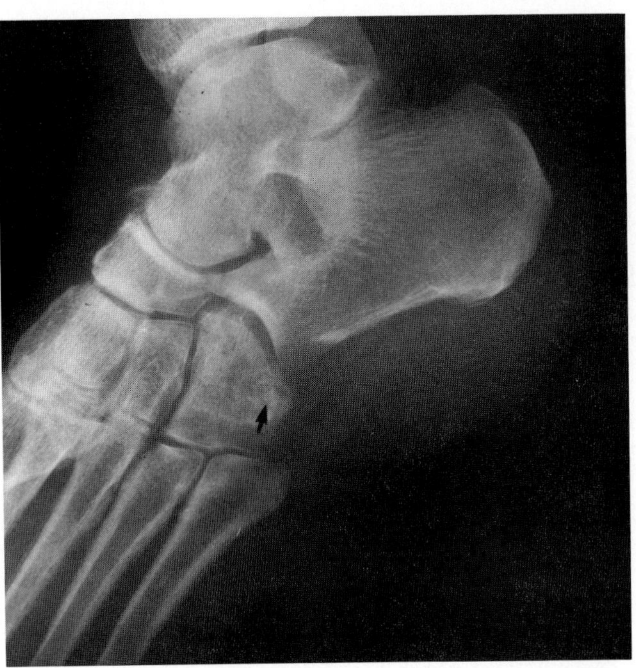

Fig. 8-62 Lateral midfoot injury with an impaction fracture of the cuboid (arrow).

sion fractures (Fig. 8-63). With crush injuries there is no consistent pattern of injury.[221,226]

Isolated fractures of the tarsal bones without associated joint involvement are uncommon.[213] These injuries are especially unusual in children and can only be diagnosed when associated subluxation or dislocation has been excluded.[219–221]

Eichenholtz and Levene[214] described several categories of navicular fracture. In their study, 47% of navicular fractures were avulsions, 29% involved the body, and 24% were tuberosity fractures. Stress fractures are discussed below. Avulsion fractures are caused by twisting or eversion forces, with fragments avulsing as a result of the pull of the talonavicular capsule or anterior fibers of the deltoid. These fractures should not be confused with the well-marginated cortex seen on secondary ossification centers. Tuberosity fractures are also, in a sense, avulsion fractures because again either the posterior tibial tendon or the anterior deltoid fibers are implicated during eversion of the foot.[221] Most body fractures are associated with fracture-dislocations of the midfoot.[221] In children the normal irregularity of the navicular ossification center should not be confused with fracture. Confusion can be avoided by comparison radiographs with the normal extremity and by careful consideration of clinical findings.[219]

Isolated fractures of the cuneiforms and cuboid are uncommon in children and adults.[219,221]

Imaging of the midfoot begins with routine AP, lateral, and oblique views of the foot. In many cases, subtle subluxations, avulsion fractures, or undisplaced fractures are difficult to identify. Main and Jowett[226] reported a delay in diagnosis in more than 41% of patients when routine views were used. One should carefully study the soft tissues. Swelling or hemorrhage that causes distortion of the fat planes may provide a valuable clue to the location of a fracture or subtle subluxation. The articular surfaces of all bones should be parallel (Fig. 8-64).

If routine views are normal or if a questionable area is identified, further studies should be performed. Fluo-

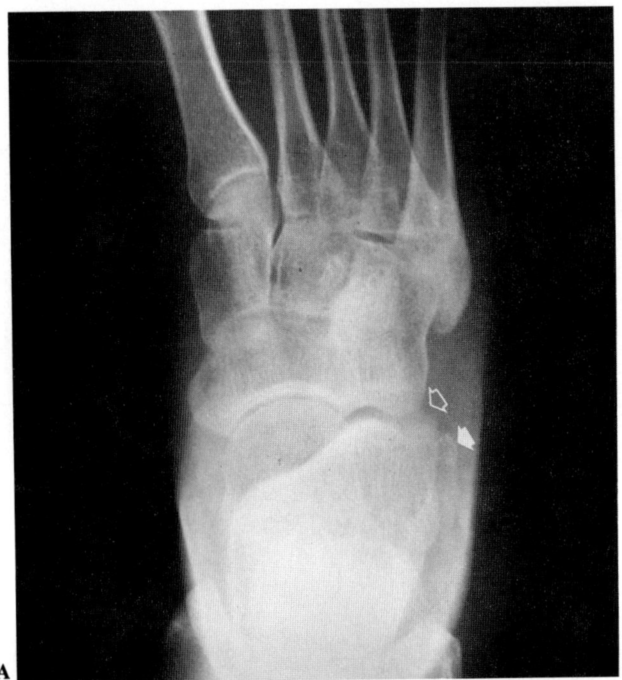

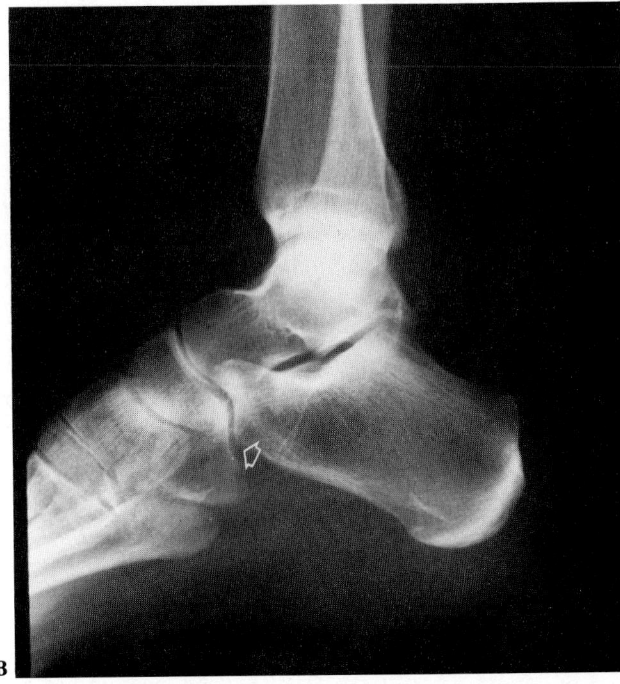

Fig. 8-63 Plantar injury with subluxation (open arrows) and calcaneal avulsion fracture (closed arrow) seen on AP (**A**) and lateral views (**B**).

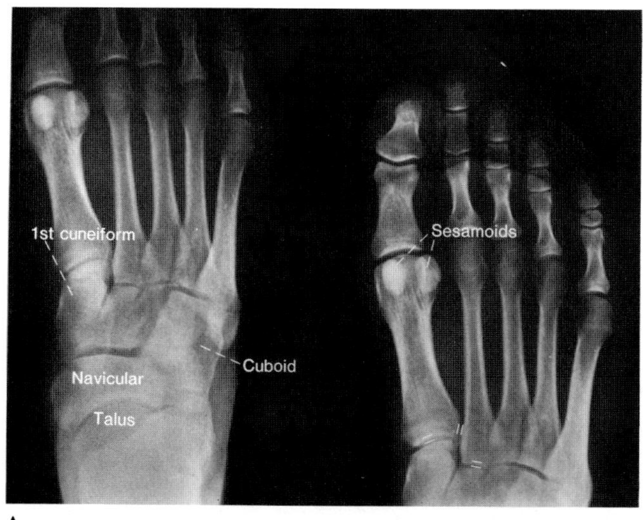

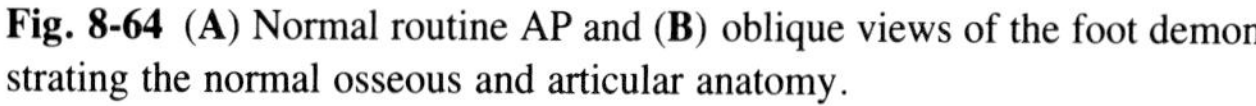

A

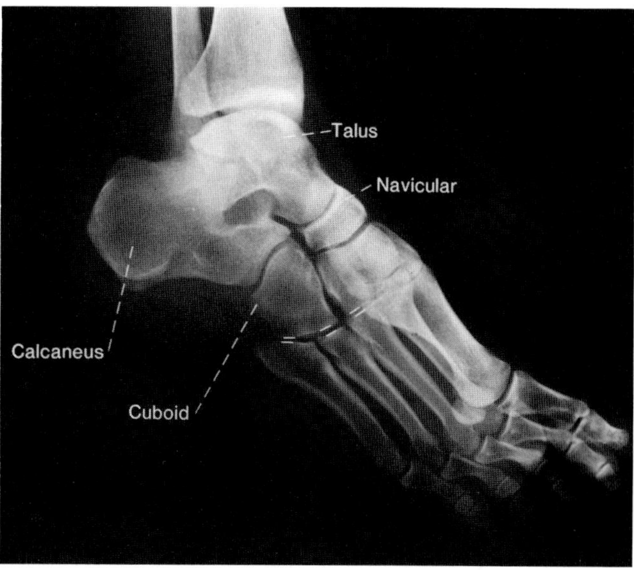

B

Fig. 8-64 (**A**) Normal routine AP and (**B**) oblique views of the foot demonstrating the normal osseous and articular anatomy.

roscopically positioned spot films may be useful in the acute setting and can be performed quickly. Trispiral tomography or CT is especially useful in detection of subtle fractures and articular abnormalities.[218]

Tarsometatarsal Fracture-Dislocations

Tarsometatarsal fracture-dislocations are commonly referred to as Lisfranc injuries. This injury is based on the description of amputation through these joints by a surgeon of the same name during the Napoleonic Wars.[208–210] There is uncertainty as to whether Lisfranc ever described the dislocation, but the joint has become known as Lisfranc's joint because of his surgical description.[212] The injury is uncommon, accounting for less than 1% of fracture-dislocations.[207,215,217]

The four lateral metatarsals (two through five) are connected at the bases by transverse metatarsal ligaments. This is not the case at the base of the first and second metatarsal. Here the transverse ligament is absent. The second metatarsal is situated in a mortise formed by the medial and lateral cuneiform, and its ligamentous support is via the transverse ligament laterally and the medial and second cuneiforms proximally (Fig. 8-65).[207,208,231] The oblique ligament from the medial cuneiform to the base of the second metatarsal is implicated in avulsion fractures of the second metatarsal base. The plantar ligaments and tendons provide more support than the dorsal soft tissues, which explains why most dislocations occur dorsally.[208] The dorsalis pedis artery passes between the proximal first and second metatarsals as it enters the plantar aspect of the foot to form the plantar arch. Therefore, it is susceptible to injuries of fracture-dislocations in this region.[221]

The mechanism of injury is similar in children and adults.[230] Typically, the injury occurs with forced plantar flexion of the forefoot with or without associated rotation (Fig. 8-66).[230,231] This can occur during a fall, such as from an upper bunk (bunkbed fracture in children), or with landing on the toes, which forces the forefoot into plantar flexion. Other mechanisms include falls with the forefoot fixed or compression of the foot due to a heavy object striking the heel when the individual is kneeling (Fig. 8-66). The injury that

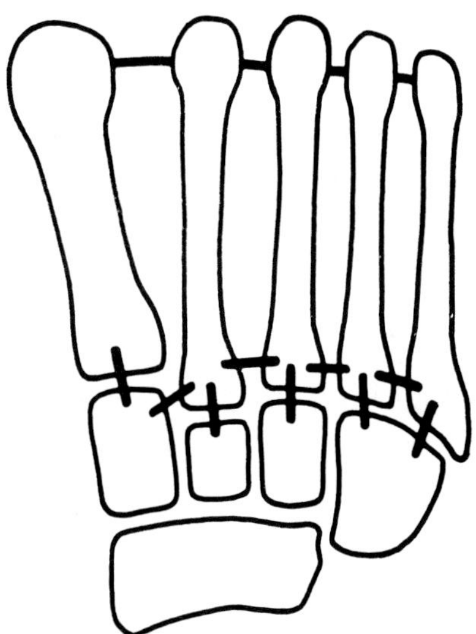

Fig. 8-65 Illustration of bony and ligamentous anatomy of the tarsometatarsal joints. There is no transverse ligament between the first and second metatarsals. The second metatarsal base is situated in a mortise formed by the cuneiforms. *Source:* Reprinted with permission from Wiley JJ, Tarsometatarsal joint injuries in children, *Journal of Pediatric Orthopedics* (1981;1: 255–260), Copyright © 1981, Raven Press.

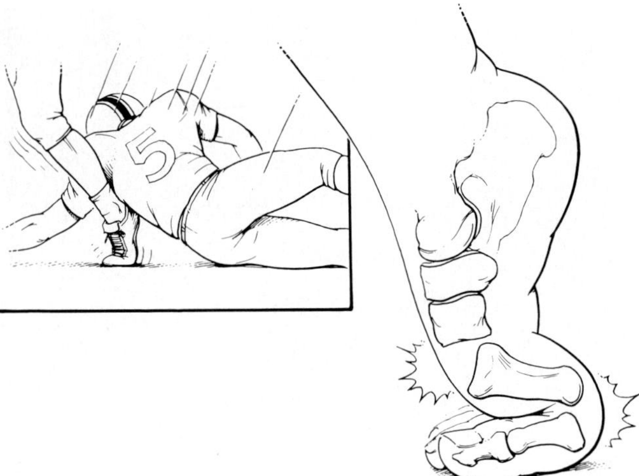

Fig. 8-66 Illustration of the mechanism of Lisfranc injuries in athletes.

occurs takes several different patterns.[207,208,221] The homolateral pattern (total incongruity) occurs when all five metatarsals are displaced. The displacement is almost always in the lateral direction (Fig. 8-67). The alignment of both the first and the second metatarsal bases is abnormal. Fractures of the second metatarsal are common in this pattern because of its position in the mortise formed by the cuneiforms (Fig. 8-66).[207,208,220,230,232] Partial incongruity occurs when the first metatarsal fractures at the base and the shaft displaces medially with associated lateral displacement of the second through fifth metatarsals.[220] A third pattern of injury (divergent) occurs when the base of the first metatarsal subluxes or dislocates medially and the second metatarsal or a combination of the second through fifth metatarsals displaces laterally.[207,208,220,230] The significance of this injury is the associated cuneiform and navicular fracture. Rarely, an isolated tarsometatarsal dislocation can occur.[225]

Radiographic evaluation must start with careful evaluation of the tarsometatarsal relationships. Routine views of the foot are usually sufficient for diagnosis of obvious fracture-dislocations of the tarsometatarsal joint (Fig. 8-67). Subtle ligament injuries may be easily overlooked, however. These injuries may spontaneously reduce, so that nonstress radiographs may appear normal. On the AP view the medial margin of the second metatarsal base should align with the margin of the second cuneiform (Fig. 8-66). The space between the first and second metatarsal bases should be assessed, but this is less useful than the foregoing relationship.[216] The lateral margins of the first metatarsal and cuneiform should align, however. The medial base of the fourth metatarsal should align with the medial margin of the cuboid (Fig. 8-66). The bases of the remaining metatarsals are more difficult to evaluate because of bony overlap and the overlapping tuberosity of the fifth metatarsal. The metatarsal bases should be parallel to the tarsal articular surfaces, however.[216,227,228] On the lateral view the second metatarsal and cuneiform should be aligned such that an uninterrupted line can be drawn along their dorsal surfaces.

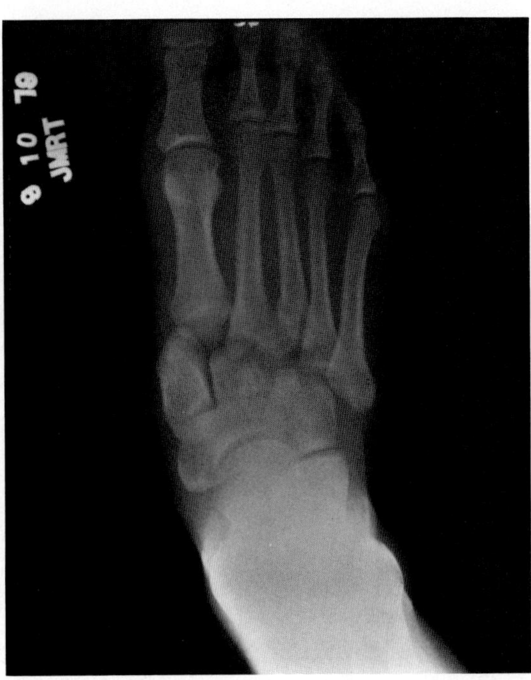

Fig. 8-67 AP view of the foot demonstrating total incongruity with lateral dislocation of all five metatarsals.

In children, care must be taken that subtle fractures of the first metatarsal base are not overlooked. This injury is associated with ligamentous disruption, and the subtle first metatarsal fracture may be the only clue radiographically (Fig. 8-68). Comparison views with the uninvolved foot are useful in children.[222]

On occasion, fluoroscopically positioned spot views or stress views may be indicated to detect subtle ligament injury. Conventional tomography or CT can also be useful to evaluate more fully the bony relationships and to exclude cuneiform and navicular fractures.[218]

Metatarsal and Phalangeal Fractures

Metatarsal fractures are common in adults and children. Injuries are usually the result of direct trauma (being stepped on by an opponent). Twisting or shearing injuries, however, may also lead to fracture.[208,219,221] The neck of the metatarsal is weaker than the shaft, which explains the higher incidence of fractures at this location, especially in children.[219] Patients generally present with pain, swelling, and ecchymosis over the injured metatarsals. Fractures may be incomplete (torus or greenstick) in children (Fig. 8-69). In adults, complete fractures are most common.[208,219]

Fractures of the fifth metatarsal base are common in children and adults. Two basic fracture patterns with different prognoses can be distinguished. Avulsion of the proximal tuberosity is most common. This is due to an abrupt pull of the peroneus brevis. The adductor digiti minimi and lateral cord of the plantar fascia also insert on the fifth metatarsal base.[219]

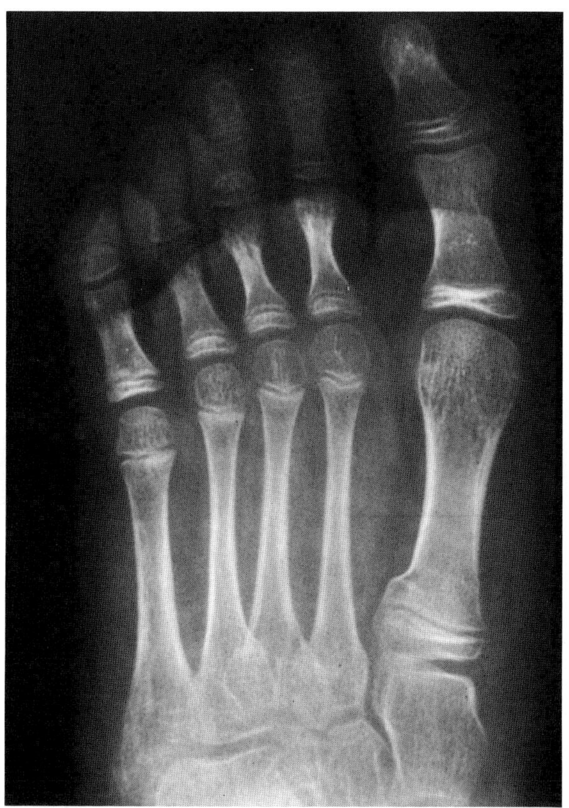

Fig. 8-68 Lisfranc injury with a subtle torus fracture of the first metatarsal base.

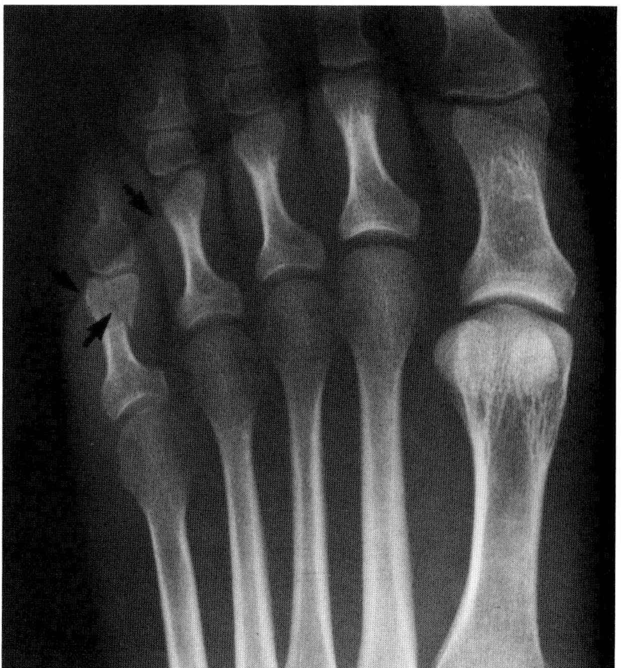

Fig. 8-69 Oblique intraarticular fracture of the fifth proximal phalanx. The skin fold (arrows) should not be mistaken for a fracture line.

This fracture must be distinguished from the normal tuberosity in children (Fig. 8-70). The growth plate runs parallel to the shaft, whereas fractures will be perpendicular to the shaft (Fig. 8-70B). Avulsion of the epiphyses is uncommon, but if avulsion is suspected comparison with the normal extremity should be performed. Differentiation of this fracture from the os peroneum or os vesalianum is usually not difficult because of the smooth cortical margins of the latter.

The second type of fifth metatarsal base fracture is often referred to as the Jones fracture.[223,224,229] This fracture involves the proximal diaphysis or metaphysis (Fig. 8-71). Treatment of this fracture can be difficult and may require internal fixation.[211]

Phalangeal fractures occur when the bare toe strikes a hard object or when a heavy object lands on the toe. Most fractures are minimally displaced. Care must be taken to evaluate all radiographs, or these fractures may be overlooked. It is important to determine whether fractures are intraarticular (Fig. 8-69).

Dislocations of the metatarsophalangeal and interphalangeal joints may be isolated or associated with fracture. Metatarsophalangeal dislocations are usually due to hyperextension with the proximal phalanx forced dorsally over the metatarsal, tearing the plantar capsule.[208] The great toe is most commonly involved. Medial and lateral dislocations are

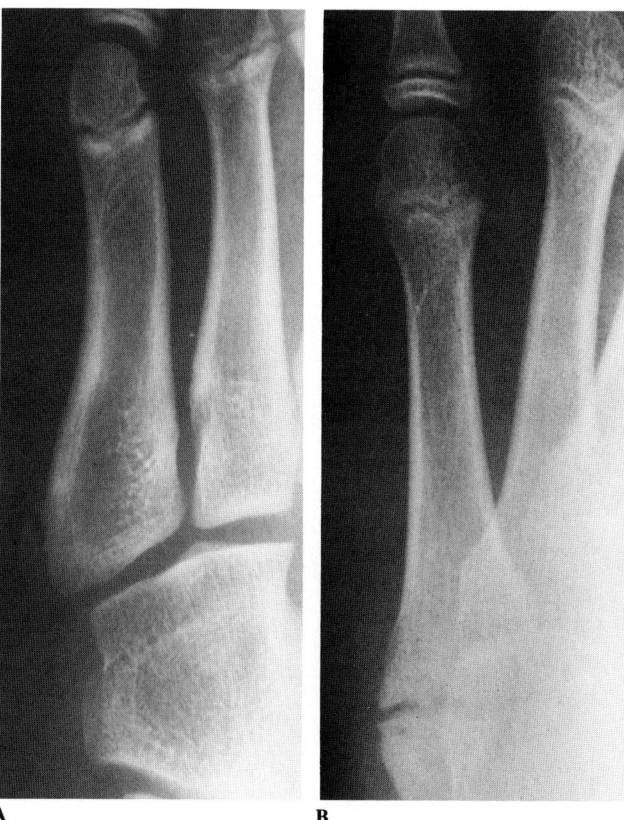

A B

Fig. 8-70 (**A**) Normal AP view of the fifth metatarsal. The epiphysis and physis are parallel to the shaft. (**B**) Transverse fracture of the fifth metatarsal base.

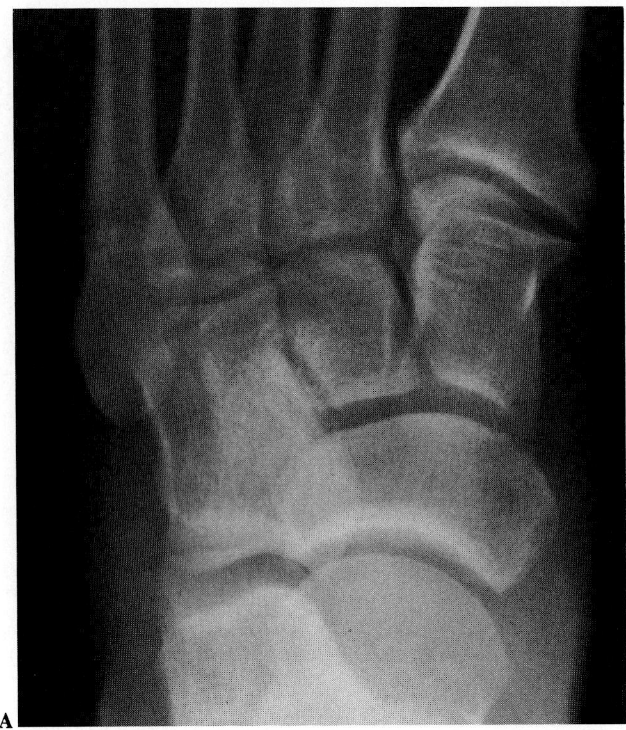

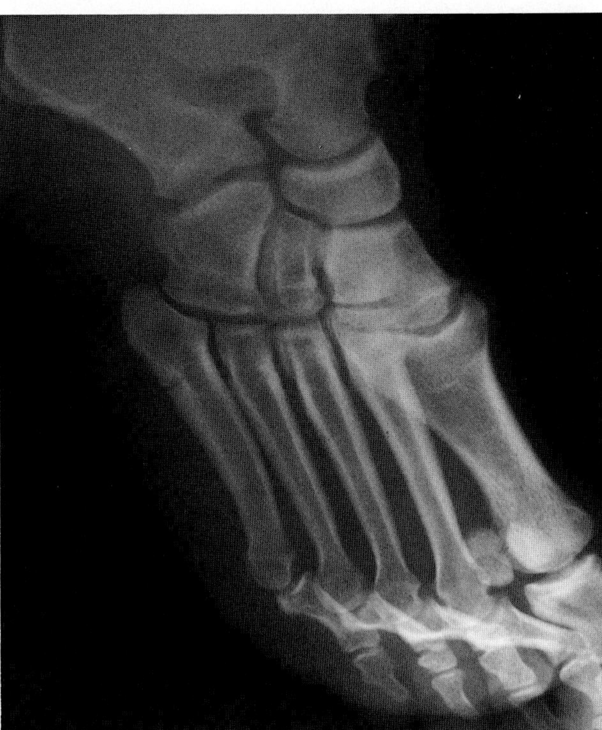

Fig. 8-71 (**A**) AP and (**B**) oblique views of the foot demonstrating a Jones fracture.

less common (Fig. 8-72). Similar forces lead to dislocations of the interphalangeal joints.

AP, oblique, and lateral radiographs of the foot are routinely obtained. The AP and oblique views are most useful because bony overlap makes evaluation more difficult on the lateral view (Fig. 8-71). The lateral view is useful in determining fracture angulation and the direction of dislocations. After reduction of dislocations, it is important to obtain the same views to be certain that there is no associated fracture or soft tissue interposition (wide joint space). Tomography is useful on occasion, especially for sesamoid fractures (Fig. 8-73).[233]

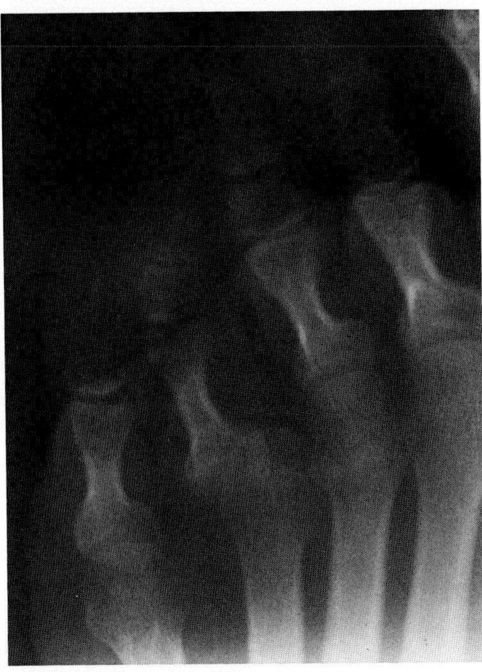

Fig. 8-72 AP view of the foot demonstrating lateral dislocation of the fourth metatarsophalangeal joint.

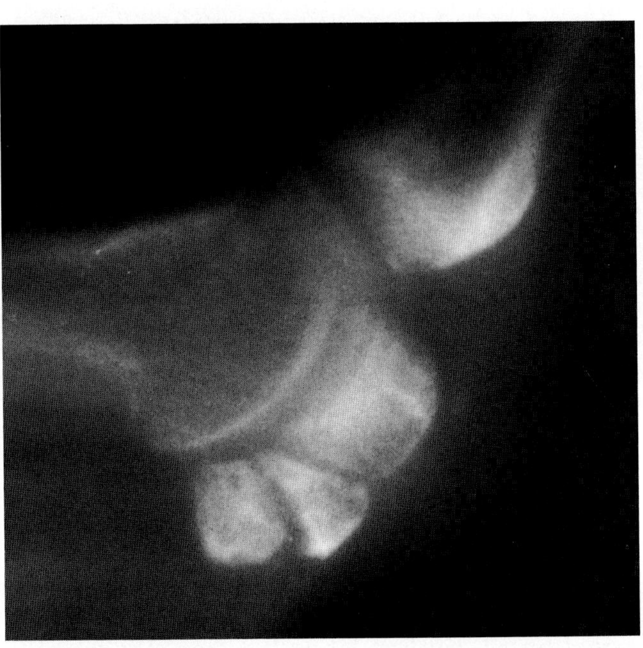

Fig. 8-73 Lateral tomogram demonstrating a sesamoid fracture.

STRESS FRACTURES

Stress fractures are discussed thoroughly in Chapter 12. These injuries are particularly common in the foot and can involve the calcaneus, midfoot, and metatarsals. Radionuclide scans are useful for detection of early stress fractures and for localizing subtle fractures for radiographic evaluation (Fig. 8-32).[223]

REFERENCES

Introduction

1. Backx FJG, Erich WBM, Kemper ABA, Verbeek ALM. Sports injuries in school-aged children. *Am J Sports Med.* 1989;17:234–240.

2. Cass JR, Morrey BF. Ankle instability: current concepts, diagnosis and treatment. *Mayo Clin Proc.* 1984;59:165–170.

3. Garrick JG, Requa RK. The epidemiology of foot and ankle injuries. *Clin Sports Med.* 1988;7:29–36.

4. Halpern B, Thompson N, Curl WW, Andrews JR, Hunter SC, Boring JR. High school football injuries: identifying the risk factors. *Am J Sports Med.* 1987;15:113–117.

5. Kuist M, Kujala UM, Heinonen OJ, et al. Sports-related injuries in children. *Int J Sports Med.* 1989;10:81–86.

6. Matheson GO, MacIntyre JG, Taugton JE, Clement DB, Lloyd-Smith R. Musculoskeletal injuries associated with physical activity in older adults. *Med Sci Sports Exerc.* 1989;21:379–385.

7. Mattalino AJ, Deese M, Campbell ED. Office evaluation and treatment of lower extremity injuries in the runner. *Clin Sports Med.* 1989; 8:461–475.

8. Paty JG. Diagnosis and treatment of musculoskeletal running injuries. *Semin Arthritis Rheum.* 1988;18:48–60.

9. Rothenberger LA, Chang JI, Cable TA. Prevalence and types of injuries in aerobic dancers. *Am J Sports Med.* 1988;16:403–407.

10. Wong JC, Gregg JR. Knee, ankle and foot problems in the preadolescent and adolescent athlete. *Clin Podiatr Med Surg.* 1986;3:731–745.

Anatomy

11. Anderson JE. *Grant's Atlas of Anatomy.* 8th ed. Baltimore: Williams & Wilkins; 1983.

12. Berquist TH. *MRI of the Musculoskeletal System.* New York: Raven; 1990.

13. Berquist TH. *Radiology of the Foot and Ankle.* New York: Raven; 1989.

14. Burman MS, Lapidus DW. The functional disturbances caused by inconsistent bones and sesamoids of the foot. *Arch Surg.* 1931;22:936–975.

15. Clemente CD. *Gray's Anatomy of the Human Body.* 13th ed. Philadelphia: Lea & Febiger; 1985.

16. Dunn AW. Anomalous muscles simulating soft tissue tumors of the lower extremities. *J Bone Joint Surg Am.* 1965;47:1397–1400.

17. Georgen TG, Danzig LA, Resnick D, Owen CA. Roentgen evaluation of the tibiotalar joint. *J Bone Joint Surg Am.* 1977;59:874–877.

18. Hollinshead HW. *Anatomy for Surgeons.* 3rd ed. New York: Harper & Row; 1982;3.

19. Jahss MH. *Disorders of the Foot.* Philadelphia: Saunders; 1982.

20. Jonsson K, Fredin HO, Cederlund CG, Bauer M. Width of the normal ankle joint. *Acta Radiol.* 1984;25:147–149.

21. Kelikian H, Kelikian AS. *Disorders of the Ankle.* Philadelphia: Saunders; 1985.

22. Lauge-Hansen N. Fractures of the ankle. Analytical historical survey as basis of a new experimental roentgenologic and clinical investigation. *Arch Surg.* 1948;56:259–317.

23. Lauge-Hansen N. Fractures of the ankle. II. Combined experimental-surgical and experimental-roentgenological investigation. *Arch Surg.* 1950;60:959–985.

24. Leung RC, Wong WL. The vessels of the 1st metatarsal web space. An operative and radiographic study. *J Bone Joint Surg Am.* 1983; 65:235–238.

25. McDougall A. The os trigonum. *J Bone Joint Surg Br.* 1955; 37:256–265.

26. Morrey BF, Cass JR, Johnson KA, Berquist TH. The foot and ankle. In: Berquist TH, ed. *Imaging of Orthopedic Trauma.* 2nd ed. New York: Raven; 1991:453–577.

27. Mukherjee SK, Pringle RM, Baxter AD. Fracture of the lateral process of the talus. *J Bone Joint Surg Br.* 1974;56:263–273.

28. O'Rahilly R. A survey of tarsal and carpal anomalies. *J Bone Joint Surg Am.* 1953;35:626–641.

29. Resnick D. Radiology of the talocalcaneal articulations. *Radiology.* 1974;111:581–586.

30. Steel M, Johnson KA, Dewitz MA. Radiographic measurements of the normal adult foot. *Foot Ankle.* 1980;1:151–158.

31. Sutherland DH, Cooper L, Daniel D. The role of plantar flexors in normal walking. *J Bone Joint Surg Am.* 1980;62:354–363.

32. Venning P. Radiologic studies of variation in ossification of the foot. III. Cone shaped epiphysis of the proximal phalanges. *Am J Phys Anthropol.* 1961;19:131–136.

33. Weissman SD. *Radiology of the Foot.* Baltimore: Williams & Wilkins; 1983.

Soft Tissue Trauma

34. Abraham E, Sternaman JE. Neglected rupture of the peroneal tendon causing recurrent sprains of the ankle. *J Bone Joint Surg Am.* 1979; 61:1247–1248.

35. Ala-Ketola L, Peranen J, Kovivisto E, Puupera M. Arthrography in the diagnosis of ligament injuries and classifications of ankle injuries. *Radiology.* 1977;125:63–68.

36. Andrews JR. Overuse syndromes of the lower extremity. *Clin Sports Med.* 1983;2:137–148.

37. Baxter DE, Thigpen CM. Heel pain. Operative results. *Foot Ankle.* 1984;5:16–25.

38. Berkowitz JF, Kier R, Radicel S. Plantar fasciitis: MR imaging. *Radiology.* 1991;179:665–667.

39. Berquist TH. *MRI of the Musculoskeletal System.* New York: Raven; 1990.

40. Berquist TH. *Radiology of the Foot and Ankle.* New York: Raven; 1989.

41. Black HM, Brand RL, Eichelberger MR. An improved technique for the evaluation of ligamentous injury in severe ankle sprains. *Am J Sports Med.* 1978;6:276–282.

42. Blanchard KS, Finlay DBL, Scott DJA, Ley CC, Siggins D, Allen MJ. A radiological analysis of lateral ligament injuries of the ankle. *Clin Radiol.* 1986;37:247–251.

43. Blei CL, Nirschl RP, Grant EG. Achilles tendon: US diagnosis of pathologic conditions. *Radiology.* 1986;159:765–767.

44. Bonutti PM, Bell GR. Compartment syndrome of the foot. *J Bone Joint Surg Am.* 1986;68:1449–1450.

45. Brand RL, Collins MDF. Operative management of ligamentous injuries to the ankle. *Clin Sports Med.* 1982;1:117–130.

46. Brown JE. The sinus tarsi syndrome. *Clin Orthop.* 1960;18:231–233.

47. Cass JR, Morrey BF. Ankle instability: current concepts, diagnosis, and treatment. *Mayo Clin Proc.* 1984;59:165–170.

48. Church CC. Radiographic diagnosis of acute peroneal tendon dislocation. *AJR.* 1977;129:1065–1068.

49. Cox JS, Hewes TF. Normal talar tilt angle. *Clin Orthop.* 1979; 140:37–41.

50. Daffner RH, Riemer BL, Lupetin AR, Dash N. Magnetic resonance imaging in acute tendon ruptures. *Skeletal Radiol.* 1980;15:619–621.

51. Davies JAK. Peroneal compartment syndrome secondary to rupture of the peroneus longus. *J Bone Joint Surg Am.* 1979;61:783–784.

52. Dezwart DF, Davidson JSA. Rupture of the posterior tibial tendon associated with ankle fractures. *J Bone Joint Surg Am.* 1983;65:260–261.

53. Dokter G, Lundaw LA. The accessory soleus muscle: symptomatic soft tissue tumor or accidental finding. *Neth J Surg.* 1981;33:146–149.

54. Dory MA. Arthrography of the ankle joint in chronic instability. *Skeletal Radiol.* 1986;15:291–294.

55. Edwards GS, DeLee JC. Ankle diastasis without fracture. *Foot Ankle.* 1984;4:305–312.

56. Evans GA, Frenyo SD. The stress-tenogram in diagnosis of ruptures of the lateral ligament of the ankle. *J Bone Joint Surg Br.* 1979;61:347–351.

57. Fetto JF. Anatomy and physical examination of the foot and ankle. In: Nicholas JA, Hershman EB, eds. *The Lower Extremity and Spine in Sports Medicine.* St Louis, MO: Mosby; 1986:371–395.

58. Fornage BD. Achilles tendon: US examination. *Radiology.* 1986;159:759–764.

59. Funk DA, Cass JA, Johnson KA. Acquired adult flatfoot secondary to posterior tibial-tendon pathology. *J Bone Joint Surg Am.* 1986;68:95–102.

60. Garth WP. Flexor hallucis tendonitis in a ballet dancer. *J Bone Joint Surg Am.* 1981;63:1489.

61. Gilula LA, Oloff L, Caputi R, Destouet JM, Jacobs A, Solomon MA. Ankle tenography: a key to unexplained symptomatology. Part II: diagnosis of chronic tendon disabilities. *Radiology.* 1984;151:581–587.

62. Goergen TG, Resnick D. Arthrography of the ankle and hindfoot. In: Dalinka MK, ed. *Arthrography.* New York: Springer-Verlag; 1980:137–153.

63. Horsfield D, Murphy G. Stress views of the ankle joint in lateral ligament injury. *Radiography.* 1985;51:7–11.

64. Inglis AE, Scott N, Sculo TP, Patterson AH. Rupture of the tendo Achilles: an objective assessment of surgical and non-surgical treatment. *J Bone Joint Surg Am.* 1976;58:990–993.

65. Johannsen A. Radiologic diagnosis of lateral ligament lesion of the ankle. *Acta Orthop Scand.* 1978;49:295–301.

66. Jozsa L, Kvist M, Balint BJ, et al. The role of recreational sport activity in Achilles tendon rupture. *Am J Sports Med.* 1959;17:338–343.

67. Kelikian H, Kelikian AS. *Disorders of the Ankle.* Philadelphia: Saunders; 1985.

68. Kier R, McCarthy S, Dietz MJ, Rudicel S. MR appearance of painful conditions of the ankle. *RadioGraphics.* 1991;11:401–414.

69. Kleiger B. The posterior tibiotalar impingement syndrome in dancers. *Bull Hosp Joint Dis Orthop Inst.* 1987;47:203–210.

70. Kleinman M, Gross AE. Achilles tendon rupture following steroid injection. *J Bone Joint Surg Am.* 1983;65:1345–1347.

71. Kvist M, Jozsa L, Jarvinen MJ, Kvist H. Chronic Achilles paratendonitis in athletes. *Pathology.* 1987;19:1–11.

72. Laine HR, Harjula ALJ, Peltokallio P. Ultrasonography as a differential diagnostic aid in achillodynia. *J Ultrasound Med.* 1987;6:351–362.

73. Larson E. Experimental instability of the ankle: a radiographic investigation. *Clin Orthop.* 1986;204:193–200.

74. Leach RE. Leg and foot injuries in racquet sports. *Clin Sports Med.* 1988;4:359–370.

75. Leach RE, Jones R, Silva T. Rupture of the plantar fascia in athletes. *J Bone Joint Surg Am.* 1978;60:537–539.

76. Lillich JS, Baxter DE. Common forefoot problems in runners. *Foot Ankle.* 1986;7:145–151.

77. Liou J, Totty WG. Magnetic resonance imaging of ankle injuries. *Top Magn Resonance Imaging.* 1991;3:1–22.

78. Mann RA, Thompson FM. Rupture of the posterior tibial tendon causing flat foot. *J Bone Joint Surg Am.* 1985;67:556–561.

79. Marinacci AA. Neurological deficit syndromes of the tarsal tunnel. *Bull Los Ang Neurol Soc.* 1968;33:90–100.

80. Marshall P. The rehabilitation of overuse foot injuries in athletes and dancers. *Clin Podiatr Med Surg.* 1989;6:639–655.

81. Mattalino AJ, Deese M, Campbell ED. Office evaluation and treatment of lower extremity injuries in runners. *Clin Sports Med.* 1989; 8:461–475.

82. McConkey JP, Favero KJ. Subluxation of the peroneal tendons within the peroneal tendon sheath. *Am J Sports Med.* 1987;15:511–513.

83. Morrey BF, Cass TR, Johnson KA, Berquist TH. Foot and ankle. In: Berquist TH, ed. *Imaging of Orthopedic Trauma.* New York: Raven; 1991.

84. Morti R. Dislocation of the peroneal tendon. *Am J Sports Med.* 1977;5:19–22.

85. Murr S. Dislocation of the peroneal tendon with marginal fracture of the lateral malleolus. *J Bone Joint Surg Br.* 1965;43:563–565.

86. Newmark H, Olken SM, Mellon WS, Malhotra AK, Halls J. A new finding in radiographic diagnosis of Achilles tendon rupture. *Skeletal Radiol.* 1982;8:223–224.

87. O'Connor D. Sinus tarsi syndrome. A clinical entity. *J Bone Joint Surg Am.* 1958;40:720.

88. Paty JG. Diagnosis and treatment of musculoskeletal running injuries. *Semin Arthritis Rheum.* 1988;18:48–60.

89. Rettig AC, Shelbournek D, Beltz HF, Robertson DW, Afken P. Radiographic evaluation of foot and ankle injuries in athletes. *Clin Sports Med.* 1987;6:905–919.

90. Romanus B, Lundahl S, Stener B. Accessory soleus muscle: a clinical and radiographic presentation of 11 cases. *J Bone Joint Surg Am.* 1986; 68:731–734.

91. Rosenberg ZS, Feldman F, Singson RD. Peroneal tendon injuries: CT analysis. *Radiology.* 1986;161:743–748.

92. Rosenberg ZS, Feldman F, Singson RD, Price GJ. Peroneal tendon injury associated with calcaneal fractures. CT findings. *AJR.* 1987; 149:125–129.

93. Rzonci EG, Baylis WJ. Common sports injuries to the foot and leg. *Clin Podiatr Med Surg.* 1988;5:591–612.

94. Sauser DD, Nelson RC, Lavine MH, Wu CW. Acute injuries of the lateral ligaments of the ankle: comparison of stress radiography and arthrography. *Radiology.* 1983;148:653–657.

95. Schweigel JF, Knickerbacker WJ, Cooperberg P. A study of ankle instability utilizing ankle arthrography. *J Trauma.* 1977;17:878–881.

96. Simon RR, Hoffman JR, Smith M. Radiographic comparison of plain films on second- and third-degree ankle sprains. *Am J Emerg Med.* 1986;4:387–389.

97. Smart GW, Taunton JE, Clement DB. Achilles tendon disorders in runners. A review. *Med Sci Sports Exerc.* 1980;12:231–243.

98. Smith RW, Reischl SF. Metatarsophalangeal joint synovitis in athletes. *Clin Sports Med.* 1988;7:75–88.

99. Spiegel PK, Staples OS. Arthrography of the ankle joint: problems in diagnosis of acute lateral leg injuries. *Radiology.* 1975;114:587–590.

100. Stein RE. Rupture of the posterior tibial tendon in closed ankle fractures. *J Bone Joint Surg Am.* 1985;67:493–494.

101. Szczukowski M, St Pierre RK, Fleming LL, Somogyi J. Computerized tomography in the evaluation of peroneal tendon dislocation. A report of two cases. *Am J Sports Med.* 1983;11:444–447.

102. Tehranzadeh J, Stoll DA, Gabriele OM. Case report 271: posterior migration of the os peroneum of the left foot, indicating a tear of the peroneal tendon. *Skeletal Radiol.* 1984;12:44–47.

103. Termansen NB, Hansen H, Damvolt V. Radiologic and muscular status following injury to the lateral ligaments of the ankle. *Acta Orthop Scand.* 1979;50:705–708.

104. Warren BL, Jones CJ. Predicting plantar fasciitis in runners. *Med Sci Sports Exerc.* 1987;19:71–73.

Ankle Fractures

105. Arimoto HR, Forrester DM. Classification of ankle fractures: an algorithm. *AJR*. 1980;135:1057–1063.

106. Ashhurst APC, Bromer RS. Classification and mechanism of fractures of the leg bones involving the ankle. *Arch Surg*. 1922;4:51–129.

107. Berquist TH. *Radiology of the Foot and Ankle*. New York: Raven; 1989.

108. Carothers CO, Crenshaw AH. Clinical significance of a classification of epiphyseal injuries of the ankle. *Am J Surg*. 1955;89:879–889.

109. Cone RO, Ngugen V, Flournoy JG, Guerra J. Triplane fracture of the distal tibia epiphysis: radiologic and CT studies. *Radiology*. 1984; 153:763–767.

110. Cooperman DR, Spiegel PG, Laros SG. Tibial fractures involving the ankle in children. *J Bone Joint Surg Am*. 1978;60:1040–1045.

111. Crenshaw AH. Injuries of the distal tibial epiphysis. *Clin Orthop*. 1965;41:98–107.

112. DeZwart DF, Davidson JSA. Rupture of the posterior tibial tendon associated with fractures of the ankle. *J Bone Joint Surg Am*. 1983; 65:260–262.

113. Dias LS. Fractures of the tibia and fibula. In: Rockwood CA, Wilkins KE, King RE, eds. *Fractures in Children*. Philadelphia: Lippincott; 1984;3:983–1042.

114. Dias LS, Giegerich CR. Fractures of the distal tibia epiphysis in adolescence. *J Bone Joint Surg Am*. 1983;65:438–444.

115. Dihlman W. Computed tomography of the ankle joint. *Chirurg*. 1982;53:123–126.

116. Genant HK, Kozin F, Bekerman C, McCarty DJ, Sims J. The reflex sympathetic dystrophy syndrome. *Radiology*. 1975;117:21–32.

117. Goldberg VM, Aadalen R. Distal tibial epiphyseal injuries: the role of athletics in 53 cases. *Am J Sports Med*. 1978;6:263–268.

118. Griffiths HJ. Trauma to the ankle and foot. *CRC Crit Rev Diagn Imaging*. 1979;26:45–105.

119. Kleiger B, Mankin JJ. Fracture of the lateral portion of the distal tibial epiphysis. *J Bone Joint Surg Am*. 1964;46:25.

120. Larson RL. Epiphyseal injuries in the adolescent. *Orthop Clin North Am*. 1973;4:839–851.

121. Lauge-Hansen N. Fractures of the ankle II: combined experimental-surgical once experimental roentgenologic investigations. *Arch Surg*. 1950;60:957–985.

122. Leach RE. Fractures of the tibia and fibula. In: Rockwood CA, Green DP, eds. *Fractures in Adults*. Philadelphia: Lippincott; 1984;2:1593–1663.

123. Lynn MD. The triplane distal tibial epiphyseal fracture. *Clin Orthop*. 1972;86:187–190.

124. Montague AP, McQuillan RF. Clinical assessment of apparently sprained ankle and detection of fracture. *Injury*. 1985;16:545–546.

125. Morrey BF,Cass JR, Johnson KA, Berquist TH. *Imaging of Orthopedic Trauma*. New York: Raven; 1991.

126. Olerud C. Supination-eversion ankle fractures sustained during downhill skiing. *Acta Orthop Trauma Surg*. 1985;104:129–131.

127. Ovadia DN, Beals RK. Fractures of the tibial plafond. *J Bone Joint Surg Am*. 1986;68:543–551.

128. Peiro A, Araal J, Mortos F, Mut T. Triplane distal tibial epiphyseal fracture. *Clin Orthop*. 1981;160:196–200.

129. Poplawski ZJ, Wiley AM, Murry JF. Post-traumatic dystrophy of the extremities. *J Bone Joint Surg Am*. 1983;66:642–654.

130. Rettig AC, Shelbourne KD, Beltz HF, Robertson DW, Arfken P. Radiographic evaluation of foot and ankle injuries in the athlete. *Clin Sports Med*. 1987;6:905–919.

131. Rogers LF. Radiology of epiphyseal injuries. *Radiology*. 1970;96:289–299.

132. Salter RB, Harris WR. Injuries involving the epiphyseal plate. *J Bone Joint Surg Am*. 1963;45:587–622.

133. Shelbourne KD, Fisher DA, Rettig AC, McCarroll JR. Stress fractures of the medial malleolus. *Am J Sports Med*. 1988;16:60–63.

134. Spiegel PG, Cooperman DR, Laros GS. Epiphyseal fractures of the distal ends of the tibia and fibula. *J Bone Joint Surg Am*. 1978;60:1046–1050.

135. Torg JS, Baldini FC, Zelko RR, Pavlov H, Piff TC, Dos M. Fractures of the fifth metatarsal distal to the tuberosity. *J Bone Joint Surg Am*. 1984;66:209–214.

136. Towbin R, Dimbar JS, Towbin J. Teardrop sign: plain film recognition of ankle effusion. *AJR*. 1980;134:985–990.

137. Wilson FC. Fractures and dislocations of the ankle. In: Rockwood CA, Green DP, eds. *Fractures in Adults*. Philadelphia: Lippincott; 1984;2:1665–1702.

138. Wong JC, Gregg JR. Knee, ankle and foot problems in the preadolescent and adolescent athlete. *Clin Podiatr Med Surg*. 1986;3:731–745.

139. Yde J. The Lauge-Hansen classification of malleolar fractures. *Acta Orthop Scand*. 1980;51:181–192.

140. Yde J, Kristensen KD. Ankle fractures: supination eversion fractures of stage IV. *Acta Orthop Scand*. 1980;51:981–990.

141. Yde J, Kristensen KD. Ankle fractures: supination eversion fractures stage II. Primary and late operative and non-operative treatment. *Acta Orthop Scand*. 1980;51:695–702.

Talar Fractures and Dislocations

142. Alexander AH, Lichtman DM. Surgical treatment of transchondral talar dome fractures. *J Bone Joint Surg Am*. 1980;62:646–652.

143. Berndt AL, Harty M. Transchondral fractures (osteochondritis dissecans) of the talus. *J Bone Joint Surg Am*. 1959;41:988–1020.

144. Berquist TH. *MRI of the Musculoskeletal System*. 2nd ed. New York: Raven; 1990.

145. Berquist TH. *Radiology of the Foot and Ankle*. New York: Raven; 1989.

146. Blair HC. Comminuted fractures and fracture dislocations of the body of the talus. *Am J Surg*. 1943;59:37–43.

147. Bonnin JG. *Injuries of the Ankle*. New York: Grune & Stratton; 1950.

148. Burkus JK, Sella FJ, Southwick WO. Occult injuries of the talus diagnosed by bone scan and tomography. *Foot Ankle*. 1984;4:316–324.

149. Canale ST, Belding RH. Osteochondral lesions of the talus. *J Bone Joint Surg Am*. 1980;62:97–102.

150. Canale ST, Kelly FB. Fractures of the neck and the talus. *J Bone Joint Surg Am*. 1978;60:143–156.

151. Coltart WD. Aviators astragalus. *J Bone Joint Surg Br*. 1952; 34:545–566.

152. DeLee J, Curtis R. Subtalar dislocation of the foot. *J Bone Joint Surg Am*. 1982;64:433–437.

153. DeSmet AA, Fisher DA, Burnstein MI, Graf BK, Lange RH. Value of MR imaging in staging osteochondral lesions of the talus (osteochondritis dissecans): results in 14 patients. *AJR*. 1990;154:555–558.

154. Detenbeck LC, Kelly PJ. Total dislocation of the talus. *J Bone Joint Surg Am*. 1969;51:283–288.

155. El-Koury GY, Yousefzadek DH, Mulligan GM, Moore TE. Subtalar dislocation. *Skeletal Radiol*. 1982;8:99–103.

156. Flick AB, Gould N. Osteochondritis dissecans of the talus: review of the literature and a new surgical approach for medial dome lesions. *Foot Ankle*. 1985;5:165–185.

157. Floyd FJ, Ransom RA, Dailey JM. Computed tomography scanning of the subtalar joint. *J Am Podiatr Assoc*. 1984;14:533–537.

158. Gross RH. Fractures and dislocations of the foot. In: Rockwood CA, Wilkins KE, Kuig RE, eds. *Fractures in Children*. Philadelphia: Lippincott; 1984;3:1043–1103.

159. Hawkins LG. Fractures of the lateral process of the talus. *J Bone Joint Surg Am.* 1965;47:1170–1175.

160. Hawkins LG. Fractures of the neck of the talus. *J Bone Joint Surg Am.* 1970;52:991–1002.

161. Heckman JD. Fractures and dislocations of the foot. In: Rockwood CA, Green DP, eds. *Fractures in Adults* 2nd ed. Philadelphia: Lippincott; 1984:1703–1832.

162. Hontas MJ, Haddad RJ, Schlesinger LC. Conditions of the talus in runners. *Am J Sports Med.* 1986;14:486–490.

163. Kelikian H, Kelikian AS. *Disorders of the Ankle*. Philadelphia: Saunders; 1985.

164. Kleiger B, Ahmed M. Injuries of the talus and its joints. *Clin Orthop.* 1976;121:243–262.

165. Letts RM, Gibeault D. Fractures of the neck of the talus in children. *Foot Ankle.* 1980;1:74–77.

166. Lorentzen JE, Christensen SB, Krogsoe O, Snepper O. Fractures of the neck of the talus. *Acta Orthop Scand.* 1977;48:115–120.

167. Mindell EB, Cisek EE, Kartalian G, Dziob JM. Late results of injuries of the talus. *J Bone Joint Surg Am.* 1963;45:221–245.

168. Morrey BF, Cass JR, Johnson KA, Berquist TH. Foot and ankle. In: Berquist TH, ed. *Imaging of Orthopedic Trauma and Surgery*. Philadelphia: Saunders; 1986:407–498.

169. Mukherjee SK, Pringle RM, Baxter RM. Fracture of the lateral process of the talus. *J Bone Joint Surg Br.* 1974;56:263–273.

170. Mulfinger GL, Trueta JC. The blood supply of the talus. *J Bone Joint Surg Br.* 1970;52:160–167.

171. Pennal GF. Fractures of the talus. *Clin Orthop.* 1963;30:53–63.

172. Peterson L, Goldie I, Lindell D. The arterial supply of the talus. *Acta Orthop Scand.* 1974;45:260–270.

173. Quirk R. Talar compression syndrome in dancers. *Foot Ankle.* 1982;3:65–68.

174. Resnick D. Radiology of the talocalcaneal articulations. *Radiology.* 1984;111:581–586.

175. Resnick D. Talar ridges, osteophytes and beaks: a radiologic commentary. *Radiology.* 1984;151:329–332.

176. Segal D, Waselewski S. Total dislocation of the talus. *J Bone Joint Surg Am.* 1980;62:1370–1372.

177. Seltzer SE, Weissman BN, Braunstein EM, Adams DF, Thomas WH. Computed tomography of the hind foot. *J Comput Assisted Tomogr.* 1984;8:488–497.

178. Sierra A, Potchen EJ, Moore J, Smith GH. High-field magnetic resonance imaging of aseptic necrosis of the talus. *J Bone Joint Surg Am.* 1986;68:927–928.

179. Snepper O, Christensen SB, Krogsoe O, Lorentzen J. Fracture of the body of the talus. *Acta Orthop Scand.* 1977;48:317–324.

180. Solomon MA, Gilula LA, Oloff LM, Oloff J, Compton J. CT scanning of the foot and ankle: normal anatomy. *AJR.* 1986;146:1192–1203.

181. Stephens NA. Fracture-dislocation of the talus in childhood. *Br J Surg.* 1956;43:600–604.

182. Thompson JP, Loomer RL. Osteochondral lesions of the talus in a sports medicine clinic. *Am J Sports Med.* 1984;12:460–463.

Calcaneal Fractures

183. Böhler L. Diagnosis, pathology, and treatment of fractures of the os calcis. *J Bone Joint Surg Am.* 1931;13:75–89.

184. Cave EF. Fracture of the os calcis—the problem in general. *Clin Orthop.* 1963;30:64–66.

185. Essex-Loprestie P. The mechanism, reduction technique, and results in fractures of the os calcis. *Br J Surg.* 1952;39:395–419.

186. Gellman M. Fractures of the anterior process of the calcaneus. *J Bone Joint Surg Am.* 1931;13:877–879.

187. Gilmer PW, Herzenberg J, Frank JL, Silverman P, Morteney S, Goldner JL. Computerized tomographic analysis of acute calcaneal fractures. *Foot Ankle.* 1986;6:184–193.

188. Gross RH. Fractures and dislocations of the foot. In: Rockwood CA, Wilkins KE, King RE, eds. *Fractures in Children*. Philadelphia: Lippincott; 1984;3:1043–1103.

189. Guyer BH, Levinsuhn EM, Fredrickson BE, Bailey GL, Formikell M. Computed tomography of calcaneal fractures: anatomy, pathology, dosimetry, and clinical relevance. *AJR.* 1985;145:911–919.

190. Heckman JD. Fractures and dislocations of the foot. In: Rockwood CA, Green DP, eds. *Fractures in Adults*. Philadelphia: Lippincott; 1984;2:1703–1832.

191. Heger L, Wolff K. Computed tomography of the calcaneus: normal anatomy. *AJR.* 1985;145:123–129.

192. Isbister JF. Calcaneofibular abutment following crush fracture of the calcaneus. *J Bone Joint Surg Br.* 1974;56:274–278.

193. Lance EM, Corey EJ, Wade PA. Fractures of the os calcis. *J Trauma.* 1964;4:15–56.

194. Morrey BF, Cass JF, Johnson KA, Berquist TH. Foot and ankle. In: Berquist TH, ed. *Imaging of Orthopedic Trauma*. Philadelphia: Saunders; 1991:453–577.

195. Norfay JF, Rogers LF, Adams GP, Graves HC, Herser WJ. Common calcaneal avulsion fracture. *AJR.* 1980;134:119–123.

196. Pablot SM, Daneman A, Strurger DA, Carroll N. The value of computed tomography for early assessment of comminuted calcaneal fractures. *J Pediatr Orthop.* 1985;5:435–438.

197. Renfrew DL, El-Khoury GY. Anterior process fractures of the calcaneus. *Skeletal Radiol.* 1985;14:121–125.

198. Rettig AC, Shelbourne KD, Beltz HF, Robertson DW, Arfken P. Radiographic evaluation of foot and ankle injuries in athletes. *Clin Sports Med.* 1987;6:905–919.

199. Rosenberg ZS, Feldman F, Surgson RD. Intra-articular calcaneal fractures: computed tomographic analysis. *Skeletal Radiol.* 1987;16:105–113.

200. Ross SDK, Sowerby RR. The operative treatment of fractures of the os calcis. *Clin Orthop.* 1985;199:132–143.

201. Rowe CR, Sakillarides HT, Freeman PA. Fractures of the os calcis. A long term follow-up study in 146 patients. *JAMA.* 1963;184:920–924.

202. Schmidt TL, Weiner DS. Calcaneal fractures in children. An evaluation of the nature of injury in 56 children. *Clin Orthop.* 1982;171:150–155.

203. Segal D, Marsh JL, Leiter B. Clinical application of computerized axial tomography scanning of calcaneal fractures. *Clin Orthop.* 1985;199:114–123.

204. Slatis P, Kroduoto O, Santavista S, Laasonen EM. Fractures of the calcaneus. *J Trauma.* 1979;19:939–943.

205. Stephenson JR. Displaced fractures of the os calcis involving the subtalar joint: the key role of the superomedial fragment. *Foot Ankle.* 1983;4:91–101.

206. Trott AW. Fractures of the foot in children. *Orthop Clin North Am.* 1976;7:677–686.

Midfoot and Forefoot Injuries

207. Aitken AP, Paulsen D. Dislocation of the tarso-metatarsal joints. *J Bone Joint Surg Am.* 1963;45:246–260.

208. Anderson LD. Injuries of the forefoot. *Clin Orthop.* 1977;122:18–27.

209. Bonutti PM, Bell GR. Compartment syndrome of the foot. *J Bone Joint Surg Am.* 1986;68:1449–1450.

210. Cain PR, Seligson D. Lisfranc's fracture-dislocation with intercuneiform dislocation. *Foot Ankle.* 1981;2:156–160.

211. Carp L. Fracture of the fifth metatarsal bone with special reference to delayed union. *Ann Surg.* 1927;86:308–320.

212. Cassebaum WH. Lisfranc fracture dislocations. *Clin Orthop*. 1963;30:116–129.

213. Dick IL. Impacted fracture of the tarsal navicular. *Proc R Soc Med*. 1941;35:760.

214. Eichenholtz SN, Levene DB. Fracture of the tarsal navicular bone. *Clin Orthop*. 1964;34:142–157.

215. English TA. Dislocation of the metatarsal bone and adjacent toe. *J Bone Joint Surg Br*. 1964;46:700–704.

216. Foster SC, Foster RR. Lisfranc's tarsometatarsal fracture dislocation. *Radiology*. 1976;120:79–83.

217. Gissane W. A dangerous type of fracture of the foot. *J Bone Joint Surg Br*. 1951;33:535–538.

218. Goiney RC, Connell DG, Nichols DM. CT evaluation of tarsometatarsal fracture-dislocation injuries. *AJR*. 1985;144:985–990.

219. Gross RH. Fractures and dislocation of the foot. In: Rockwood CA, Wilkins KE, King RE, eds. *Fractures in Children*. Philadelphia: Lippincott; 1984:1043–1103.

220. Hardcastle PH, Reschauer R, Kutscha-Lissberg E, Schoffman W. Injuries of the tarsometatarsal joint: incidence, classification, and treatment. *J Bone Joint Surg Br*. 1982;64:349–356.

221. Heckman JD. Fractures of the foot and ankle. In: Rockwood CA, Green DP, eds. *Fractures*. Philadelphia: Lippincott; 1984:1703–1832.

222. Johnson GF. Pediatric Lisfranc injury: "bunkbed" fracture. *AJR*. 1981;137:1041–1044.

223. Jones R. Fracture of the base of the fifth metatarsal bone by indirect violence. *Ann Surg*. 1902;35:697–700.

224. Kavanaugh JH, Borower TD, Mann RV. The Jones' fracture revisited. *J Bone Joint Surg Am*. 1978;60:776–782.

225. Macy NJ, DeVoer P. Mid-tarsal dislocation of the first ray. *J Bone Joint Surg Am*. 1983;65:265–266.

226. Main BJ, Jowett RL. Injuries of the mid-tarsal joint. *J Bone Joint Surg Br*. 1975;57:89–97.

227. Nielsen S, Agnholt J, Christensen H. Radiologic findings in lesions of the ligamentum bifurcatum of the mid foot. *Skeletal Radiol*. 1987; 16:114–116.

228. Norfray JF, Feline RA, Steinberg RI, Galinski AW, Gilula LA. Subtleties of Lisfranc fracture-dislocations. *AJR*. 1981;137:1151–1156.

229. Torg JS, Balduini FC, Zelko RR, Povlov LT, Peff TC, Das M. Fractures of the base of the fifth metatarsal distal to the tuberosity. *J Bone Joint Surg Am*. 1984;66:209–214.

230. Wiley JJ. Tarso-metatarsal joint injuries in children. *J Pediatr Orthop*. 1981;1:255–260.

231. Wiley JJ. The mechanism of tarsometatarsal joint injuries. *J Bone Joint Surg Br*. 1971;53:474–482.

232. Wilppula E. Tarsometatarsal fracture-dislocation. *Acta Orthop Scand*. 1973;44:335–345.

233. Zinman H, Keret Q, Reis ND. Fracture of the medial sesamoid bone of the hallux. *J Trauma*. 1981;21:581–582.

Chapter 9

Shoulder and Arm

INTRODUCTION

Upper extremity sports injuries occur less frequently than those in the lower extremity. Soft tissue injuries are most common and occur in contact sports as well as noncontact activities.[1,2,9,14] Baseball, football, swimming, tennis, weightlifting, and archery are frequently associated with shoulder injuries.[1–16] The type of injury varies with the activity. Table 9-1 lists common injuries associated with those sports.

Clinical history and physical examination suggest the diagnosis in many cases. Proper use of arthrography, magnetic resonance imaging (MRI), and other radiographic techniques, however, is essential in confirming the diagnosis and characterizing the extent of injury.

ANATOMY

The shoulder is anatomically complex, and a review of certain anatomic features is helpful in understanding how to perform imaging procedures and interpret radiographic findings.

Osteology

The clavicle is a slightly curved (S-shaped) bone that lies ventral to the shoulder girdle (Fig. 9-1). It is one of the first bones to ossify.[17,20] The medial epiphysis does not unite until the end of the second decade; this should not be mistaken for a fracture. There are no secondary ossification centers distally. The clavicle articulates with the acromion distally and, rarely, with the coracoid.[21,24] Medially the pestle-shaped portion of the clavicle articulates with the sternum and first rib. The midportion of the clavicle is tubular, and the distal portion is relatively flat.[17,20,24] The dorsal surface of the clavicle is roughened proximally and distally. The trapezius and deltoid muscles insert distally, and the sternocleidomastoid and pectoralis major muscles insert proximally (Fig. 9-1). Inferiorly the conoid and trapezoid bands of the coracoclavicular ligament attach as the clavicle bows dorsally. They insert on the conoid tubercle and trapezoid ridge, respectively.[19,20,24]

The scapula is dorsal to the chest wall. The wing (body) of the scapula is a large, flat, triangular bone that is almost entirely covered with muscles dorsally and ventrally (Fig. 9-2). The

Table 9-1[2,6,8,11] Common Shoulder Lesions in Athletes

Acromioclavicular arthritis
Rotator cuff impingement
Biceps tendinitis
Glenoid labral tears
Instability
Bursitis
Thoracic outlet syndrome
Muscle tears

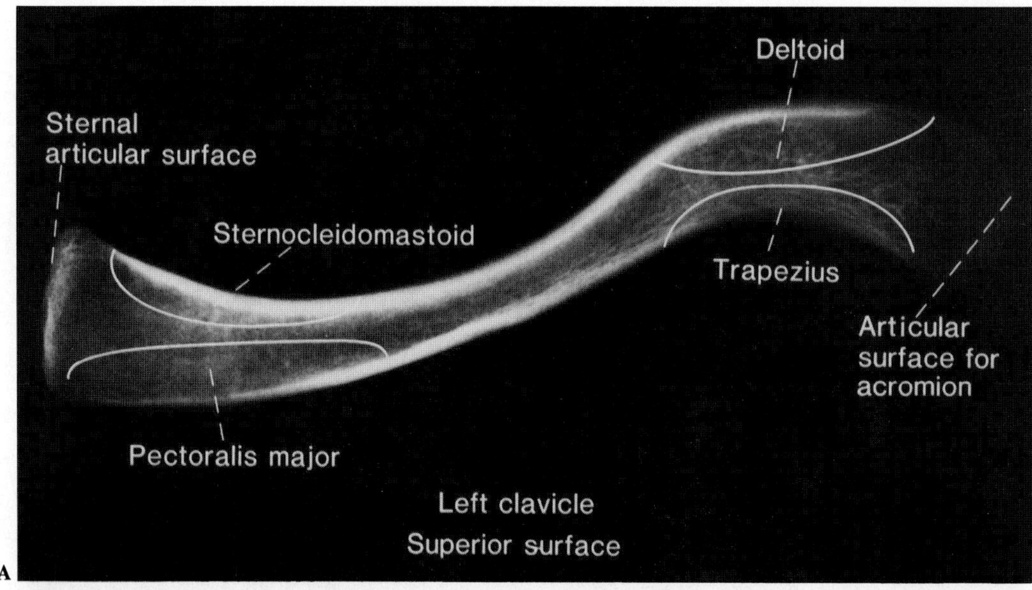

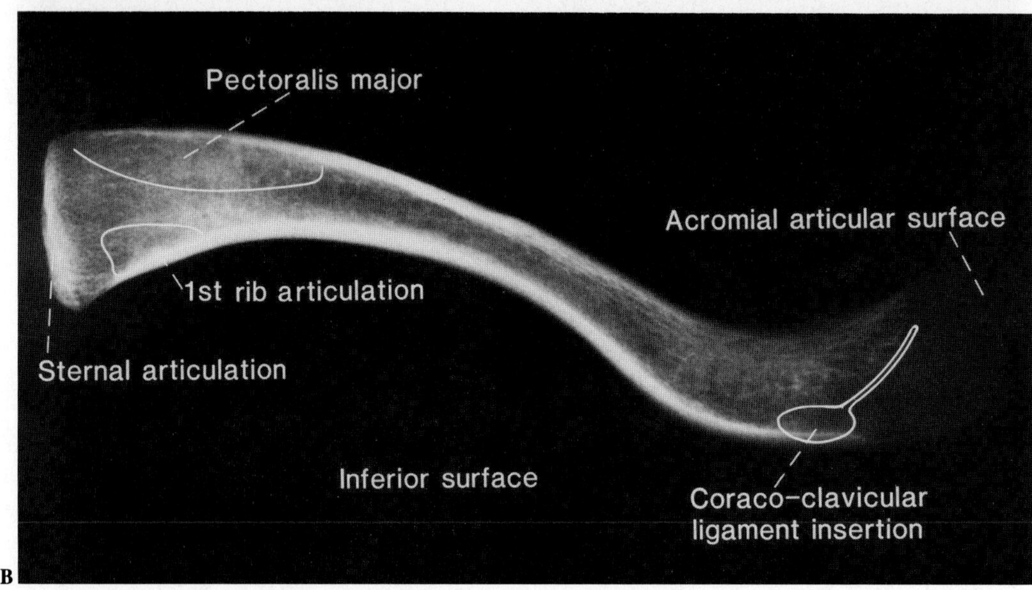

Fig. 9-1 Specimen radiographs of the clavicle seen superiorly (**A**) and inferiorly (**B**) demonstrating the osseous anatomy and muscle attachments. *Source:* Reprinted from *Imaging of Orthopedic Trauma* ed 2 by TH Berquist, 1991, Raven Press, © Mayo Foundation.

subscapularis covers the ventral surface. Dorsally the supraspinatus takes its origin above the spine of the scapula and the infraspinatus below (Figs. 9-2 and 9-5). The teres major and minor arise from the inferior scapula. The triceps originates from a tubercle just below the glenoid (Fig. 9-2A). This tubercle is usually easily visible radiographically. The supraglenoid tubercle is located just superior to the glenoid and serves as the origin of the long head of the biceps brachii. When seen en face, the glenoid lies at the junction of the scapular body with the scapular spine lying posteriorly and the coracoid anteriorly (Fig. 9-2B). This forms a Y with the glenoid at the junction of the limbs.[19,20,24]

There are several secondary ossification centers that should not be confused with fractures. These include the superior glenoid, inferior glenoid, acromial, coracoid, and infrascapular. These ossification centers usually fuse in the second decade.[19,29] The glenoid ossification centers may be a source of confusion when diagnosing patients with shoulder instability.

The humeral head is nearly hemispheric and has four times the surface area of the glenoid.[24,27,28,32] The anatomic neck is located at the margin of the articular surface and lies in an oblique plane running superiorly from medial to lateral zones (Fig. 9-3). The surgical neck lies more inferiorly, below the tuberosities.[24]

The greater tuberosity is located laterally below the anatomic neck. This structure is seen in profile with the shoulder externally rotated (Fig. 9-3). There are three facets on the greater tuberosity for insertion of three of the muscles of the rotator cuff.[23,24] The insertion for the supraspinatus is most

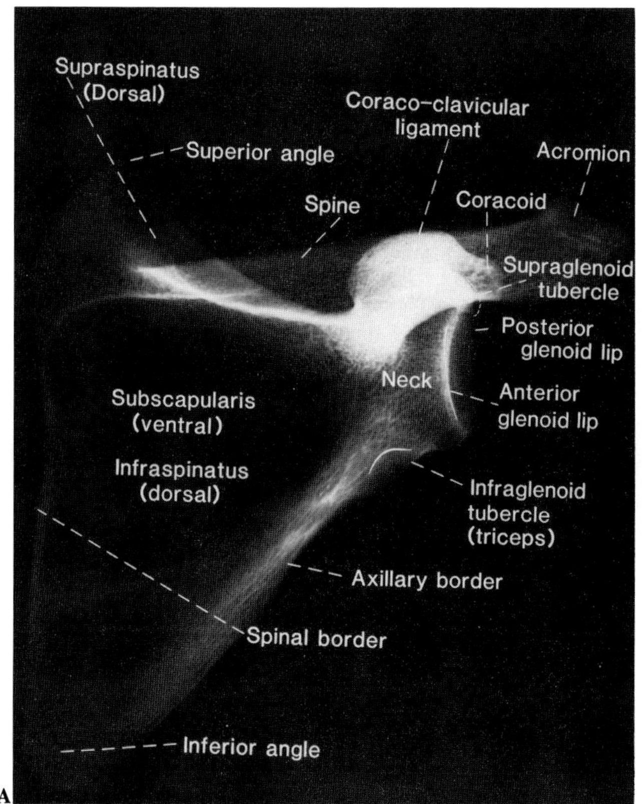

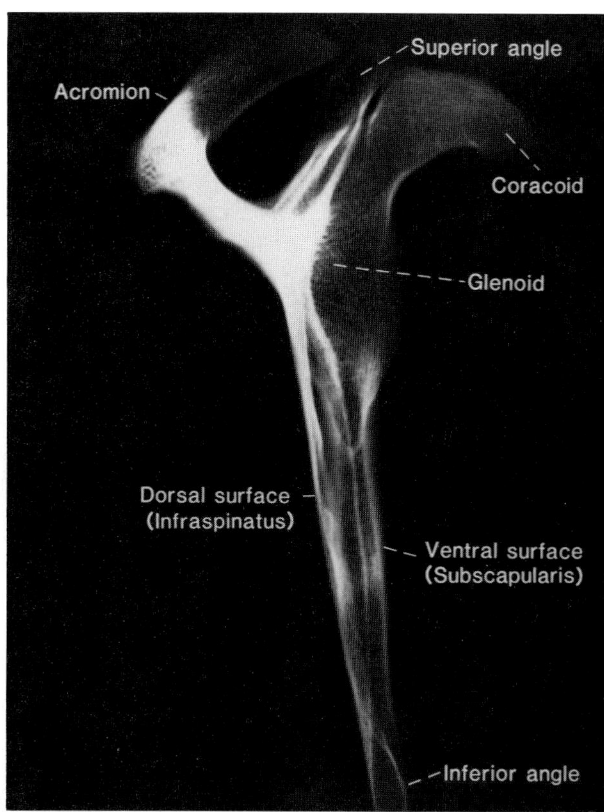

Fig. 9-2 Specimen radiographs of the scapula seen from (**A**) the anteroposterior (AP) and (**B**) lateral projections. *Source:* Reprinted from *Imaging of Orthopedic Trauma* ed 2 by TH Berquist, 1991, Raven Press, © Mayo Foundation.

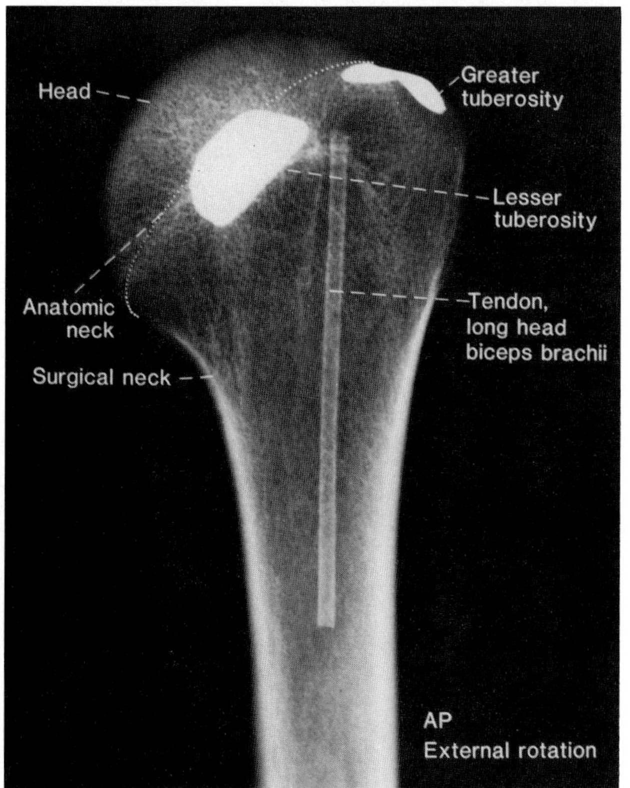

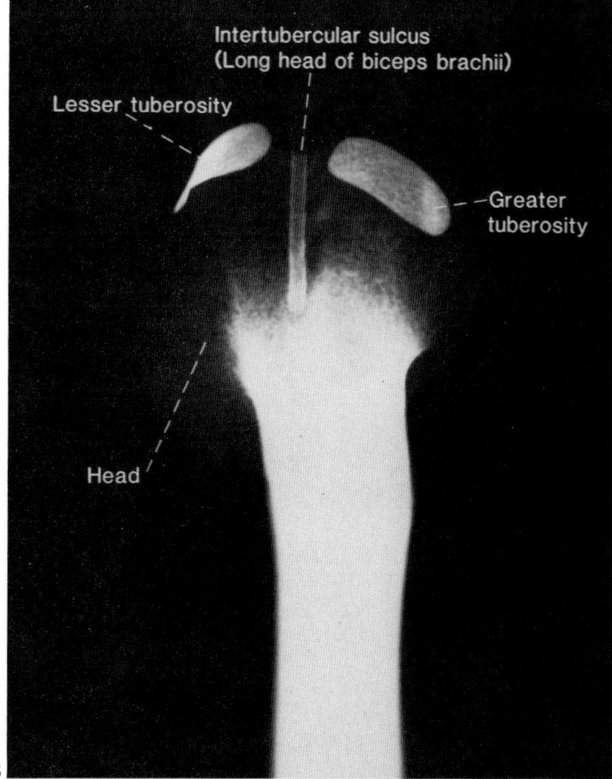

Fig. 9-3 Specimen radiographs demonstrating the anatomy of the upper humerus in external rotation (**A**) and axially (**B**). *Source:* Reprinted from *Imaging of Orthopedic Trauma* ed 2 by TH Berquist, 1991, Raven Press, © Mayo Foundation.

anterior, lying near the intertubercular sulcus. The infraspinatus and teres minor insert just posterior to the supraspinatus (Fig. 9-3). The intertubercular sulcus lies between the greater and lesser tuberosities. Radiographically this groove normally measures about 11 mm in width and 4.6 mm in depth.[17,19] The tendon of the long head of the biceps brachii runs through this groove.[17,19,20] The lesser tuberosity lies medial to the intertubercular sulcus and serves as the insertion for the subscapularis (Fig. 9-3).

Articular Anatomy

Glenohumeral Joint

The glenohumeral joint is a ball-and-socket (spheroidal) joint.[17,18,20] The normally shallow glenoid cavity is much smaller than the humeral head.[27,28] The cavity is deepened by a fibrocartilaginous labrum, which extends around the entire peripheral margin of the glenoid cavity (Fig. 9-4).

The synovium-lined capsule attaches proximally to the glenoid labrum and extends peripherally to the anatomic neck of the humerus.[17,20,26] The total capsular volume is nearly twice that of the humeral head.[27] The capsule is stronger anteriorly and inferiorly and is reinforced by surrounding muscles, tendons, and ligaments (Fig. 9-4). Superiorly reinforcement is achieved by the rotator cuff muscles, specifically the supraspinatus (Fig. 9-5). Inferiorly there is support of the glenoid attachment by the triceps brachii, which originates from the infraglenoid tubercle. Anterior reinforcement is provided by the subscapularis tendon. Posteriorly the teres minor and infraspinatus are adjacent to the capsule (Fig. 9-5).[17,18,24] Superiorly the tendon of the long head of the biceps brachii arises from the supraglenoid tubercle and labrum. The tendon crosses the superior joint and exits through the intertubercular sulcus (Fig. 9-3).[19,24] This sulcus is formed by the greater and lesser tuberosities. The roof of the groove is covered by the transverse humeral ligament. The biceps tendon is covered by a synovial sheath that extends several centimeters beyond the normal capsule to about the level of the surgical neck.[17,18,20,24]

Additional support is provided by four ligament complexes: the coracohumeral ligament, which arises from the coracoid to insert in the greater and lesser tuberosities; the superior glenohumeral ligament, which originates just below the coracohumeral ligament and blends with the capsule as it inserts in the lesser tuberosity; the middle glenohumeral ligament, which arises from the anterior glenoid and crosses inferiorly to the superior glenohumeral ligament to insert in the lower portion of the lesser tuberosity; and the inferior glenohumeral ligament, which arises from the anterior glenoid and inserts in the region of the surgical neck below the middle glenohumeral ligament.[17,19,20,25,27] Stability supplied by the capsule and ligaments is augmented considerably by the rotator cuff (Figs. 9-4 and 9-5).[26]

There may be numerous bursae about the shoulder, but most do not communicate with the joint, and they are not always constant (Table 9-2). The most important are the subscapularis, subdeltoid, subcoracoid, and subacromial. The subscapularis bursa is situated anteriorly beneath the coracoid

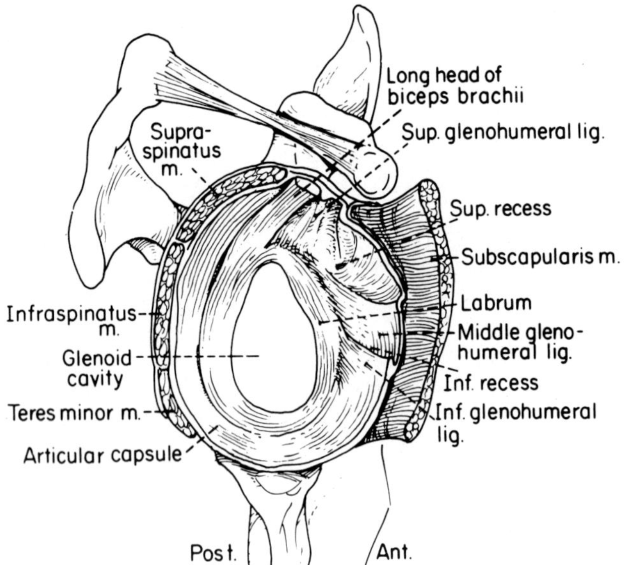

Fig. 9-4 Illustration of glenoid en face. *Source:* Reprinted from Morrey BF and Choa EY in *Clinical Biomechanics: A Case History Approach* (p26) by J Black and JH Dumpleton (eds) with permission of Churchill Livingstone, © 1981.

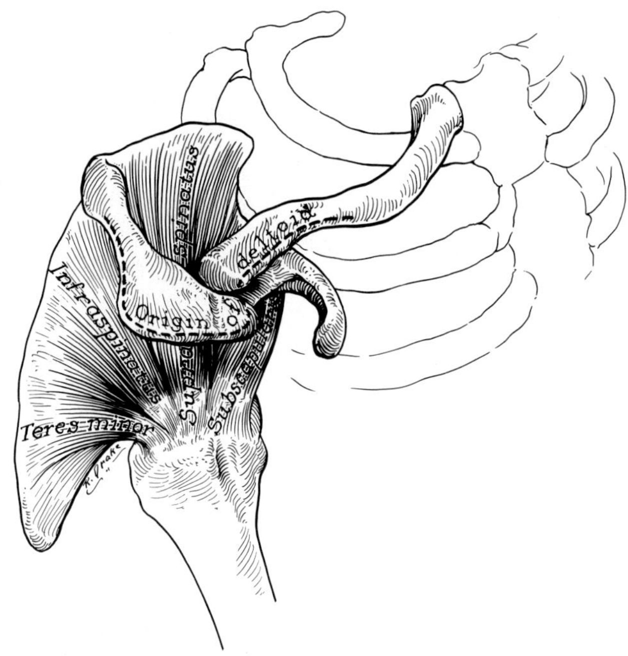

Fig. 9-5 Illustration demonstrating the muscles of the rotator cuff. *Source:* Courtesy of Mark B. Coventry, Mayo Clinic, Rochester, Minnesota.

Table 9-2 Shoulder Bursae

Bursa	*Location*	*Normal Joint Communication*
Subscapular	Between subscapularis tendon and capsule	Yes
Infraspinatous	Between capsule and infraspinatus tendon	Inconstant
Subdeltoid	Between deltoid and rotator cuff	No
Subacromial	Between acromion and rotator cuff (usually contiguous with subdeltoid)	No
Subcoracoid	Between coracoid and subscapularis (may be contiguous with subacromial)	No
Coracobrachialis	Between coracobrachialis and subscapularis	No
Latissimus dorsi	Between latissimus dorsi and teres major	No
Teres major	Between teres major and humeral insertion	No
Pectoralis major	Between pectoralis major and humeral insertion	No

Source: Reprinted from *Imaging of Orthopedic Trauma* ed 2 by TH Berquist, 1991, Raven Press, © Mayo Foundation.

process and lies dorsal to the subscapularis tendon. The infraspinatus bursa communicates with the posterior joint and lies between the capsule and the infraspinatus tendon. This is not always present.[17,20,24] Communication with the tendon sheath of the long head of the biceps is almost always present in the normal shoulder.[19,20,24] A large bursa lies between the rotator cuff and acromion. It is composed of subdeltoid, subacromial, and subcoracoid portions.[20,24] This does not communicate with the capsule if the rotator cuff is intact.[20,24,30,31]

Acromioclavicular Joint

The acromioclavicular joint is a synovial joint that joins the distal clavicle and the medial portion of the acromion. An intraarticular disc is occasionally present.[20] Both gliding and rotary motion (scapula) are possible.[20,25,27] The capsule of the joint is supported by the superior and inferior acromioclavicular ligaments; major support is derived from the coracoclavicular ligament (trapezoid and coracoid ligaments), however. Rarely, a joint is present between the coracoid and clavicle.[21]

Sternoclavicular Joint

The medial articular portion of the clavicle forms a gliding synovial joint with the manubrium and the cartilaginous portion of the first rib. The clavicular surface is larger than the articular surface of either the manubrium or the first rib.[20,28] Ligamentous support includes the interclavicular ligament superiorly, the costoclavicular ligament inferiorly, and the anterior and posterior sternoclavicular ligaments. An articular disc extends from the upper clavicle to the cartilage of the first rib, dividing the joint into medial and lateral compartments.[19,20,24]

Neurovascular Anatomy

The relationships of the neurovascular structures to the clavicle and sternoclavicular joint deserve mention.

The subclavian artery and vein pass posterior to the sternoclavicular joint. The second portion of the artery passes posterior to the scalenus anterior, which inserts into the upper portion of the first rib (Fig. 9-6). The brachial plexus (C5–T1 ventral roots) descends to join the vessels at this point. The axillary artery, a continuation of the subclavian artery, begins at the lateral margin of the first rib and extends to the distal border of the teres major. The neurovascular structures pass between the midclavicle and first rib through the axilla and along the medial aspect of the upper humerus. The major blood supply to the humerus and surrounding musculature is derived from branches of the axillary artery. These include the anterior and posterior humeral circumflex, clavicular, acromial, and deltoid branches from the thoracoacromial axis.[17,20,24]

Fracture-dislocations of the sternoclavicular joint and glenohumeral joint may result in neurovascular complications.[19] These are discussed in more detail later in this chapter.

Biomechanics

The glenohumeral configuration and supporting structures of the shoulder allow uniquely complex motion.[22,23,26,27,31,32] The muscles involved in glenohumeral motion are the rotator cuff, deltoid, pectoralis major, latissimus dorsi, and teres major.[31] Motion occurs primarily at the glenohumeral joint. Motion also occurs in the acromioclavicular and sternoclavicular joints, however.[27] Glenohumeral motion is responsible for 120° of the 180° abduction arc. More than 120° of abduction requires scapular and clavicular motion. If the humerus cannot externally rotate, motion is restricted owing to impingement of the greater tuberosity on the acromion. With full abduction (180°), the scapula is capable of rotating 60°. The major muscles producing full abduction are the deltoid, supraspinatus, trapezius, and serratus anterior.[18,20,32]

The biomechanics of abduction have been stressed owing to common clinical problems involving the rotator cuff (tears and impingement).[18,25] This movement can be studied fluoroscopically as a part of shoulder arthrography. The shoulder is also capable of flexion, extension, adduction, and rotation.[20] The main flexors are the pectoralis major and anterior deltoid fibers, with some contribution coming from the biceps brachii.[18,20] Extension is accomplished with fibers from the posterior deltoid, teres major, and latissimus dorsi. Adduction is achieved by contraction of the subscapularis, infraspinatus, teres minor, pectoralis major, latissimus dorsi, and teres

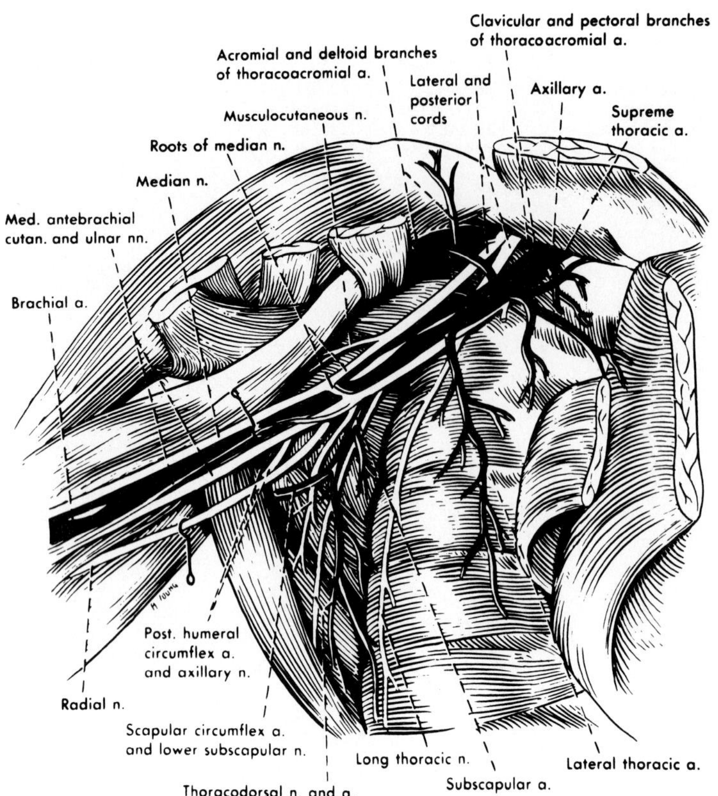

Fig. 9-6 Illustration of the neurovascular anatomy of the shoulder. *Source:* Reprinted from *Anatomy for Surgeons, Vol 3, The Back and Limbs*, ed 3, by HW Hollinshead, 1982, JB Lippincott.

major.[20] External rotation is powered by the infraspinatus and teres minor, and internal rotation is powered by the pectoralis major, latissimus dorsi, teres major, and subscapularis.[20,24]

IMAGING TECHNIQUES

Routine Radiography

Numerous routine and special views have been described for evaluating the shoulder and humerus.[34–36,54,57,60] This section discusses the routine screening evaluation plus special views that may be useful for evaluating the injured athlete.

The most useful three views for evaluating the shoulder in acute trauma include the true anteroposterior (AP) in external rotation, axillary, and scapular Y or Neer views (Fig. 9-7).[36,54,60,90] Routine views of the humerus include an AP view of the entire humerus in internal and external rotation and in certain cases a transthoracic view.[34–36]

The true AP view of the shoulder requires rotating the patient posteriorly 40° to see the glenohumeral joint tangentially. In the supine position the patient can be supported with a wedge or bolster. In the upright position the patient simply may be rotated (Fig. 9-7A). The scapular Y view or 60° anterior oblique view is obtained by elevating the shoulder or rotating the patient anteriorly 60°. This view (Fig. 9-7C) demonstrates a Y configuration, with the Y being formed by the wing of the scapula, scapular spine, and coracoid. The glenoid is at the limbs of the Y with the humeral head centered over it.[34–36] The axillary view (Fig. 9-7B) generally requires abduction of the involved arm by 90°. Only mild abduction may be sufficient to allow the axillary view to be obtained, however.[34,35]

Localized views of the scapula, clavicle, and acromioclavicular and sternoclavicular articulations are discussed later as they apply to specific injuries in those locations. Certain special views that are of value in detecting both osseous and soft tissue injury bear further discussion here.

The views already discussed represent the general alternatives for investigation of the shoulder and humerus. The humerus is generally radiographed in the AP and lateral projections.[34,35]

On occasion it may be desirable to obtain radiographs of the bicipital groove. With the extremity in the anatomic position, the groove is positioned approximately 15° lateral to the midportion of the anterior aspect of the humeral head. Fisk[52] suggested one method of visualizing this groove. An alternative position has the involved side elevated slightly with cushion support. The cassette is positioned above the shoulder with the hand in an anatomic position. The central beam is centered on the upper aspect of the humeral head.[34–36] This view offers a projection of the length of the groove. The upper angle of the groove is better shown in the Fisk projection (Fig. 9-8).[52]

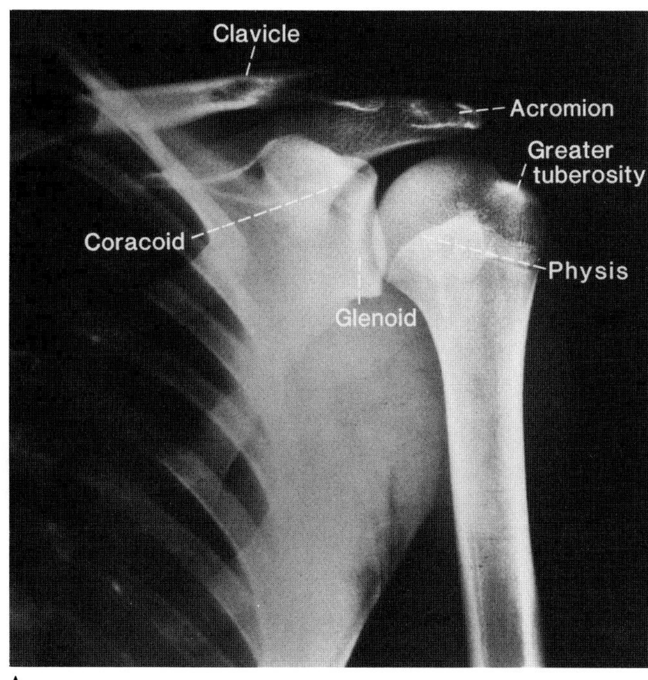

A

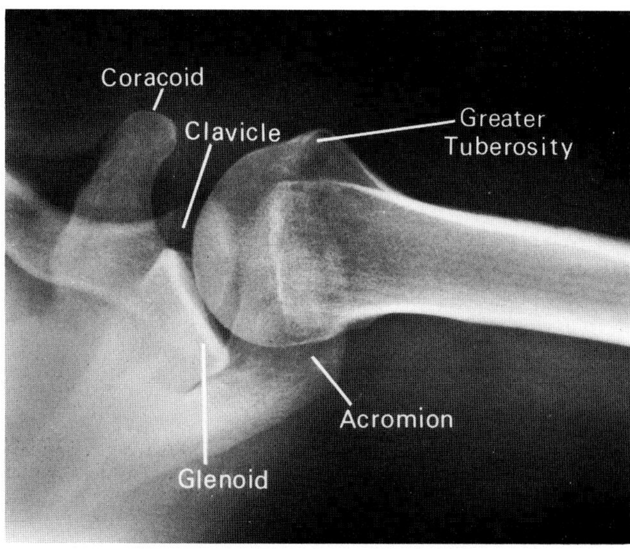

B

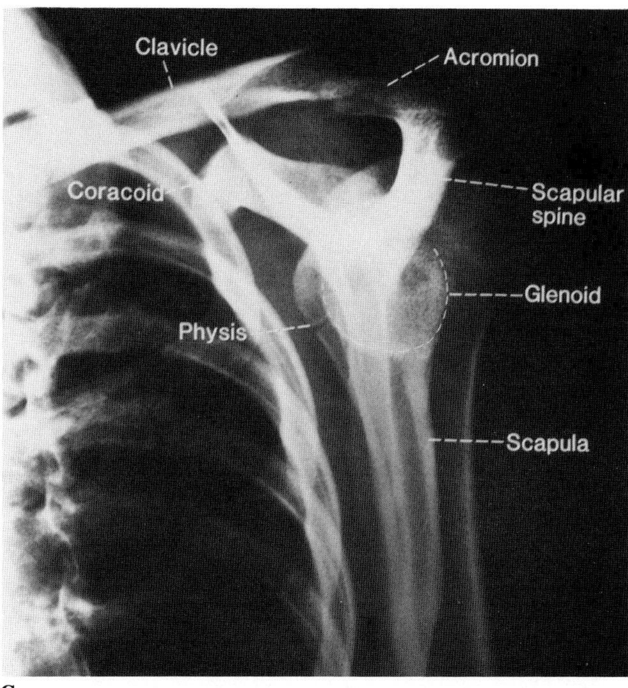

C

Fig. 9-7 Radiographs of the shoulder demonstrating the anatomy displayed on (**A**) AP, (**B**) axillary, and (**C**) scapular Y views.

A number of views have been developed to augment the evaluation of chronic shoulder instability.[36,46] These views are designed to visualize a bony or calcific reaction, a fracture of the anterior glenoid rim, or a compression fracture of the posterior aspect of the humeral head (the Hill-Sachs lesion).[68] In the acute anterior dislocation the Hill-Sachs deformity is seen on the AP view and is usually characteristic (Fig. 9-9). On occasion the humeral head can be seen to be indented posteriorly and impacted on the anterior glenoid rim, which becomes the genesis of the humeral head defect. The anterior nature of this dislocation can be confirmed with axillary or anterior oblique radiographs (Fig. 9-10).[36,47,50]

In the nonacute setting, the diagnosis of continuing shoulder instability may be difficult. Hill and Sachs[68] suggested using an AP radiograph with the arm in marked internal rotation to visualize the humeral impaction-fracture. Rokous et al[89] suggested a modified axillary view (the West Point axillary) to define glenoid lesions. The patient is prone with the arm abducted 90° and rotated so that the forearm hangs off the X-ray table and is pointed directly at the floor. The X-ray tube is positioned with the central ray projecting 25° from the horizontal and 25° medially. This technique demonstrates the anteroinferior glenoid rim to better advantage than the standard axillary view. The fixed arm position and rotation usually also demonstrate the Hill-Sachs lesion when it is present. In the 63 patients with chronic subluxation of the shoulder studied by Rokous et al,[89] 53 (84%) demonstrated abnormalities of the glenoid rim. No cases of acute anterior dislocation demonstrated this abnormality, but 6 of 19 cases (32%) with recurrent anterior dislocation did have this lesion.

Hall and colleagues[63] described a view developed by Stryker known as the Stryker notch view. The patient is supine with the hand adjacent to or on top of the head and the elbow directed vertically. The central beam is angled 10° cephalad and centered on the coracoid (palpable). In patients with recurrent anterior dislocation, Hall and colleagues[63] could identify the humeral head lesion in 18 of 20 shoulders (90%; Fig. 9-11).

More recently, additional views have been described to identify shoulder subluxation, instability, Hill-Sachs lesions,

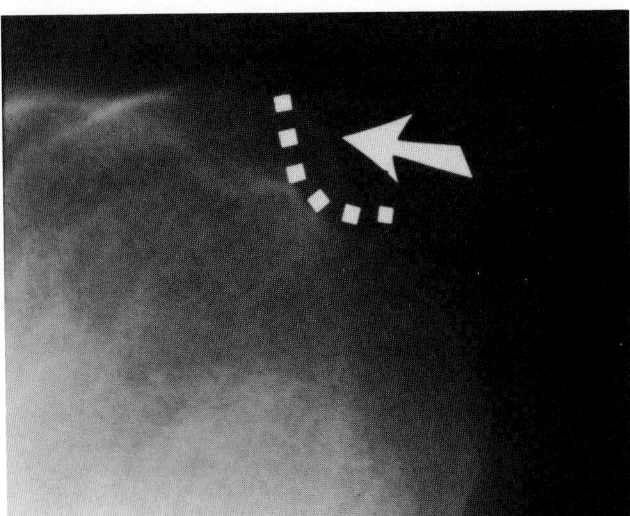

Fig. 9-8 Bicipital groove view (arrow) with normal margins (dotted line).

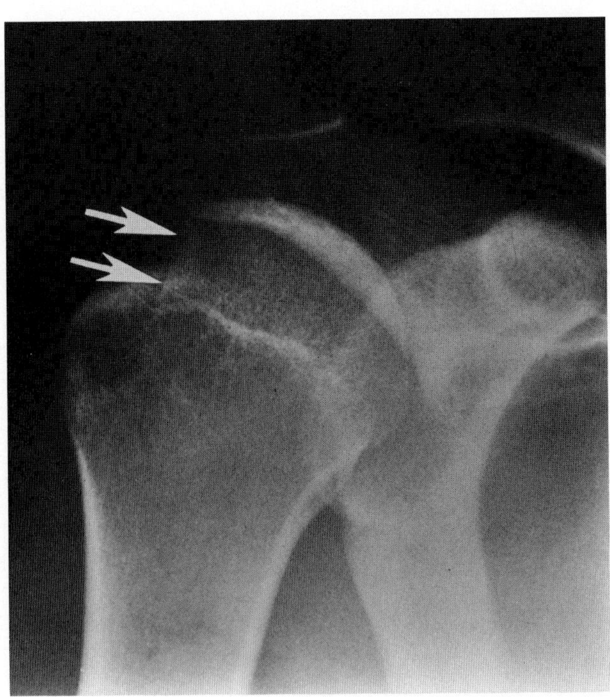

Fig. 9-9 AP view of the shoulder demonstrating squaring of the humeral head (arrows) due to a Hill-Sachs deformity.

and glenoid lesions.[56,75] The apical oblique view is obtained with the patient seated or supine with the injured shoulder against the cassette and the opposite shoulder rotated 45° anteriorly (Fig. 9-12).[56] The central beam is directed 45° caudally through the shoulder with the scapula parallel to the beam because of the adducted position of the extremity.[56] This view provides a coronal profile of the glenohumeral joint that is ideal for detection of intraarticular fractures, dislocations, instability, Hill-Sachs deformities, and glenoid injuries.[56]

Detection of acromial abnormalities is useful in diagnosis of impingement.[36,73] Routine radiographs may demonstrate chronic changes such as sclerosis, irregularity of the greater

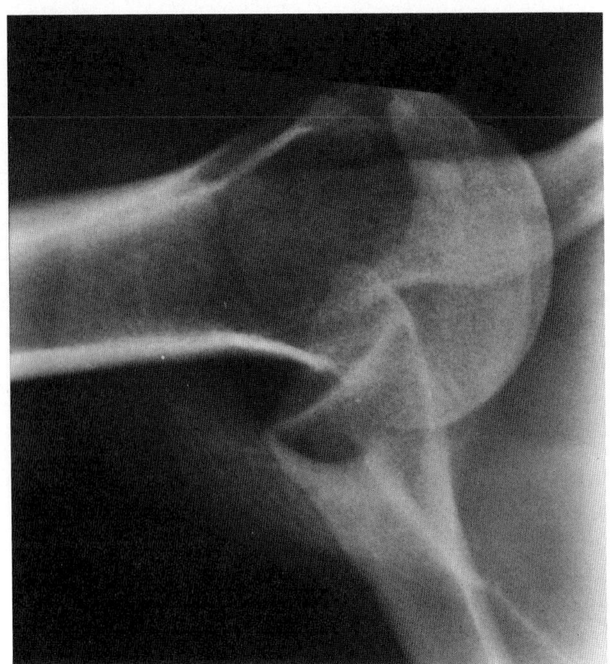

Fig. 9-10 Axillary view of the right shoulder demonstrating an anterior dislocation.

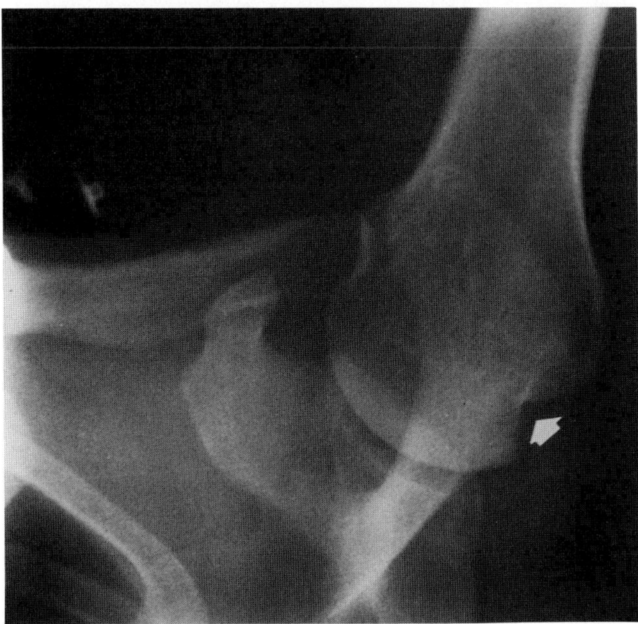

Fig. 9-11 Stryker notch view demonstrating the Hill-Sachs lesion (arrow).

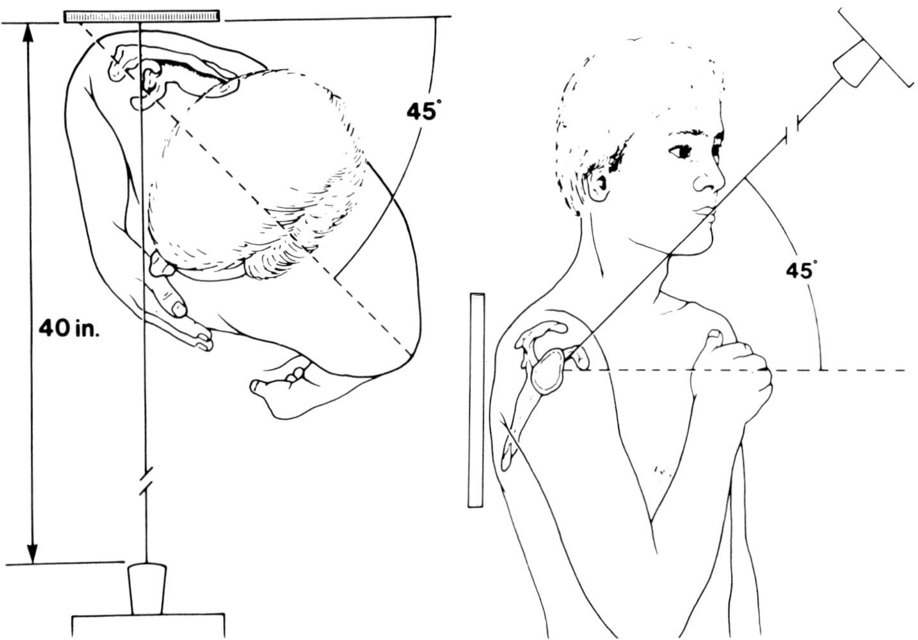

Fig. 9-12 Illustration of positioning for apical oblique view. *Source:* Reprinted with permission from Garth WP, Slappey CE and Ochs CW. Roentgen demonstration of instability of the shoulder: the apical oblique projection in *Journal of Bone and Joint Surgery* (1984;66A:1450–1453), Copyright © 1984, Journal of Bone and Joint Surgery.

tuberosity, acromioclavicular joint changes, and superior subluxation of the humeral head.[36,73] Acromial changes can be viewed by angling the beam 30° caudally on the AP view or by angling the tube 5° with the same position used for the scapular lateral view (Fig. 9-13).[73,75,85]

In patients who are being evaluated for recurrent anterior shoulder instability, multiple views are necessary to outline all the bone pathology because one single view does not always depict both Hill-Sachs and glenoid lesions. In these situations, the basic AP views in internal and external rotation are supplemented by a West Point axillary and a Stryker notch view. With these two additional views, it is unlikely that important findings will be missed. Fluoroscopy is also useful to obtain optimal positioning in selected cases.[36]

Tomography

Tomography is seldom indicated in the shoulder, but it may be a useful adjunct to routine radiography and special views. This is especially true for the medial third of the clavicle and the sternoclavicular joint because thoracic contents may obscure alterations in bone structure or joint relationships. Shoulder pain is often traumatic or degenerative in origin, but small neoplasms such as an osteoid osteoma may cause difficulty in diagnosis. Radioisotope scans can localize the lesion, allowing selection of a tomographic projection to define the lesion.[36]

Combined arthrography and tomography may better define structures outlined by the contrast material.[36] Arthrotomography is discussed later in this chapter along with arthrography.

Ultrasonography

The role of sonography for evaluating shoulder disorders continues to evolve.[38,51,57,80] In early studies, features consistently associated with tendon tears included abnormal motion patterns of the supraspinatus with arm rotation and persistently disrupted echoes within the tendon substance. Cuff tears typically follow four patterns: focal cuff thinning, nonvisualization, discontinuity in echo patterns, and a central echogenic band in the substance of the rotator cuff.[69,80] Large tears are imaged as regions of diminished echo density.[38,64]

As experience with sonography of the shoulder has expanded, its use for evaluation of both the biceps tendon and the rotator cuff has gained acceptance. Axial and longitudinal scans to evaluate these structures are quite successful in experienced hands. Middleton et al[80] reported both sensitivity and specificity to be 91% for detection of rotator cuff tears. Errors related to ultrasound are usually due to operator technique or lack of familiarity with normal anatomy.[80] This is documented by variation in accuracy reports, which range from 63% to 94%.[69,80,81]

Computed Tomography

Radiographic evaluation of the sternoclavicular joint and medial clavicular region may be difficult because of overlying structures.[65,67,76] Computed tomography (CT) is useful for overcoming these difficulties.[36,65,67,76] Scapular spine or body lesions may also be further defined with this technique.[88]

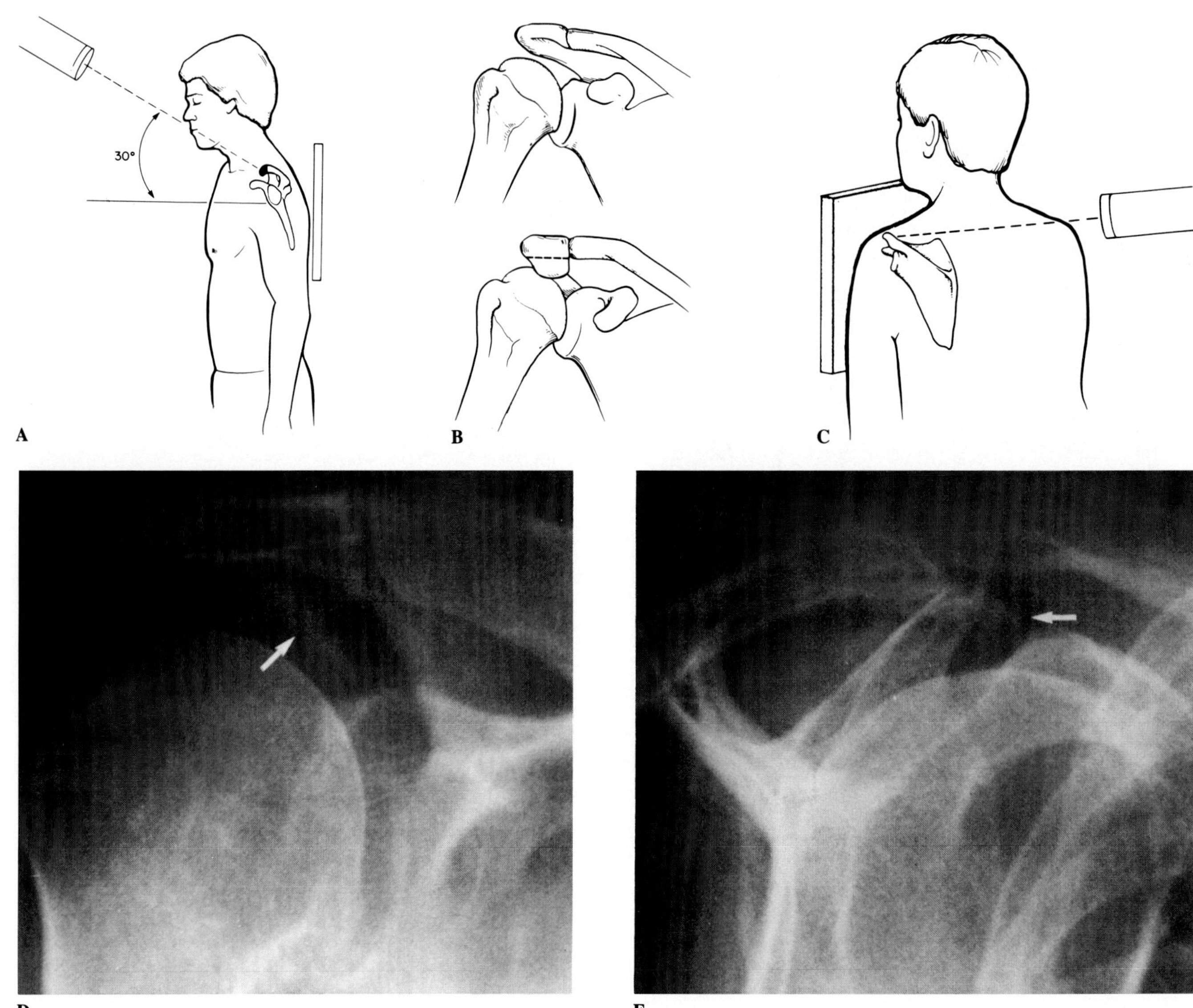

Fig. 9-13 (**A**) Patient positioned for 30° caudally angled AP view to demonstrate the anterior acromion. (**B**) Typical AP view is normal (top), but the subacromial abnormality is seen on the angled view (bottom). (**C**) Position for supraspinatus outlet view. (**D**) Appearance of a spur (arrows, **D** and **E**) on the 30° angled view depicted in **A**. (**E**) Supraspinatus view demonstrated in **C**. *Source:* Reprinted with permission from Kilcoyne RF, Reddy PK, Lyons F and Rockwood CA, Optimal plain film imaging of shoulder impingement syndrome, *American Journal of Roentgenology* (1989;153:795–797), Copyright © 1989, American Roentgen Ray Society.

CT has proved to be especially useful for better definition of glenoid fractures and more complex fractures because often the shoulder views are not adequate to make a decision about the need for surgery (Fig. 9-14).[36] Combined with arthrography, CT is useful for evaluating instability and glenoid labral lesions.[91–93] CT arthrography is discussed more completely later.[41,45]

Shoulder Arthrography

Proper choice of arthrographic technique requires an awareness of the patient's clinical problem (eg, rotator cuff tear, adhesive capsulitis, or impingement syndrome) as well as an understanding of the plain film findings. Despite the introduction of MRI, shoulder arthrography is still often used to evaluate tears of the rotator cuff and other shoulder pathology.[36,41,79,87,91,93] Subtle changes in the shoulder may also be detected, especially with double-contrast techniques and by combining arthrographic techniques with CT or conventional tomography.[58,62,66,72,82]

In a series of 552 shoulder arthrograms performed at the Mayo Clinic, 38% of patients were referred with pain and diminished range of motion. The majority of these patients were suspected to have rotator cuff lesions. An additional 19% were referred with definite clinical evidence of cuff tears. Thus 57% of the arthrograms were performed with cuff disease specifically in mind.[36]

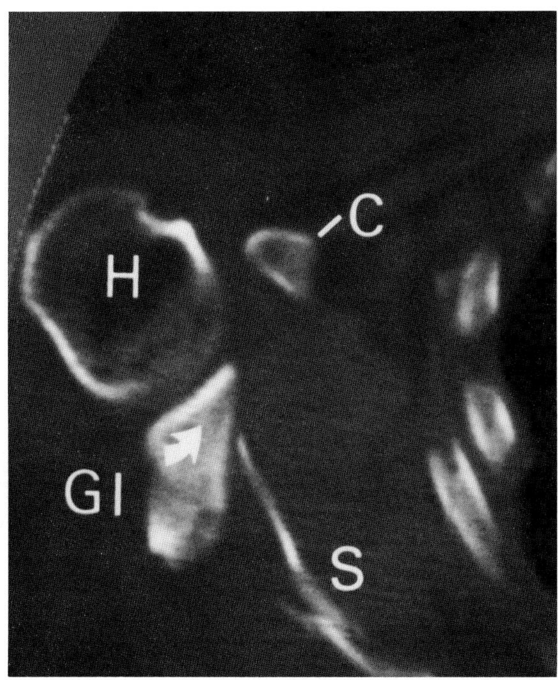

Fig. 9-14 Computed tomography (CT) image of the shoulder after complex scapular fracture. H, Humerus; C, coracoid; Gl, glenoid; S, scapula.

Knowledge of the patient's suspected problem and careful evaluation of routine radiographs can assist one in proper performance of the arthrogram and in the choice of filming sequence or CT for the best definition of the patient's problem.[36,41,91–93]

Review of plain film findings on 552 patients undergoing shoulder arthrography has provided extensive data regarding these findings.[36] Previous reports of plain film findings in patients with rotator cuff tears describe superior subluxation of the humeral head (distance from the humeral head to the acromion, ≤7 mm), reversal of the normal acromial convexity, sclerosis or cystic changes in the greater tuberosity, and bony eburnation of the glenoid or humeral head inferomedially.[48,55] The last finding (hypertrophic spurring involving the humeral head inferomedially) is not a reliable indicator of rotator cuff tearing and can be seen with many chronic shoulder problems.[36,48] DeSmet[48] reported plain film abnormalities in 90.4% of 42 patients with rotator cuff tears. Our review of 552 arthrograms at the Mayo Clinic revealed 145 complete and 38 partial tears of the rotator cuff. As would be expected, changes on plain radiographs were much more common with complete chronic cuff tears. Patients with acute cuff tears (no associated fractures) less frequently demonstrate bony abnormalities on plain films.[36]

Superior subluxation of the humeral head causes a reduction of the distance between the acromion, which is normally convex inferiorly, and the humeral head. Consistency in measurement is essential if one is to utilize this measurement properly. We measure all cases in external rotation. This measurement is virtually always greater than 1 cm in normal individuals (Fig. 9-15).

In the patients with rotator cuff tears the acromiohumeral distance was less than 1 cm in 95% of cases, with 65% measuring less than 0.7 cm (Fig. 9-15).[36] The small percentage of cases with 1-cm measurements and rotator cuff tears were young patients with small cuff tears.

Changes in the greater tuberosity were evident in 90% of patients with compete cuff tears.[36] These findings included cystic changes, sclerosis, and small erosions (Fig. 9-16).

Subtle changes on the inferior surface of the acromion or distal clavicle were present in 75% of patients with complete cuff tears[36] (Fig. 9-15). These findings were also noted in a

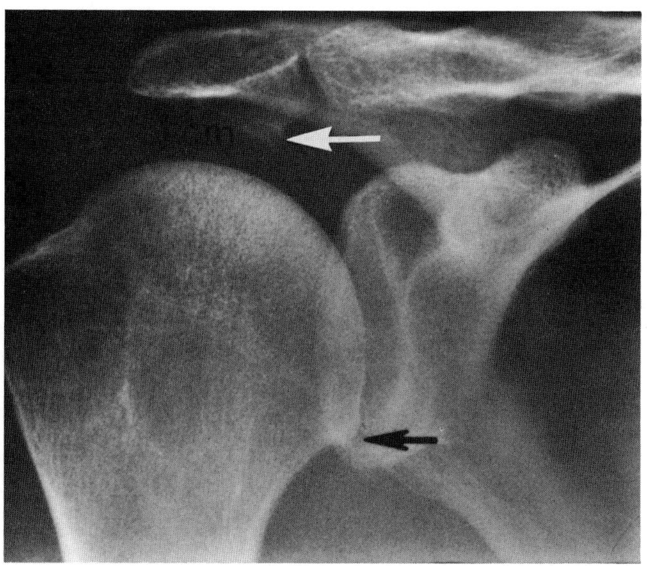
A

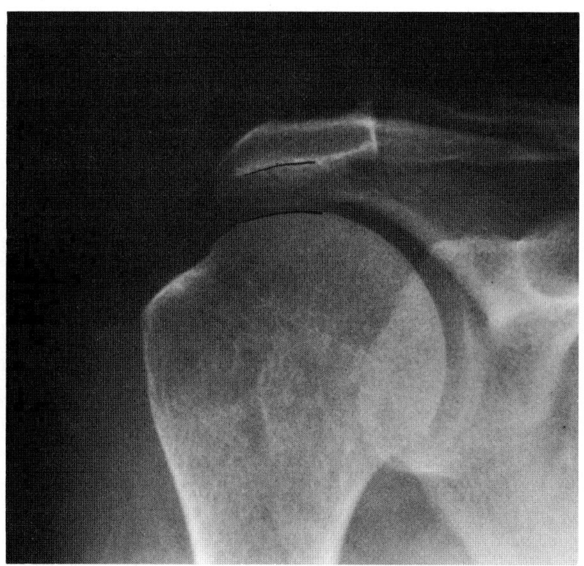
B

Fig. 9-15 Routine AP views of the shoulder in external rotation. **(A)** Normal humeral acromial distance (1 cm) with subacromial spurring (upper arrow) and an inferior glenoid spur (lower arrow). **(B)** Chronic rotator cuff tear with reduced humeroacromial distance.

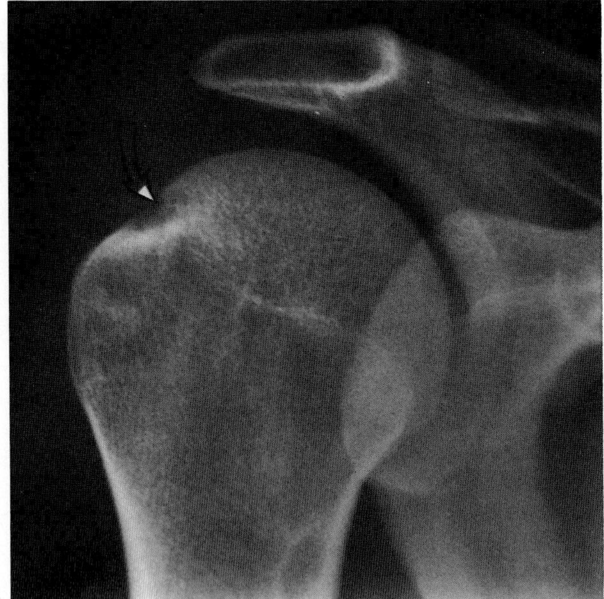

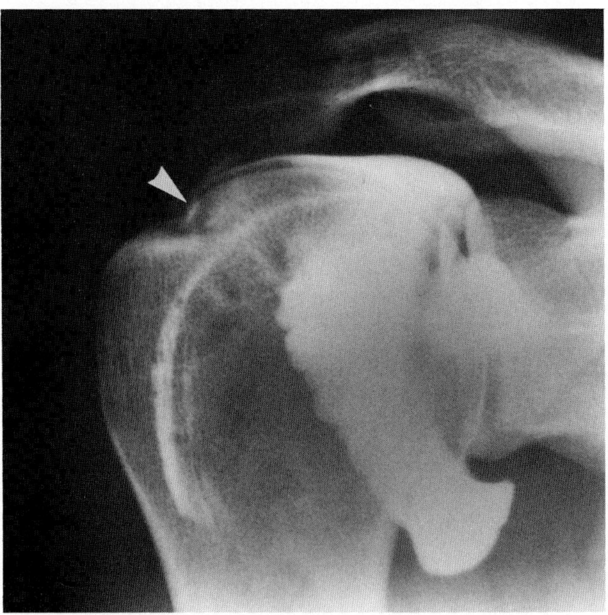

Fig. 9-16 (**A**) Routine view of the shoulder demonstrating erosion (arrow) of the greater tuberosity. (**B**) Single-contrast arthrogram demonstrating a partial tear (arrow) peripherally.

large percentage of patients with impingement syndrome. Therefore, such changes are less specific for a rotator cuff tear than changes in the greater tuberosity or superior subluxation of the humeral head.[36]

Eburnation along the glenoid rim and spurring of the inferomedial aspect of the humeral head were present in 25% of patients (Fig. 9-15), but this finding can also be seen with degenerative arthritis and in adhesive capsulitis.[36] Other views should also be reviewed for findings suggesting instability or previous dislocation (eg, Hill-Sachs lesions or Bankart deformity).

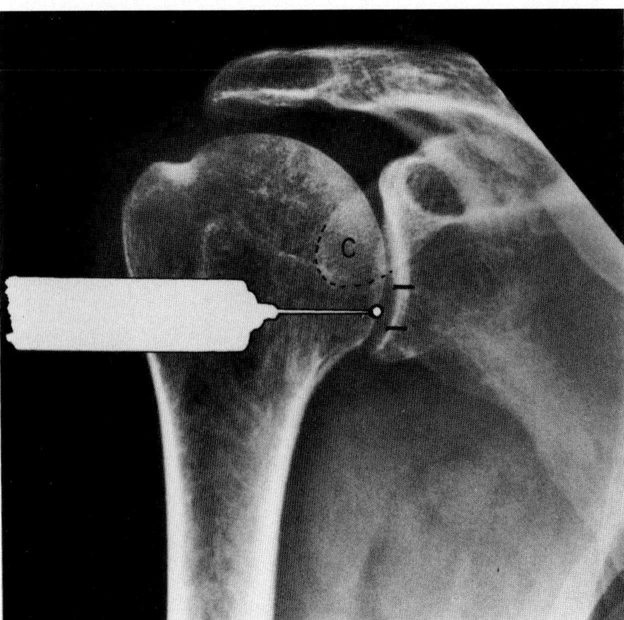

Fig. 9-17 Needle position for entering the glenohumeral joint. C, Coracoid. *Source:* Reprinted from *Imaging of Orthopedic Trauma* ed 2 by TH Berquist, 1991, Raven Press, © Mayo Foundation.

Technique

Shoulder arthrography is performed on a fluoroscopic table with an overhead tube and a small ($\leq$6 mm) focal spot. This provides better geometry than conventional fluoroscopic equipment, resulting in better film quality.[36]

With the patient in the supine position, the arm to be examined is externally rotated. A scout film is obtained to be certain that the radiographic technique is optimum. The technical quality of the films taken after injection is crucial, and preinjection scout films minimize the problem of inadequate technique and the need for repeat injections.

After optimum radiographic technique is established, the patient is prepared for the procedure with a 5-minute surgical scrub and subsequent application of povidone-iodine (Betadine) to the skin in the area to be injected. A 5-mL syringe with 1% lidocaine (Xylocaine) and a 25-gauge needle are used to mark the site of injection. The site is chosen over the glenohumeral joint below the coracoid and approximately at the junction of the middle and distal thirds of the glenoid articular surface (Fig. 9-17). A wheal is made in the skin over the joint entrance point. The soft tissues are also infiltrated with lidocaine. We err toward the medial margin of the humeral head. This ensures intraarticular positioning of the needle. The needle enters the joint or strikes the humeral head. With this technique the glenoid labrum is avoided.[36]

The injection is made with fluoroscopic guidance to be certain that the needle is properly positioned. If it is properly positioned, the contrast material flows away from the needle around the humeral head. An extensive literature is available concerning variations in this technique.[58,61,66,72,82]

If single-contrast technique is utilized, 6 to 10 mL of diatrizoate meglumine (Hypaque-M-60) is injected. Low-osmolality, nonionic agents are now available that may be more tolerated than ionic agents. Too much contrast material obscures detail, rendering the arthrogram less informative. With experience one can judge capsular volume early and avoid excessive amounts of contrast material. In double-contrast examinations, 4 mL of contrast material and then 10 to 15 mL of air are injected, depending upon the capsule size. Again, too much contrast material defeats the purpose of a double-contrast examination. The injection must be observed fluoroscopically. If contrast material is seen to leak into the subacromial bursa during the injection, the exact site of a rotator cuff tear can be visualized.[36]

After the injection the patient is exercised under fluoroscopic control, and any symptoms and radiographic changes are carefully noted. The relationship of the head and tuberosities to the acromion and coracoid can be examined if impingement is suspected clinically. The patient is then fluoroscopically positioned for tangential AP views of the glenohumeral joint. Films are taken in external and internal rotation. The tangential projection allows better evaluation of the articular cartilage.

The patient is then moved to a different radiographic suite, and the remainder of the films are performed. With a routine single-contrast examination, axillary, upright weight-bearing, and scapular lateral (Y) views are obtained in addition to the internal and external rotation views.[36] Bicipital groove views are obtained if symptoms dictate. If routine film findings lead one to suspect a rotator cuff tear but none is found on the initial arthrograms, further exercise and occasionally reinjection are performed to prevent false-negative studies.[36]

If a double-contrast examination is performed, the same views are obtained. Axillary views are taken in the prone and supine position, however, to demonstrate the glenoid labrum to better advantage. Conventional tomography or CT is occasionally necessary to evaluate the labrum and other subtle changes, especially in patients with previous dislocations or chronic shoulder instability.[36,41,45,79,87,91–93]

Double-contrast technique is best if CT or conventional tomography is used. Lesions are less frequently obscured, and injection of air allows more time for imaging.[58,66,87] Single-contrast examinations are effective for demonstrating cuff tears and are the study of choice for adhesive capsulitis. The synovium, articular cartilages, and labrum, however, are often obscured with single-contrast technique (Fig. 9-18). The biceps tendon is also more difficult to evaluate. Extravasation of contrast material may be noted from the biceps tendon sheath and subscapularis bursa in normal individuals (Fig. 9-19). Subtle changes, specifically tendon pathology or labral injuries, are more easily assessed with double-contrast technique (Fig. 9-20).[36,58,61]

Rotator Cuff Tears

The most common indication for shoulder arthrography is evaluation of patients with suspected tears in the rotator cuff. Many patients with rotator cuff tear have a history of trauma. The incidence is higher in patients older than 50 years of

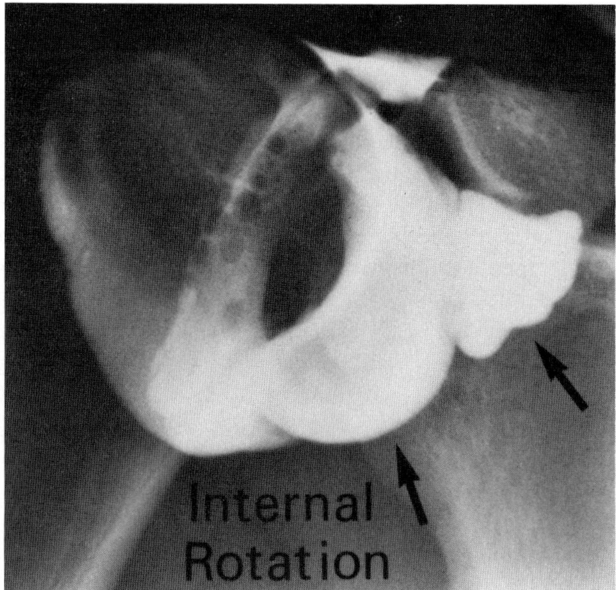

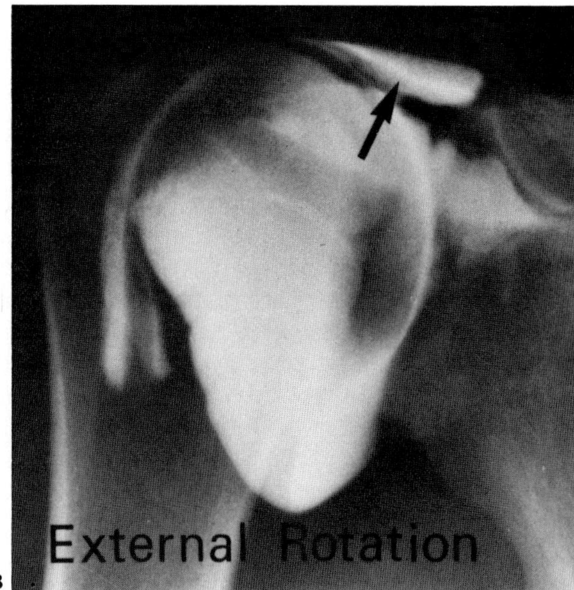

Fig. 9-18 Normal single-contrast arthrogram in internal (**A**) and external (**B**) rotation. Note that the articular cartilage and labrum are not clearly seen. Contrast medium over the biceps tendon (arrows) should not be confused with a tear.

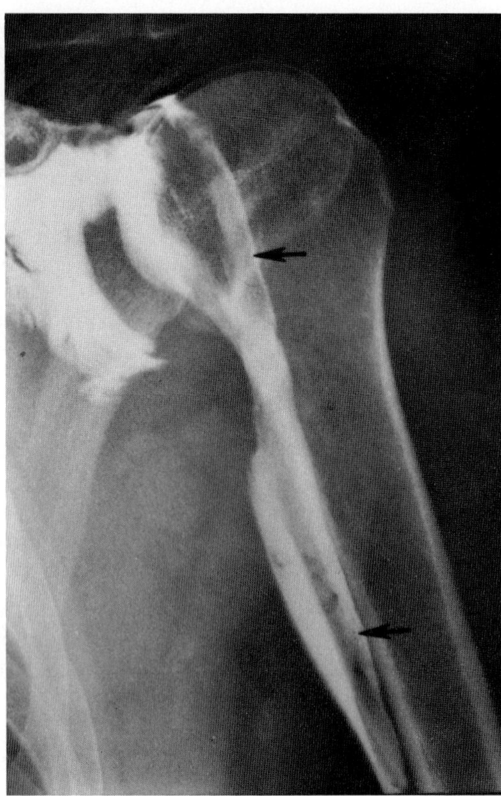

Fig. 9-19 Single-contrast arthrogram with normal extravasation of contrast agent along the biceps tendon (arrows).

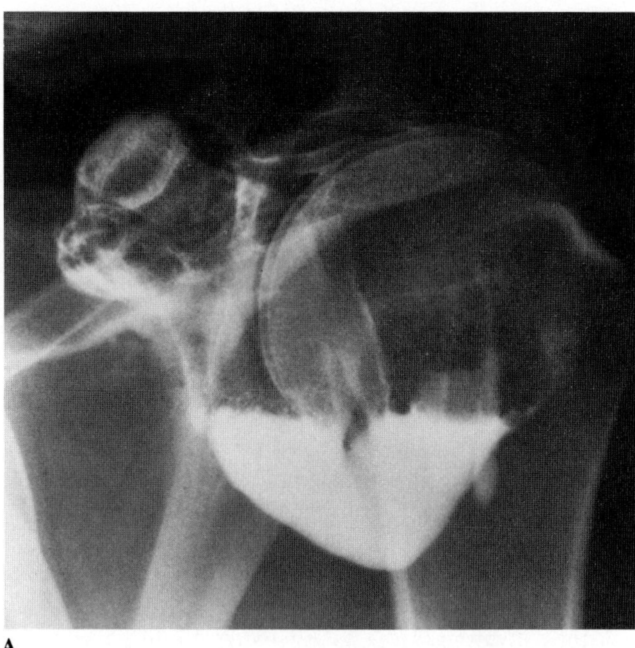

A

Fig. 9-20 Double-contrast arthrogram. (**A**) Upright external rotation views.

age.[42,79,84] In our experience at the Mayo Clinic (552 cases), 91% of the patients were older than 40 years of age.[36]

In our study all but 9% of the cases were chronic tears, with a history of trauma within 2 years being reported in more than 60% of patients. Of the 552 arthrograms reviewed, 145 revealed complete tears of the cuff as demonstrated by communication of the glenohumeral joint with the subacromial bursa (Fig. 9-21).[36]

The most important views are the AP views with internal and external rotation (Fig. 9-21). Almost all rotator cuff tears start in or are confined to the supraspinatus tendon. With external rotation of the shoulder, this tendon is the most lateral compared with the other tendons of the rotator cuff. In rotator cuff tears, upward subluxation is most severe on this view because the amount of tendon between the humeral head and the acromion is least. In the external rotation view, the distance from the edge of the humeral head cartilage to the tendon edge as defined by the contrast material is significant. This will depict the medial to lateral length of the tear. The extent of the tear in a posterior direction, or alternatively the width of the tear, is assessed on the internal rotation view. When the shoulder is internally rotated, the infraspinatus becomes more lateral and lies under the acromion as seen on the AP view. If the upper surface and undersurface of the tendon are well outlined and complete to the tendon insertion, the tear has not extended to any degree into the infraspinatus and is thus a small or medium-sized tear. If the tendon is not well outlined on both surfaces but another tendon gap is seen, the tear has extended into the infraspinatus and is at least large in size. If the axillary view shows a normal posterior capsule pouch, the tear is large, but if the posterior pouch is also obliterated, as mentioned previously, the tear probably extends to include the posterior aspect of the infraspinatus also and is global or massive in size. Finally, an anterior oblique view should be obtained to confirm observations of the extent of the tendon tearing.[36,58,61]

In patients with partial tears the arthrogram reveals extravasation of contrast material into a portion of the cuff without filling of the subacromial bursa (Fig. 9-16). Partial thickness tearing of the rotator cuff usually occurs in the supraspinatus. This can be seen as an extension of contrast material into the tendon substance but not into the bursa. If the contrast material extends past the end of the cartilage surface laterally, a portion of the tendon attachment is torn or has degenerated. These findings may be clarified by using a traction view in the upright position. Such findings also suggest that a careful evaluation is necessary because a component of the impingement syndrome related to anterior acromial osteophyte formation may well be present. Figure 9-22 points out the importance of multiple views in assessing the rotator cuff. The AP views were normal in this case.

In our experience at the Mayo Clinic, 85% of complete tears involved the supraspinatus near its insertion into the greater tuberosity; the adjacent infraspinatus was also involved in 39% of the cases. Tears in the subscapularis and teres minor were much less common, occurring in only 12% of the patients.[36]

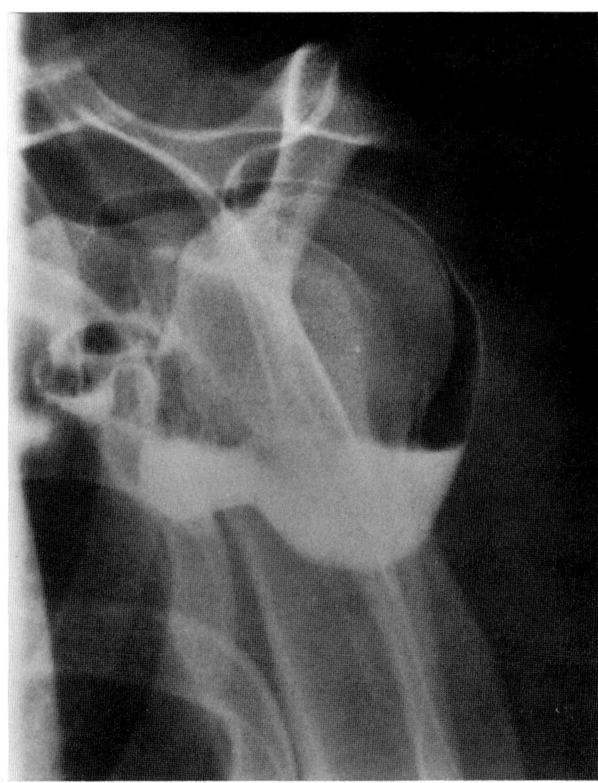

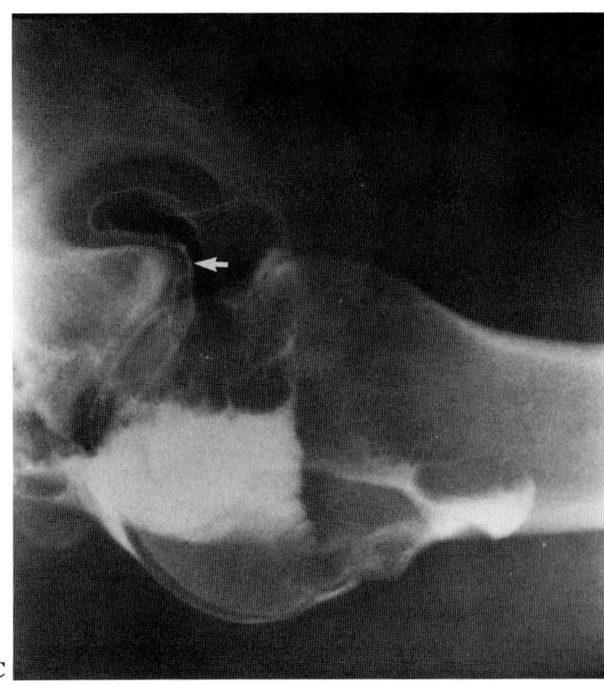

Fig. 9-20 contd (**B**) scapular Y view, and (**C**) prone axillary view. Note the clearly defined labrum (arrow in C) and articular cartilage.

In our study the accuracy rate did not differ significantly when double-contrast techniques were compared to single-contrast techniques. Partial tears were more readily detected with double-contrast techniques, however. The latter allow one to evaluate the size of the tear and the appearance of the tendon ends. These findings may aid the surgeon in determining the best treatment.[58,61] We find that in tears 1 to 2 cm in length evaluation of the tendon ends is of value but that in

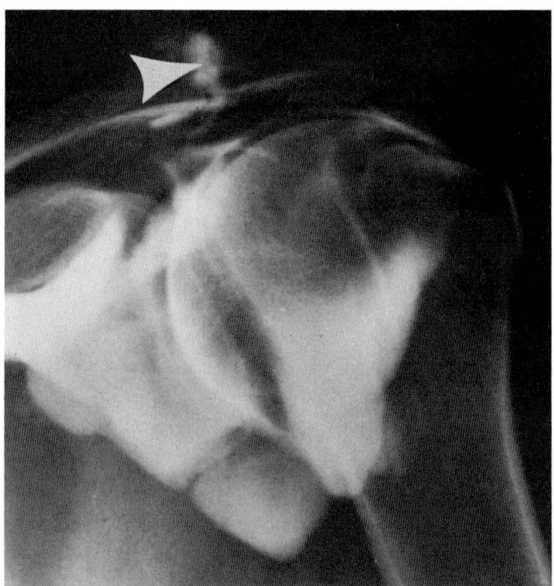

Fig. 9-21 External rotation view of a single-contrast arthrogram demonstrating a rotator cuff tear. Note that contrast medium also enters the acromioclavicular joint (arrowhead).

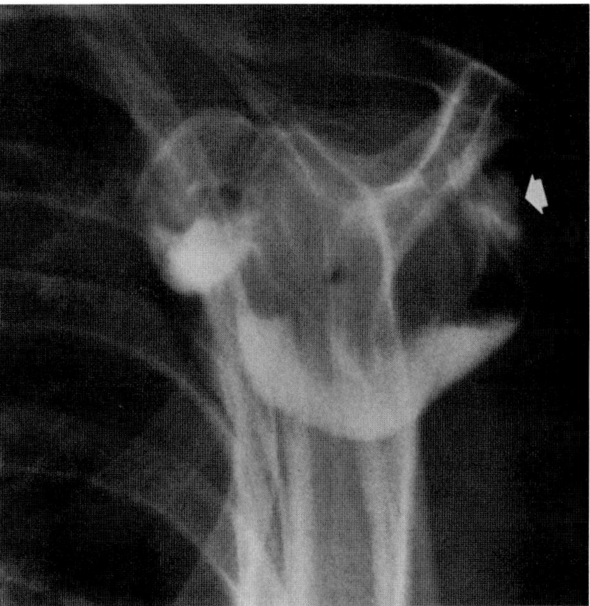

Fig. 9-22 Double-contrast arthrogram demonstrating a partial posterior rotator cuff tear (arrow) not evident on the other routine views.

larger chronic tears with extensive plain film findings the tendon ends are more difficult to visualize owing to scarring. In patients with superior subluxation and an acromiohumeral distance of 5 mm or less, we have found double-contrast technique to add little to the diagnosis. Also, in this setting, unless surgery is contemplated, we see little need to perform the arthrogram in the first place. Double-contrast arthrography is not utilized before arthroscopy because the air hinders the arthroscopist.

Adhesive Capsulitis

The term *adhesive capsulitis* was coined by Neviaser in 1953.[84] Patients present with pain and variable degrees of reduction in the range of motion of the involved shoulder. The etiology is unclear, but it has been stated that the condition may be due to capsular thickening or adhesions involving the capsule, biceps, and subacromial bursa.[36,59,84] Regardless of the etiology, however, arthrography is an effective diagnostic tool.[33,36]

The most common arthrographic feature is decreased capsular volume with reduced size of the axillary recess and subscapular bursa (Fig. 9-23). Other findings include a small axillary recess, lymphatic filling, synovitis, and irregularity of the capsular insertions.[36,59,84] Patients may complain of shoulder discomfort after only a small amount of contrast material has been injected.[33,36,59,84] After 2 to 4 mL of contrast material is injected it may become apparent that the capsule volume is only minimally reduced. Double-contrast technique adds little to the diagnosis.

The biceps tendon sheath fails to fill in 20% of patients with adhesive capsulitis.[36,61] The significance of this finding is uncertain, but biceps adhesions have been described by several investigators.[36,86]

Once the diagnosis is established, the arthrogram may then become a therapeutic tool to distend the contracted capsule and to relieve, at least temporarily, the patient's symptoms (Fig. 9-23).[36,59,84] This can be accomplished by gradually distending the capsule with a mixture of contrast material and 1% lidocaine (Xylocaine) or bupivacaine and betamethasone. The injection volume is gradually increased until the capsule ruptures; at this point further injection is unnecessary. The extravasation usually occurs along the subscapularis. This is followed by a set of assisted exercises with a gradually increasing range of motion. For this technique to be used, other precipitating or continuing sources of pain must be excluded. Unless formal manipulation accompanies the procedure, the amount of success one will have in gaining more movement is uncertain. Our experience has shown that the most success occurs in patients with mild to moderate reduction in capsular volume. In patients with a rotator cuff tear, dilatation is of little value because the capsule will decompress into the subacromial bursa.

Biceps Tendon Abnormalities

Arthrography, if properly utilized, may aid in diagnosis of biceps tendon abnormalities. Again, plain film evaluation is important. A bicipital groove view should be obtained in cases of clinically suspected biceps tendon lesions. The bony appearance of the groove may provide some clue to the diagnosis. Cone and colleagues[43] noted an average medial wall angle of 48°. The average width was 11 mm and the depth 4.6 mm. Medial wall bone spurs and spurs in the groove were noted in 33% and 8%, respectively, of the cases in their series. If the angle approaches 90°, constriction and tenosynovitis is said to be a diagnostic consideration. Angles less than 30° may be associated with subluxation of the biceps tendon.[43,86]

The main difficulty in detecting biceps tendon abnormalities arthrographically is the lack of consistent filling of this tendon sheath. Only when the tendon sheath is filled can evaluation of the tendon be accomplished. This is most accurate with double-contrast technique and bicipital groove views combined with weight-bearing internal and external rotation views.[36,61,72,82] The number of tendon sheaths filled does not differ significantly with single- or double-contrast technique, but the detail, especially in the intracapsular portion, is much improved with the double-contrast technique.[36,61] Positive findings include complete or partial tears noted by absence of the tendon in the sheath, irregularity of the tendon, or distortion of the sheath (Fig. 9-24). Subluxation of the tendon is best seen on the bicipital groove view, but it can also be detected by failure of the tendon to change position properly on internal and external rotation views.[36,43,61]

Although routine arthrography can be used to study the biceps tendon, there are now more suitable alternatives. Ultrasonography, CT arthrography, and MRI are excellent techniques. Axial images are easily obtained, and the anatomy of the tendon is more clearly displayed.[37,40]

Articular Cartilage and Labral Abnormalities

Arthrography is also valuable in evaluating the articular cartilage, glenoid labrum, and synovium. Cartilaginous lesions can be detected before they are obvious on plain films.[36,61] More commonly, the arthrogram is utilized in patients with shoulder instability. Evaluation of the glenoid labrum for Bankart lesions and the humeral head for Hill-Sachs deformities may indicate dislocations.[41,79,87,91–93] The capsule may be generous as well, indicating an additional factor contributing to the instability.[94]

In evaluating the glenoid labrum and articular cartilage, double-contrast arthrography provides much greater detail. Care must be taken not to utilize more than 4 mL of positive contrast medium or large portions of the articular cartilage may be obscured.[36]

We prefer both supine and prone axillary views as well as fluoroscopically positioned internal and external rotation views for the best evaluation of the labrum and articular cartilage. In patients with shoulder instability, better detail is offered by CT. Despite the introduction of MRI, many clinicians still prefer double-contrast CT (Fig. 9-25).[36,41,79,87] CT images are obtained after conventional images. Axial scans at 3- to 5-mm intervals are obtained with the patient supine and the arm in neutral position (Fig. 9-25).[36] With this technique the

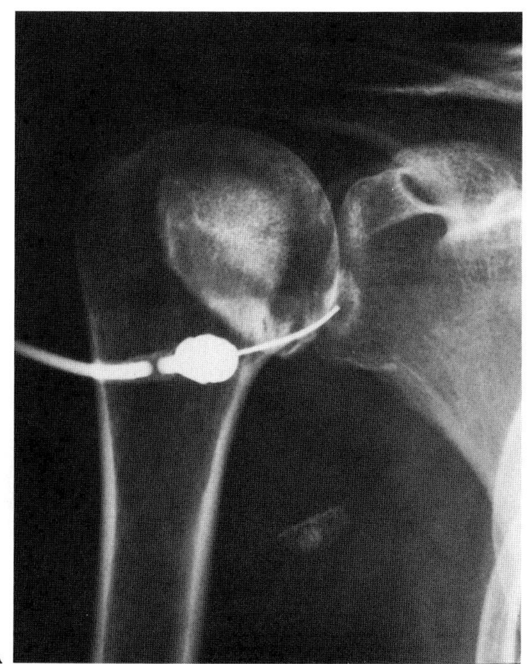

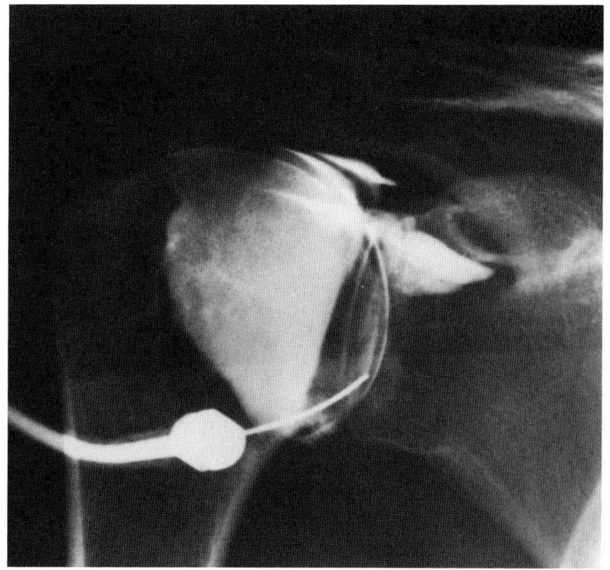

Fig. 9-23 Adhesive capsulitis. (**A**) Initial injection demonstrates marked reduction in capsular volume. (**B** and **C**) Gradual distention with contrast material, bupivacaine, and betamethasone. (**D**) Capsule has ruptured medially. The patient had marked improvement with complete recovery after physical therapy.

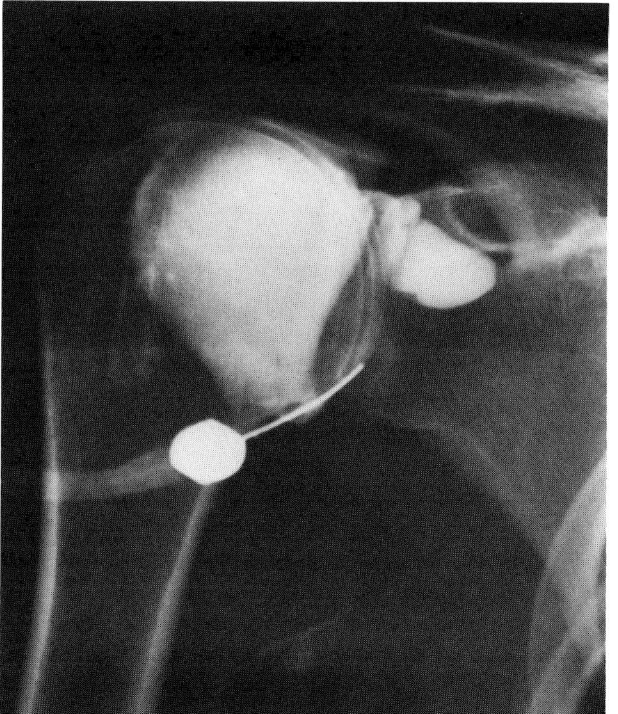

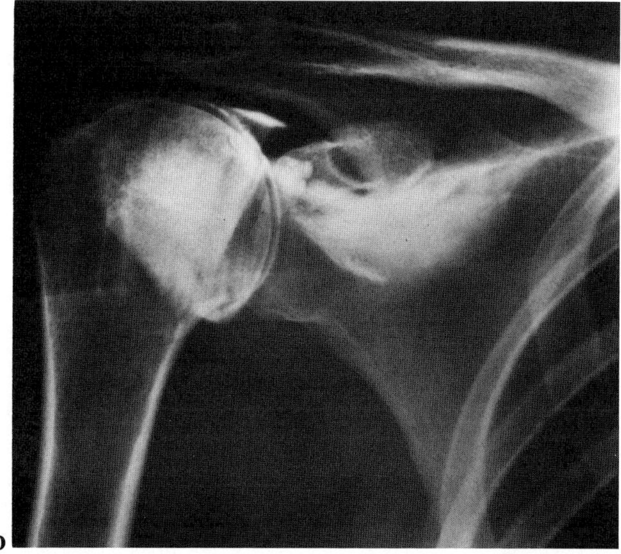

accuracy for evaluating the labrum and capsule approaches 100%.[66] Deutsch et al[49] reported a sensitivity of 96% and an accuracy of 86%. Callaghan et al[41] reported a specificity of 100% for labral injuries and Hill-Sachs lesions. The ability to evaluate the biceps tendon is obvious.

Double-contrast examination with a scapular lateral view or CT is also crucial to evaluate capsule size and to detect any changes in the configuration of the anterior, posterior, and inferior recesses of the capsule (Fig. 9-22). With anterior dislocations the capsule may be stripped from the glenoid, resulting in a generous anterior capsule and loss of the separation between the axillary recess and subscapularis bursa.[36] For any significance to be attached to this, the arm must be in external rotation because it is common for this confluence to occur without instability when the arm is internally rotated. Partial or complete rotator cuff tears may also be detected in association with chronic instability. Evaluation of patients with previous trauma or surgery may be aided by an upright

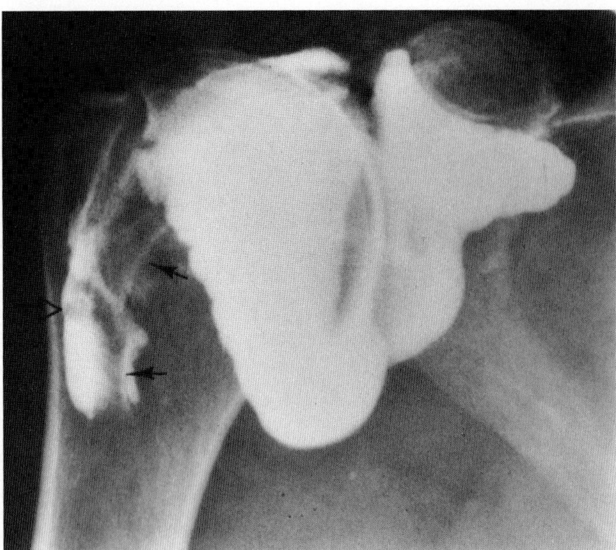

Fig. 9-24 External rotation view of a single-contrast arthrogram demonstrating subluxation of the biceps tendon (arrows) with a loose body (open arrow) in the tendon sheath.

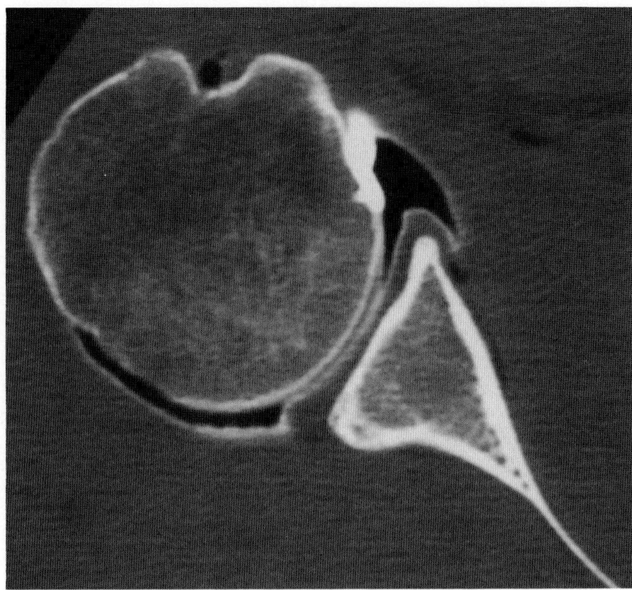

Fig. 9-25 Normal double-contrast CT arthrogram demonstrating the normal glenoid labrum.

weight-bearing view, which assists in determining the degree of laxity.[36]

Loose bodies may be sufficiently ossified to be detected on routine radiographs. CT arthrography can be helpful, however, especially when the loose bodies are in such unusual locations as the biceps tendon sheath.[41] Care must be taken not to mistake air bubbles for loose bodies. If the arthrogram is specifically requested for the detection of osteocartilaginous fragments, single-contrast examinations may be more useful.[36]

Bursography

We utilize bursography infrequently, and to date the indications are still somewhat unclear. This technique may become more efficacious in the future, however, and certainly radiologists and orthopaedists should be familiar with injection or aspiration of this bursa.

The subacromial bursa is a caplike structure between the rotator cuff and the acromion with subdeltoid, subacromial, and subcoracoid portions. The normal bursa may be difficult to inject accurately.[36,55,78]

The patient is placed on the fluoroscopic table in the supine position. The anterior shoulder is prepared with povidone-iodine (Betadine) solution as in arthrographic technique. The bursography set is the same as the tray used for arthrography. A 5-mL syringe with a 25-gauge needle is used to mark the subacromial region, and a wheal is made in the skin with 1% lidocaine (Xylocaine). The soft tissues are also anesthetized. After injection of the local anesthetic, a 1½-inch 22-gauge needle is advanced vertically and slightly superiorly under the acromion. When the undersurface of the acromion is reached, the needle can be withdrawn 1 to 2 mm, and the tip should be in the subacromial bursa. Any fluid should be aspirated at this time and sent for the appropriate laboratory studies. Three milliliters of diatrizoate meglumine (Hypaque-M-60) and 5 mL or more of room air are used to distend the bursa. This promotes better elevation of the synovium and upper surface of the cuff, allowing these as well as any extrinsic ligamentous or bony deformities of the bursa to be evaluated (Fig. 9-26). Radiographs are obtained in internal and external rotation as well as axillary and scapular positions. The scapular lateral view allows the most advantageous study of the acromial and coracoid relationships to the bursa.[36]

After the radiographic study, diagnostic or therapeutic injection with bupivacaine or lidocaine and betamethasone may be performed, thus adding to the versatility of the study.[36,78]

Acromioclavicular Arthrography

Radiographic approach to the acromioclavicular joint, although not as commonly employed as glenohumeral arthrography, may be of diagnostic and therapeutic value.

Patients to be studied are prepared in the usual manner with sterile technique. The joint can be entered superiorly or anteriorly (Fig. 9-27) after injection of local anesthetic. Fluoroscopic guidance ensures proper positioning. One milliliter to 2 mL of diatrizoate meglumine can be injected. This amount of contrast material normally should not extend beyond the capsule. Extension of contrast material medially toward the coracoid indicates coracoclavicular ligament injury. Commu-

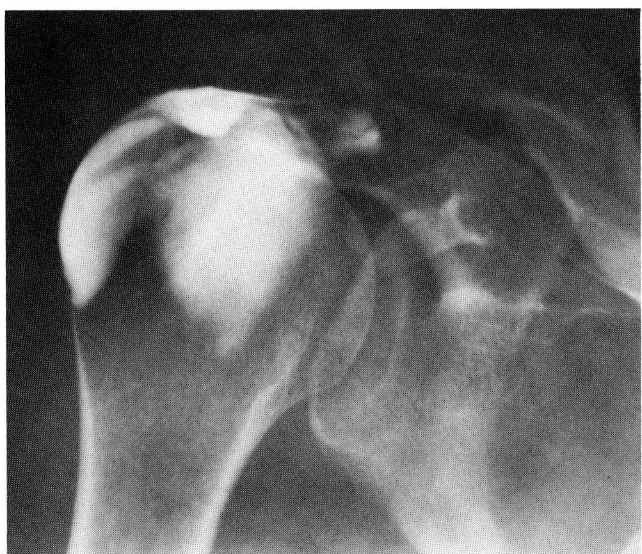

Fig. 9-26 Normal subacromial bursogram.

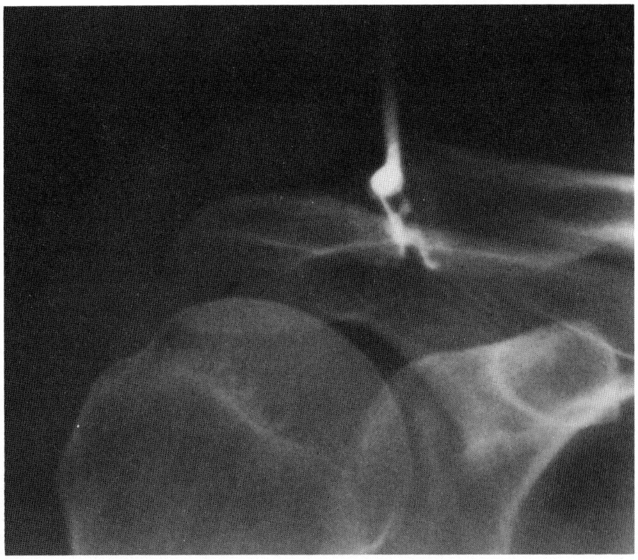

Fig. 9-27 Normal acromioclavicular arthrogram.

nication with the subacromial bursa is not uncommon in patients with chronic impingement or rotator cuff disease.[36]

Magnetic Resonance Imaging

Techniques for MR examination of the shoulder region vary with clinical symptoms. New software and coil techniques have greatly enhanced the ability of MR examinations to evaluate patients with shoulder symptoms. A particularly important development is the ability to obtain off-axis, small–field of view images in the shoulder region. This allows the patient to be examined in a more comfortable position with the arm at the side. Larger patients may need to be rotated slightly with the uninvolved arm above the head for proper positioning in the gantry. Off-axis, small–field of view images with the surface coil still represent the most optimal technique in these patients. In some cases the body coil with a smaller field of view can be utilized, but image quality is usually suboptimal.[37,39,70,71]

MRI is particularly suited for evaluation of the shoulder because it is capable of detecting lesions in the rotator cuff as well as other abnormalities in the glenohumeral joint, acromioclavicular joint, and associated periarticular soft tissues.[37,77,88]

The technique described in this chapter, consisting of axial, coronal, and sagittal T2- and T1-weighted sequences, is well suited for evaluating patients with suspected rotator cuff tears (Fig. 9-28). Patients with stage I disease (Fig. 9-29) or tendinitis have an intact rotator cuff. There is increased signal intensity within the supraspinatus tendon, however. This is generally most obvious on T2-weighted sequences but can be seen as an area of intermediate signal intensity (gray) on T1-weighted sequences. This increased signal intensity is probably due to edema, inflammation, and hemorrhage in the tendon. During this stage of rotator cuff disease, the subacromial bursa is generally not distended with fluid, and the normal fat plane between the rotator cuff and deltoid is clearly demonstrated. In contrast to MR images, arthrograms would be normal during this stage of rotator cuff disease. Histologic changes during this phase of rotator cuff disease show inflammation and mucoid degenerative changes within the tendon.[88,94,96]

Additional osseous and articular changes in the acromioclavicular joint may also be evident in patients at this time.[44] These are easily demonstrated on coronal and sagittal images, which usually demonstrate expansion, either fibrocartilaginous or osseous, of the subacromial joint with deformity of the adjacent supraspinatus muscle.[59,94,95]

The ability to demonstrate early changes in the rotator cuff is important in treatment planning, specifically in developing surgical criteria for management of patients with impingement syndrome. Patients who fail to respond to conservative therapy in this setting may require acromioplasty and excision of the coracoacromial ligament to prevent stage II and III disease.[83]

In patients with complete rotator cuff tears it is important to identify the ends of the tendons and to calculate as closely as possible the size of the tear.[36,37] Coronal and sagittal images are usually sufficient in this regard, and again T2-weighted sequences provide the best contrast distinction between the dark tendon and the high-intensity signal of the fluid between the ends of the torn tendon (Fig. 9-30). In addition to demonstration of the tear, appreciation of the tendon thickness is also important. In chronic disease the tendon is often significantly thinned. Additional findings include fluid in the subacromial

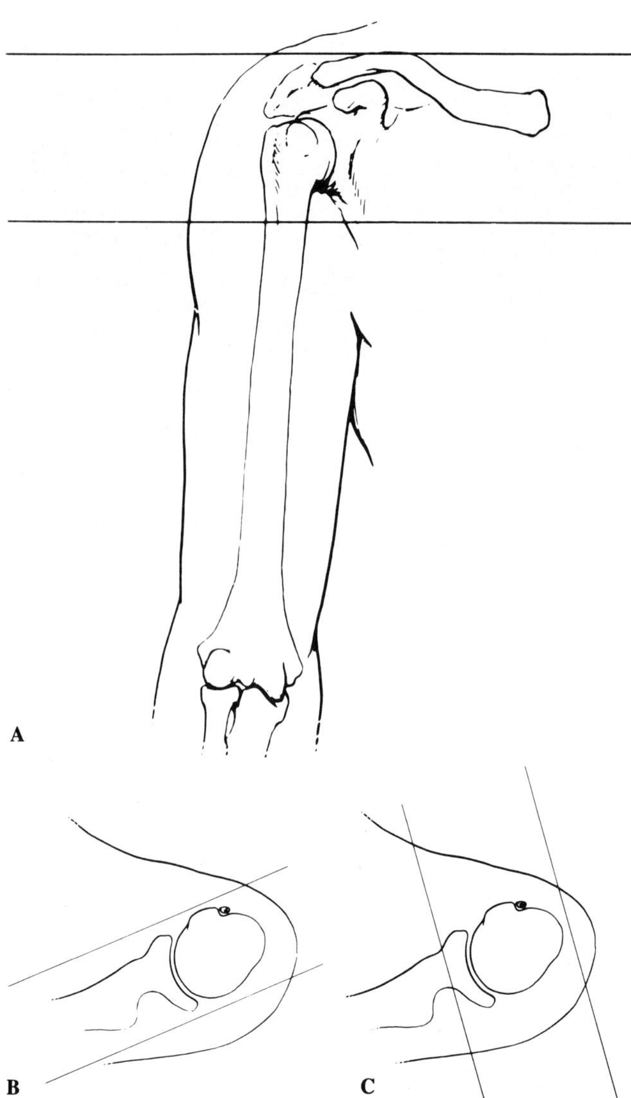

Fig. 9-28 (**A**) Illustration of coronal anatomy and sections selected for axial magnetic resonance imaging (MRI) planes. (**B**) Illustration of planes for coronal MR images. (**C**) Illustration of planes for sagittal images.

and subdeltoid bursae and obliteration of the normal subdeltoid fat stripe. It is not unusual in advanced disease to see communication from the glenohumeral joint through a tear into the subacromial bursa with continued extension into the acromioclavicular joint. In addition, cystic or ganglionlike lesions may appear on the dorsal aspect of the acromioclavicular joint in patients with advanced chronic rotator cuff tears. These patients may also demonstrate atrophy and retraction of the supraspinatus muscle along with the secondary osseous changes previously described.[88,94–96]

Experience with MRI is more limited with incomplete rotator cuff tears.[37,53] Incomplete tears may occur superiorly or inferiorly and are demonstrated as areas of increased signal intensity involving only a partial thickness of the tendon, usually in a linear fashion perpendicular to the course of the

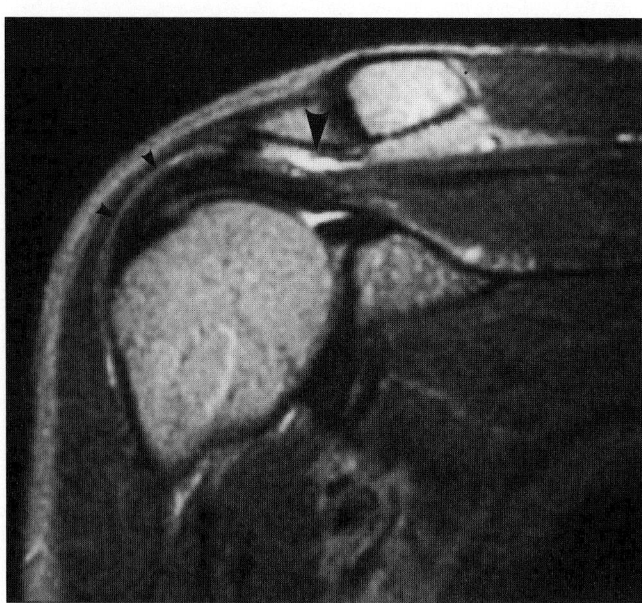

Fig. 9-29 Coronal T2-weighted image of the shoulder demonstrating increased signal (large arrowhead) in the subacromial bursa. The tendon is thick with increased signal intensity as a result of a stage I injury. The subdeltoid fat plane (small arrowheads) is intact.

tendon (Fig. 9-31). These findings may be difficult to differentiate from those of tendinitis. In this setting, double-contrast arthrography with weight-bearing views may still be the most effective in identifying subtle tears of the inferior surface of the tendon.[36,37] Superior defects would require bursography, however, which is a more difficult technique to perform.[78] Therefore, it is apparent that at some point MRI will also be the technique of choice in this regard.[37,94,96]

On the basis of the work of Kneeland[74] and Zlatkin[94,96] and their colleagues, diagnostic criteria for MRI have been developed. Criteria are based on changes involving the rotator cuff as well as secondary signs involving the subacromial and subdeltoid fat planes and bursae. The grading system is as follows: A normal tendon with normal signal intensity and morphology is considered grade 0. Grade 1 tendons have increased signal but normal width and morphology. A grade 2 tendon shows increased signal intensity with changes in morphology such as tendon thinning or irregularity. Grade 3 tendons have discontinuity with increased signal in the region of tendinous disruption that is best appreciated on T2-weighted images (Fig. 9-30).[94,96]

Zlatkin and Dalinka[94] and Zlatkin et al[96] reported the accuracy of shoulder MRI with these criteria. Sensitivity, specificity, and accuracy of 91%, 88%, and 89%, respectively, for all tears, partial and complete, were demonstrated. MRI was also noted to be more sensitive than arthrography in diagnosis of small anterior supraspinatus tendon tears.

It is important to compare the results of MRI with those of other accepted imaging techniques, specifically arthrography, bursography, and ultrasonography. Both single- and double-

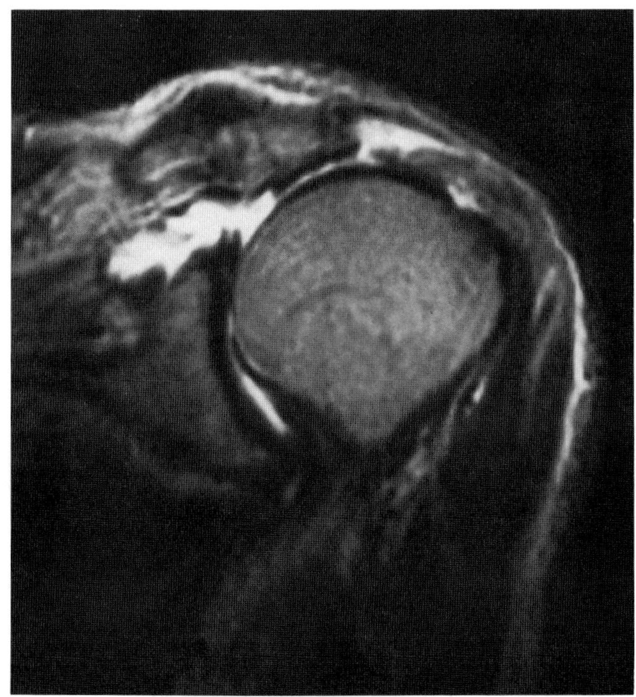

Fig. 9-30 Coronal MR image demonstrating marked superior subluxation of the humeral head. There is a large cuff tear with retraction of the supraspinatus tendon.

contrast arthrography has been accurate in detection of rotator cuff tears. Unless arthrography is combined with bursography, however, partial superior tears and impingement are difficult to diagnose.[36,55,78] Bursography is invasive and difficult to perform unless the procedure is performed by an experienced examiner.[55,78]

Burk et al[39] compared the results of arthrography, MRI, and ultrasound in a group of 38 patients referred for suspected rotator cuff tears. Both MRI and double-contrast arthrography demonstrated sensitivities of 92% and specificities of 100% for normal cuffs. Diagnosis of cuff tears was equal with both techniques. Ultrasound was 63% sensitive for diagnosis of cuff tears and demonstrated a specificity of only 50% for intact rotator cuffs. Others have reported ultrasound to have an accuracy of 87% to 94% for diagnosis of rotator cuff tears;[80] importantly, the negative predictive value of ultrasonography was 95%. In the operated group, however, the specificity of ultrasound was only 73% compared to 100% for arthrography.[40]

Arthrography is an accurate (98%) but invasive technique for diagnosis of rotator cuff tears, but it is of little value in evaluating impingement.[36,61] Ultrasound is accurate in some physicians' hands but has not achieved the wide acceptance of MRI or arthrography because of the experience required by examiners and its difficulty in achieving acceptance in the orthopaedic community. Physicians not involved in performing and interpreting ultrasound find the image difficult to evaluate. MRI is noninvasive and provides a method of screening for many osseous and soft tissue abnormalities. Although refinements are still in progress, it appears to be the noninvasive technique of choice for evaluating impingement and rotator cuff pathology.

Imaging of Capsular Abnormalities

The capsular structures of the shoulder consist of the synovial membrane, the capsule, the associated glenohumeral ligaments, the glenoid labrum, and associated bursae and recesses.[36,94,96] The subscapularis muscle and tendon are also closely applied to the anterior capsule. Imaging of the shoulder capsule has conventionally been accomplished with either conventional or CT arthrography.[36,41] Contrast arthrography provides valuable information regarding the size and integrity of the capsule and also allows intraarticular injections of anesthetic and/or a combination of anesthetic and steroid compounds to treat and diagnose certain shoulder disorders.[36,61]

Capsular volume is difficult to evaluate with noncontrast MRI because the degree of distention of the capsule cannot be evaluated unless contrast material of some type is injected.[53] Recently, gadolinium-DTPA has been advocated as an MR

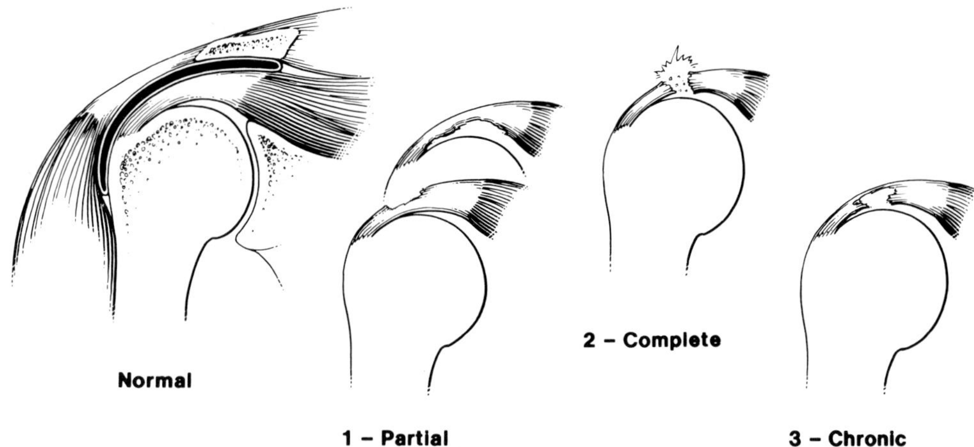

Fig. 9-31 Illustration of normal, partial thickness (inferior and superior), full thickness, and chronic rotator cuff tears.

arthrography contrast agent. To date, however, there has not been enough significant experience to understand clearly its implications in MRI of the shoulder. Certainly fluoroscopically monitored injections of contrast material are much more efficacious than MR arthrography at this point. Therefore, patients who are being evaluated for subtle changes in the synovial lining or for changes in capsular volume such as adhesive capsulitis are still studied to better advantage with conventional arthrography or arthrography combined with CT or conventional tomography.

Disruption of the shoulder capsule can be detectable by arthrography or MRI. Loss of integrity of the capsule or its adjacent or associated ligaments can be identified on MRI as poorly defined areas of increased signal intensity adjacent to the capsule on T2-weighted sequences (Fig. 9-32). Capsular lesions are most easily evaluated in the axial and coronal planes.

Recurrent shoulder dislocations are a common problem in orthopaedic practice.[36,42] Originally, it was believed that the Bankart lesion (glenoid labral tear or osteochondral fracture of the inferior labrum) was the main lesion causing recurrent anterior dislocation. More recently the entire anterior capsule mechanism has been implicated.[37,94,96] Type 2 and 3 capsular insertions are more often associated with instability (Fig. 9-33).[95]

Until recently, arthrography with CT has been the technique of choice for evaluating the glenoid labrum.[36,66,87] T2-Weighted or gradient-echo sequences can be used to evaluate the glenoid labrum as well. Conventional axial and coronal images (Fig. 9-34) will demonstrate the entire labrum, but it may be optimal to use radial GRASS interleaved (GRIL) sequences, similar to those described in the knee, to view the labrum tangentially. Currently, most software does not provide the capability to select multiple off-axis radial GRIL images.

Normally the glenoid labrum has a triangular shape and appears black (low intensity) on spin-echo and gradient-echo sequences (Fig. 9-34). There are some variations in the appearance of the labrum because it is generally sharper anteriorly and slightly more rounded posteriorly (Fig. 9-34).[37,77] Disruptions of the labrum are seen as linear areas of high signal intensity on MR images. Complete avulsion or total absence of the labrum is easily identified. Degenerative changes within the labrum that do not communicate with the articular surface, similar to those changes described in the knee, may also be evident. The clinical significance of these is probably similar to that of changes in the knee meniscus, and therefore a glenoid labrum tear should not be suggested unless there is a clear linear defect that articulates with the articular surface of the labrum or a labral detachment (Fig. 9-35). Tears are most commonly identified anteriorly; therefore, if GRIL techniques are not available, the axial plane is usually best suited to identify these lesions.[37,77,94,96]

Subtle osseous abnormalities, including avascular necrosis and fractures, can also be detected with MRI (Fig. 9-36), making it an ideal screening technique in athletes with shoulder disorders.[37,40]

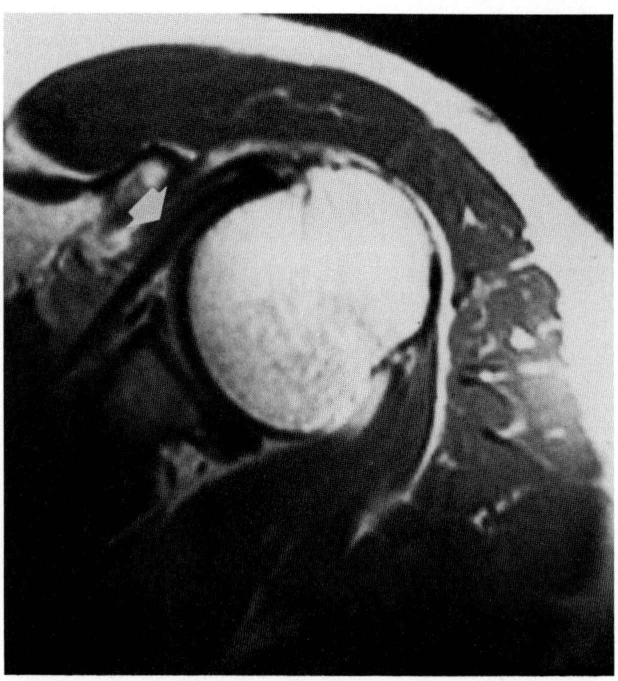

A

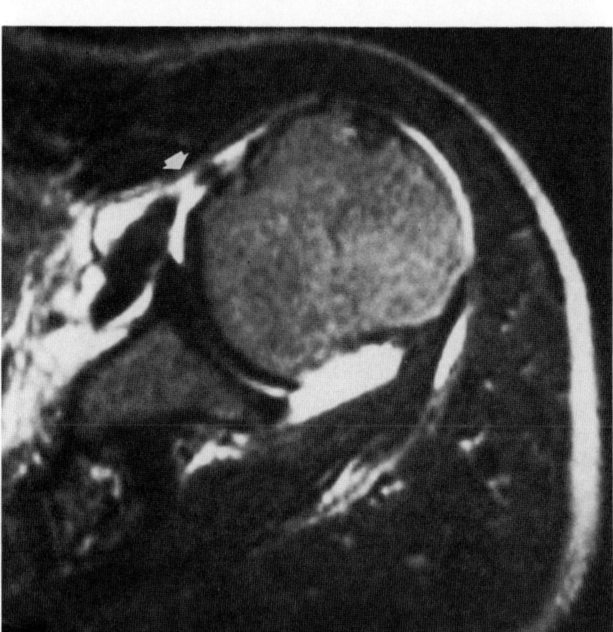

B

Fig. 9-32 (**A**) Normal subscapularis tendon (arrow) and (**B**) torn tendon (arrow) demonstrated on axial MR images.

FRACTURES, DISLOCATIONS, AND OSSEOUS INJURIES

Fractures of the Proximal Humerus

Fractures of the proximal humerus usually occur in older patients.[104] If one considers all fractures, about 5% involve

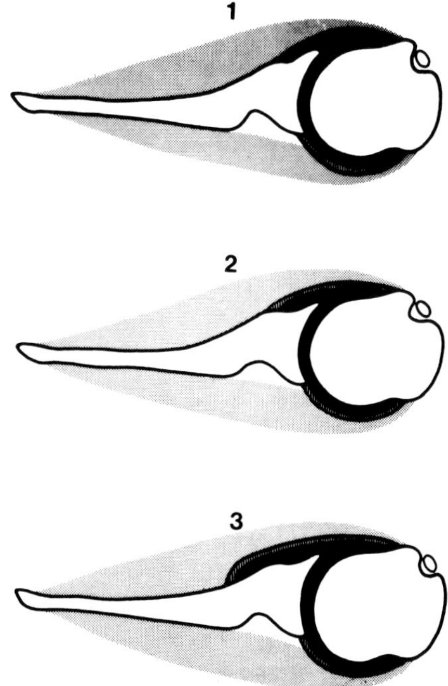

Fig. 9-33 Illustrations of variations in the anterior capsular attachments. Type 1, in or near the anterior glenoid labrum; 2, along the scapular neck; type 3, medial to the glenoid neck. *Source:* Reprinted with permission from Zlatkin MD, Dalinka MK and Kressel HY, Magnetic resonance imaging of the shoulder, *Magnetic Resonance Quarterly* (1989;5:3–22), Copyright © 1989, Raven Press.

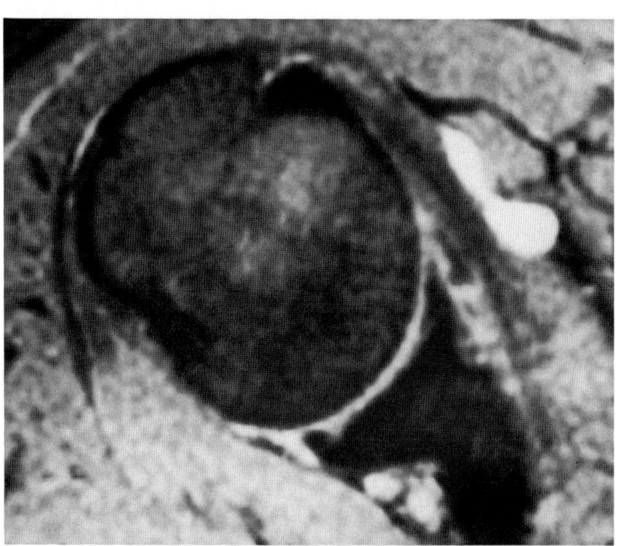

Fig. 9-34 Normal axial gradient echo image of the glenoid labrum.

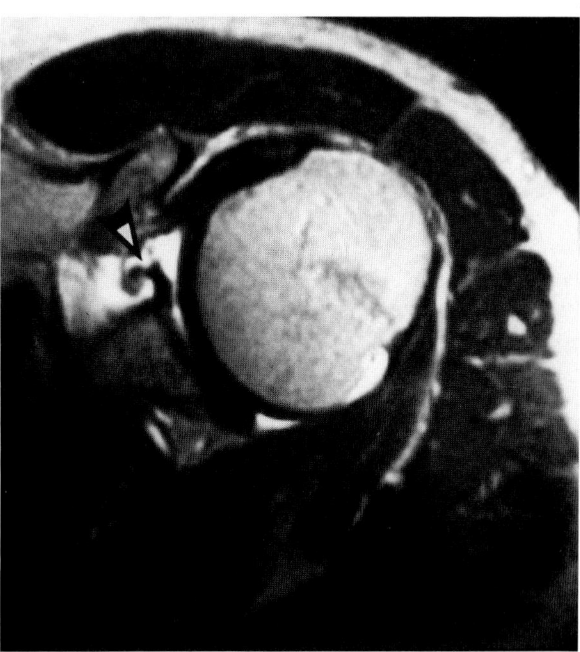

Fig. 9-35 Partial detachment of the anterior labrum (arrowhead) on a T2-weighted MR image (SE 2000/60).

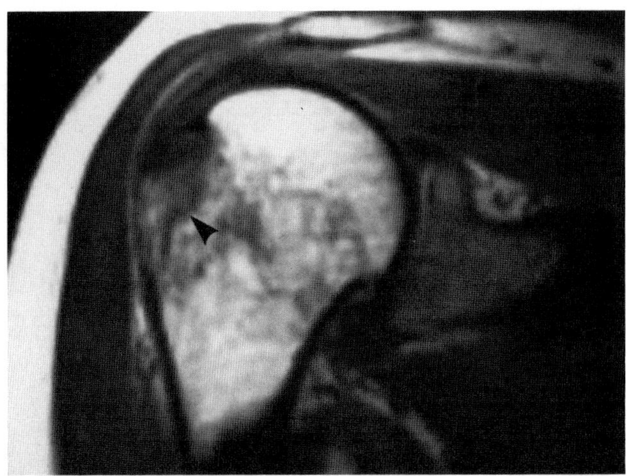

Fig. 9-36 Coronal T1-weighted MR image (SE 500/20) demonstrating an undisplaced greater tuberosity fracture (arrowhead).

the proximal humerus.[114,140] In older patients, the fracture most often occurs after minor trauma, such as a fall. In younger individuals and athletes, the skeletal strength is greater than that provided by ligaments, so that dislocations usually occur instead of fractures.[125,140] When fractures occur in this age group, they usually result from a fall with the elbow flexed and wrist dorsiflexed. Eighty percent of humeral fractures in children (<16 years old) involve the proximal epiphysis.[112]

Fractures of the proximal humerus tend to follow the physeal lines that divide the humerus into four parts: the humeral head, lesser tuberosity, greater tuberosity, and shaft (Fig. 9-37).[104,128] Neer[136] proposed the most widely accepted classification for adult fractures of the proximal humerus. This classification is based on the number of fragments and the degree of displacement or angular deformity. If

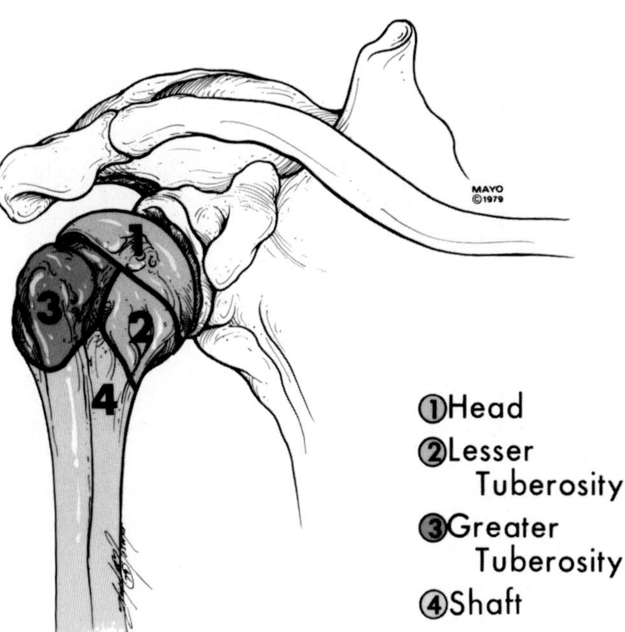

Fig. 9-37 Illustration of the four major fragments used to describe proximal humeral fractures. *Source:* Reprinted from *Imaging of Orthopedic Trauma* ed 2 by TH Berquist, 1991, Raven Press, © Mayo Foundation.

there is 1 cm of displacement between the fragments or greater than 45° of angular malposition, the fragment is considered displaced (Fig. 9-38).[109,122,128,129,135]

The majority of proximal humeral fractures (80% to 85%) are undisplaced.[128,136] Fractures most commonly involve the surgical neck.[104,136] The rotator cuff, capsule, and periosteum assist in maintaining the position of the fragments.[140] A two-part fracture indicates that one fragment is displaced more than 1 cm or angulated more than 45° (Fig. 9-38). Three-part fractures have two displaced or angulated fragments. With four-part fractures, all fragments are displaced. Isolated fractures of the tuberosities are rare unless there is an associated dislocation (Fig. 9-39).[116,132]

The Salter-Harris or Neer-Horowitz[139] classification can be applied to proximal humeral fractures in children. In the latter, grade I fractures are displaced by less than 5 mm, grade II fractures by one-third the width of the humeral shaft (Fig. 9-38), grade III fractures by two-thirds the width of the humeral shaft, and grade IV fractures by more than two-thirds the width of the humeral shaft.[139]

As a general rule, with two-part displacement closed manipulation restores acceptable position. Immobilization with a sling or Velpeau immobilizer is followed by early exercise to avoid adhesive capsulitis.[136] Open reduction is occasionally attempted to restore position. Open reduction is generally required for adult three- and four-part fractures.

Humeral shaft fractures are also unusual in the young athlete. Nevertheless, direct trauma in contact sports or repetitive trauma in throwing sports (eg, in a baseball pitcher or quarterback) may lead to humeral shaft fractures.[119] Fractures due to direct trauma are likely to be transverse or oblique. Throwing fractures are frequently spiral in nature.[119] Proximal and humeral shaft fractures are frequently displaced as a result of muscle forces (Fig. 9-40).

Accurate radiographic evaluation of the shoulder can be obtained with the shoulder trauma series (40° posterior oblique in external rotation, axillary view, and scapular view). AP and lateral views are usually adequate to define humeral shaft

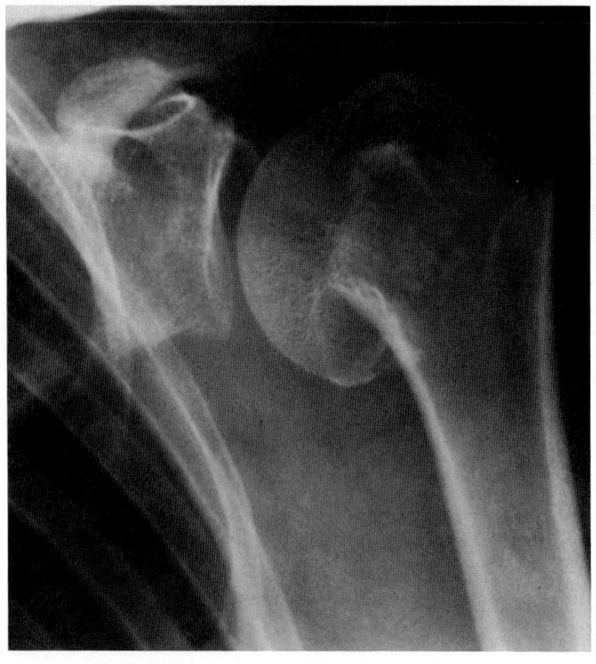

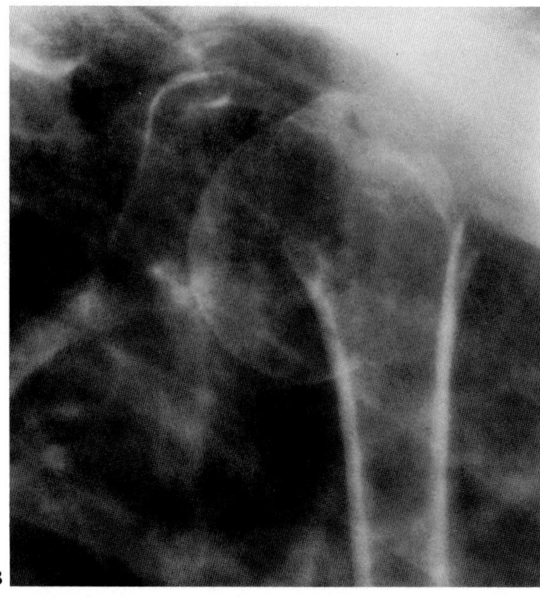

Fig. 9-38 (**A**) AP and (**B**) transthoracic views of a physeal fracture of the proximal humerus.

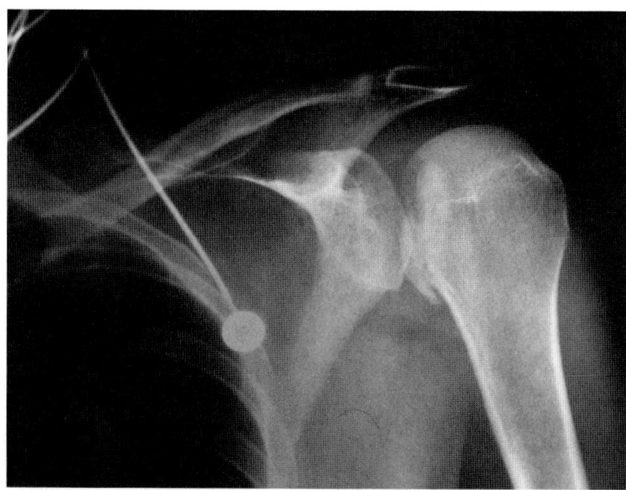

Fig. 9-39 AP view of the shoulder demonstrating an isolated tuberosity fracture associated with posterior dislocation.

fractures.[104] Proper classification requires experience. Because the majority of fractures are undisplaced, it is not surprising that interobserver errors are higher with three- and four-part fractures.[129] CT is useful to ensure proper classification and for accurate assessment of fragment position before therapy.[109,128,129]

Isolated avulsion fractures of the humerus are uncommon.[104] Avulsion of the lesser tuberosity by the subscapularis tendon, however, has been reported (Fig. 9-39). This is a significant injury because the anterior buttressing effect of the subscapularis muscle is lost, leading to anterior instability.[116,132] The fracture is usually obvious on routine trauma views, but CT is useful when the origin of the fragment is in question.[128]

Glenohumeral Dislocations

Dislocations of the glenohumeral joint occur more frequently than dislocations at any other articulation. They account for 50% of all dislocations.[140,147] Most dislocations are anterior (97%). Posterior dislocations occur in 2.0% to 4.3% of patients, and superior and inferior dislocations are rare.[115,140,156]

Anterior Dislocations

Most anterior dislocations (96%) are due to trauma, usually resulting from a fall with the arm in abduction and external rotation. Rarely, the dislocation is due to direct posterolateral trauma. In adolescence, dislocations in boys outnumber those in girls by 5:1.[126,140] As the humeral head dislocates, it is forced anteriorly and inferiorly against the capsule, glenohumeral ligaments, and subscapularis. These structures provide the majority of the shoulder's anterior stability. The posterolateral aspect of the humeral head comes in contact with the glenoid rim, which may result in an associated impaction fracture. This was described by Hill and Sachs and bears their name, the Hill-Sachs deformity.[124] This lesion occurs in 67% to 76% of cases.[104] Associated lesions of the anteroinferior glenoid rim reportedly occur less frequently, appearing in approximately 50% of cases.[104,140]

Most anterior dislocations are obvious on the conventional AP radiograph. Nevertheless, a routine trauma series is most accurate (40° posterior oblique, axillary, and Y views) for complete assessment of the dislocation and associated fractures. Dislocations are described according to their location. In order of decreasing frequency, dislocation may be subcoracoid (Fig. 9-41), subglenoid, subclavicular, or intrathoracic.[104,140]

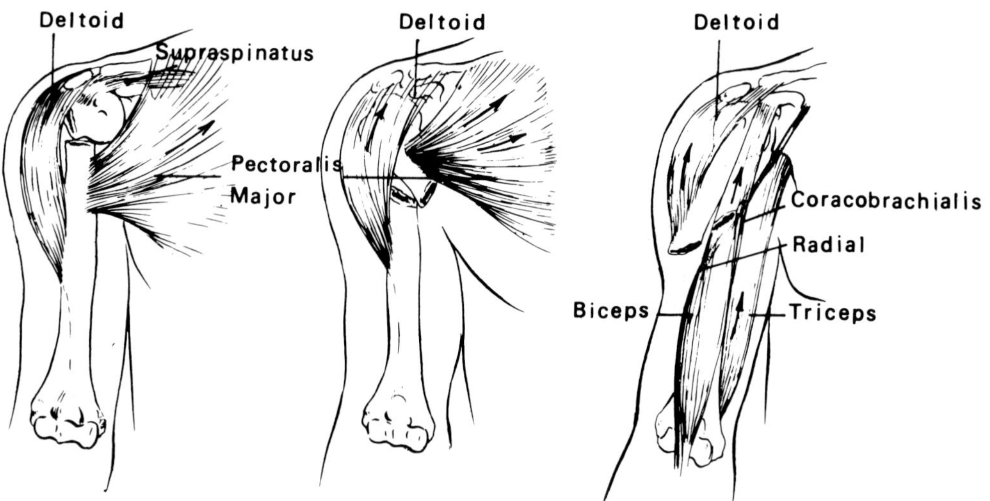

Fig. 9-40 Illustration of muscle forces (arrows) on humeral fractures. *Source:* Reprinted from *Fractures in Adults*, Vol 1, ed 3 (p 844) by CA Rockwood and DP Green with permission of JB Lippincott, © 1984.

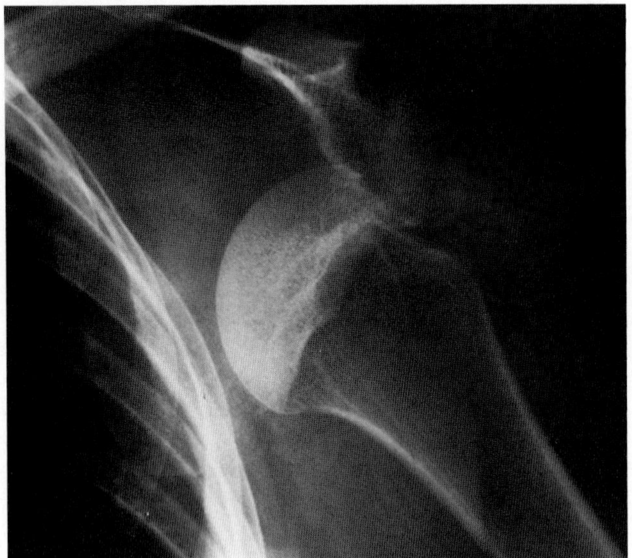

Fig. 9-41 AP view of the shoulder demonstrating an anterior dislocation with an associated greater tuberosity fracture.

After closed reduction, the radiographic trauma series, except for the axillary view, should be repeated. The radiographs must be carefully studied to ensure adequate reduction and to exclude associated fractures (greater tuberosity, Hill-Sachs, or glenoid rim). For example, if the anterior dislocation results in the humeral head lying medial to the coracoid, reduction may be more difficult. Interposition of the tendon of the long head of the biceps may occur with this type of dislocation, making reduction difficult or impossible. Displacement of the biceps tendon should also be considered in dislocations with large greater tuberosity fractures because the bicipital groove may be involved (Fig. 9-42).[127] Fractures of the greater tuberosity occur in up to 15% of anterior dislocations (Fig. 9-43). Rarely, coracoid fractures occur with anterior dislocation.[103]

Additional views, described earlier in this chapter, are useful in detecting subtle Hill-Sachs deformities and glenoid rim fractures. The Stryker notch view is easy to duplicate and accurate for Hill-Sachs deformities in 90% of patients with recurrent dislocation.[121] AP internal rotation views will detect Hill-Sachs deformity in 50% of patients with recurrent dislocation. Glenoid rim fractures may be obvious on routine axillary or West Point views (Fig. 9-44).[100,104] Labral injuries, however, may be present with no obvious bony changes. Therefore, double-contrast arthrography, with or without CT, or arthrotomography may be indicated in patients with recurrent dislocations. MRI is also useful in this setting.

Treatment of anterior dislocation can usually be accomplished with closed reduction. Exceptions include patients with soft tissue interposition, subacromial greater tuberosity displacements, and large (>5 mm) glenoid rim fractures. Glenoid fractures can lead to recurrent dislocation or traumatic arthritis.[99,130,134,140,154] Internal fixation is considered in these patients.[104,126]

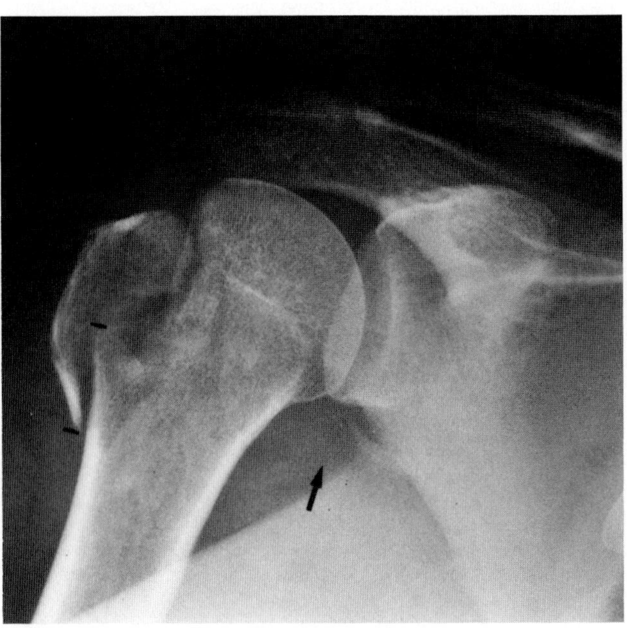

Fig. 9-42 Postreduction AP view after anterior dislocation with fractures of the greater tuberosity and inferior labrum (arrow).

Posterior Dislocations

Only about 2.0% to 4.3% of shoulder dislocations are posterior.[118,133,140,154] In sports, the injury usually occurs during falls with the arm adducted and internally rotated or with direct trauma to the anterior shoulder.[104,140,155]

Clinically, the patient's arm may be held in slight abduction and internal rotation. External rotation is blocked. The diagnosis is missed clinically in many patients.[123,140]

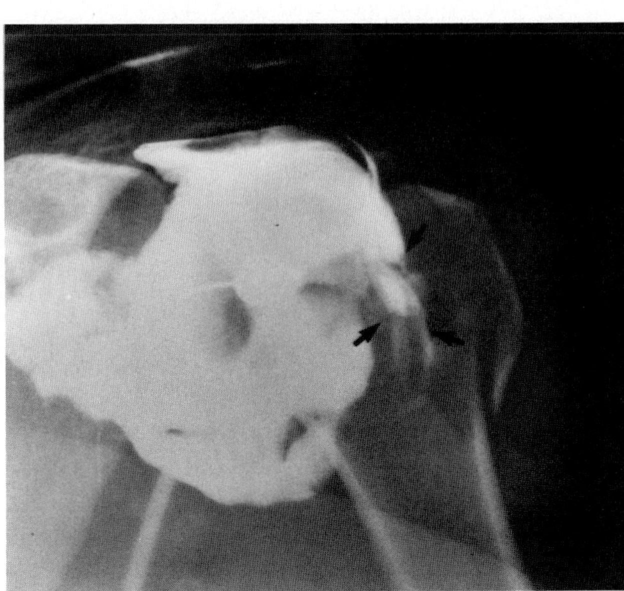

Fig. 9-43 Postdislocation arthrogram showing a ruptured capsule with entrapped biceps tendon (arrows) between the humerus and greater tuberosity fracture.

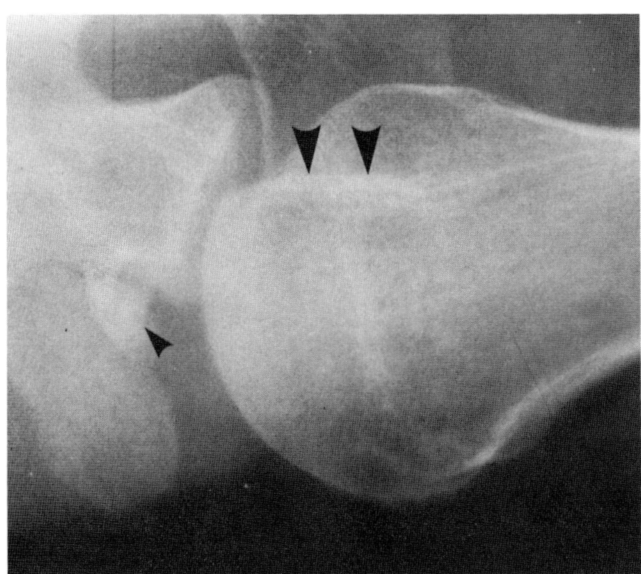

Fig. 9-44 West Point view demonstrating an obvious labral fracture (single arrowhead) and Hill-Sachs deformity (double arrowheads).

The injury may be easily overlooked on the conventional AP view. There are, however, several signs present:[110]

- the humeral head is fixed in internal rotation (100%)
- the joint may appear abnormally widened or narrowed
- the usual half-moon overlap of the humeral head and glenoid may be absent or distorted (55%)
- a trough line may appear in the humeral head, representing a compression fracture of the anterior aspect of the humeral head (75%)
- there may be an associated fracture of the lesser tuberosity (25%)

Routine use of the 40° posterior oblique, AP, scapular Y, and axillary views (trauma series) should prevent missed diagnoses of posterior dislocation. The Y view is particularly useful because the relationship of the humeral head to the glenoid is easy to see. Also, the view can be obtained without moving the arm (Fig. 9-45). Rather than memorize the various signs on the conventional AP view, we suggest the use of these alternative views for more accurate diagnoses.

Fractures of the lesser tuberosity and, less commonly, of the glenoid as well as posterior capsule tears with rim fractures are associated with posterior dislocations (Fig. 9-39).[136]

Posterior dislocations can usually be treated with closed reduction.[115] The incidence of recurrence is much lower than that with anterior dislocations,[136] but the incidence of arthrosis is higher.[139]

Superior and Inferior Dislocations

Superior and inferior dislocations (luxatio erecta) are rare.[115,140] Superior dislocations overlie the acromion or

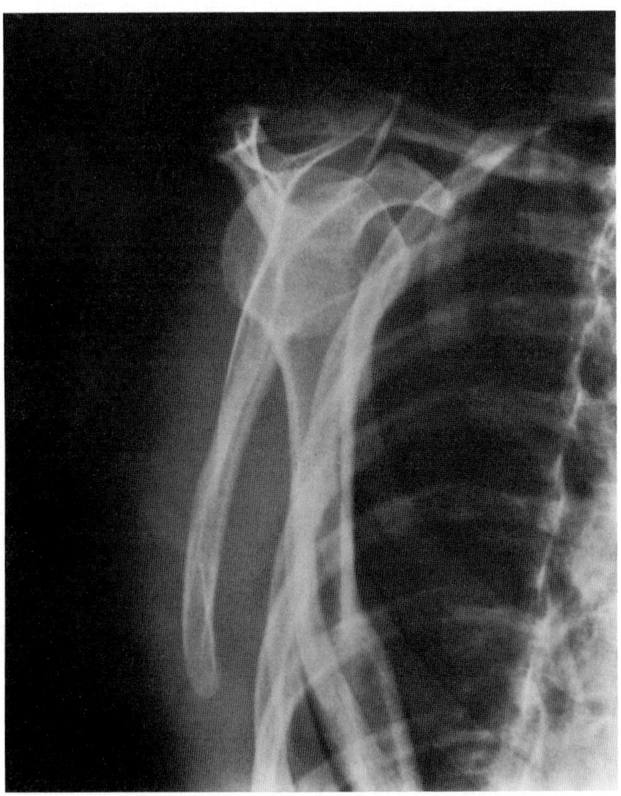

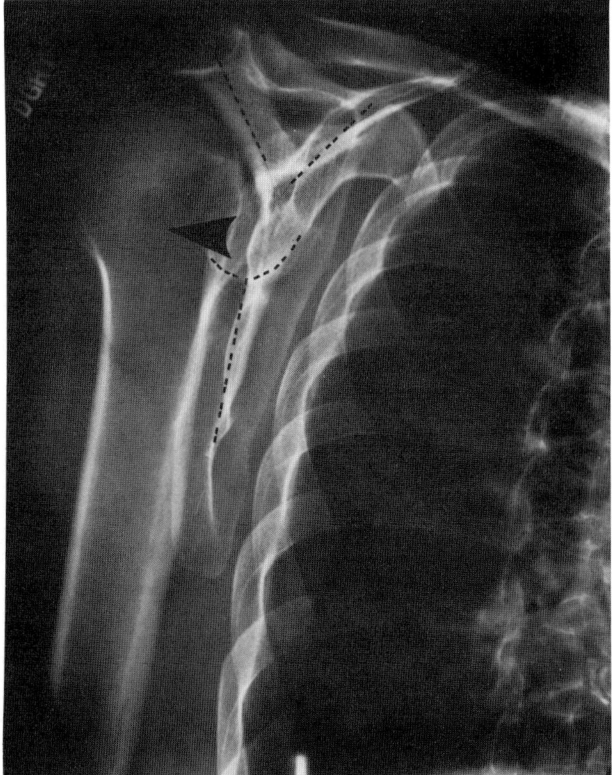

Fig. 9-45 (**A**) Normal scapular Y view and (**B**) posterior dislocation (arrow).

clavicle on the AP view. This dislocation is usually due to a severe upward force on the adducted arm.[115] With luxatio erecta, the humerus becomes parallel to the spine of the scapula, and the arm is abducted. Downey et al[115] reported this type of dislocation in 0.5% of all dislocations. This injury is due to force on the flexed arm (above the head). As a result, the humeral head is forced downward. Inferior subluxation may be associated with humeral fractures, glenoid fractures, capsular tears, or brachial plexus injury.[156] These types of dislocations can usually be managed initially with closed reduction, but more injuries and rotator cuff tears may be present.

Complications of Glenohumeral Dislocations

Complications of glenohumeral dislocations and fracture-dislocations are more common than complications of proximal humeral fractures. Associated fractures and recurrent dislocations are the most common problems.[140] Other associated fractures include those of the greater tuberosity (15%) and, less frequently, the coracoid as well as lesser tuberosity or subscapularis avulsions.[116,132]

Recurrence is a common problem after anterior dislocations. This is more common in young athletes (55% of those younger than 22 years) compared to older patients (12% of those older than 30 years).[126] Delayed arthrosis is also common after dislocations; the incidence increases after posterior dislocation.[148] Rupture of the capsule and tears of the rotator cuff may occur either acutely or with recurrent dislocations. CT, arthrography, or MRI is important in the evaluation of patients with suspected soft tissue or cartilaginous injury after dislocation.[105,108,143]

Neurovascular injury may occur in the axillary region after dislocations. Vascular injuries include laceration, thrombosis, intimal laceration, and false aneurysms of the axillary artery.[104,140] Axillary artery injuries may be overlooked initially owing to collateral circulation. Peripheral pulses may be present even with significant axillary artery injury. Early diagnosis with selective angiographic techniques is essential to determine the extent of injury. Amputation rates after axillary artery occlusion have been reported to be as high as 43%.[104]

The axillary nerve crosses the subscapularis anteriorly.[140] Stretching or compression can occur, especially with anterior dislocations. Complete disruption is uncommon, and loss of function is rare.[104,140]

Acromioclavicular Dislocations

Dislocations of the acromioclavicular joint (12%) occur less commonly than glenohumeral dislocations (85%).[98,104] The mechanism of injury is usually a fall in which force is directed to the point of the shoulder (Fig. 9-46). Dislocations due to indirect forces directed superiorly through the humeral head have also been reported.[140]

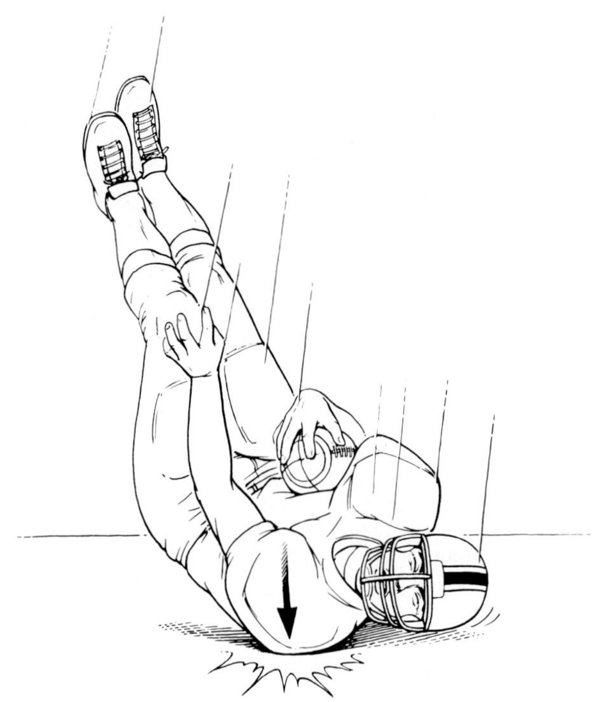

Fig. 9-46 Illustration of mechanism of injury to the acromioclavicular joint. Generally a fall on the point of the shoulder is implicated.

Allman[97] classified adult acromioclavicular joint injuries (types I to III) on the basis of the degree of ligament injury (Fig. 9-47). Rockwood[145] added three additional categories (types IV to VI), but these rarely occur in athletes (Fig. 9-47). In children (younger than 15 or 16 years old), this classification does not apply. The ligaments are usually intact, and the clavicle displaces out of the periosteal sleeve (Fig. 9-48).[112] Radiographic changes in type I and type II injuries may be subtle. The radiographs are normal in type I. Generally, radiographs of the shoulder will overpenetrate the acromioclavicular joint. Therefore, it is best to obtain well-coned views centered on the joint with the tube angled 15° to the head. This will reduce the amount of bony overlap. Weight-bearing views are essential to diagnose type II lesions and to differentiate type II from type III injuries (Fig. 9-49).[102,140,143,144] In type III injuries, the coracoclavicular ligaments are torn if the distance between the upper aspect of the coracoid and the undersurface of the clavicle is greater than 50%, or increased by more than 5 mm, compared with the normal shoulder (Figs. 9-47 and 9-49).[102,112,140,153]

Treatment of most type I and II injuries is successful with closed methods. Occasionally, closed reduction fails with type II lesions, and late distal clavicle excision is necessary. Internal fixation is more often necessary with type III adult injuries.[140,145]

Adjacent fractures can accompany acromioclavicular dislocation (Fig. 9-50). In our experience at the Mayo Clinic, the coracoid and clavicle are fractured most frequently. Intraarticular acromial fractures may also occur.[104]

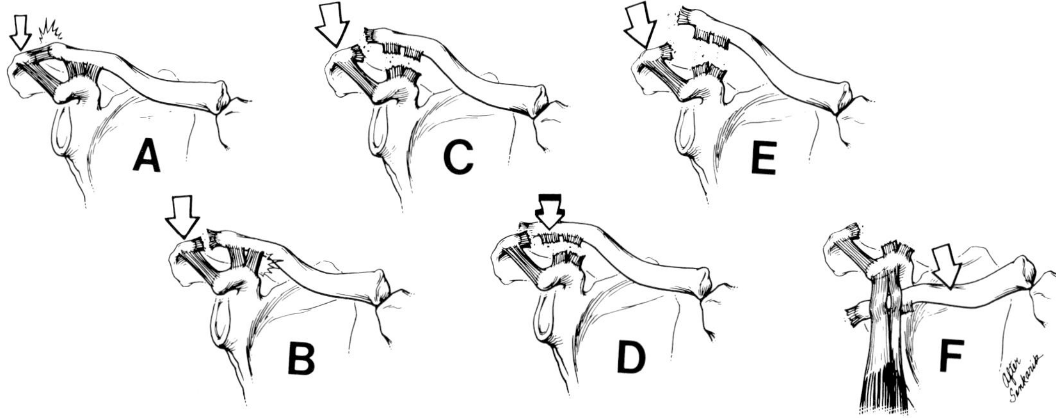

Fig. 9-47 Acromioclavicular joint injury.[144,145] (**A**) Type I, sprain of acromioclavicular ligaments. (**B**) Type II, disruption of acromioclavicular ligaments with intact coracoclavicular ligaments. (**C**) Type III, disruption of both acromioclavicular and coracoclavicular ligaments. (**D**) Type IV, disruption of both acromioclavicular and coracoclavicular ligaments with posterior displacement of the clavicle. (**E**) Type V, disruption of both acromioclavicular and coracoclavicular ligaments with superior elevation of the distal clavicle. (**F**) Type VI, anterior entrapment.

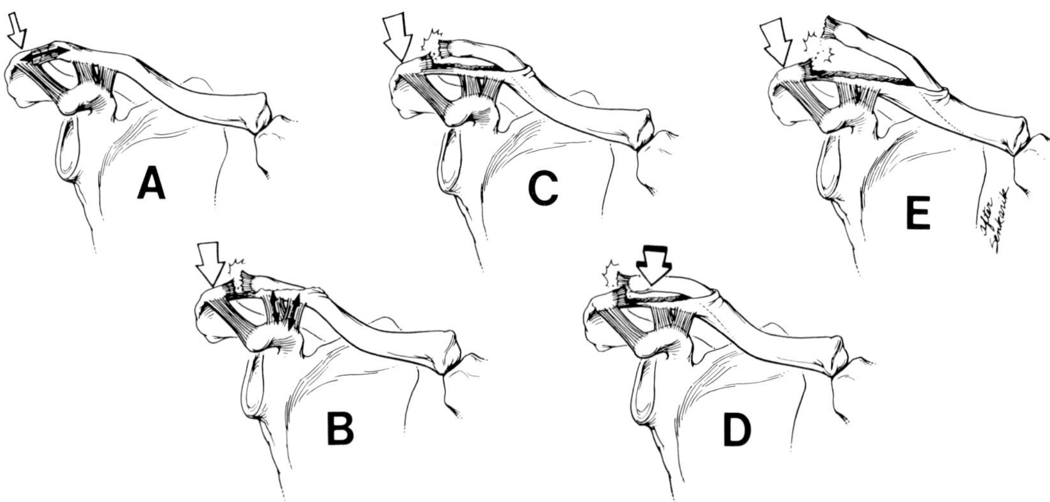

Fig. 9-48 Acromioclavicular joint injury in children.[144] (**A**) Type I, acromioclavicular sprain. (**B**) Type II, disruption of the acromioclavicular ligaments and partial tear of the periosteal sleeve. (**C**) Type III, disruption of acromioclavicular ligaments with elevation of the distal clavicle. (**D**) Disruption of acromioclavicular ligaments with posterosuperior clavicle displacement. (**E**) Ligaments intact, gross superior displacement of the clavicle out of the periosteal sleeve.

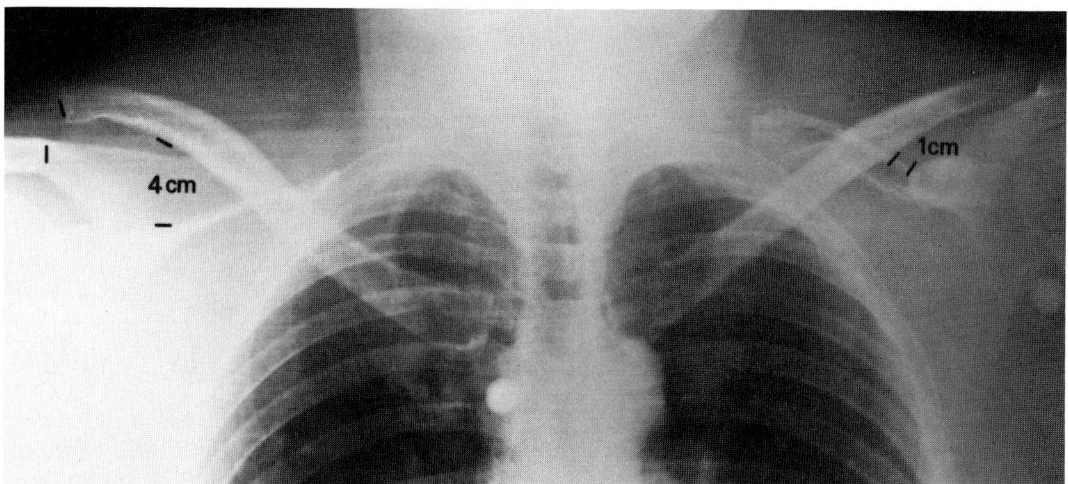

Fig. 9-49 Weight-bearing views of both shoulders taken on a transverse coned-down 14 × 7 film. There is a grade III separation on the right.

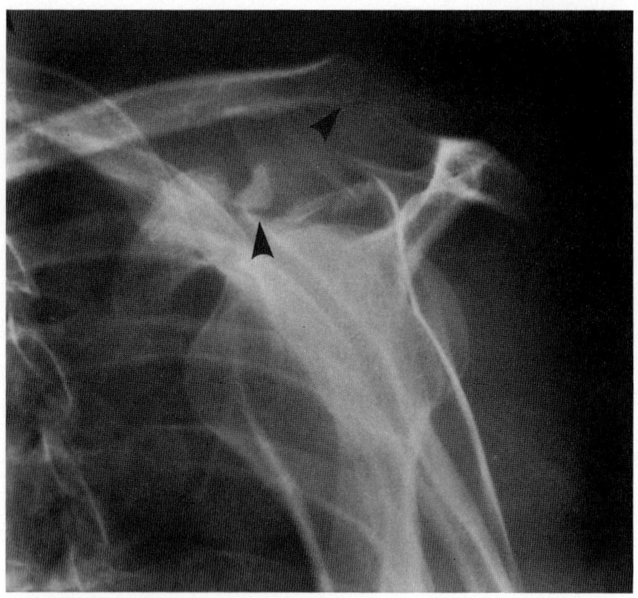

Fig. 9-50 Scapular Y view demonstrating an acromioclavicular separation (upper arrowhead) and coracoid fracture (lower arrowhead).

Sternoclavicular Dislocations

Dislocations of the sternoclavicular joint are uncommon.[111,149] Dislocation usually results from indirect trauma to the shoulder. Posterolateral forces transmitted medially cause anterior dislocation. Direct anterior trauma can occur in sports such as football. This causes posterior dislocation.[140,145] Anterior dislocations occur much more frequently than posterior dislocations (Fig. 9-51).[140,145]

Anterior dislocations may be easily palpable. Posterior dislocations can be more difficult to diagnose clinically owing to swelling. Early diagnosis is necessary because reduction after 48 hours is difficult.[107,151] In addition, posterior dislocations may be potentially fatal injuries because of involvement of the trachea and great vessels.

Allman[97] classified sternoclavicular dislocations in the same manner as acromioclavicular dislocations. Type I injuries cause only slight tearing of the sternoclavicular ligament. In type II lesions the sternoclavicular ligament is torn, and type III injury results in tears of both the sternoclavicular and the costoclavicular ligaments. In the last situation, either anterior or posterior dislocation occurs.[97]

Radiographic evaluation of this injury is difficult. Overlying structures often cause confusion (Fig. 9-52).[104,107,111,142] Conventional tomography or, more appropriately, CT is the technique of choice.[104,107] Actually, CT provides sufficient images for accurately evaluating subluxations as well as complete dislocations (Fig. 9-53). Subtle changes in the joint are much more obvious with CT than with routine films or tomography. The direction of displacement is also more obvious. An additional advantage of CT is the ability to assess the trachea, great vessels, and adjacent soft tissues.

Clavicle Fractures

Clavicle fractures are common, especially in children.[112,137,140,144,145] The injury usually is caused by a fall

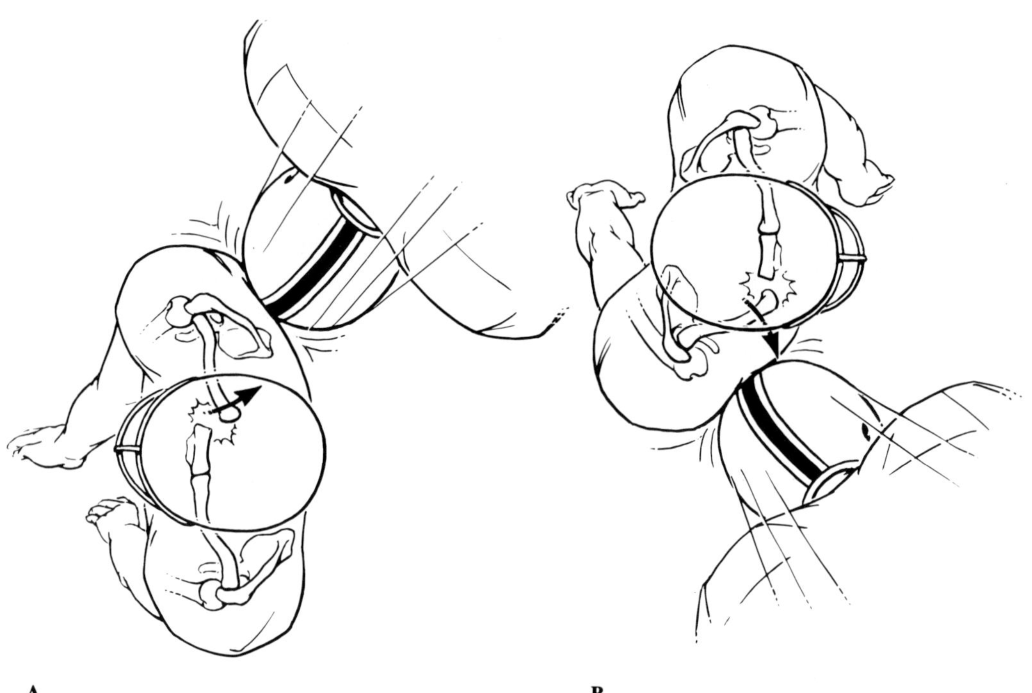

Fig. 9-51 Illustration of the mechanism of injury in sternoclavicular dislocations. (**A**) Posterior, (**B**) anterior.

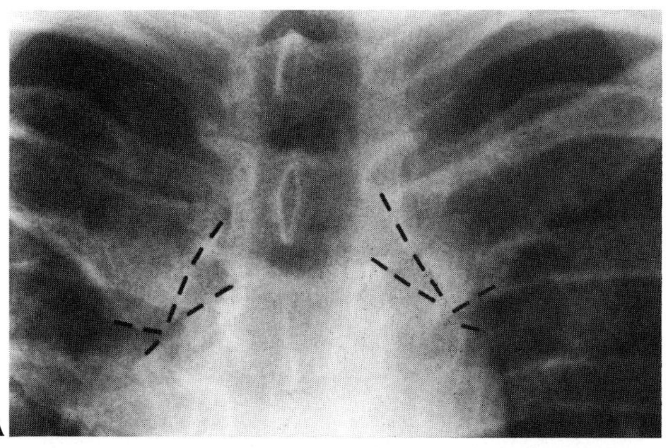

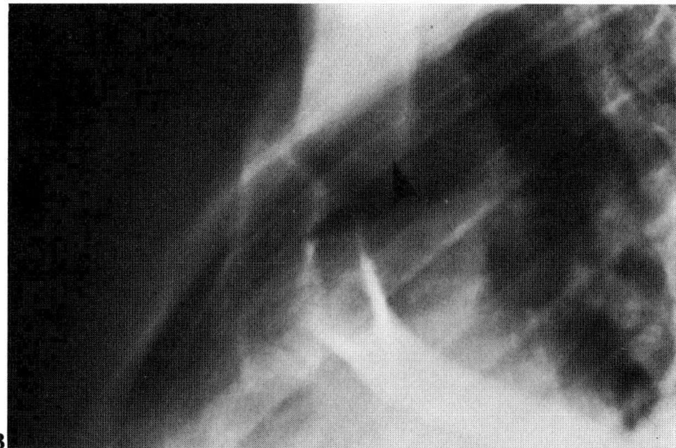

Fig. 9-52 (**A**) Posteroanterior and (**B**) lateral views showing the difficulty in defining the sternoclavicular joint. The Heinig view (**B**) shows posterior displacement of the clavicle (arrowhead).

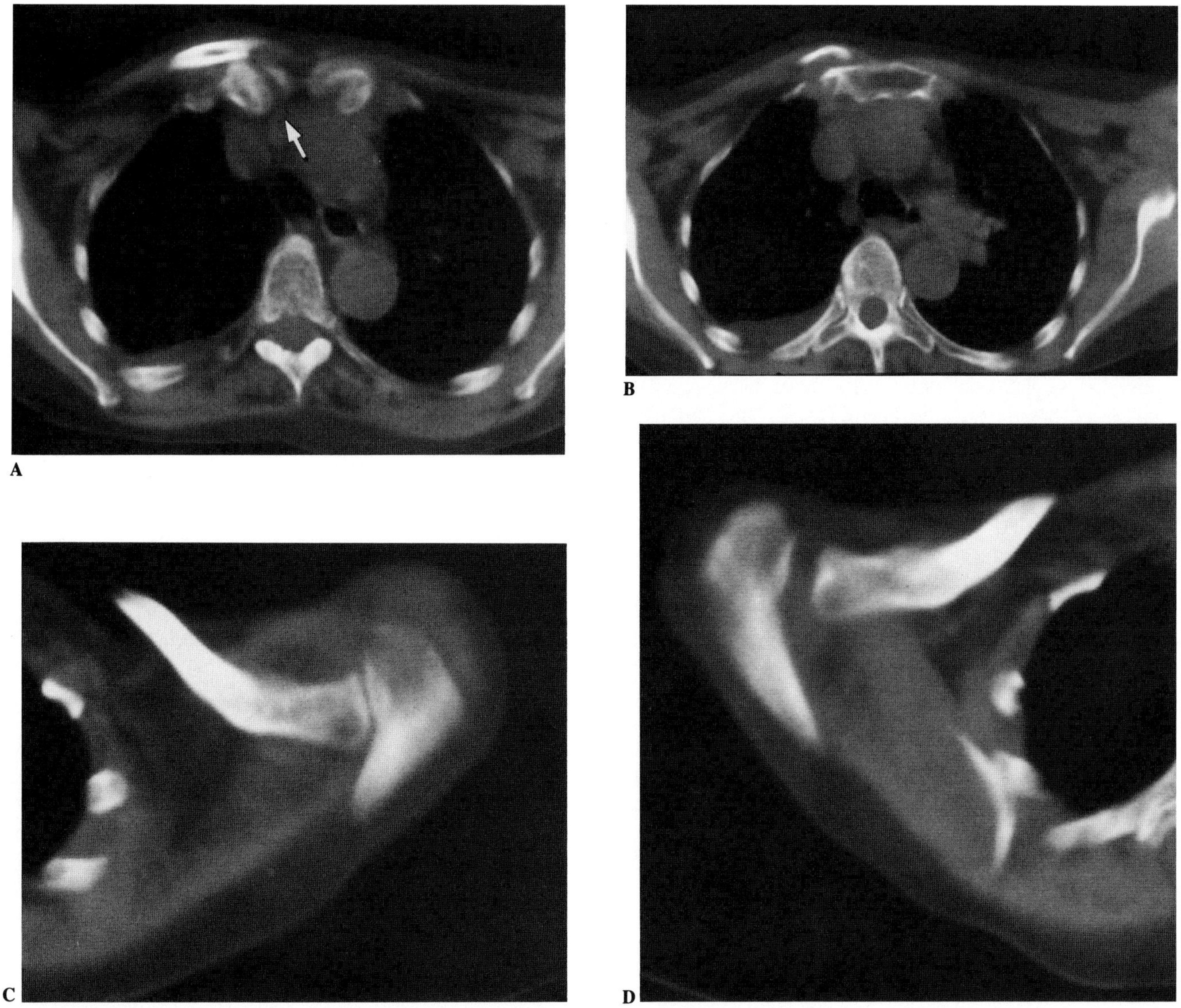

Fig. 9-53 CT images of a sternoclavicular fracture-dislocation and grade II separation. (**A**) The sternoclavicular joint (arrow) is subluxed, and (**B**) there is an associated fracture. (**C**) The left acromioclavicular joint is normal. (**D**) The right acromioclavicular joint is widened.

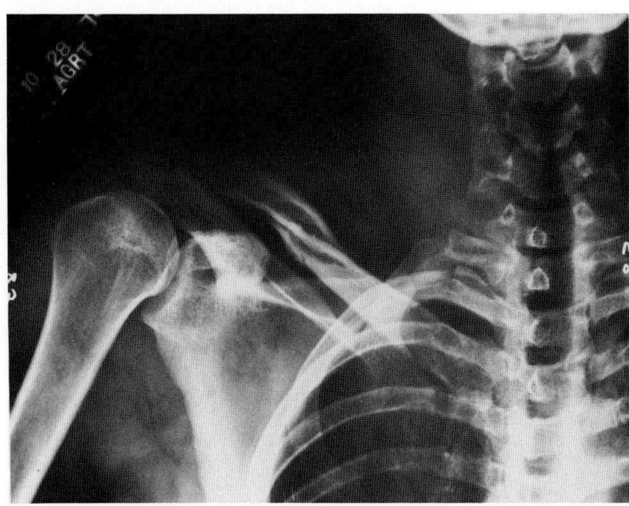

Fig. 9-54 Angled AP view (20° cephalad) demonstrating a fracture of the midclavicle. This was not evident on the straight AP view.

on the outstretched hand. The lateral force directed through the shoulder results in fracture of the midclavicle (Fig. 9-54). Less frequently direct trauma to the clavicle or shoulder results in fracture.

Fractures of the middle third of the clavicle are most common (80%).[97,138,145] Allman[97] classified clavicle fractures anatomically. Group I fractures involve the middle third of the clavicle. Displacement of these fractures is common. The sternocleidomastoid elevates the proximal fragment, and the weight of the arm tends to lower the distal fragment. This results in a superior tented radiographic appearance (Fig. 9-55). Group II fractures involve the distal clavicle (lateral to the coracoclavicular ligament; Fig. 9-56). These fractures make up 15% of clavicle fractures.[97,145] Group III fractures (5%) involve the medial clavicle.[104]

Radiographic evaluation of the middle and distal clavicle is not difficult. AP or oblique views of the clavicle, with the tube angled 15° or more to the head, will allow good visualization of the middle and distal clavicle (Fig. 9-54). The angulation projects the clavicle above the chest. A coned-down 15° angled view is best to overcome the problem of overpenetrating the acromioclavicular joint. Subtle midclavicle fractures may be overlooked. If symptoms dictate, a 40° cephalad angle may make detection less difficult (Fig. 9-54). Evaluation of the proximal clavicle is more difficult. Forty-degree angled views and oblique views are usually adequate if the fracture is displaced. In selected cases, especially undisplaced fractures, CT may be necessary.[104]

Most clavicle fractures can be treated with closed reduction and shoulder support (sling, figure-of-8 bandage, etc).[111,140,145] Group II fractures of the distal clavicle may require internal fixation. Resection of the distal clavicle may be required in patients with persistent symptoms.

Significant complications are less common with clavicle fractures than with glenohumeral fracture-dislocations. Malunion of midclavicle fractures or excessive callus formation does occur. This may result in compression of the adjacent neurovascular structures between the clavicle and first rib.[112,144]

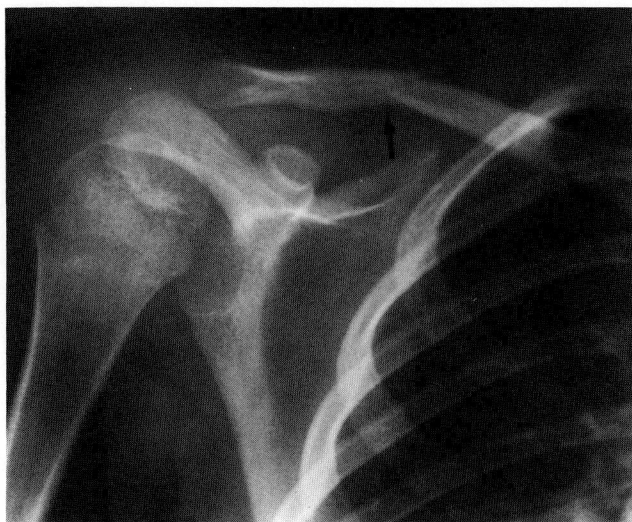

Fig. 9-55 Slightly elevated fracture of the midclavicle (arrow) in a child. This injury occurred during a fall in soccer.

Nonunion occurs in only 1% to 2% of cases. Osteoarthritis may occur after intraarticular fracture.[104] This is more common at the acromioclavicular joint. Posttraumatic osteolysis may be seen in the distal clavicle. Patients present with continued pain and weakness after trauma. Erosive changes develop on the distal clavicle; these are visible on the radiograph. Involvement may progress to the level of the coracoclavicular ligaments. Changes may be due to synovial hyperplasia, but this is uncertain. After treatment with immobilization some degree of bone healing occurs, although the joint often remains widened.[104,117]

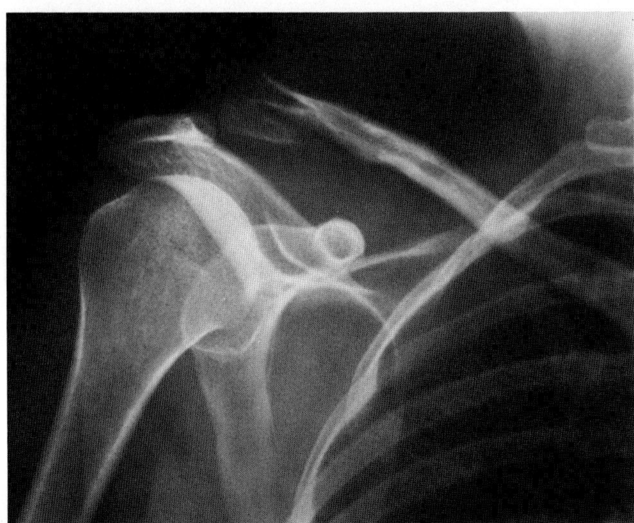

Fig. 9-56 Fracture of the distal clavicle with associated ligament injuries.

Scapular Fractures

Fractures of the scapula are uncommon (1% of all fractures).[104,112,144] Injury to the body of the scapula is caused by direct force. The scapula is well protected by an envelope of muscles. Therefore, considerable force is required to cause the fracture, and displacement of body fractures is usually not significant. Fractures of the body of the scapula are rare in athletes.

Fractures of the body may extend to the glenoid articular surface. Most commonly, glenoid fractures are associated with dislocations. Varriale and Adler,[154] however, have described glenoid fractures that are not associated with dislocation. Fractures may be undisplaced, displaced, or bursting. Detection of glenoid fractures is crucial because, if displaced, they lead to traumatic arthritis. Scapular Y, West Point, and axillary views are most useful in demonstrating these fractures.[99,104] Avulsion fractures of the infraglenoid tubercle are due to forceful triceps contraction. This fracture may also lead to recurrent dislocation, especially if a portion of the rim is involved.[140]

Fractures of the acromion usually are due to a direct blow from above. Stress fractures, however, may also occur in association with dislocations and rotator cuff tears.[113] Radiographic diagnosis is not difficult in most cases. The axillary and Y views are particularly useful in the diagnosis of subtle acromial fractures (Fig. 9-50).

Fractures of the coracoid process may be due to direct trauma or avulsion.[103,104,131] Muscular origins of the coracoid include the coracobrachialis, short head of the biceps, and pectoralis minor.[146] Most fractures occur at the base. Displacement is usually prevented by ligament attachment.

Repeated trauma in trapshooters may result in a coracoid stress fracture.[104,106,150,151] Radiographic evaluation of coracoid fractures should include the scapular Y view and the axillary view (Fig. 9-57).[120,151] In addition, weight-bearing views should be considered. Fractures of the coracoid are associated with acromioclavicular dislocation.

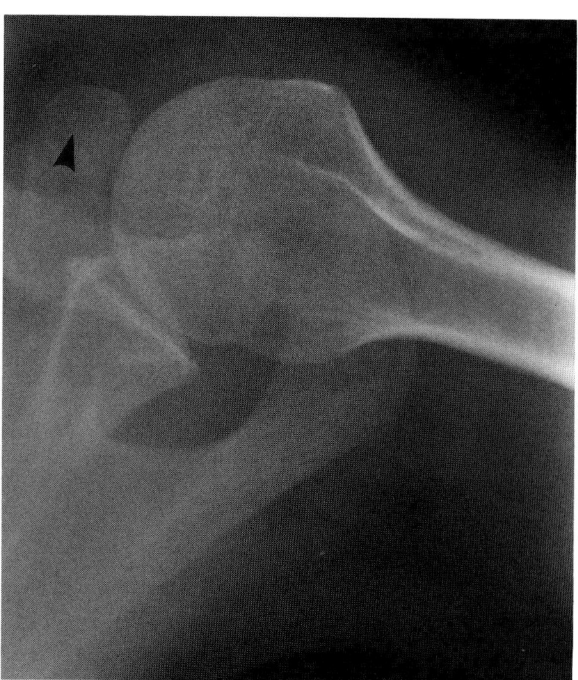

Fig. 9-57 Axillary view of the shoulder demonstrating an undisplaced coracoid fracture (arrowhead).

Miscellaneous Osseous Conditions

Several additional conditions have been described that result in shoulder pain. Posttraumatic osteolysis of the clavicle was mentioned above.[104,117]

Osteochondritis dissecans is most common in the knee and then in the ankle, hip, and elbow.[104,152] Rarely, the condition may also affect the glenoid. The lesion is not difficult to identify if it is located away from the inferior labrum. In this setting, confusion with a Bankart lesion may occur. True AP (40° posterior oblique) and axillary views are most useful. CT or MRI, however, is most useful for staging and complete evaluation of this unusual lesion.[104,152]

Little league shoulder is a condition described in young baseball pitchers. The condition is due to repeated trauma and was believed to be a growth plate fracture. Barnett[101] prefers the term *proximal humeral epiphyseolysis*. The involved epiphysis is irregular and widened; these changes are similar to those noted with slipped capital femoral epiphysis (Fig. 9-58). Changes are usually readily apparent on AP views of the shoulder. Patients present with pain when throwing. Healing occurs with rest. The condition must be differentiated from impingement syndrome.[101]

Blocker's exostosis (Fig. 9-59) is due to contusion or repetitive trauma to the region of the deltoid insertion on the humerus. Trauma to this region is common in offensive linemen and others involved in blocking during football plays. Repeated trauma can lead to painful periostitis and adjacent soft tissue injury.[141] If the area is not properly protected, an organized exostosis that extends anterolaterally from the humerus (Fig. 9-59) may occur. Conservative therapy with protection of the area during the early stages is the best method of therapy.[141]

SOFT TISSUE TRAUMA

Certain aspects of soft tissue trauma have been discussed above. Soft tissue injuries are common in athletes, however, and certain conditions deserve further attention, specifically as they apply to imaging evaluation.

Rotator Cuff and Capsular Injuries

Shoulder injuries are particularly common in tennis, swimming, and throwing sports such as base-

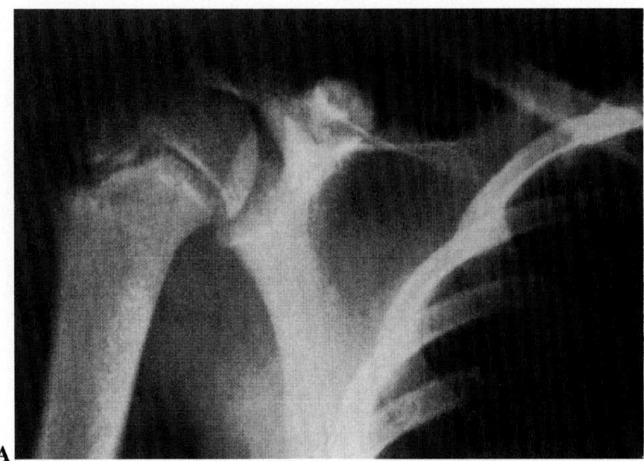

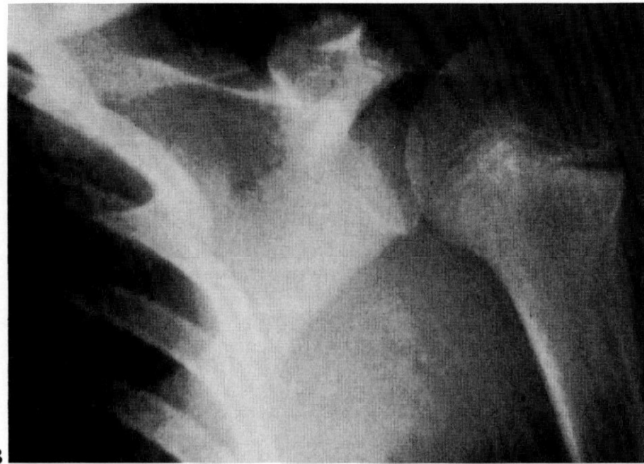

Fig. 9-58 AP views of the shoulder in a little league pitcher with epiphyseolysis. Note the irregularity of the involved physis (**A**) compared to the normal shoulder (**B**). *Source:* Reprinted with permission from Barnett LS, Little league shoulder syndrome: proximal humeral epiphyseolysis in adolescent baseball pitchers, *Journal of Bone and Joint Surgery* (1985;67A:495–496), Copyright © 1985, Journal of Bone and Joint Surgery.

ball.[157,165,171,175,176,193,195,206,209] Forty percent to 80% of competitive swimmers develop shoulder symptoms.[186,196,209] Symptoms are most common in swimmers after 6 to 8 years of competition. The butterfly, freestyle, and backstroke techniques are implicated most frequently.[167,209] In addition, up to 65% of baseball players develop rotator cuff injuries.[195]

The arm and shoulder in these sports have similar motions. The arm is abducted and externally rotated, stretching the anterior capsule and muscles with maximal contraction posteriorly. When the player is striking a tennis ball or throwing a ball, the shoulder moves from abduction and external rotation into forward flexion and internal rotation.[178,185,186,192,203,206] When the arm is abducted and externally rotated, the cuff and subacromial bursa are impinged between the humerus and acromion.[183,184] In addition to impingement, biceps tendinitis and instability may be present.[165,206] The latter is probably due to repetitive capsular stretching. Rotator cuff tears and labral injuries are uncommon in young athletes (younger than 20 years of age).[186]

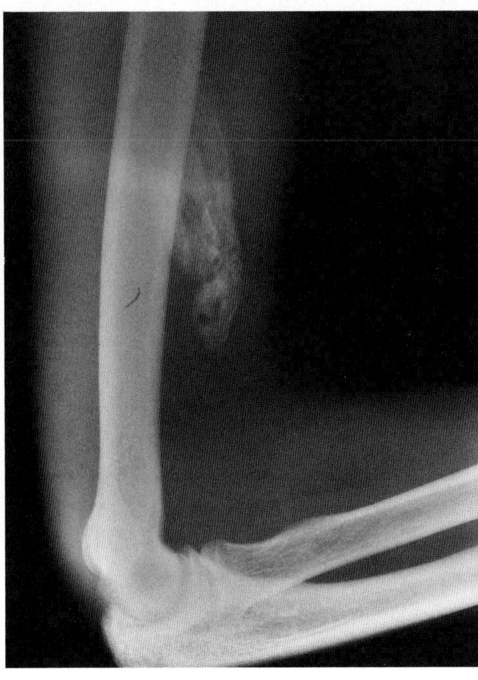

Fig. 9-59 Blocker's exostosis. There is mature ossification of the soft tissues anterior to the mid-humerus. *Source:* Courtesy of Bernard F Morrey and Michael J Stuart, Dept. of Orthopedic Surgery, Mayo Clinic, Rochester, Minnesota.

Athletes engaged in the above activities usually present with shoulder pain. Pain may be generalized, but more often the symptoms are anterior or lateral.[192] Symptoms may be related to impingement and/or associated biceps tendinitis.[184]

The arch of the shoulder is formed by the clavicle, acromioclavicular joint, anterior acromion, and coracoacromial ligament (Fig. 9-60). The subacromial bursa allows smooth motion between the arch and the humeral head.[186,192] Abnormalities in the structures of this arch may lead to impingement. Three stages of impingement have been described (Fig. 9-61).[186,202] Stage 1 changes occur in young athletes (12 to 25 years old) and include edema and hemorrhage. These changes occur most commonly in the critical zone just medial to the supraspinatus insertion.[158,169] Stage 2 changes occur in older athletes (25 to 40 years) after years of repetitive microtrauma. Fibrosis of the subacromial bursa, thickening of the coracoacromial ligament, and subtle acromial or greater tuberosity changes may be evident. Stage 3 changes typically occur in patients 40 years old or older. Further degeneration and rotator cuff tears occur.[157–159,186,192,204,205]

Related conditions such as instability may have similar presentations. Athletes may describe a dead arm, which is probably related to repetitive capsular stretching.[186]

A related condition, tennis shoulder, is a postural change in the exercised extremity and results in drooping of the shoulder and scoliotic changes in the thoracic spine. This condition is

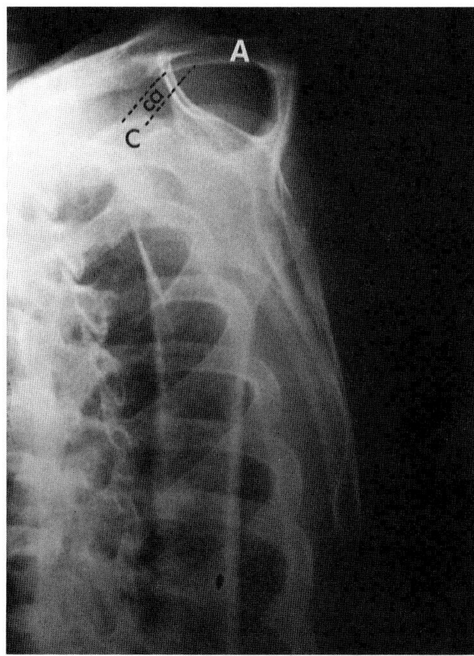

Fig. 9-60 Scapular Y view demonstrating the acromion (A), coracoid (C), and coracoacromial ligament (ca) in relation to the humeral head.

due to repetitive stretching of the trapezius, levator scapulae, and rhomboideus minor and major, which allows the shoulder to drop. There is also an increase in the muscle and osseous mass of the extremity, which contributes to the postural change.[202]

Imaging of athletes with shoulder pain should ideally identify abnormalities in bone, muscle, ligaments, and tendons. Multiple techniques have been used to identify capsular abnormalities and rotator cuff injuries.[159–162,168,172,173] Routine radiographs provide useful secondary signs of cuff and capsular abnormalities. Superior subluxation of the humeral head reducing the humeroacromial distance to less than 7 mm indicates rotator cuff injury.[159] Changes in the acromion, acromioclavicular joint, and greater tuberosity are also useful (Figs. 9-15 and 9-16).[168,188,205] Hypertrophic changes in the acromioclavicular joint, subacromial sclerosis and spur formation, and erosions or sclerosis of the greater tuberosity are useful findings.[166,188] Special views described earlier, including the apical oblique view, fluoroscopy, and the scapular Y view, are useful in this regard.[177,189,201,205]

Arthrography was once the gold standard for evaluating the rotator cuff and capsule. Although MRI has gained wide acceptance, arthrography, especially with CT, is still a valuable technique. Partial and complete tears can be accurately diagnosed with routine arthrography (Fig. 9-62). On multiple views or CT the capsule volume and other abnormalities can also be identified.[174,179,208,211] Sonography is also useful for evaluating the rotator cuff, but it is less useful as an overall screening technique for shoulder disorders.[172,180,197,212]

MRI, as previously discussed, is an effective technique for evaluating patients with suspected impingement, rotator cuff tears, and capsular abnormalities.[159,191] Utilization of T2-weighted sequences in the coronal, sagittal, and axial planes provides valuable information regarding the cuff, capsule, arch of the shoulder, and surrounding soft tissues.[161,162,169,181,182]

Changes suggesting cuff disease and impingement on routine films or bursography can be even more accurately assessed with MRI.[175,207] Bone, articular, and soft tissue changes can all be identified.[159,169,207] Changes in the acromion and the acromioclavicular and coracoacromial ligaments are obvious (Fig. 9-63). The shape of the acromion may be significant; it may be flat (type I), gently curved (type II), or hooked anteriorly (type III; Fig. 9-64). The last is associated with rotator cuff disease.[169]

Signal intensity changes and variations in thickness are most useful in assessment of the rotator cuff.[159,161,162,207] The double-echo T2-weighted spin-echo sequence (SE

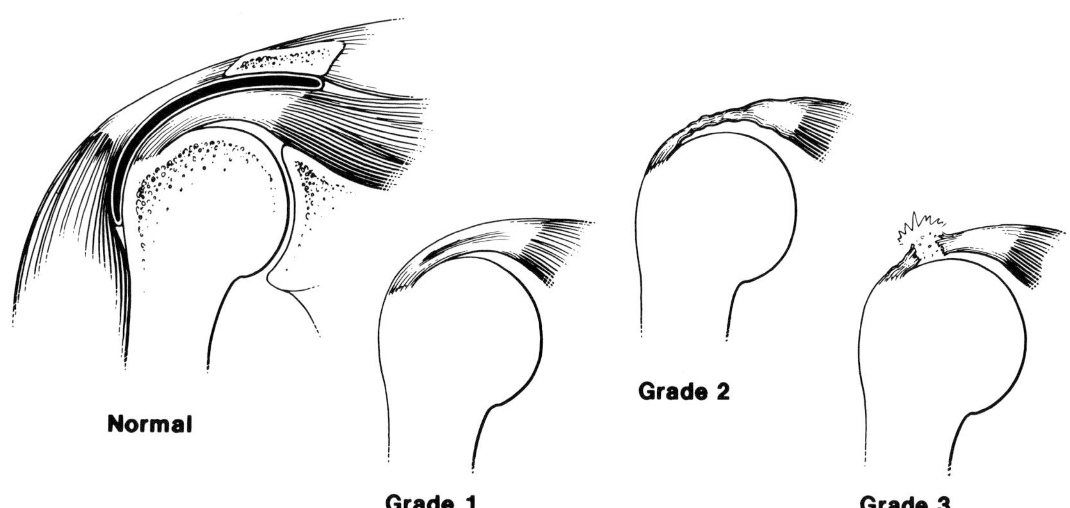

Fig. 9-61 Illustration of normal, grade 1 (edema/hemorrhage), grade 2 (thinning and fibrosis), and grade 3 (cuff tear) rotator cuff injuries.

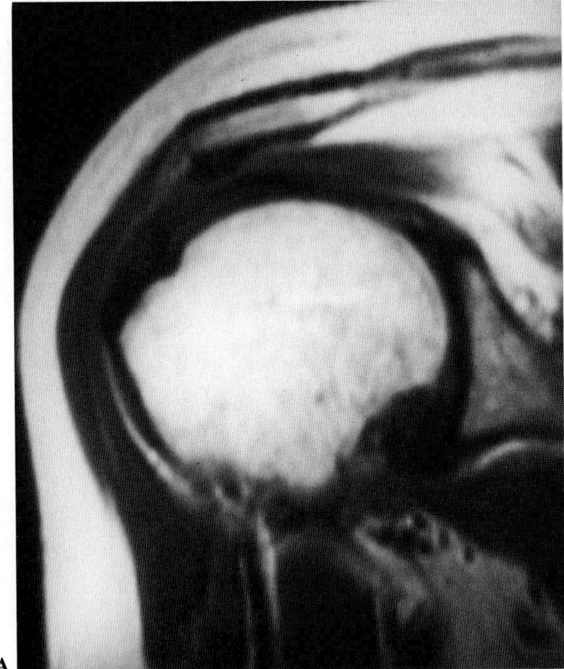

A

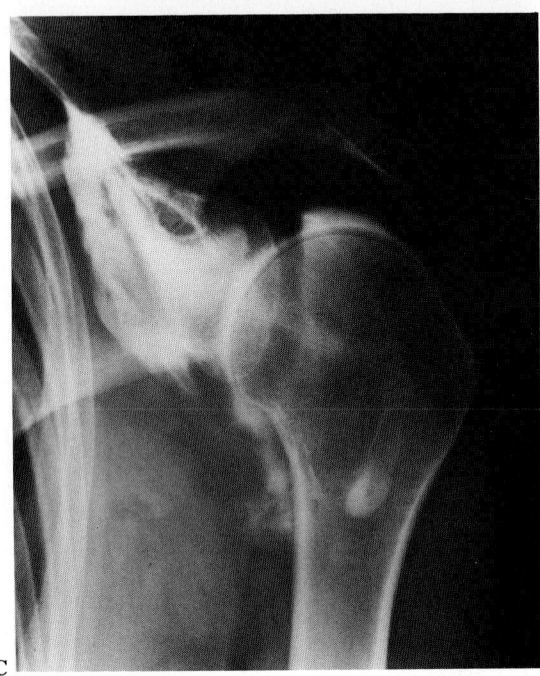

C

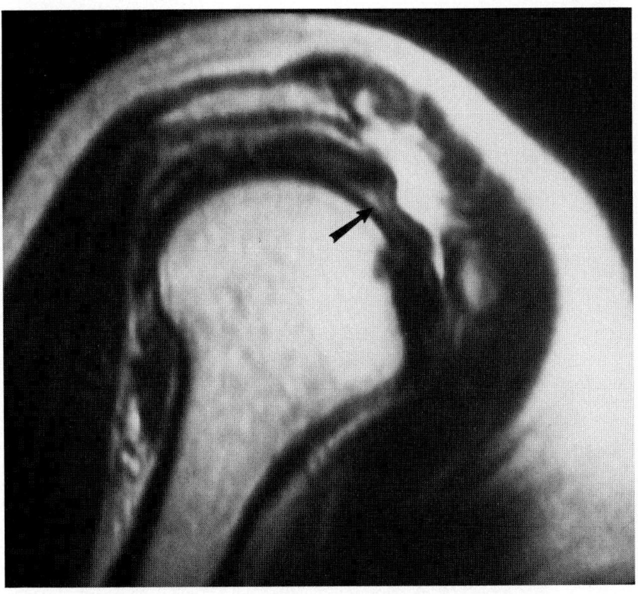

B

Fig. 9-62 Evaluation of a pitcher with chronic shoulder pain. (**A**) Coronal (SE 500/20) MR image demonstrates impingement due to a subacromial fibroosseous spur. (**B**) Sagittal T2-weighted MR image (SE 2000/60) shows fluid in the subacromial bursa with slight thinning and increased signal in the cuff (arrow). There may be a cuff tear. (**C**) Stress arthrogram shows no evidence of a cuff tear. The diagnosis was bursitis with impingement.

2000/80,20) is most useful, but gradient-echo techniques may also be used.[159,169] Chronic cuff disease or tendinitis manifests as slight variation in thickness with mild increased signal intensity on the first echo and little or no increase in signal intensity on the second echo. Partial tears are seen as areas of increasing intensity on the second echo that do not fully involve the tendon. The most specific sign of a full thickness tear is fluid or high signal with no cuff evident (Fig. 9-65).[169] The axial view is also useful when small cuff tears are present and involve areas other than the supraspinatus (Fig. 9-66).[159,169] Secondary signs of rotator cuff tears include supraspinatus muscle retraction, irregularity of the superior margin of the cuff, cuff thinning, indistinct subdeltoid flat plane, and fluid in the subacromial bursa (Fig. 9-67).[159,169] The last can be seen with bursitis alone. Specificity and sensitivity of MRI in evaluating cuff disease are both approximately 90%.[169,207]

Biceps Injuries

Biceps injury or tendinitis is frequently associated with rotator cuff disease.[163–165,183,197,198] The biceps tendon passes adjacent to the superior labrum as it crosses the joint and enters the biceps groove between the greater and lesser tuberosities (Fig. 9-3). Biceps tendon injuries include inflammation or overuse syndromes, subluxation, dislocation, and rupture.[163,165,184,195] Injuries occur most frequently in swimmers and throwing athletes.[165,195]

Patients usually present with anterior shoulder pain.[184] Pain may also be more generalized because it is frequently associated with impingement. These symptoms may mask underlying instability. Therefore, imaging should provide information about stability, impingement, and the biceps tendon. Sonography is useful for evaluating the cuff and biceps tendon.[197,199,200] MRI or CT arthrography is preferred

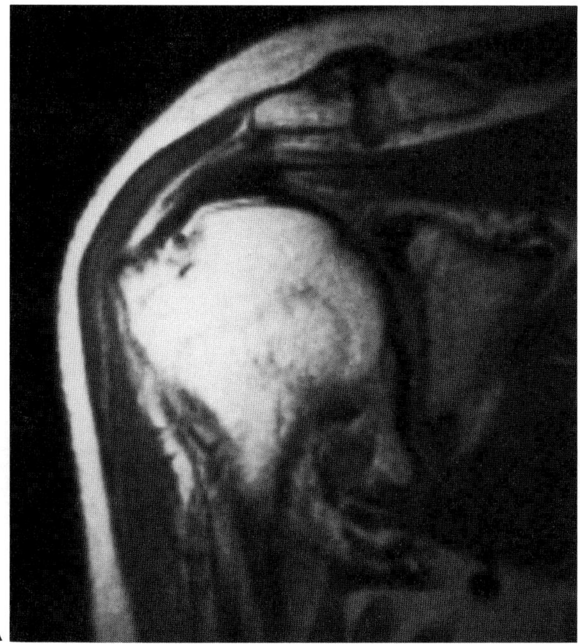

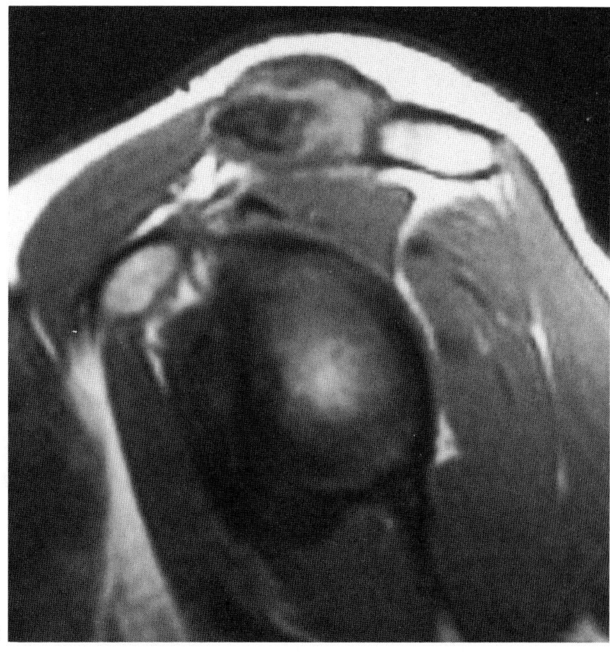

Fig. 9-63 MR images demonstrating secondary changes associated with impingement or cuff disruption. (**A**) Coronal T1-weighted MR image (SE 500/20) demonstrating erosive changes in the greater tuberosity (arrow). (**B**) Sagittal MR image demonstrating hypertrophy of the acromioclavicular joint with impingement.

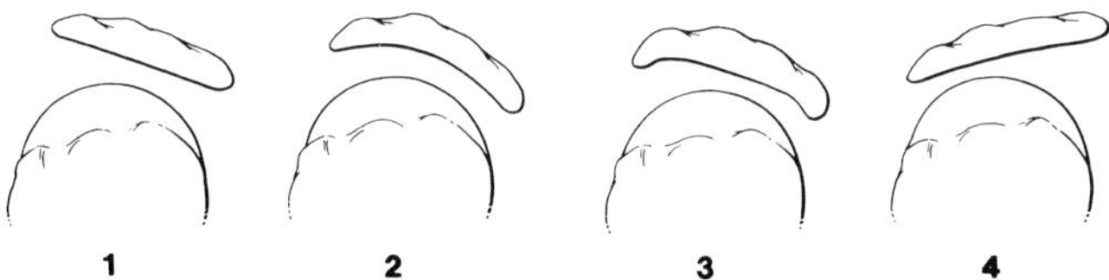

Fig. 9-64 Illustration of acromial configurations. 1, Type I: straight; 2, type II: curved; 3, type III: hooked; 4, type IV, anterior angulation.

in practice at the Mayo Clinic, however. The biceps tendon is demonstrated on coronal and axial images. T2-Weighted axial images are most useful. Tendon size, position, and disruption can be identified (Fig. 9-68). Subluxation may require gradient-echo imaging in internal and external rotation to detect subtle changes (Fig. 9-69).[159]

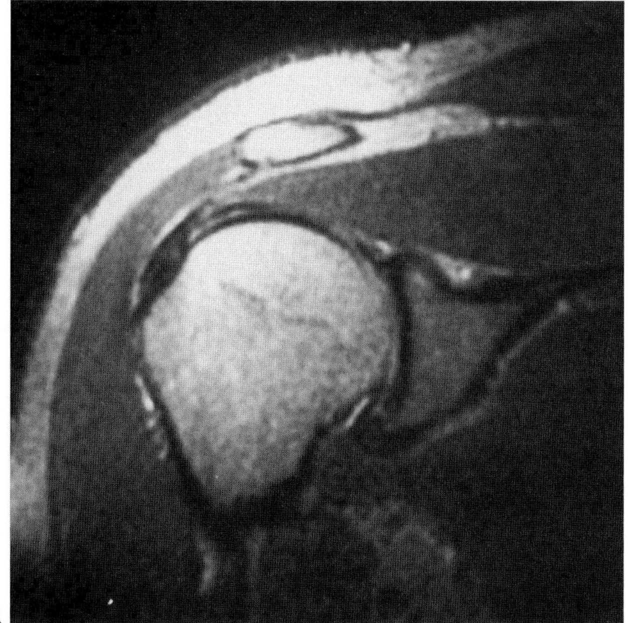

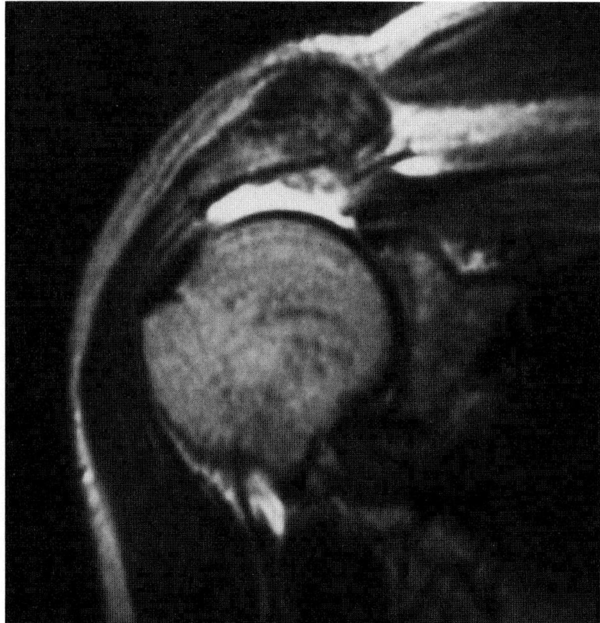

Fig. 9-65 MR appearance of cuff disease. (**A**) Coronal (SE 2000/80) MR image demonstrates thinning and slightly increased signal in the rotator cuff. No definite tear can be identified. (**B**) Coronal (SE 2000/70) image demonstrates a large tear with fluid separating the tendon ends.

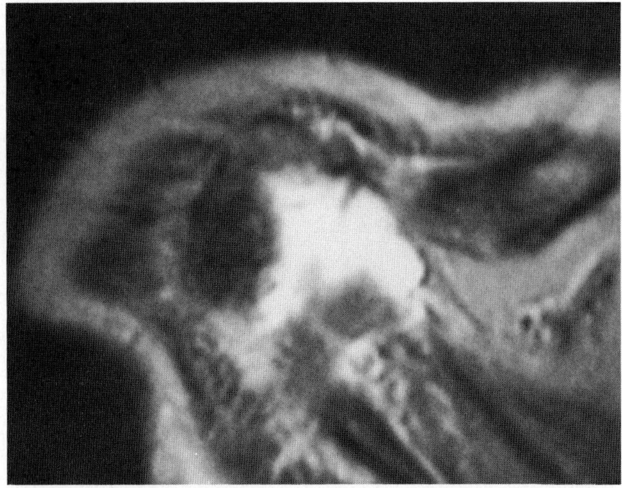

A

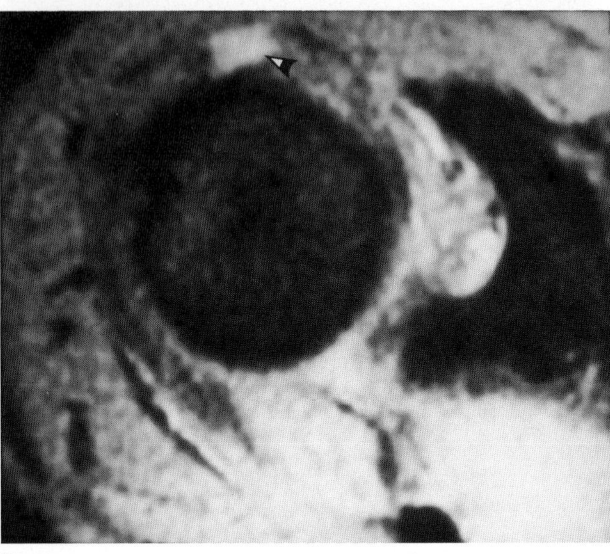

B

Fig. 9-66 Axial MR images of the shoulder. (**A**) Large supraspinatus tear. (**B**) Small peripheral tear (arrowhead).

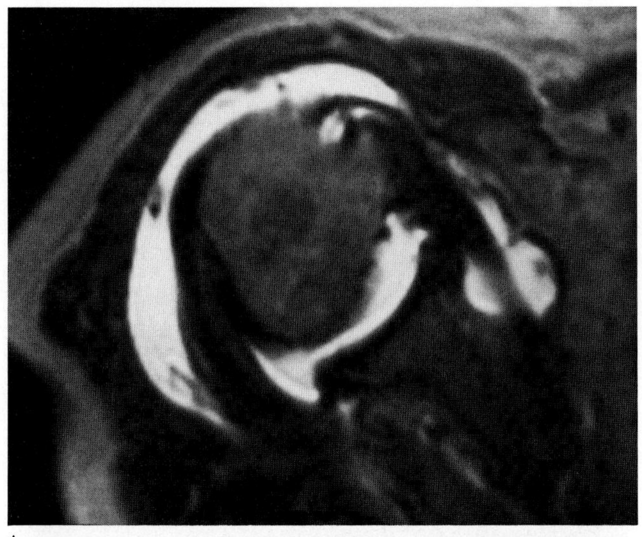

A

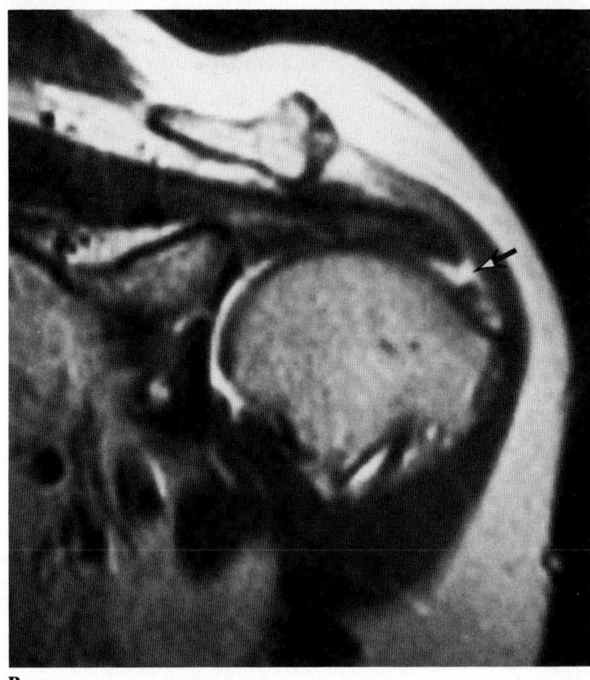

B

Fig. 9-67 (**A**) Axial (SE 2000/80) MR image demonstrating a large amount of fluid and synovitis in the subdeltoid bursa. (**B**) Coronal (SE 2000/80) MR image demonstrating a complete tear (arrow).

Bursitis

There are numerous bursae about the shoulder (Table 9-2). Most do not communicate with the shoulder joint. Inflammation of these structures is not uncommon. The subacromial and subdeltoid bursae are most often involved (Fig. 9-62), as they are in the early phases of impingement.

The scapulothoracic bursa is located at the inferomedial angle of the scapula and can become inflamed in throwing athletes, especially baseball pitchers.[184] Pain in this region and, on occasion, a palpable mass should suggest the diagnosis.

Imaging with sonography may demonstrate a fluid-filled lesion if the scapula does not interfere. MRI may be required to confirm the nature of the lesion and to exclude other pathology.[159]

Muscle Tears

Muscle tears in the upper extremity do not occur nearly as frequently as in the lower extremity. Nevertheless, this injury

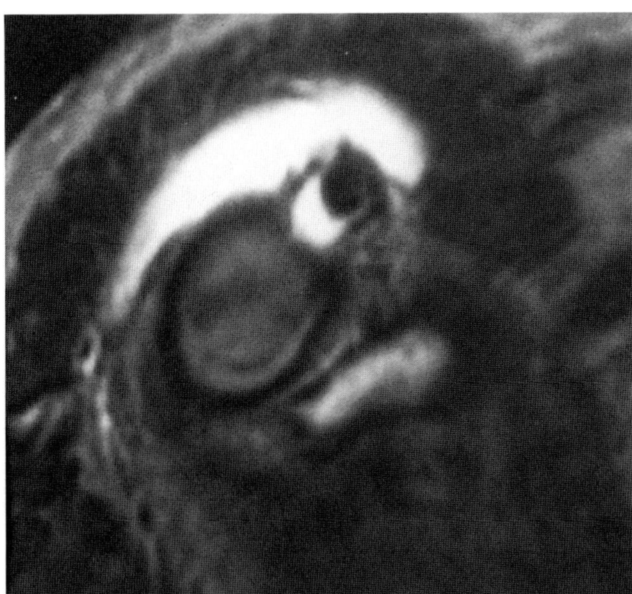

Fig. 9-68 Axial (SE 2000/80) MR image demonstrating a subdeltoid effusion and biceps tendon sheath inflammation.

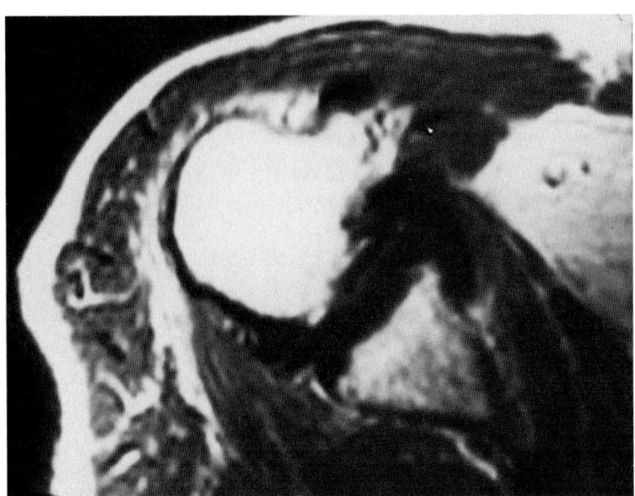

Fig. 9-69 Axial MR image demonstrating thickening and subluxation of the biceps tendon.

has been described in weight lifters and offensive linemen in football.[187,190] Pectoralis muscle tears occur in weight lifters and triceps tears in linemen.[159,187] The latter are probably related to pushing off during blocking.

Patients present with pain, weakness of the involved muscle, and ecchymosis. MRI is preferred to detect and stage the injury.[159,210] T2-Weighted images in two planes are most useful; these ensure greater accuracy in assessing the extent of injury.

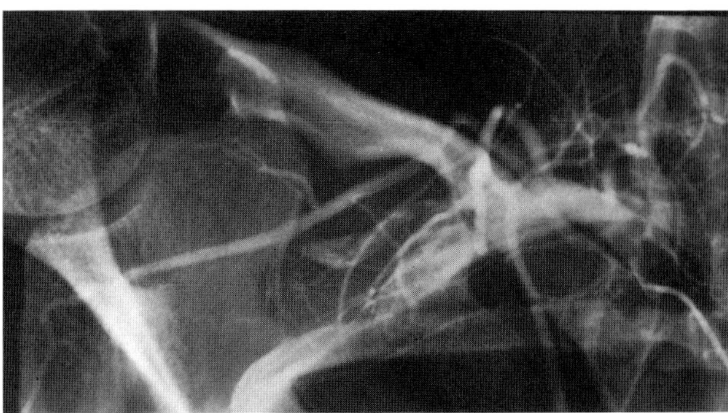

Fig. 9-70 Angiogram demonstrating thoracic outlet syndrome.

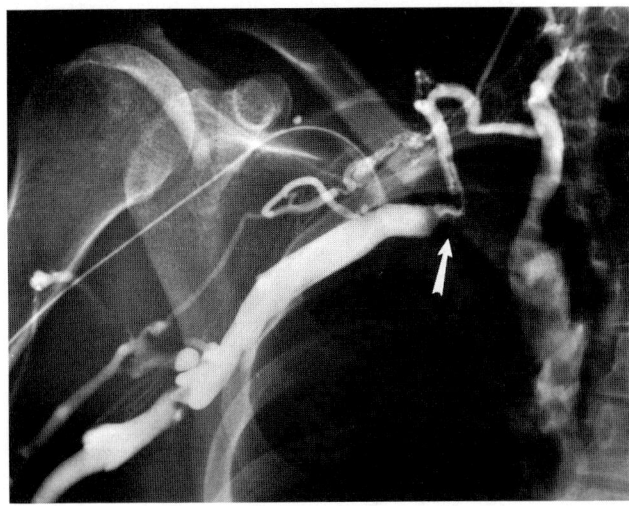

Fig. 9-71 Venogram demonstrating subclavian vein thrombosis (arrow) in a weight-lifter. *Source:* Courtesy of H.J. Williams, Dept. of Diagnostic Radiology, Mayo Clinic Jacksonville, Jacksonville, Florida.

Neurovascular Injuries

Neurovascular injury, as an isolated event, is unusual. Injuries do occur as complications of shoulder dislocation and in athletes with thoracic outlet syndrome (Fig. 9-70). Nerve entrapment due to soft tissue injury or anomalies may occur.[170,194] MRI is preferred to evaluate the latter. Angiography or venography may be required to evaluate outlet syndrome and other vascular injuries (Fig. 9-71).

REFERENCES

Introduction

1. Axe MJ. Evaluation and treatment of common throwing injuries of the shoulder and elbow. *Del Med J*. 1987;59:593–598.

2. Ciullo JV, Stevens GG. The prevention and treatment of injuries to the shoulder in swimming. *Sports Med*. 1989;7:182–204.

3. Fukuda H, Neer CS II. Archer's shoulder. *Orthopedics*. 1988; 11:171–174.

4. Garth WP, Allman FL, Armstrong WS. Occult anterior subluxation of the shoulder in noncontact sports. *Am J Sports Med.* 1987;15:579–585.

5. Garth WP, Leberte MA, Cool TA. Recurrent fractures of the humerus in a baseball pitcher. *J Bone Joint Surg Am.* 1988;70:305–306.

6. Jobe FW, Bradley JP. The diagnosis and nonoperative treatment of shoulder injuries in athletes. *Clin Sports Med.* 1989;8:419–438.

7. Johnson JE, Sim FH, Scott SG. Musculoskeletal injuries in competitive swimmers. *Mayo Clin Proc.* 1987;62:289–304.

8. Jones MW, Matthews JP. Rupture of pectoralis major in weight lifter. *Injury.* 1988;19:219.

9. Lehman RC. Shoulder pain in the competitive tennis player. *Clin Sports Med.* 1988;7:309–327.

10. Mann DL, Little N. Shoulder injuries in archery. *Can J Sports Sci.* 1989;14:85–92.

11. McCarthy WJ, Yao JST, Schafer MF, et al. Upper extremity arterial injury in athletes. *J Vasc Surg.* 1989;9:317–327.

12. McLeod WD, Andrews JR. Mechanisms of shoulder injury. *Phys Ther.* 1986;66:1901–1904.

13. McMaster WC. Anterior glenoid labrum damage: a painful lesion in swimmers. *Am J Sports Med.* 1986;14:383–387.

14. Nirschl RP. Prevention and treatment of elbow and shoulder injuries in the tennis player. *Clin Sports Med.* 1988;7:289–308.

15. Priest JD. The shoulder of the tennis player. *Clin Sports Med.* 1988; 7:387–402.

16. Richardson AB. Orthopedic aspects of competitive swimming. *Clin Sports Med.* 1987;6:639–645.

Anatomy

17. Anderson JE. *Grant's Atlas of Anatomy.* 8th ed. Baltimore: Williams & Wilkins; 1983.

18. Basmajian JV. The surgical anatomy and function of the arm-trunk mechanism. *Surg Clin North Am.* 1963;43:1471–1482.

19. Berquist TH. *Imaging of Orthopedic Trauma.* 2nd ed. New York: Raven; 1991.

20. Clemente CD. *Gray's Anatomy of the Human Body.* 13th ed. Philadelphia: Lea & Febiger; 1985.

21. Cockshott P. The coracoclavicular joint. *Radiology.* 1979;131:313.

22. Depalma AF. *Surgery of the Shoulder.* Philadelphia: Lippincott; 1973.

23. Hitchcock HH, Bechtol CO. Painful shoulder. *J Bone Joint Surg Am.* 1948;30:263–273.

24. Hollinshead WH. *Anatomy for Surgeons.* 3rd ed. New York: Harper & Row; 1982;3.

25. Lucas DB. Biomechanics of the shoulder joint. *Arch Surg.* 1973; 107:425–432.

26. Mitchell MJ, Caesey G, Berthoty DP, Sartoris DJ, Resnick D. Peribursal fat plane in the shoulder: anatomic study and clinical experience. *Radiology.* 1988;168:699–704.

27. Neer CS, Rockwood CA. Fractures and dislocations of the shoulder. In: Rockwood CA, Green DP, eds. *Fractures in Adults.* 2nd ed. Philadelphia: Lippincott; 1984:1:675–985.

28. Post M. *The Shoulder: Surgical and Nonsurgical Management.* Philadelphia: Lea & Febiger; 1978.

29. Prodromas CC, Ferry JA, Schiller AL, Zarino B. Histologic studies of the glenoid labrum from fetal life to old age. *J Bone Joint Surg Am.* 1990; 72:1344–1348.

30. Saha AK. Dynamic instability of the glenohumeral joint. *Acta Orthop Scand.* 1973;44:668–670.

31. Saha AK. *Theory of Shoulder Mechanism.* Springfield, IL: Thomas; 1961.

32. Turkel SJ, Pono MW, Marshall JL, Girgis FG. Stabilizing mechanisms preventing anterior dislocation of the glenohumeral joint. *J Bone Joint Surg Am.* 1981;63:1208–1217.

Imaging Techniques

33. Andrew L, Lundberg BJ. Treatment of rigid shoulders by joint distention arthrography. *Acta Orthop Scand.* 1965;36:45–53.

34. Ballinger PW. *Merrill's Atlas of Roentgenographic Positions and Standard Radiographic Procedures.* 5th ed. St Louis, MO: Mosby; 1982.

35. Bernau A, Berquist TH. *Orthopedic Positioning in Diagnostic Radiology.* Baltimore: Urban & Schwarzenberg; 1983.

36. Berquist TH. *Imaging of Orthopedic Trauma.* 2nd ed. New York: Raven; 1991.

37. Berquist TH. *MRI of the Musculoskeletal System.* New York: Raven; 1990.

38. Brandt TD, Cardone BW, Grant TH, Post M, Weiss CA. Rotator cuff sonography: a reassessment. *Radiology.* 1989;173:323–327.

39. Burk LD, Karasick D, Kurtz AB, et al. Rotator cuff tears: prospective comparison of MR imaging with arthrography, sonography and surgery. *AJR.* 1989;153:87–92.

40. Burk LD, Torres JL, Marone PJ, Mitchell DG, Rifkin MD, Karasick D. MR imaging of shoulder injuries in professional baseball players. *J Magn Resonance Imaging.* 1991;1:385–389.

41. Callaghan JJ, McNiesh LM, Dehaven JP, Savory GG, Polly DW. A prospective comparison of double contrast computed tomography, arthrography and arthroscopy of the shoulder. *Am J Sports Med.* 1988;16:13–20.

42. Cofield RH. Rotator cuff disease of the shoulder. *J Bone Joint Surg Am.* 1985;67:974–979.

43. Cone RO III, Danzig L, Resnick D, Goldman AB. The bicipital groove: radiographic, anatomic and pathologic study. *AJR.* 1983;141: 781–788.

44. Cone RO III, Resnick D, Danzig L. Shoulder impingement syndrome: radiographic evaluation. *Radiology.* 1984;150:29–33.

45. Danzig L, Resnick D, Greenway G. Evaluation of unstable shoulders by computed tomography. *Am J Sports Med.* 1982;10:138–141.

46. DeSmet AA. Anterior oblique projection in radiography of the traumatized shoulder. *AJR.* 1980;134:514–518.

47. DeSmet AA. Axillary projection in radiography of the nontraumatical shoulder. *AJR.* 1980;143:511–514.

48. DeSmet AA. Diagnosis of rotator cuff tear on routine radiographs. *J Can Assoc Radiol.* 1977;28:54–57.

49. Deutsch AL, Resnick D, Mink JH, et al. Computed and conventional arthrotomography of the glenohumeral joint: normal anatomy and clinical experience. *Radiology.* 1984;153:603–609.

50. Fagerland M, Ahlgren O. Axial projection of the humeroscapular joint. *Acta Radiol.* 1981;22:203.

51. Farrin PU, Jaroma H, Harju A, Soimakallio S. Shoulder impingement syndrome: sonographic evaluation. *Radiology.* 1990;176:845–849.

52. Fisk C. Adaptation of the technique for radiography of the bicipital groove. *Radiol Technol.* 1965;37:47.

53. Flannigan B, Kursunoglu-Brahme S, Synder S, Karzel R, Delpizzo W, Resnick D. MR arthrography of the shoulder: comparison with conventional MR imaging. *AJR.* 1990;155:829–832.

54. Flinn RM, MacMilan CL, Campbell DR. Optimal radiography of the acutely injured shoulder. *J Can Assoc Radiol.* 1983;34:128–132.

55. Fuduka H, Mikasa M, Yumanaka K. Incomplete thickness rotator cuff tears diagnosed by subacromial bursography. *Clin Orthop.* 1987; 223:51–58.

56. Garth WP, Sloppey CE, Ochs CW. Roentgen demonstration of instability of the shoulder: the apical oblique projection. *J Bone Joint Surg Am.* 1984;66:1450–1453.

57. Genoe GA, Mueller J. Normal shoulder variations in technetium-99m polyphosphate bone scan. *South Med J*. 1974;67:659–663.

58. Ghelman B, Goldman AB. Double-contrast shoulder arthrogram: evaluation of rotator cuff tears. *Radiology*. 1977;124:251–254.

59. Gilula LA, Schoenecker PL, Murphy WA. Shoulder arthrography as a treatment modality. *AJR*. 1978;131:1047–1048.

60. Golding FC. The shoulder: the forgotten joint. *Br J Radiol*. 1962; 34:149–158.

61. Goldman AB, Dines DM, Warren RF. *Shoulder Arthrography: Technique, Diagnosis, and Clinical Correlation*. Boston: Little, Brown; 1982.

62. Hall FM. Morbidity from shoulder arthrography. *AJR*. 1981; 136:56–62.

63. Hall RH, Isaac F, Booth CR. Dislocation of the shoulder with special reference to accompanying small fractures. *J Bone Joint Surg Am*. 1959; 41:489–493.

64. Harcke AT, Grissom LE, Furkelstein MS. Evaluation of the musculoskeletal system with sonography. *AJR*. 1988;150:1253–1261.

65. Hatfield MK, Gross BH, Glazer GM, Mortel W. Computed tomography of the sternum and its articulation. *Skeletal Radiol*. 1984;11:197–203.

66. Haynor DR, Shuman WP. Double contrast CT arthrography of the glenoid labrum and shoulder girdle. *RadioGraphics*. 1984;4:411–421.

67. Heinig CF. Retrosternal dislocation of the clavicle: early recognition, X-ray diagnosis, and management. *J Bone Joint Surg Am*. 1968;50:830.

68. Hill NH, Sachs MD. The grooved defect of the humeral head. A frequently unrecognized complication of dislocation of the shoulder joint. *Radiology*. 1940;35:690.

69. Holder J, Fretz CJ, Terrier F, Gerber C. Rotator cuff tears: correlation of sonographic and surgical findings. *Radiology*. 1988;169:791–794.

70. Holt RG, Helms CA, Steinback L, Neumann C, Munk PL, Genant HK. Magnetic resonance imaging of the shoulder: rationale and current applications. *Skeletal Radiol*. 1990;19:5–14.

71. Iannotti JP, Zlatkin MB, Esterhai JL, Kressel HY, Dalinka MK, Spindler KP. Magnetic resonance imaging of the shoulder. *J Bone Joint Surg Am*. 1991;73:17–29.

72. Kilcoyne RF, Matsen FA II. Rotator cuff measurement by arthropneumotomography. *AJR*. 1983;140:315–318.

73. Kilcoyne RF, Reddy PK, Lyons F, Rockwood CA. Optimal plain film imaging of shoulder impingement syndrome. *AJR*. 1989;153:795–797.

74. Kneeland JB, Middleton WD, Carrera GF, et al. MR imaging of the shoulder: diagnosis of rotator cuff tears. *AJR*. 1987;149:333–337.

75. Korngut PJ, Salazar AM. The apical oblique view of the shoulder: its usefulness in acute trauma. *AJR*. 1987;149:113–116.

76. Lee FA, Gwinn JL. Retrosternal dislocation of the clavicle. *Radiology*. 1974;110:631.

77. Legan JM, Burkhard TK, Goff WB II, et al. Tear of the glenoid labrum: MR imaging of 88 arthroscopically confirmed cases. *Radiology*. 1991;179:244–246.

78. Lie S, Most WA. Subacromial bursography. *Radiology*. 1982; 144:626–630.

79. Mahvash R, Murkoff J, Bonamo J, et al. Computed tomography arthrography of shoulder instabilities in athletes. *Am J Sports Med*. 1988; 16:352–361.

80. Middleton WD, Reinus WR, Totty WG, Melson GL, Murphy WA. Ultrasonographic evaluation of the rotator cuff and biceps tendon. *J Bone Joint Surg Am*. 1986;68:440–450.

81. Middleton WD, Reinus WR, Totty WG, Melson GL, Murphy WA. US of the biceps tendon apparatus. *Radiology*. 1985;157:211–215.

82. Mink JH, Richardson H, Grant TT. Evaluation of the glenoid labrum by double-contrast arthrography. *AJR*. 1979;133:883–887.

83. Neer CS II. Anterior acromioplasty for chronic impingement syndrome in the shoulder. *J Bone Joint Surg Am*. 1972;54:41–50.

84. Neviaser JS. Adhesive capsulitis of the shoulder joint. *J Bone Joint Surg Am*. 1953;27:211.

85. Newhouse KE, El-Khoury GY, Nepala JV, Montgomery WJ. The shoulder impingement view: a fluoroscopic technique for detection of subacromial spurs. *AJR*. 1988;151:539–541.

86. O'Donoghue DH. Subluxing biceps tendon in athletes. *J Sports Med*. 1973;1:20–29.

87. Rafii M, Firooznia H, Bonamo JJ, Minkoff J, Golumbo C. Athlete shoulder injuries: CT arthrographic findings. *Radiology*. 1987;162:559–564.

88. Rafii M, Firooznia H, Sherman O, et al. Rotator cuff lesions: signal patterns in MR imaging. *Radiology*. 1990;177:817–823.

89. Rokous JR, Feagin JA, Abbott HG. Modified axillary roentgenogram. *Clin Orthop*. 1972;82:84–86.

90. Rubin SA, Gray RL, Green WR. The scapular "Y": a diagnostic aid in shoulder trauma. *Radiology*. 1974;110:725–736.

91. Shuman WB, Kilcoyne RF, Matsen RA, Rogers JJ, Mack LA. Double contrast computed tomography of the glenoid labrum. *AJR*. 1983; 141:581–584.

92. Surgson RD, Feldman F, Bigliani L. CT arthrographic patterns in recurrent glenohumeral instability. *AJR*. 1987;149:749–753.

93. Surgson RD, Feldman F, Bigliani LU, Rosenberg ZS. Recurrent shoulder dislocation after surgical repair. Double contrast CT arthrography. *Radiology*. 1987;162:425–428.

94. Zlatkin MD, Dalinka MK. The glenohumeral joint. *Top Magn Resonance Imaging*. 1989;1:1–13.

95. Zlatkin MD, Dalinka MK, Kressel HY. Magnetic resonance imaging of the shoulder. *Magn Resonance Q*. 1989;5:3–22.

96. Zlatkin MD, Iannotti JP, Roberts MC, et al. Rotator cuff disease: diagnostic performance of MR imaging. *Radiology*. 1989;172:223–229.

Fractures, Dislocations, and Osseous Injuries

97. Allman FL. Fractures and ligamentous injuries of the clavicle and its articulations. *J Bone Joint Surg Am*. 1967;49:774–784.

98. Arner O, Sandahl U, Orhling H. Dislocation of the acromioclavicular joint: a review of the literature and report of 56 cases. *Acta Chir Scand*. 1957;113:140–152.

99. Aston JW Jr, Gregory CF. Dislocation of the shoulder with significant fracture of the glenoid. *J Bone Joint Surg Am*. 1973;55:1531–1533.

100. Bankart ASB. Recurrent or habitual dislocation of the shoulder joint. *Br Med J*. 1923;2:1132–1133.

101. Barnett LS. Little league shoulder syndrome: proximal humeral epiphyseolysis in adolescent baseball pitchers. *J Bone Joint Surg Am*. 1985; 67:495–496.

102. Bearden JM, Hughston JC, Whatley GS. Acromioclavicular dislocation: method of treatment. *J Sports Med*. 1973;1:5–7.

103. Benchetrit E, Friedman B. Fracture of the coracoid process associated with subglenoid dislocation of the shoulder. *J Bone Joint Surg Am*. 1979; 61:295–298.

104. Berquist TH. *Imaging of Orthopedic Trauma*. 2nd ed. New York: Raven; 1991.

105. Berquist TH. *MRI of the Musculoskeletal System*. 2nd ed. New York: Raven; 1990.

106. Boyer DW Jr. Trapshooter's shoulder: stress fracture of the coracoid process. *J Bone Joint Surg Am*. 1975;57:862.

107. Buckerfield CT, Castle ME. Acute traumatic retrosternal dislocation of the clavicle. *J Bone Joint Surg Am*. 1984;66:379–384.

108. Callaghan JJ, McNiesh LM, Dehaven JP, Savory CG, Polly DW. A prospective comparison study of double contrast computed tomography, arthrography and arthroscopy of the shoulder. *Am J Sports Med*. 1988; 16:13–20.

109. Castagno AA, Shuman AA, Kilcoyne RF, Haynor DR, Morris ME, Matsen FA. Complex fractures of the proximal humerus: role of CT in treatment. *Radiology*. 1987;165:759–762.

110. Cisternino SJ, Rogers LF, Stuffleban BC, Kruglik GD. The trough line: a radiographic sign of posterior dislocation. *AJR*. 1978;130:951–954.

111. Cope R, Riddervold HO. Posterior dislocation of the sternoclavicular joint: report of 2 cases with emphasis on the radiologic management and early diagnosis. *Skeletal Radiol*. 1988;17:247–258.

112. Dameron TB, Rockwood CA. Fractures and dislocations of the shoulder. In: Rockwood CA, Wilkins KE, King RE, eds. *Fractures in Children*. Philadelphia: Lippincott; 1984;3:577–623.

113. Dennis DA, Ferlic DC, Clayton ML. Acromial stress fractures associated with cuff-tear arthrography. *J Bone Joint Surg Am*. 1986;68:937–940.

114. DePalma AF, Cantilli RA. Fractures of the upper end of the humerus. *Clin Orthop*. 1961;20:73–93.

115. Downey EF Jr, Cartes DJ, Bower AC. Unusual dislocations of the shoulder. *AJR*. 1983;140:1207–1210.

116. Earwaker J. Isolated avulsion fracture of the lesser tuberosity of the humerus. *Skeletal Radiol*. 1990;19:121–125.

117. Erickson SJ, Kneeland BJ, Komorowski RA, Knudson GJ, Carreru GF. Post-traumatic osteolysis of the clavicle: MR features. *J Comput Assisted Tomogr*. 1990;14:835–837.

118. Fronek J, Warren RF, Bowin M. Posterior subluxation of the glenohumeral joint. *J Bone Joint Surg Am*. 1989;71:205–216.

119. Garth WP, Leberte MA, Cool TA. Recurrent fractures of the humerus in a baseball pitcher. *J Bone Joint Surg Am*. 1988;70:305–306.

120. Goldberg RP, Vicks B. Oblique angled view for coracoid fractures. *Skeletal Radiol*. 1983;9:195.

121. Hall RH, Isaac E, Booth CR. Dislocation of the shoulder with special reference to accompanying small fractures. *J Bone Joint Surg Am*. 1959; 41:489–494.

122. Hawkins RJ, Bell RH, Gurr K. The three-part fracture of the proximal part of the humerus. *J Bone Joint Surg Am*. 1986;68:1410–1414.

123. Hawkins RJ, Neer CS II, Mendoza FX. Locked posterior dislocation of the shoulder. *J Bone Joint Surg Am*. 1987;69:9–18.

124. Hill AA, Sachs MD. The grooved defect of the humeral head—a frequently unrecognized complication of dislocations of the shoulder joint. *Radiology*. 1940;35:690.

125. Horak J, Nilsson BE. Epidemiology of fractures of the upper end of the humerus. *Clin Orthop*. 1975;112:250–253.

126. Hovelius L. Anterior dislocation of the shoulder in teenagers and young adults. *J Bone Joint Surg Am*. 1987;69:393–399.

127. Janecki CJ, Barnett DC. Fracture-dislocation of the shoulder with biceps tendon interposition. *J Bone Joint Surg Am*. 1979;61:142.

128. Kilcoyne RF, Shuman WP, Matsen FA III, Rockwood CA. The Neer classification of displaced proximal humeral fracture: spectrum of findings on plain radiographs and CT scans. *AJR*. 1990;154:1029–1033.

129. Kristiansen B, Andersen ULS, Olsen CA, Vanmarken J. The Neer classification of fractures of the proximal humerus. An assessment of interobserver variation. *Skeletal Radiol*. 1988;17:420–422.

130. Kummel BM. Fracture of the glenoid causing chronic dislocation of the shoulder. *Clin Orthop*. 1970;69:189–191.

131. Mariani PP. Isolated fracture of the coracoid process in an athlete. *Am J Sports Med*. 1980;8:129.

132. McAuliffe TB, Dowd GS. Avulsion of the subscapularis tendon. *J Bone Joint Surg Am*. 1987;69:1454–1455.

133. McLaughlin HL. Posterior dislocations of the shoulder. *J Bone Joint Surg Am*. 1952;34:584–590.

134. McLaughlin HL, MacLellan DI. Recurrent anterior dislocation of the shoulder. II. A comparative study. *J Trauma*. 1967;7:191–201.

135. Neer CS II. Anterior acromioplasty for the chronic impingement syndrome in the shoulder: a preliminary report. *J Bone Joint Surg Am*. 1972; 54:41.

136. Neer CS II. Displaced proximal humeral fractures. Part I. Classification and evaluation. *J Bone Joint Surg Am*. 1970;52:1077–1089.

137. Neer CS II. Fractures of the distal clavicle with detachment of the coracoclavicular ligament in adults. *J Trauma*. 1963;3:99–110.

138. Neer CS II. Fractures of the distal third of the clavicle. *Clin Orthop*. 1968;58:43–50.

139. Neer CS, Horowitz BS. Fractures of the proximal humeral epiphyseal plate. *Clin Orthop*. 1968;41:24–31.

140. Neer CS II, Rockwood CA. Fractures and dislocations of the shoulder. In: Rockwood CA, Green DP, eds. *Fractures in Adults*. 2nd ed. Philadelphia: Lippincott; 1984;1:675–985.

141. O'Donoghue DH. *Treatment of Injuries to Athletes*. 4th ed. Philadelphia: Saunders; 1984.

142. Paterson DC. Retrosternal dislocation of the clavicle. *J Bone Joint Surg Br*. 1961;43:90–92.

143. Rafii M, Minkoff J, Bonamo J, et al. Computed tomography arthrography of shoulder instabilities in athletes. *Am J Sports Med*. 1988; 16:352–361.

144. Rockwood CA. Fractures and dislocations of the ends of the clavicle, scapula, and glenohumeral joint. In: Rockwood CA, Wilkins KE, King RE, eds. *Fractures in Children*. Philadelphia: Lippincott; 1984;3:624–682.

145. Rockwood CA. Subluxations and dislocations about the shoulder. In: Rockwood CA, Green DP, eds. *Fractures in Adults*. 2nd ed. Philadelphia: Lippincott; 1984;1:922–985.

146. Rowe CR. Fractures of the scapula. *Surg Clin North Am*. 1963; 43:1565–1571.

147. Rowe CR. Shoulder girdle injuries. In: Cave EF, ed. *Trauma Management*. Chicago: Year Book Medical; 1974:399–453.

148. Ruberstein JD, Ebraheim NA, Kellam JF. Traumatic scapulothoracic dissociation. *Radiology*. 1985;157:297–298.

149. Salvatore J. Sternoclavicular joint dislocation. *Clin Orthop*. 1968; 58:51–55.

150. Sandrock AR. Another sports fatigue fracture: stress fracture of the coracoid process of the scapula. *Radiology*. 1975;117:274.

151. Selesnick FH, Jablow M, Frank C, Post M. Retrosternal dislocation of the clavicle. Report of 4 cases. *J Bone Joint Surg Am*. 1984;66:287.

152. Shanley DJ, Mulligan ME. Osteochondrosis dissecans of the glenoid. *Skeletal Radiol*. 1990;19:419–421.

153. Väätäinen U, Pirinen A, Mäkelä A. Radiological evaluation of the acromioclavicular joint. *Skeletal Radiol*. 1991;20:115–116.

154. Varriale PL, Adler ML. Occult fracture of the glenoid without dislocation. *J Bone Joint Surg Am*. 1983;65:688.

155. Vastamaki M, Solonen KA. Posterior dislocations and fracture-dislocations of the shoulder. *Acta Orthop Scand*. 1980;51:479–484.

156. Yosipovitch Z, Tikva P, Goldberg I. Inferior subluxation of the humeral head after shoulder injury. *J Bone Joint Surg Am*. 1989;71:751–753.

Soft Tissue Trauma

157. Anderson TE. Shoulder injuries in the athlete. *Primary Care*. 1984; 11:129–136.

158. Axe MJ. Evaluation and treatment of common throwing injuries of the shoulder and elbow. *Del Med J*. 1987;59:593–598.

159. Berquist TH. *MRI of the Musculoskeletal System*. 2nd ed. New York: Raven; 1990.

160. Buirski G. Magnetic resonance imaging in acute and chronic rotator cuff tears. *Skeletal Radiol*. 1990;19:109–111.

161. Burk LD, Karasick D, Mitchell DG, Rifkin MD. MR Imaging of the shoulder: correlation with plain radiography. *AJR*. 1990;154:549–553.

162. Burk LD, Torres JL, Marone PJ, Mitchell DG, Rifkin MD, Karasick D. MR Imaging of shoulder injuries in professional baseball players. *J Magn Resonance Imaging*. 1991;1:385–389.

163. Cervilla V, Schweitzer ME, Ho C, Motta A, Kerr R, Resnick D. Medial dislocation of the biceps brachii tendon: appearance on MR imaging. *Radiology*. 1991;180:523–526.

164. Chan TW, Dalinka MK, Kneeland JB, Chervrot A. Biceps tendon dislocation: evaluation with MR imaging. *Radiology*. 1991;179:649–652.

165. Ciullo JV, Stevens GG. The prevention and treatment of injuries to the shoulder in swimming. *J Sports Med*. 1989;7:182–204.

166. Cofield RH. Rotator cuff disease of the shoulder. *J Bone Joint Surg Am*. 1985;67:974–979.

167. Cofield RH, Simonet WT. The shoulder in sports. *Mayo Clin Proc*. 1984;59:157–164.

168. Cone RO III, Resnick D, Danzig L. Shoulder impingement syndrome: radiographic evaluation. *Radiology*. 1984;150:29–33.

169. Crues JV III, Fareed DO. Magnetic resonance imaging of shoulder impingement. *Top Magn Resonance Imaging*. 1991;3:39–49.

170. DeMaio M, Drez D, Mullins RC. The inferior transverse scapular ligament as a possible cause of entrapment neuropathy of the nerve to the infraspinatus. *J Bone Joint Surg Am*. 1991;73:1061–1063.

171. Dennis DA, Ferlic DC, Clayton ML. Acromial stress fractures associated with cuff tear arthropathy. *J Bone Joint Surg Am*. 1986;68:937–940.

172. Farin PU, Jaroma H, Jarju A, Sormakallis S. Shoulder impingement syndrome. Sonographic evaluation. *Radiology*. 1990;176:845–849.

173. Flannigan B, Kursunoglu-Brahme S, Snyder S, Karsel R, DelRizzo W, Resnick D. MR Arthrography of the shoulder: comparison with conventional MR imaging. *AJR*. 1990;155:829–832.

174. Fuduka H, Mikasa M, Yamanaka K. Incomplete thickness rotator cuff tears diagnosed by subacromial bursography. *Clin Orthop*. 1987; 223:51–58.

175. Fuduka H, Neer CS II. Archer's shoulder. *Orthopedics*. 1988; 11:171–174.

176. Garth WP, Allman FL, Armstrong WS. Occult anterior subluxation of the shoulder in noncontact sports. *Am J Sports Med*. 1987;15:579–585.

177. Garth WP, Sloppery CE, Ochs CW. Roentgenographic demonstration of instability of the shoulder: the apical oblique projection. *J Bone Joint Surg Am*. 1984;66:1450–1453.

178. Harryman DT, Sidles JA, Clark JK, McQuade KJ, Gibb TD, Matsen FA. Translation of the humeral head on the glenoid with passive motion. *J Bone Joint Surg Am*. 1990;72:1334–1343.

179. Haynor DR, Shuman WP. Double contrast CT arthrography of the glenoid labrum and shoulder girdle. *RadioGraphics*. 1984;4:411–422.

180. Holder J, Fretz CJ, Terrier F, Gerber C. Rotator cuff tears: correlation of sonographic and surgical findings. *Radiology*. 1988;169:791–794.

181. Holt RG, Helms CA, Steinbach L, Neumann C, Mink PL, Genant HK. Magnetic resonance imaging of the shoulder: rationale and current applications. *Skeletal Radiol*. 1990;19:5–14.

182. Iannotti JP, Zlatkin MB, Esterhai JL, Kressel HY, Dalinka MR, Spindler KP. Magnetic resonance imaging of the shoulder. *J Bone Joint Surg Am*. 1991;73:17–29.

183. Jobe FW. Impingement problems in athletes. *Instr Course Lect*. 1989;38:205–209.

184. Jobe FW, Bradley JP. Diagnosis and nonoperative treatment of shoulder injuries in athletes. *Clin Sports Med*. 1989;8:419–438.

185. Jobe FW, Bradley JP. Rotator cuff injuries in baseball. *Sports Med*. 1988;6:378–387.

186. Johnson JE, Sims FH, Scott SG. Musculoskeletal injuries in competitive swimmers. *Mayo Clin Proc*. 1987;62:289–304.

187. Jones MW, Matthews JP. Rupture of pectoralis major in weight lifters. *Injury*. 1988;19:219.

188. Kilcoyne RF, Reddy PK, Lyons F, Rockwood CA. Optimal plain film imaging of shoulder impingement syndrome. *AJR*. 1989;153:795–797.

189. Kornguth PJ, Salazar AM. The apical oblique view of the shoulder: its usefulness in acute trauma. *AJR*. 1987;149:113–116.

190. Kretzler HH, Richardson AB. Ruptures of the pectoralis major muscle. *Am J Sports Med*. 1989;17:453–458.

191. Legan JM, Burkhard TK, Goff WB, et al. Tears of the glenoid labrum: MR imaging of 88 arthroscopically confirmed cases. *Radiology*. 1991;179:241–246.

192. Lehman RC. Shoulder pain in the competitive tennis player. *Clin Sports Med*. 1988;7:309–327.

193. Mann DL, Littke N. Shoulder injuries in archery. *Can J Sports Sci*. 1989;14:85–92.

194. McCarthy WJ, Yao JS, Schafer MF, et al. Upper extremity arterial injury in athletes. *J Vasc Surg*. 1989;9:317–327.

195. McLeod WD, Andrews JR. Mechanism of shoulder injuries. *Phys Ther*. 1986;66:1901–1904.

196. McMaster WC. Anterior glenoid labrum damage: a painful lesion in swimmers. *Am J Sports Med*. 1986;14:383–387.

197. Middleton WD, Reinus WR, Totty WG, Melson GL, Murphy WA. Ultrasonographic evaluation of the rotator cuff and biceps tendon. *J Bone Joint Surg Am*. 1986;68:440–450.

198. Middleton WD, Reinus WR, Totty WG, Melson GL, Murphy WA. US of the biceps tendon apparatus. *Radiology*. 1985;157:211–215.

199. Misamore GW, Woodeward C. Evaluation of degenerative lesions of the rotator cuff. *J Bone Joint Surg Am*. 1991;73:704–706.

200. Nelson MC, Leather GP, Nirschl RP, Pettrone FA, Freedman MT. Evaluation of the painful shoulder. *J Bone Joint Surg Am*. 1991;73:707–716.

201. Newhouse KE, El-Khoury GY, Nepola JV, Montgomery WJ. The shoulder impingement view: a fluoroscopic technique for detection of subacromial spurs. *AJR*. 1988;151:539–541.

202. Nirschl RP. Prevention and treatment of elbow and shoulder injuries in the tennis player. *Clin Sports Med*. 1988;7:289–308.

203. Noah J, Gidumal R. Rotator cuff injuries in the throwing athlete. *Orthop Rev*. 1988;17:1091–1096.

204. Norwood LA, Barrack R, Jacobson KE. Clinical presentation of complete tears of the rotator cuff. *J Bone Joint Surg Am*. 1989;71:499–505.

205. Ozaki J, Fujimoto S, Nakagawa Y, et al. Tears of the rotator cuff of the shoulder associated with pathologic changes in the acromion. *J Bone Joint Surg Am*. 1988;70:1224–1230.

206. Priest JD. The shoulder of the tennis player. *Clin Sports Med*. 1988; 7:387–402.

207. Rafii M, Firooznia H, Sherman O, et al. Rotator cuff lesions: signal patterns at MR imaging. *Radiology*. 1990;177:817–823.

208. Rafii M, Minkoff J, Bonamo J, et al. Computed tomography arthrography of shoulder instability in athletes. *Am J Sports Med*. 1988;16:352–361.

209. Richardson AB. Orthopedic aspects of competitive swimming. *Clin Sports Med*. 1987;6:639–644.

210. Shellock FG, Fukunaga T, Mink JH, Edgerton VR. Exertional muscle injury: evaluation of concentric vs eccentric actions with serial MR imaging. *Radiology*. 1991;179:659–664.

211. Singson RD, Feldman F, Bigliani L. CT arthrographic patterns in recurrent glenohumeral instability. *AJR*. 1987;149:749–753.

212. Vick CW, Bell SA. Rotator cuff tears: diagnosis with sonography. *AJR*. 1990;154:121–123.

Chapter 10

Elbow and Forearm

INTRODUCTION

Elbow and forearm injuries can occur in contact and non-contact sports. Elbow injuries are most common in throwing and racquet sports.[1,2,4,6] Elbow pain in tennis players occurs in up to 50% of players older than 30 years.[4] It occurs with increasing frequency in pitchers with increasing number of years of activity. Elbow pain in pitchers occurs in 20% of 8- to 12-year-olds, 45% of 13- to 14-year-olds, and 58% of athletes in high school and college baseball programs.[3] Most of these injuries are overuse injuries resulting in damage to tendons, but growth plate fractures, osteochondritis dissecans, bursitis, and ulnar nerve injuries also occur.[4–7] Fractures and dislocations are usually due to more significant acute trauma. This chapter reviews the anatomy, mechanisms of injury, and imaging techniques for bone and soft tissue sports injuries of the elbow and forearm.

ANATOMY

A thorough knowledge of the bone and soft tissue anatomy of the elbow and forearm is essential to evaluate properly the clinical and imaging features of sports injuries.

Osseous Anatomy

The distal humerus expands to form the medial and lateral supracondylar columns; these stabilize the articular surface, which comprises the capitellum and trochlea (Fig. 10-1).[12,17] The proximal radius and ulna articulate respectively with the capitellum and trochlea. The proximal radius is composed of a disc-shaped radial head (Fig. 10-1), which articulates with the capitellum.[13] The proximal ulna consists of the sigmoid notch, with an arc of approximately 180°, which is rotated posteriorly to articulate with the trochlea (Fig. 10-2). On the anteroposterior (AP) view the distal humerus forms a valgus angle, thus explaining the normal 10° to 13° carrying angle (Fig. 10-1).[9,17]

The elbow articulation is one of the most congruent in the body.[18] As such, the cartilage thickness varies inversely with the congruence.[19] The articular surfaces are covered with hyaline cartilage, although this may not be continuous in the sigmoid or trochlear notch of the ulna.[17] The articular capsule of the elbow is thin anteriorly and posteriorly, with additional support being provided anteriorly by the brachialis muscle and posteriorly by the triceps muscle.[13] Supplementary support medially and laterally is provided by the collateral ligaments. The medial collateral ligaments are dominated by the anterior ulnar collateral ligament.[12] The posterior ulnar collateral ligament is taut only in flexion.[17] The medial collateral ligament originates along the inferior margin of the epicondyle. Therefore, disruption of the epicondyle indicates disruption of the medial collateral ligament complex.[14] The lateral collateral ligament extends from the epicondyle distally to the annular ligament and ulna.[13,17]

The capsule of the elbow (Fig. 10-3) attaches to the humerus just above the radial and coronoid fossae and extends beyond the coronoid of the ulna to the anterior portion of the annular ligament. The posterior capsule is closely related to the triceps tendon and attaches to the humerus above the

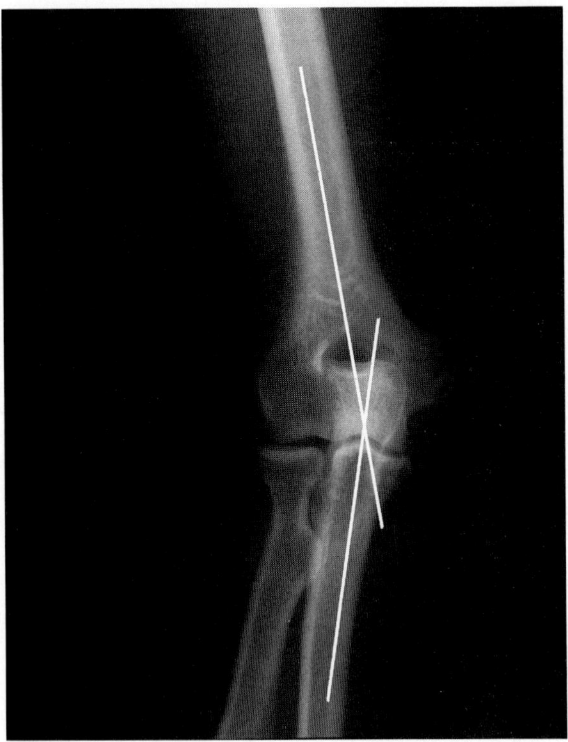

Fig. 10-1 Anteroposterior (AP) view of the elbow demonstrating the osseous anatomy. The lines delineate the normal carrying angle.

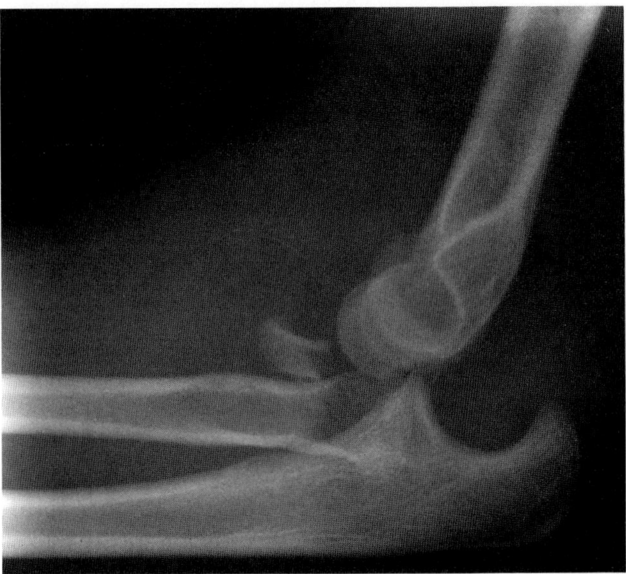

Fig. 10-2 Lateral view of the elbow after anterior fracture-dislocation. The trochlear notch of the ulna is demonstrated clearly because of the dislocation.

olecranon fossa at the upper and lateral margins of the trochlear notch of the ulna, the roughened area on the lateral side of the ulna, and the annular ligament.[13] Medially and laterally the capsule blends with the medial and lateral collateral ligaments.[13,17] The capsule is lined with synovial membrane with two prominent anterior and posterior fat pads, which are intracapsular but extrasynovial (Fig. 10-4).[13,17]

The osseous anatomy of the forearm (Fig. 10-5) is complex; the reader is referred to more extensive sources for review.[13,16,17] The radius and ulna articulate proximally and distally (Fig. 10-5, A and B). In addition, they are connected by a strong interosseous membrane that is contiguous proximally to distally except for gaps for the interosseous arteries (Fig. 10-5B).[10,15] The muscle origins and insertions on the radius and ulna are demonstrated in Figure 10-5, A and B.[13,17]

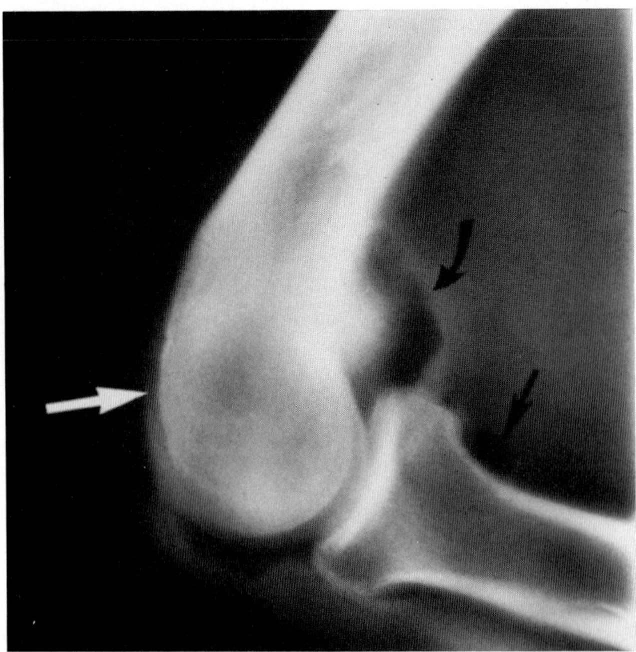

Fig. 10-3 Lateral air arthrotomogram of the elbow demonstrating the anterior capsule (curved black arrow), annular recess (straight black arrow), and posterior capsule (white arrow).

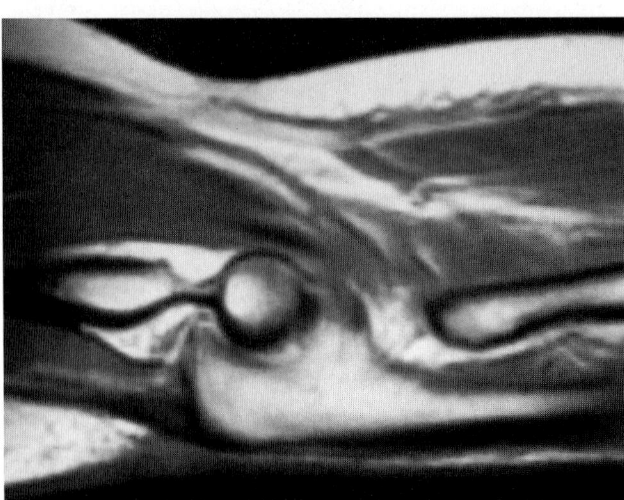

Fig. 10-4 Sagittal T1-weighted magnetic resonance (MR) image (SE 500/20) demonstrating the anterior and posterior fat pads (arrows).

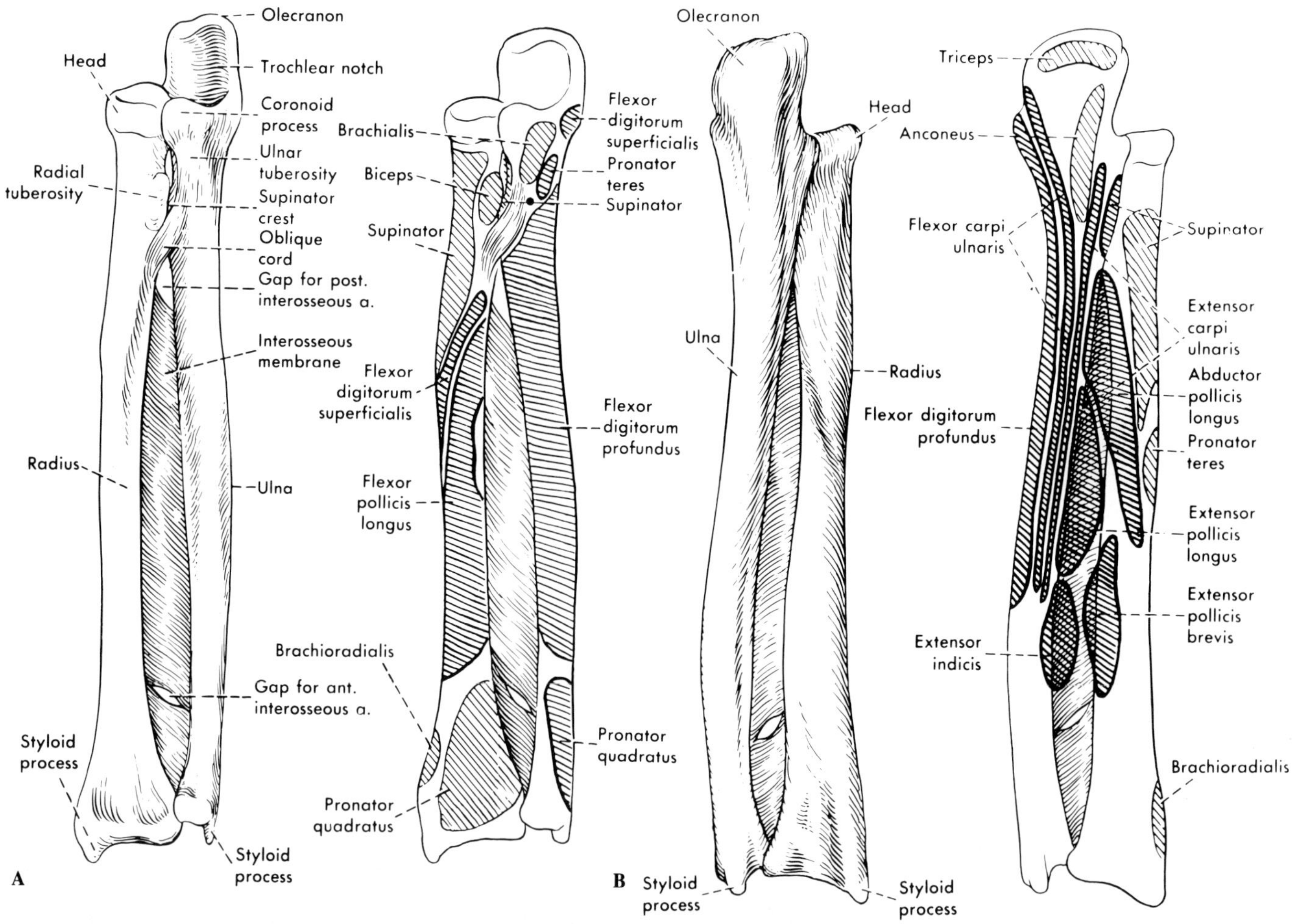

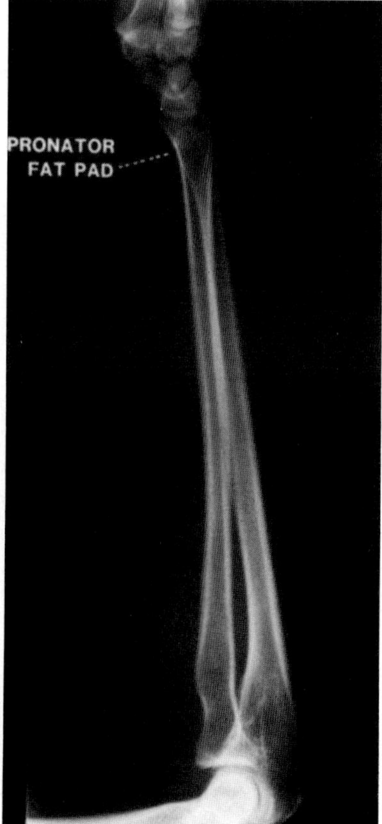

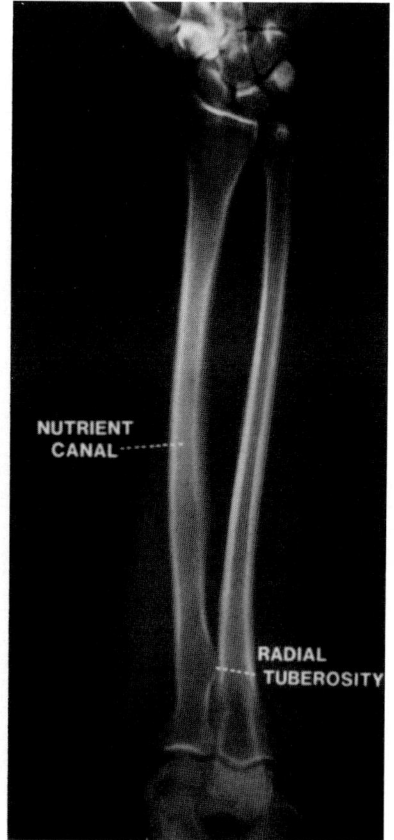

Fig. 10-5 Osseous anatomy, with muscle origins and insertions, of the radius and ulna seen anteriorly (**A**) and posteriorly (**B**). (From Hollinshead W H : The back and limbs. In: *Anatomy for Surgeons*, Vol. 3. Harper and Row, New York, 1982, with permission.) (**C**) Lateral and AP radiographs of the radius and ulna.

Muscular Anatomy

There are four base movements of the elbow and forearm. The elbow is limited to flexion and extension. Pronation and supination occurs between the radius and ulna.[8,9,13] The chief flexors of the elbow are the biceps, brachialis, and brachioradialis. The biceps crosses the elbow anteriorly and inserts on the radial tuberosity (Fig. 10-5A). The brachialis arises from the anterior humerus and passes anterior to the capsule before inserting on the proximal ulna near the coronoid. The brachioradialis arises from the distal humerus and inserts on the proximal radius.[8,13]

The primary extensors of the elbow are the triceps, especially the medial head, and the anconeus.[13] The triceps has three heads, which arise from the infraglenoid tubercle, posterior humerus, and lower posterior humerus and insert on the olecranon (Fig. 10-5B). The anconeus arises from the posterior lateral epicondyle and extends medially and distally to insert on the lateral ulna.[13]

The main pronators of the radius and ulna are the pronator teres proximally and the pronator quadratus distally. The pronator teres originates from the medial supracondylar ridge and coronoid and inserts on the lateral aspect of the mid-radius.[13,16,17] The pronator quadratus extends transversely across the distal radius and ulna (Fig. 10-5A).[13]

Supination is accomplished by the supinator and biceps brachii with minor assistance from the extensor pollicis longus, abductor pollicus longus, extensor carpi radialis longus, and brachioradialis.[13] The supinator originates from the lateral epicondyle, adjacent ligaments, and ulna and inserts on the upper lateral radius (Fig. 10-5, A and B).[13]

Most of the forearm muscles arise from the humerus and cross the elbow before inserting distally. These muscle groups and other forearm muscles affecting the wrist are discussed more fully in Chapter 11.

Neurovascular Anatomy

Knowledge of the neurovascular anatomy and the relationship of these structures to the muscles and osseous structures of the elbow and forearm is essential for evaluating neurovascular injury and nerve compression syndromes.[11,17] At the level of the distal humerus, the brachial artery is located anteromedially adjacent to its accompanying vein. The median nerve usually lies at the junction of the biceps and brachialis muscles. The ulnar nerve is positioned more posteriorly along the medial aspect of the triceps (Fig. 10-6).[13,17] At this same level, the radial nerve is most commonly seen between the brachialis and brachioradialis just anterior to the lateral aspect of the supracondylar portion of the humerus. Near the elbow, the radial nerve courses anteriorly along the margin of the brachialis and medial to the brachioradialis to a point just above the supinator, where it divides into deep and superficial branches. The superficial branch of the nerve lies anterior to the extensor carpi radialis longus, and the deep branch is either within or between the supinator and extensor digitorum posterior to the radius. The median nerve courses along the anterior aspect of the acute cubital fossa, passing beneath the flexor digitorum superficialis to lie between this muscle and the flexor digitorum profundus as it passes distally into the forearm. The ulnar nerve passes posterior to the medial epicondyle and then passes distally between the flexor digitorum profundus and flexor carpi ulnaris.[13,17]

The major vessels of the elbow and forearm are demonstrated in Fig. 10-6A. The brachial artery courses with the median nerve in the antecubital fossa before dividing into the radial and ulnar arteries. The radial artery continues distally superficial to the flexor pollicis longus as it extends into the forearm. The ulnar artery usually accompanies the median nerve along its course superficial to the flexor digitorum profundus.[13,16]

IMAGING TECHNIQUES

Routine Radiographic Techniques

A minimum of two projections is necessary to evaluate the extremity.[25,42] The AP and lateral views of the forearm (Fig. 10-5C) provide two views taken at 90° angles to fulfill this criterion. We routinely obtain AP, lateral, and both oblique views in patients with suspected elbow injury.[25,46] These views deserve further discussion.

The AP view is obtained with the patient sitting adjacent to the X-ray table or in the supine position if the injury is severe. When seated, the patient should be positioned so that the extended elbow is at the same level as the shoulder; thus the extremity is in contact with the full length of the cassette.[21,24] The AP view is of value in studying the medial and lateral epicondyles as well as the radial capitellar articular surface (Fig. 10-7). The invariant relationship of the radial head centered on the capitellum is observed. Assessment of the ulnar trochlear articular surface and at least a portion of the olecranon fossa is also possible. The normal carrying angle (5° to 20°; average, 15°) can be measured on the AP view.[25]

The lateral view is obtained by flexing the elbow 90° and placing it directly upon the cassette. Again, the beam is perpendicular to the joint. The hand must also be placed carefully in the lateral position.[21,24] This view provides good detail of the distal humerus, elbow joint, and proximal forearm. The coronoid of the ulna, which cannot be visualized readily on the AP view, and the olecranon are well visualized in the lateral projection (Fig. 10-8).

Oblique views are obtained by initially positioning the arm as one would for the usual AP film. For the medial oblique view the patient's arm is positioned with the forearm and arm (internally) rotated approximately 45°.[21,24,25] This view allows improved visualization of the trochlea, olecranon, and coronoid. The radial head is obscured by the proximal ulna (Fig. 10-9A). The lateral oblique view (Fig. 10-9B) is taken

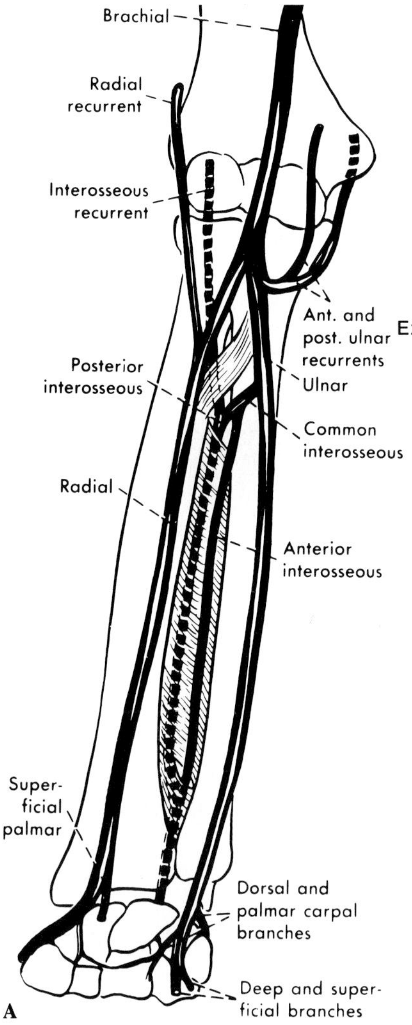

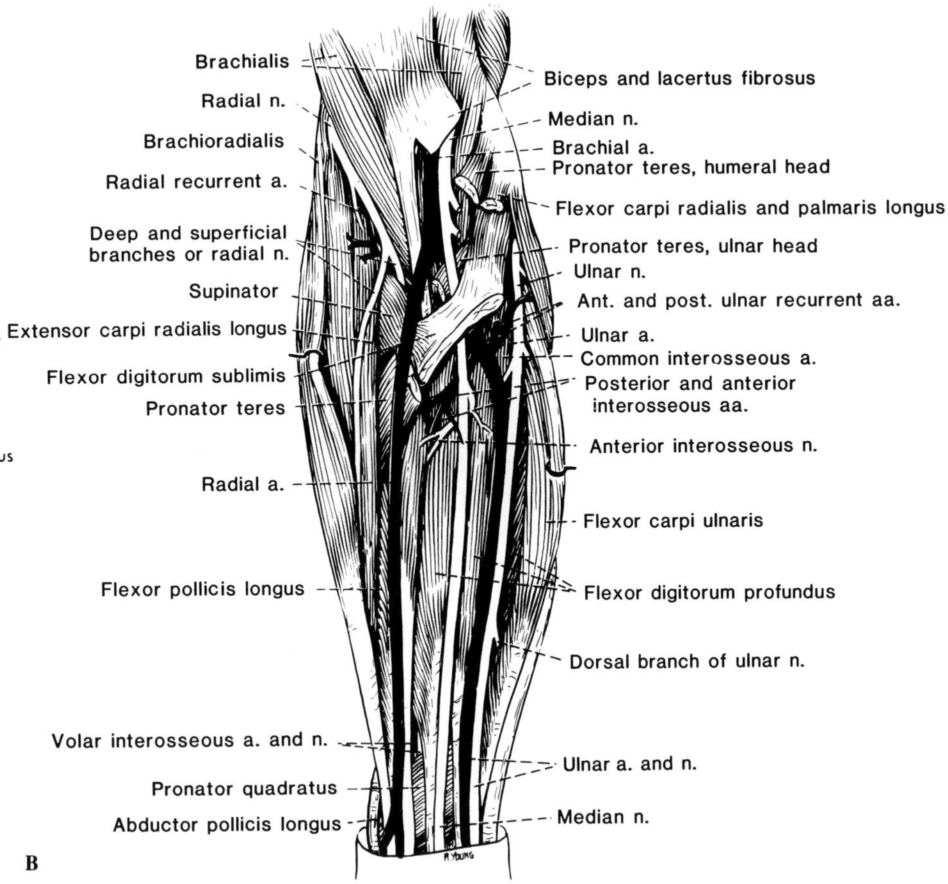

Fig. 10-6 Illustrations of the vascular (**A**) and neural (**B**) anatomy of the elbow and forearm. *Source:* Reprinted from *Anatomy for Surgeons, Vol. 3, The Back and Limbs*, ed 3 by HW Hollinshead, 1982, JB Lippincott.

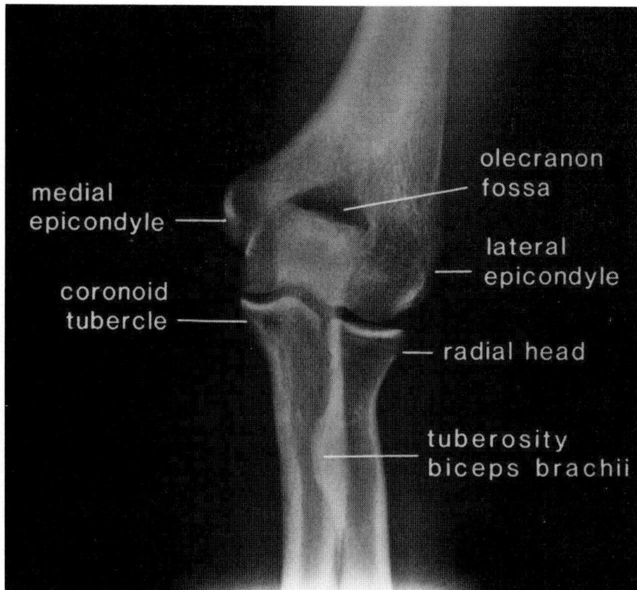

Fig. 10-7 Normal AP view of the elbow. *Source:* Reprinted from *Imaging of Orthopedic Trauma* ed 2 by TH Berquist, 1991, Raven Press, © Mayo Foundation.

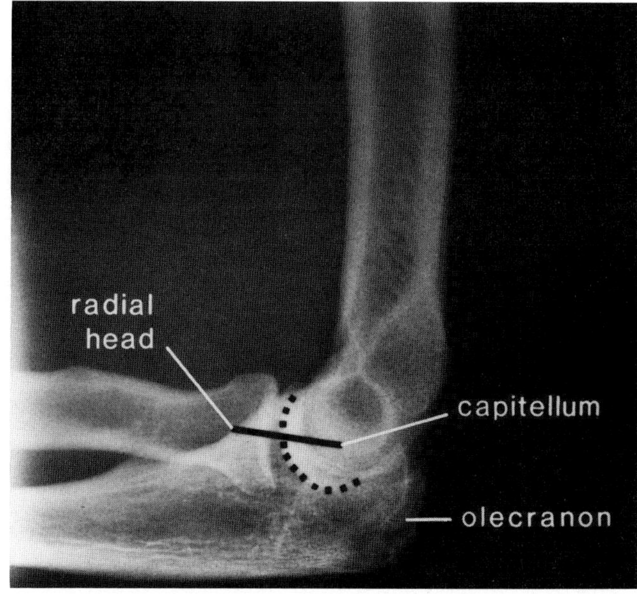

Fig. 10-8 Normal lateral view of the elbow. Solid lines indicate constate radiocapitellar relationship. *Source:* Reprinted from *Imaging of Orthopedic Trauma* ed 2 by TH Berquist, 1991, Raven Press, © Mayo Foundation.

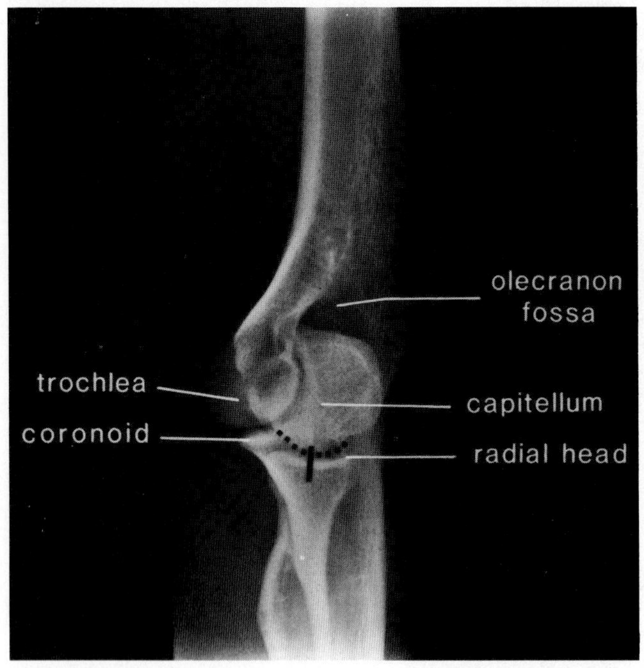

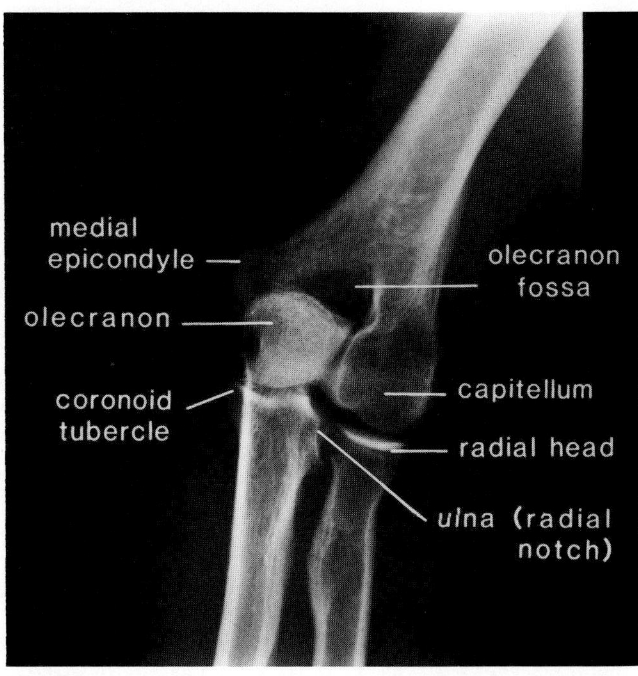

A B

Fig. 10-9 (**A**) Medial and (**B**) lateral oblique views of the elbow. Solid lines indicate constate radiocapitellar relationship. *Source:* Reprinted from *Imaging of Orthopedic Trauma* ed 2 by TH Berquist, 1991, Raven Press, © Mayo Foundation.

with the forearm, arm, and hand rotated externally. This projection provides excellent visualization of the radiocapitellar articulation, medial epicondyle, radioulnar articulation, and coronoid tubercle.[21,24,25]

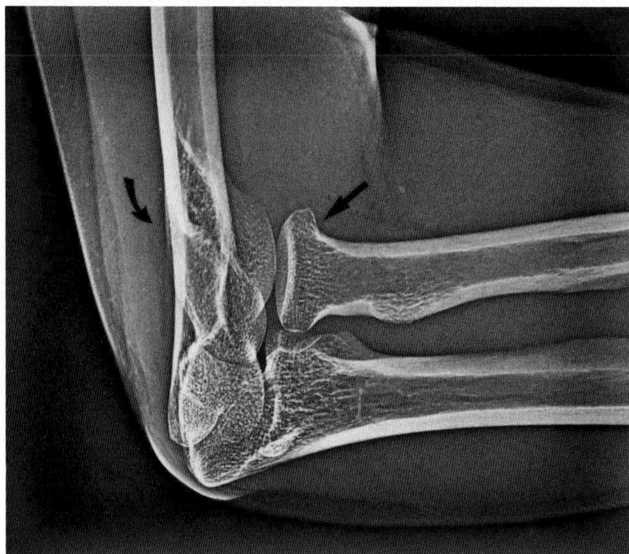

Fig. 10-10 Radial head view (xerogram) demonstrating a posterior fat pad (curved arrow) and subtle fracture (straight arrow). *Source:* Reprinted from *Imaging of Orthopedic Trauma* ed 2 by TH Berquist, 1991, Raven Press, © Mayo Foundation.

Radial head fractures are a common clinical problem in adults and often are difficult to visualize. Several other techniques may be utilized when such a lesion is suspected.[33–36,47] The radial head view (Fig. 10-10) is easily accomplished by positioning the patient as one would for a routine lateral examination and angling the tube 45° toward the joint.[33–36] This view projects the radius away from the remaining bony structures, allowing subtle changes to be detected more readily (Fig. 10-10). This view may also allow the fat pads to be visualized more easily.[25] In certain cases additional views or fluoroscopically positioned spot films may be indicated to identify subtle injuries.[25]

Assessment of the radiographic views should be complete and systematic. Certain features should be checked consistently and, if necessary, further views or modalities employed.

The relationship of the radial head to the articular surface of the capitellum is constant regardless of the view obtained (Fig. 10-11). The radius is normally bowed at the level of the tubercle. Therefore, the lines should not be extended to include this portion of the shaft. A line through the midpoint of the head and neck provides consistency.

Careful evaluation of the fat pads is essential. These structures are intracapsular but extrasynovial.[28,29,33,37,41,42,51] The anterior fat pad is normally seen on the lateral view. The posterior fat pad is obscured because of its position in the olecranon fossa. Displacement of the fat pads, particularly the posterior fat pad, is indicative of an intraarticular fracture with hemarthrosis (Fig. 10-12).[25,28,29] Norell[45] reported that 90%

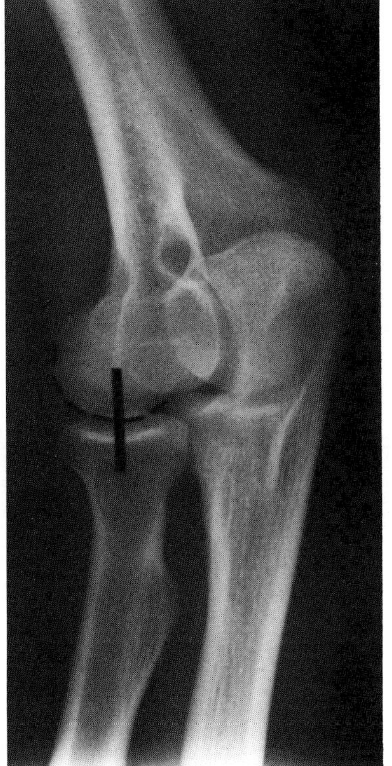

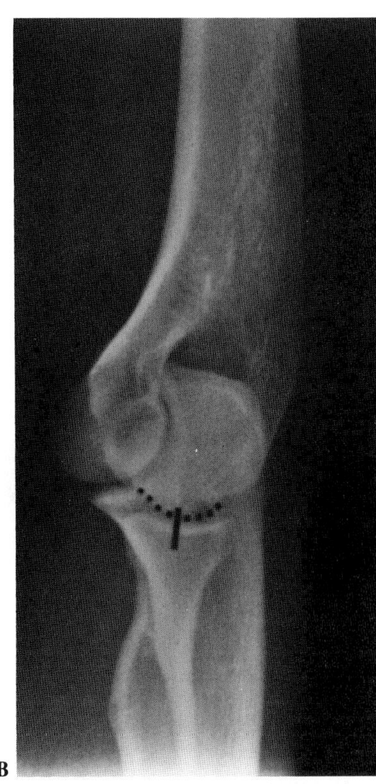

Fig. 10-11 Oblique views of the elbow demonstrating the constant relationship of the radial head (straight line) to the capitellum (broken line).

of children with posterior fat pad signs had elbow fractures. This finding is somewhat less common in the adult, but if it is present a fracture is likely. Cross-table lateral views may be more specific. A lipohemarthrosis may be evident, which is more specific for an intraarticular fracture.[20,25,55]

The supinator fat stripe lies ventral to the radial head and neck on the surface of the supinator muscle (Fig. 10-13). Fractures about the elbow will frequently displace or obliterate this structure, providing a clue to the underlying injury. Rogers and MacEwan[50] reported changes in this fat stripe in

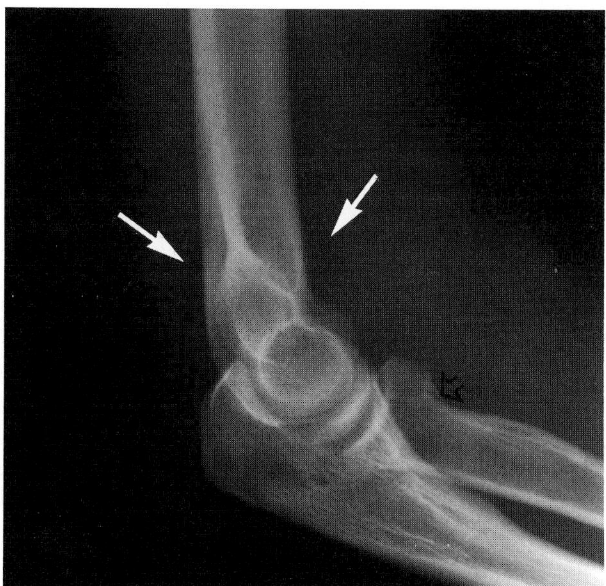

Fig. 10-12 Lateral view of the elbow showing a subtle radial head fracture (open arrow). Both fat pads (arrows) are displaced by hemarthrosis.

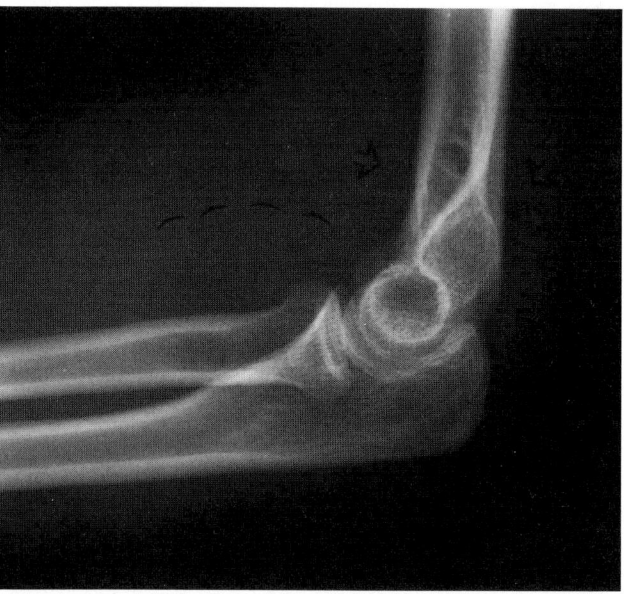

Fig. 10-13 Lateral view of the elbow with displaced fat pads (arrows) and supinator fat stripe (broken lines) in a patient with a subtle radial head fracture.

100% of fractures of the radial head and neck and in 82% of other elbow fractures.

The anterior humeral line is helpful in detecting subtle supracondylar fractures in children.[39] This line, drawn along the anterior humeral cortex, should pass through the middle third of the capitellum (Fig. 10-14).

Stress views may be required to evaluate soft tissue injury. Positioning is optimal with fluoroscopic guidance. Varus and valgus stress views should be performed on the involved elbow and normal elbow for comparison. An increase in the joint space of 2 mm compared to the normal side is abnormal (Fig. 10-15).[25]

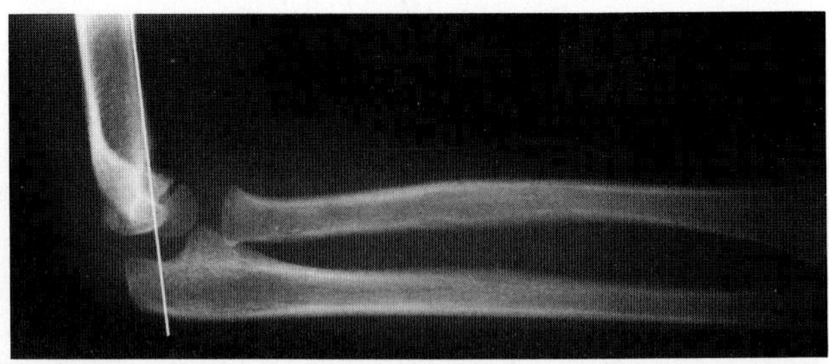

Fig. 10-14 Lateral view of the elbow and forearm in a child with a supracondylar fracture. The anterior humeral line (white line) passes posterior to the capitellum.

Special Radiographic Techniques

Several special techniques are available to assess elbow and forearm injuries that are not clearly demonstrable by routine views. These include arthrography, computed tomography (CT), conventional tomography, sonography, and magnetic resonance imaging (MRI).[22,25,26,52]

Arthrography

Elbow arthrography, although infrequently performed, is still a useful technique.[49,53] MRI may be useful in certain cases as well. Arthrography, when properly performed, can provide valuable information regarding the synovial lining, articular surfaces, and configuration of the elbow capsule. Elbow arthrography is most commonly indicated for evaluation of loose bodies or subtle synovial or articular changes.[25,40,44] Osteocartilaginous bodies may result from osteochondromatosis, osteochondritis dissecans, or osteochondral fragments from acute trauma. The articular cartilage in patients with osteochondritis dissecans is also studied effectively with elbow arthrography.[31] Arthrography is also useful for evaluating ligament or capsular tears. In our experience, as well as others', patients with chronic instability frequently demonstrate an enlarged, irregular capsule.[25,32,40,43] Elbow arthrography may reveal diminished capsular volume in patients with decreased range of motion and pain similar to changes described in adhesive capsulitis involving the shoulder.[25,43]

Multiple techniques for performing elbow arthrography have been described.[25,31,32,40,48] In most cases, we utilize double-contrast technique. This provides better detail of the articular surfaces and synovial lining of the capsule. Subtle

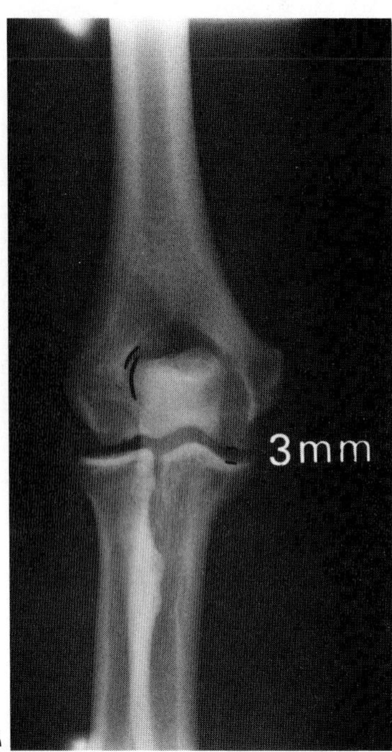

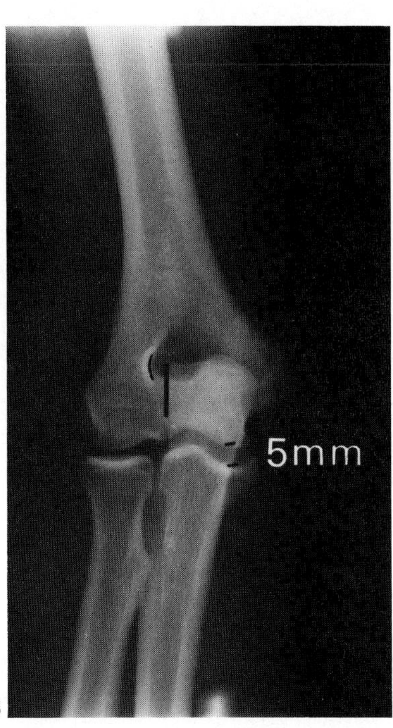

Fig. 10-15 (**A**) Normal and (**B**) stress views of the right elbow after medial ligament injury. Lines indicate change in angle. *Source:* Reprinted from *Imaging of Orthopedic Trauma* ed 2 by TH Berquist, 1991, Raven Press, © Mayo Foundation.

changes can be obscured if single-contrast studies are utilized. This method is also useful when either conventional tomography or CT is required after the injection.[52,54]

Before the procedure, fluoroscopic evaluation of the range of motion, stability, and possible loose bodies should be accomplished.[25] The elbow is prepared with sterile technique. One of two needle sites may be chosen for entering the joint. In most instances, a lateral approach into the radiocapitellar joint is chosen (Fig. 10-16). Occasionally, if a lateral injury is suspected, a posterior approach may be required. With the posterior approach, the elbow is again flexed 90°, and the medial and lateral epicondyles and olecranon are palpated. The needle is then placed at equal distances between these landmarks.[25] The needle is positioned with fluoroscopic guidance in both situations.

When the needle enters the joint space, a small amount of contrast material is introduced to check needle position. If the needle is properly located within the joint space, the contrast material will flow away from the needle tip. Contrast material will collect at the needle tip if the needle is not positioned properly. Significant resistance is also noted if the needle is not intraarticular. The joint should be aspirated before the balance of the contrast medium is injected. If fluid is present, laboratory studies (eg, culture or crystals) can be performed on a sample. Large amounts of fluid will result in dilution of the contrast medium and a suboptimal arthrogram.

Depending on the clinical setting, the injection may be performed by means of three different techniques. We most frequently use the double-contrast technique with 6 to 12 mL of air. This varies depending upon the size of the joint capsule and the patient being studied. If a significant allergy to contrast material is elicited in the patient's history, air alone may be utilized (Fig. 10-3); the detail is not ideal, however, and even with tomography the examination may be suboptimal. Single-contrast technique with 5 to 6 mL of contrast agent may be adequate in certain situations (depending on capsule size and disruptions), but this technique is rarely used.[25]

After the injection, the needle is removed and the elbow slowly exercised to avoid rupturing the capsule. This also avoids formation of excessive air bubbles. While being exercised, the elbow is studied fluoroscopically. This assists in evaluating range of motion as well as in checking for loose bodies. In addition, stress can be applied to the elbow in patients with suspected elbow instability. Routine filming includes AP, lateral, and both oblique views. Medial and lateral cross-table views (with double-contrast technique) enhance the air contrast component in the superior portion of the capsule. Routine films are followed by tomography or CT, when indicated.[25,52]

In the normal arthrogram (Fig. 10-17), the three articular compartments of the joint are readily identified (ie, radiocapitellar, ulnar-trochlear, and radioulnar). There are three recesses: anterior (coronoid), posterior (olecranon), and annular.[25,32,54] The posterior recess is particularly difficult to visualize. Tomograms in the lateral position with the elbow flexed 90° are most helpful in evaluating this region (Fig. 10-3).

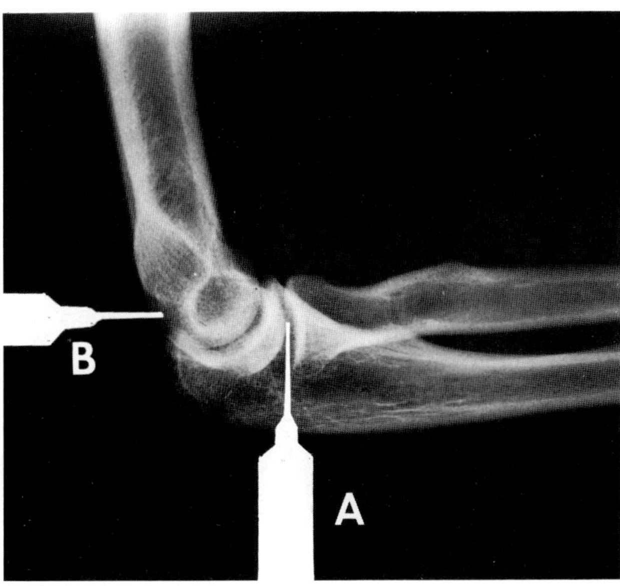

Fig. 10-16 Injection sites for elbow arthrography. (**A**) Lateral, (**B**) posterior approach. *Source:* Reprinted from *Imaging of Orthopedic Trauma* ed 2 by TH Berquist, 1991, Raven Press, © Mayo Foundation.

The normal joint capacity is 10 to 12 mL. This may decrease in cases of capsulitis or increase (to 18 to 22 mL) in patients with chronic instability or recurrent dislocations.[32]

Arthrograms in athletes are most frequently performed to evaluate chronic instability, soft tissue injury, or intraarticular abnormalities. The last are often related to articular abnormalities or loose bodies.[25,30] These so-called loose bodies may actually be free or attached. If contrast material completely surrounds the object, it may be properly considered a loose body. In certain cases tomography may be useful in detection of loose bodies and in evaluation of articular defects (Fig. 10-18).[23,25,40] Arthrography is often more definitive.

Ligament and/or capsular tears are demonstrated by extravasation of contrast material at the site of the injury (Fig. 10-19). Care must be taken not to mistake this with extravasation at the needle site. This phenomenon is frequent with capsulitis but can usually be avoided with good technique. If a lateral ligament tear is suspected, a posterior approach should be utilized. Ideally, the injection should be placed opposite the suspected tear.[25]

Magnetic Resonance Imaging

MRI of the elbow and forearm can clearly define normal bone and soft tissue anatomy and pathology.[25] Clinical information (the symptomatic region and the relationship of symptoms to flexion, extension, pronation, and supination) and the type of injury suspected are important in planning the MR examination. For a given clinical problem to be solved, the

Olecranon recess
Anterior supracondylar recess
Trochlear cartilage
Radial cartilage
Radio-ulnar articulation
Annular periradial recess

A

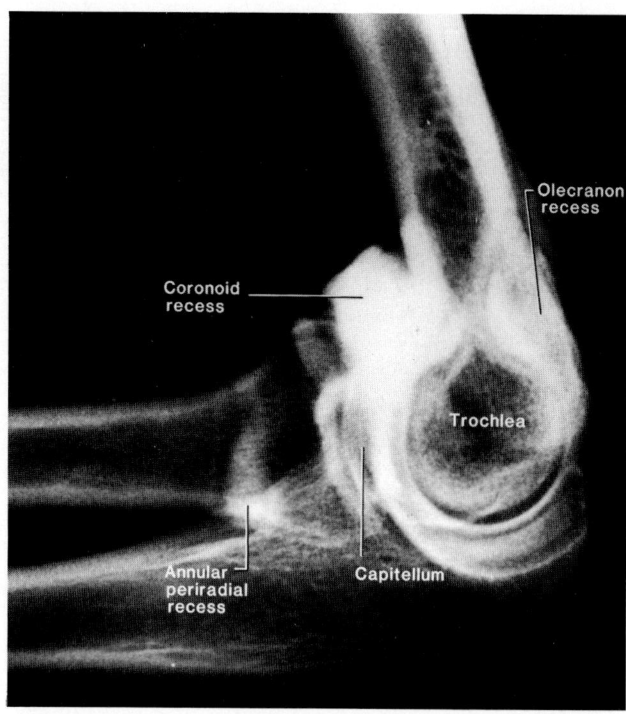

B

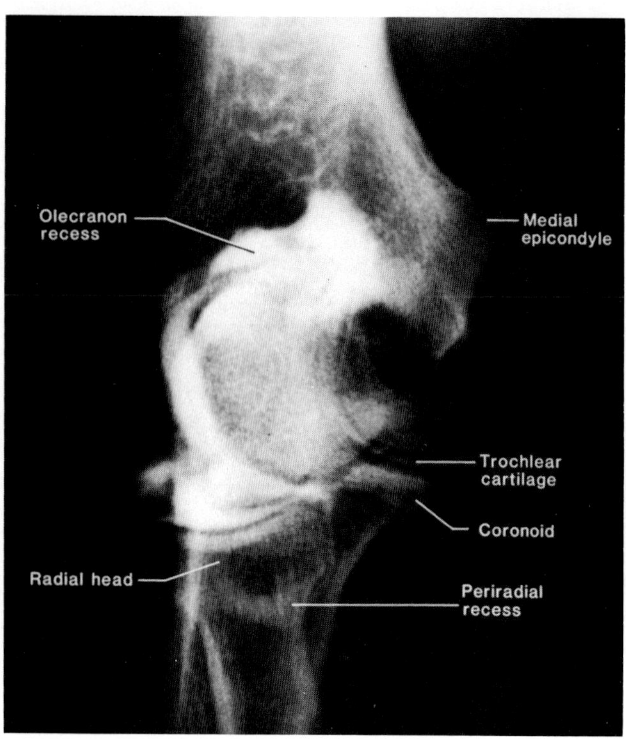

C

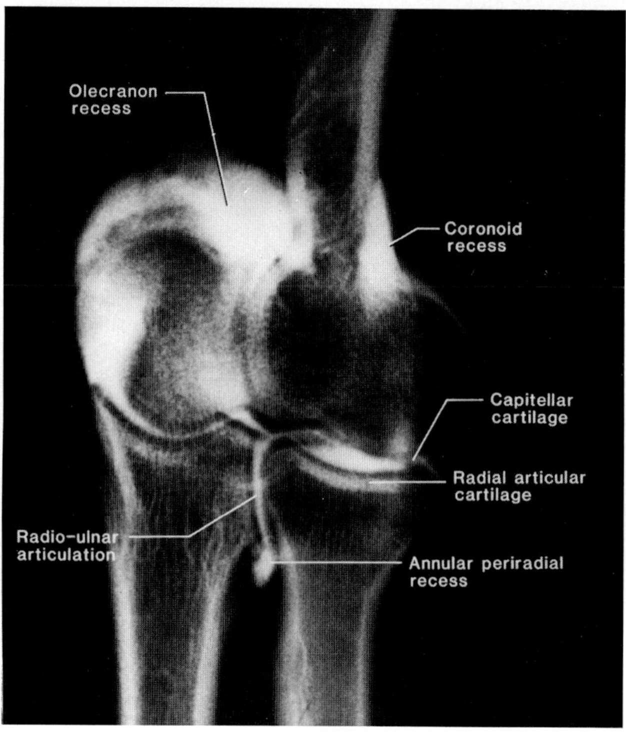

D

Fig. 10-17 Normal single-contrast arthrogram of the elbow seen on (**A**) AP, (**B**) lateral, and (**C** and **D**) oblique views. *Source:* Reprinted from *Imaging of Orthopedic Trauma* ed 2 by TH Berquist, 1991, Raven Press, © Mayo Foundation.

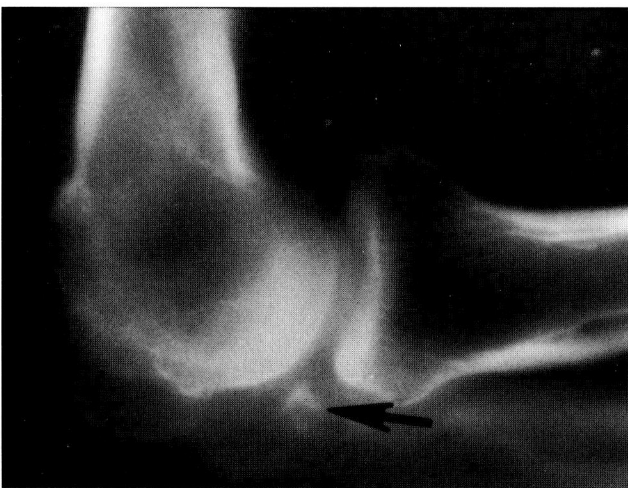

Fig. 10-18 Lateral tomogram of the elbow demonstrating an osteochondral fragment (arrow).

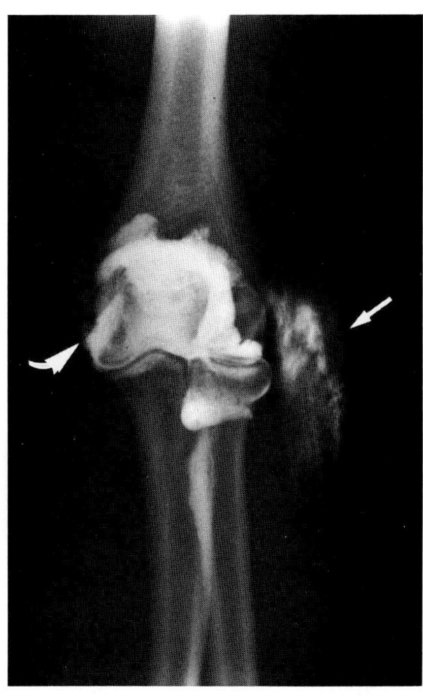

Fig. 10-19 AP arthrogram of the elbow demonstrating a lateral capsular tear (straight arrow) with chronic irregularity of the medial capsule (curved arrow).

patient must be comfortable and properly positioned and the best image planes and pulse sequences selected to optimize lesion identification and characterization.[26,27]

Patient positioning is as important with MRI as with other radiographic techniques. The types of coils available, gantry limitations, and patient size and clinical status may lead to suboptimal examinations, particularly in the upper extremity. The confining nature of the MR gantry reduces positioning options, especially for large patients. Patients are usually most comfortable when supine with the elbow extended and the arm at the side (Fig. 10-20). The circular or license plate flat coils can be used in this position. The circular coil is optimal for localized evaluation of the elbow, and the license plate coil is preferred for examination of large areas such as the forearm or elbow and forearm (Fig. 10-21). Partial-volume and circumferential coils for the upper extremity are also available. The patient can be positioned with the arm at the side only when the software allows the use of off-axis, small–field of view.[26,27]

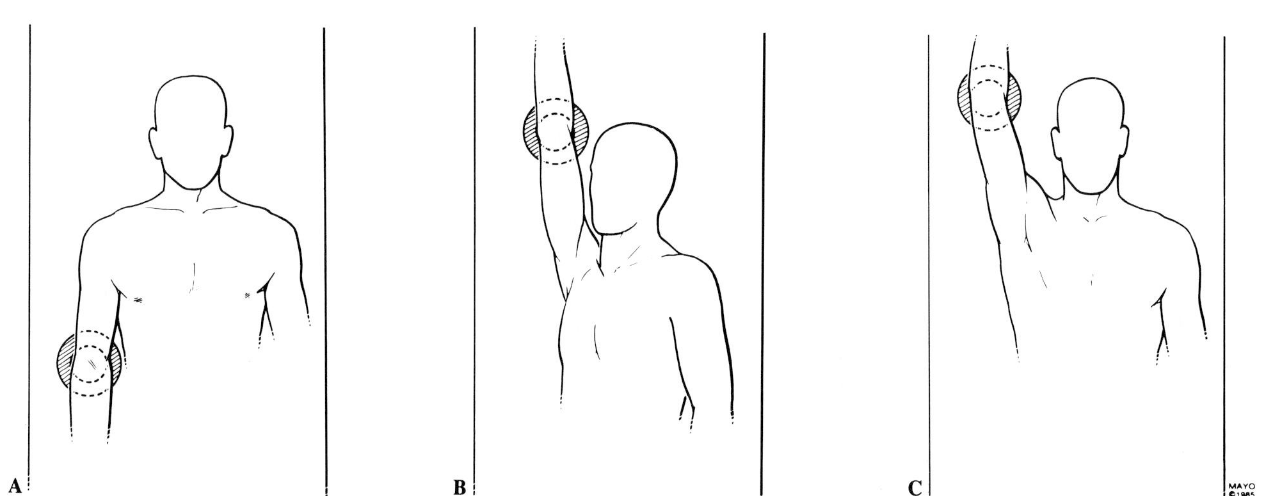

Fig. 10-20 Patient positions for MRI of the elbow. (**A**) The patient is most comfortable with the arm at the side. (**B**) Patient rotated with the arm above the head. (**C**) Patient supine with the arm above the head. *Source:* Reprinted from *Magnetic Resonance Imaging of the Musculoskeletal System* by TH Berquist, 1990, Raven Press, © Mayo Foundation.

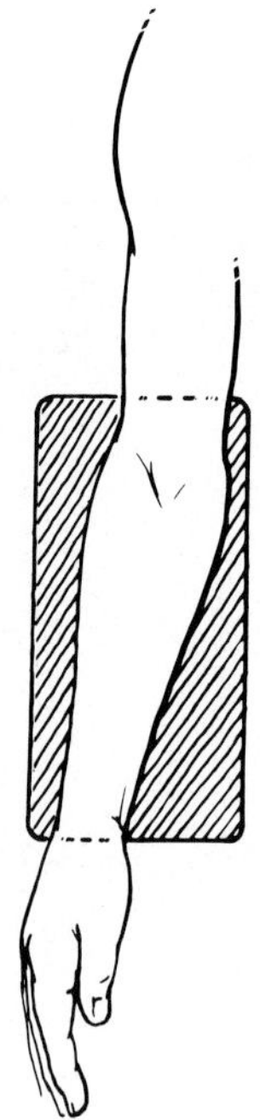

Fig. 10-21 Illustration of license plate coil for imaging of the forearm.

Different positions and coils may be required when the software does not permit off-center placement of surface coils (off-axis, small–field of view) or when patients are large. The elbow can be moved closer to the center of the magnet by rotating the patient and/or placing the elbow above the head (Fig. 10-20B). In the latter position a volume (circumferential) coil can be used. A partial-volume or circumferential coil provides more uniform signal intensity, avoiding the problem of signal drop-off seen with flat surface coils. Patient discomfort can be significant when the arm is above the head, however. As a result, images may be degraded by motion artifact. In an initial review of 200 upper extremity injuries at the Mayo Clinic, we found image degradation due to motion in 25% of cases. Motion artifact is usually not a problem when the patient is supine with the arm at the side.[26,27]

In certain situations, such as biceps insertion pathology, positioning the patient with the elbow flexed displays anatomy to better advantage (Fig. 10-22). This may be impossible with large patients. Small patients can be rotated into the oblique position with the elbow flexed at the side. Axial examinations during pronation and supination are also useful for evaluating the biceps tendon and subtle abnormalities in the radioulnar joint. Both axial and sagittal images should be obtained. When motion studies are required, it is usually best to use gradient-echo sequences (see below) and cine loop studies. Videotapes of the examination can be produced easily. This technique provides more information than static images in areas where motion is important to analyze.[25]

Many examinations of the elbow can be performed in the axial plane with T1-weighted (SE 500/20) and T2-weighted (SE 2000/20–30, 60–80) sequences. These will generally pro-

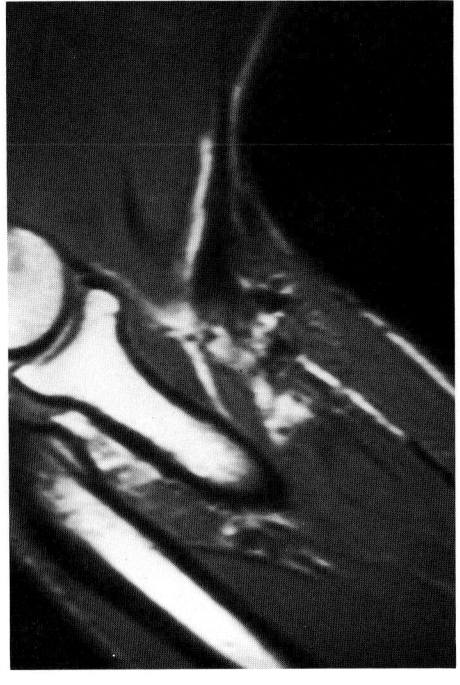

A

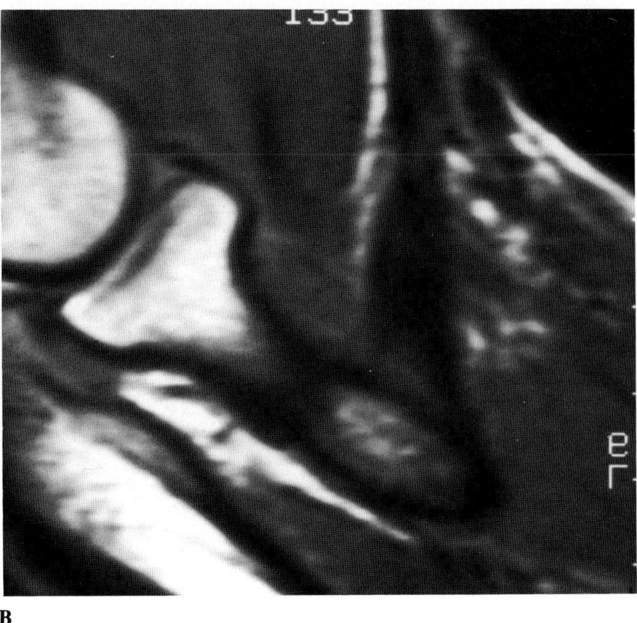

B

Fig. 10-22 Sagittal (SE 500/20) MR images of the biceps tendon. (**A**) The arm is not properly rotated. (**B**) The tendon is more easily assessed when the arm is positioned so that the entire structure can be included in the image plane.

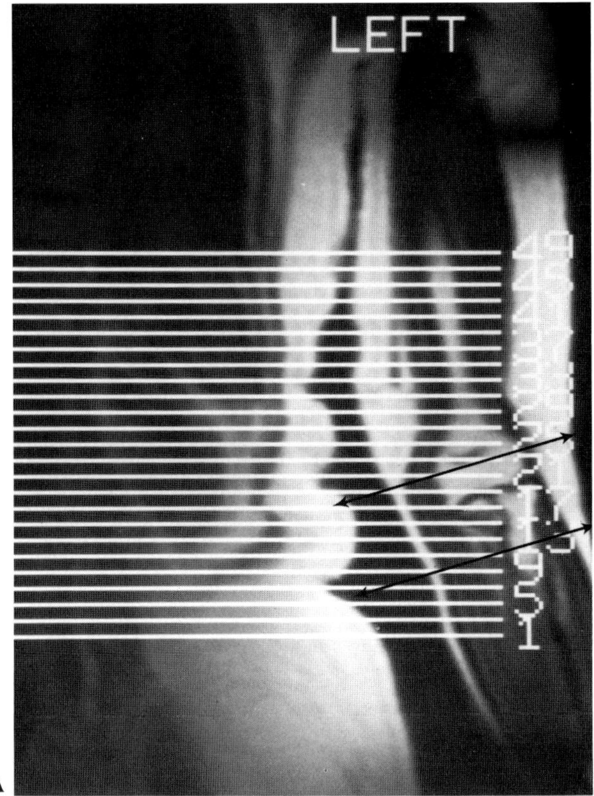

A

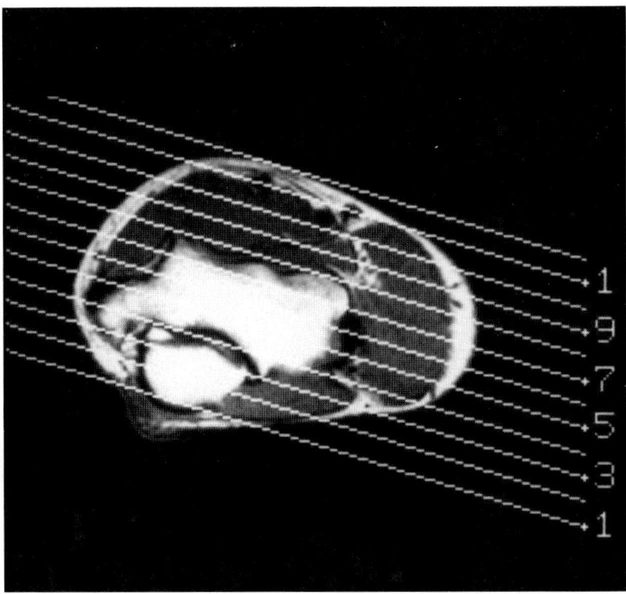

B

Fig. 10-23 (**A**) Large–field of view (42-cm) scout coronal image of the elbow. Axial images (white lines) need to be oriented properly (black lines) because of the carrying angle of the elbow or true axial sections will not be obtained. (**B**) Axial scout for coronal MR images of the elbow. The image planes should be aligned with the osseous.structures.

vide sufficient information to screen for most suspected abnormalities.[26]

In most situations a coronal scout image is obtained (Fig. 10-23). Three 1-cm thick slices are obtained with a spin-echo sequence (SE 200/20), a large field of view (32 to 40 cm), a 256 × 128 matrix, and one excitation or average. This can be accomplished in approximately 26 seconds with a 128 × 256 matrix or in 52 seconds with a 256 × 256 matrix and one excitation. The first axial images are usually performed with a T2-weighted (SE 2000/30,60 or 2000/20,80) sequence. Soft tissue contrast is superior with this pulse sequence, so that the likelihood of overlooking an abnormality is remote. Initial axial slice thicknesses vary depending upon the region of interest and the size of the suspected or palpable lesion. Large, palpable lesions can be evaluated with 1-cm thick slices and 0.25- to 0.5-cm interslice gaps. Thinner slices (3 to 5 mm, skipping 1.5 to 2.5 mm) are used when more subtle pathology is suspected. At the Mayo Clinic we typically use a 16- to 24-cm field of view, a 192 × 256 matrix, and two excitations, which provide excellent image quality. The axial T2-weighted sequence takes 12.8 minutes when these parameters are used. In the setting of trauma, the second sequence can be a gradient-echo Multiplanar GRASS (MPGR) or T2-weighted coronal or sagittal image depending on the clinical symptoms and findings on the axial images. No further studies may be needed if the examination is normal or if the lesion is clearly identified and characterized. If the nature or extent of the lesion is unclear, further image planes and sequences may be needed.[26]

Gradient-echo sequences with reduced flip angles and short repetition times provide excellent flexibility for rapid imaging in different positions. These techniques are especially useful when evaluating articular problems that require imaging of anatomic changes during flexion, extension, supination, and pronation (minimum TE/TR, flip angle, 30° to 70°; 2 to 4 Nex). Static GRASS images are particularly useful for evaluating vascular anatomy and pathology.[26,27]

Miscellaneous Techniques

On occasion, other techniques such as radionuclide scans, CT, conventional tomography, and sonography may be indicated.[25,38] Radionuclide scans are most often used to exclude subtle osseous pathology. A negative bone scan indicates that bone injury or osseous–ligament attachment injury is unlikely. Bone scans should be positive within 72 hours of the injury.[25]

Routine tomography, especially in the lateral projection, or CT may be used without intraarticular contrast agents (Fig. 10-24). More often these techniques are used in conjunction with elbow arthrography.[25]

Sonography is useful, especially for evaluation of superficial soft tissue injuries. Muscle and tendon pathology can be readily evaluated by an experienced sonographer.[22] Articular abnormalities may be evident as well but are less frequently studied with sonography.[25]

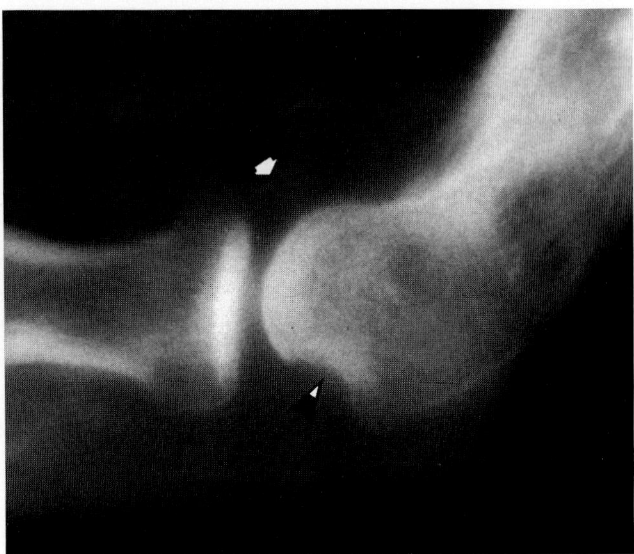

Fig. 10-24 Lateral tomogram of the elbow demonstrating an osteochondral impaction (arrowhead) with an anteriorly displaced fragment (white arrow).

SOFT TISSUE INJURIES

Soft tissue injury about the elbow is most often secondary to hyperextension or valgus stress commonly due to a fall on the outstretched hand. An associated blow directed to the posterior aspect of the elbow coincident with the fall is occasionally reported. Chronic soft tissue and articular injuries are associated with throwing sports.[59,75,85] Radiographs may be positive because tearing of the anterior capsule, stretching of the medial collateral ligament, or possibly tearing of the synovium can all result in a painful hemarthrosis. The fat pad sign will be positive, physical examination may reveal a local tenderness, and the joint will not extend fully. Many soft tissue injuries can be diagnosed clinically, but further imaging is often indicated.[60]

Ligament Injury

A brief review of the dynamic and static stabilizers of the elbow is useful in discussing ligament injuries. Lateral (varus) stability is provided by the lateral collateral ligament complex and anconeus. The medial ligament complex (anterior oblique, posterior oblique, and transverse components) provides major static support with assistance in dynamic stability from the forearm flexor group.[75]

Forces on the elbow cause compression laterally and tension medially during athletic maneuvers. Isolated ligament injuries may occur with a fall on the outstretched hand with the elbow extended.[85] Throwing sports cause similar stress to the elbow. Tears in the medial ligaments have been described in javelin throwers and pitchers.[78,83] Chronic overuse, specifically in baseball pitchers, can lead to spurring of the medial olecranon and periarticular calcifications (Figs. 10-25 and 10-26).[58]

More severe ligament disruption may lead to posterior dislocation of the elbow. Dislocation typically occurs with the elbow extended or semiextended (Fig. 10-27).[59,68,75] Initially the anterior capsule ruptures. The valgus tilt of the trochlea shifts the stress to the medial ligament complex (Fig. 10-27B), which ruptures the anterior oblique ligament. The coronoid levers under the trochlea, and the elbow dislocates posteriorly because of the dominant force and laterally because of the trochlear angle.[75] Elbow dislocation may be classified according to the position of the displaced ulna with respect to the humerus. This criterion gives rise to the following types of dislocations: posterior, posterolateral (Fig. 10-28), lateral, posteromedial, pure lateral, and anterior. The posterolateral type of dislocation is most common (80% to 90%).[62] Anterior dislocation is extremely rare. This

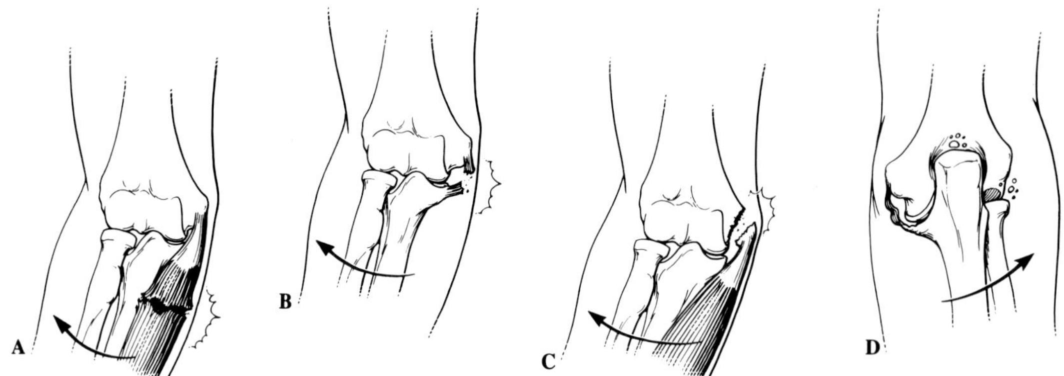

Fig. 10-25 Throwing injuries of the elbow.[58] Arrows indicate the direction of force application. (**A**) Flexor muscle injury. (**B**) Medial ligament tear. (**C**) Medial epicondyle avulsion fracture. (**D**) Ulnar spur formation with loose bodies.

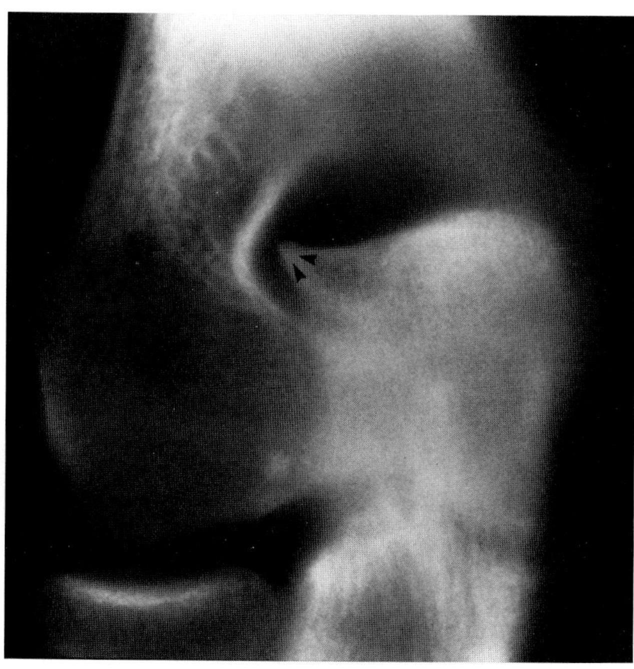

Fig. 10-26 AP view of the elbow in a pitcher with an olecranon spur (arrowheads). *Source:* Courtesy of Michael Stuart and Bernard F. Morrey, Department of Orthopedic Surgery, Mayo Clinic, Rochester, Minnesota.

classification implies little about the prognosis of such injuries, and it probably has relatively little value to the clinician. Nevertheless, it does serve to describe accurately the radiographic appearance of the displacement.[62,72,75,80]

Although the degree of dislocation varies, injury to the anterior portion of the medial collateral ligament is considered present in all cases.[80] Associated injuries are common. Fractures of the coronoid, epicondyles, or radial head occur in approximately 28% of patients with the dislocation. With these fractures, involvement of the radial head (Fig. 10-29) or coronoid is most common.[75,80]

Confirmation of ligamentous disruption can be obtained with stress views, MRI, or arthrography.[60] Stress views of the elbow are difficult to interpret because a significant valgus angulation can occur without a corresponding amount of ulnohumeral joint widening (Fig. 10-15). On the AP radiograph, the tip of the olecranon is not symmetrically aligned in the olecranon fossa.

Ideally, stress views should be performed with fluoroscopic guidance. This allows proper positioning and facilitates detection of subtle changes during the stressing maneuver. Comparison with the normal elbow is essential. A widening of the joint space greater than 2 mm above the neutral measurement may be arbitrarily considered abnormal. MRI may provide a new method of examining elbow ligament injury. The anatomic detail provided allows one to visualize the tendons and ligaments. This should allow detection of significant ligament tears. Arthrography may also be of value in detecting ligament disruption when evaluating capsule tears (Fig. 10-19).[60]

Complications of ligamentous disruption include recurrent dislocations of the elbow.[59,79] The brachial artery and median nerve may be entrapped in the joint after reduction.[62,75] The most commonly recognized radiographic complication of elbow dislocation is probably the entrapment of the medial epicondyle in the joint. This occurs in adolescents who have sustained avulsion of this structure at the time of the traumatic event.

Treatment of most soft tissue injuries about the elbow consists simply of rest and immobilization for variable periods

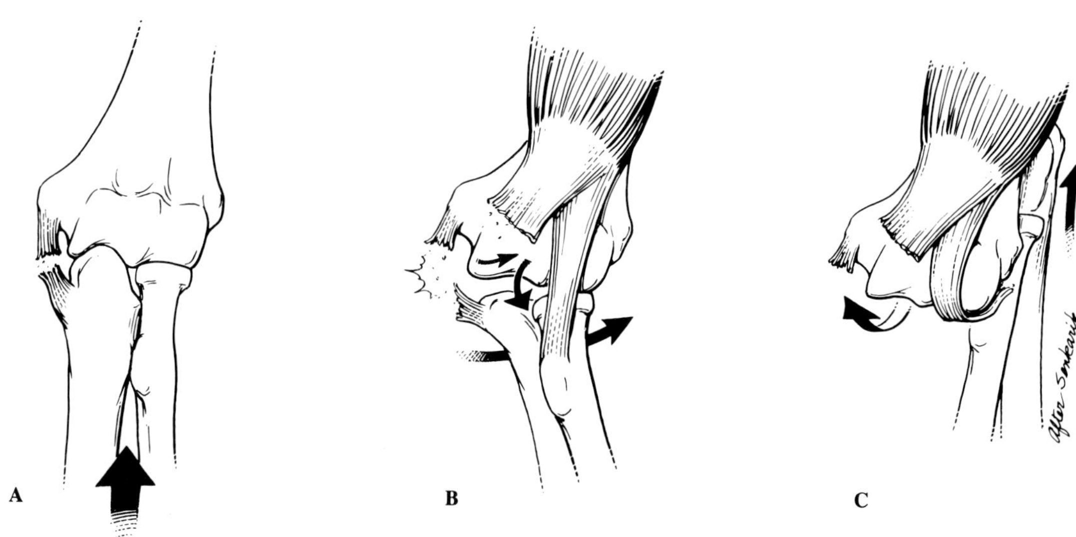

Fig. 10-27 Elbow dislocations.[124] Arrows indicate the direction of force application. (**A**) Hyperextension with medial ligament disruption. (**B**) Posterolateral ulnar displacement. (**C**) Posterior dislocation with biceps tendon trapped over the trochlea.

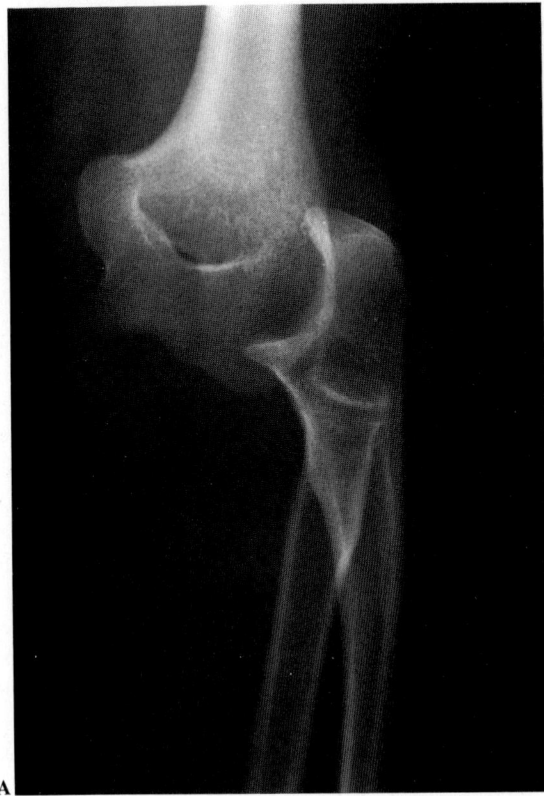

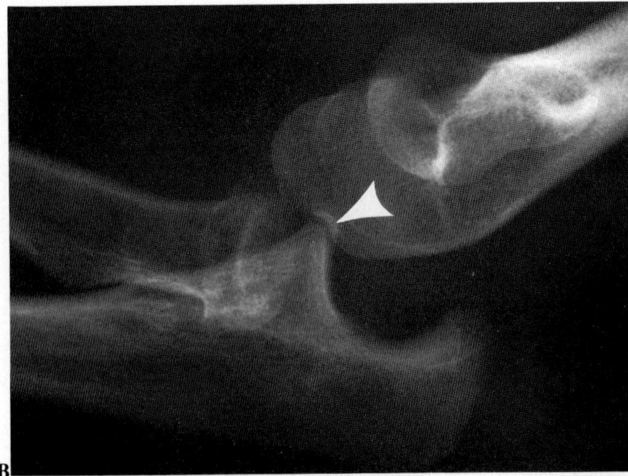

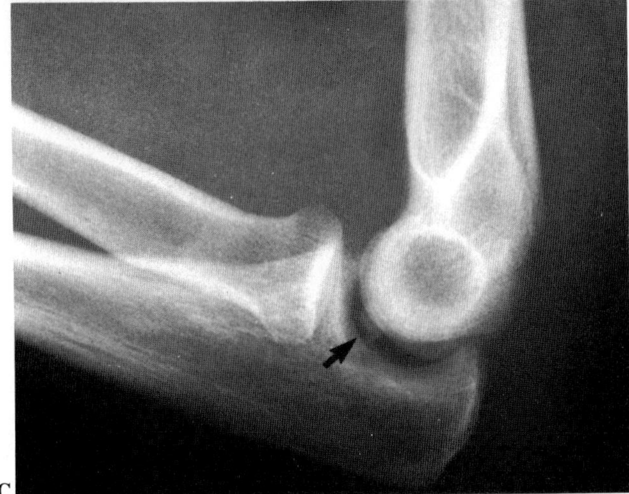

Fig. 10-28 (**A**) AP and (**B**) lateral views of the elbow after posterolateral dislocation. Note the osteochondral trochlear fracture on the lateral view (arrowhead in **B**). (**C**) Postreduction lateral view shows a fragment in the joint space (arrow) preventing complete reduction.

of time. Usually less than 2 weeks, or at most 3 weeks, of immobilization is required after dislocation because late instability occurs in only about 1% or 2% of patients and because a flexion contracture can result with prolonged immobilization.[72,79] Most clinicians recommend early motion at least through a safe or protected arc (eg, from 30° to 100°).[74]

Muscle and Tendon Injuries

Chronic overuse injuries of the medial and lateral tendons (tendinitis) are common about the elbow. Partial (second-degree strains) and complete (third-degree strains) ruptures of muscle or muscle-tendon units are uncommon.[74–76,85] Tendon injury at the elbow can be classified in a manner similar to that for rotator cuff injuries. The initial stages are inflammation, followed by fibroblastic degeneration, and finally partial or complete disruption.[77] The last is unusual.

Tendinitis may involve the medial or lateral origins at the epicondyles or, less frequently, the triceps tendon posteriorly.[77] Patients present with local pain and tenderness that

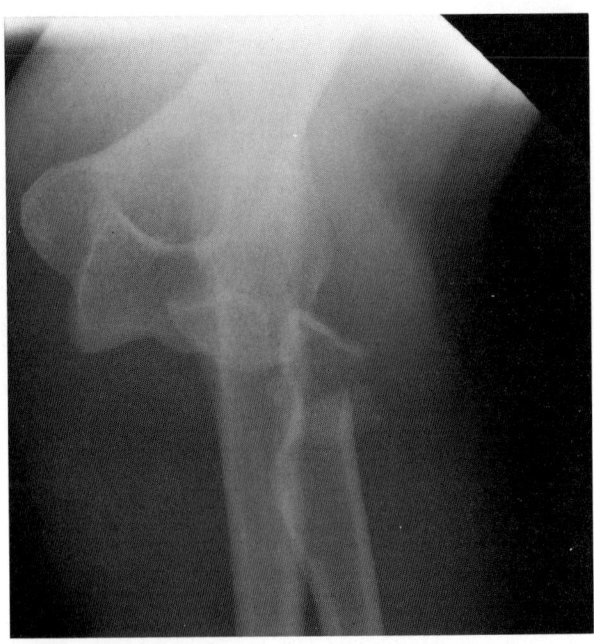

Fig. 10-29 AP view of the elbow after posterolateral dislocation with radial head fracture.

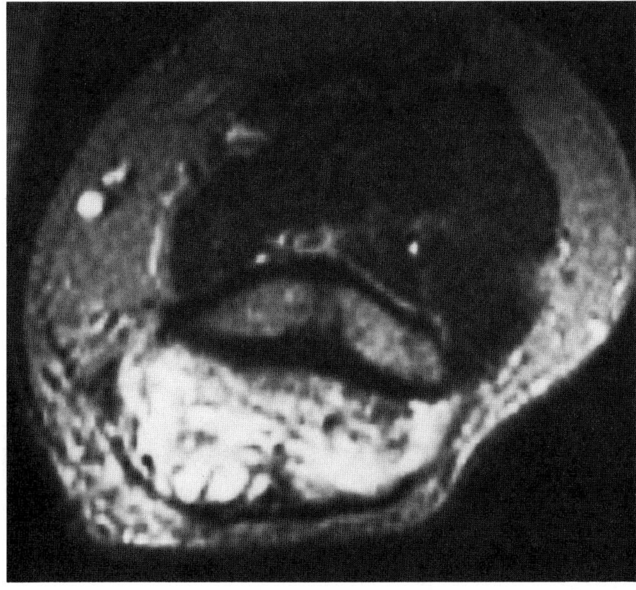

A

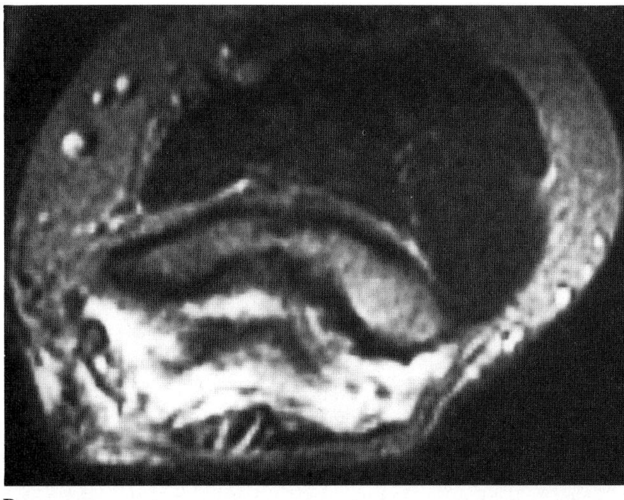

B

Fig. 10-30 Axial (**A** and **B**) and sagittal (**C** and **D**) T2-weighted MR images (SE 2000/80) of a football lineman demonstrating a triceps tendon tear (arrows) near the olecranon insertion.

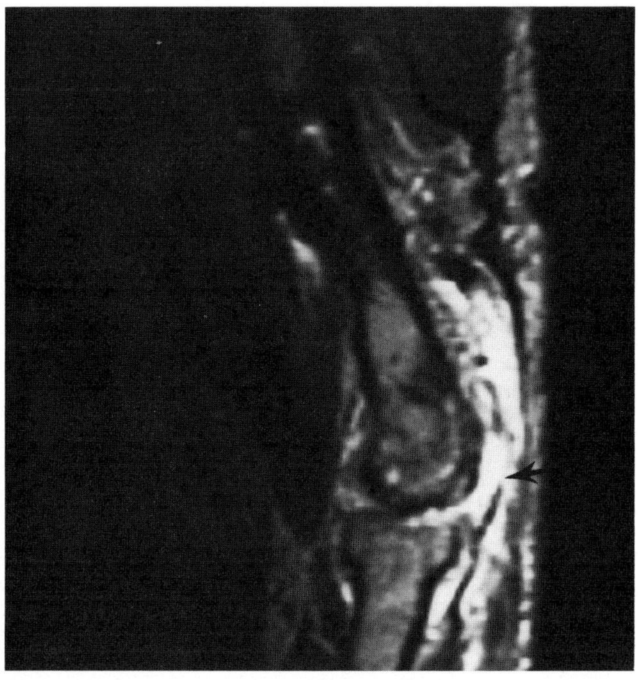

C

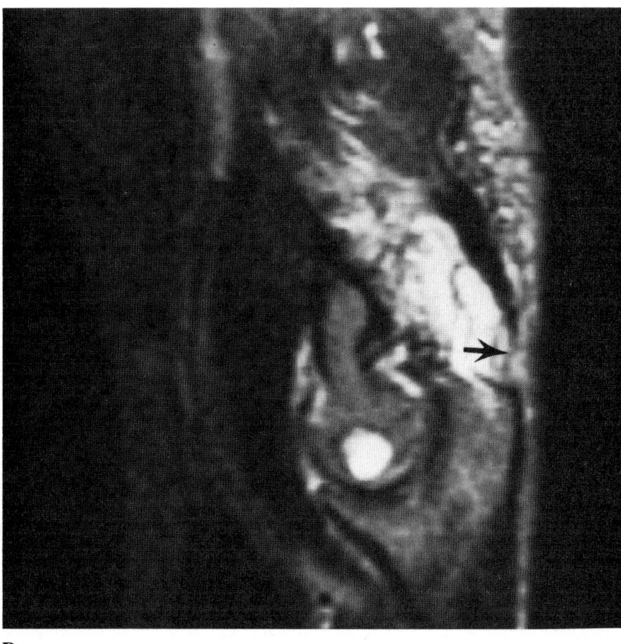

D

can also be created by contraction of the involved muscle groups. Patients with tendinitis are usually 30 to 55 years old and frequently are involved in racquet sports (tennis elbow).[57,77,85]

Lateral tendinitis involves the extensor carpi radialis brevis (100%), and extensor aponeurosis (35%). Exostosis may form on the lateral epicondyle in 20% of cases, and on occasion (approximately 1%) the radial nerve is involved.[77,85]

Medial tendinitis predominantly involves the flexor carpi radialis, but in 10% of cases the flexor carpi ulnaris is involved. Partial rupture may occur in 3% of cases.[77] Calcification of the pericondylar soft tissues may be evident on radiographs in up to 25% of patients with chronic medial epicondylitis.[77,85]

Little League elbow is a complex of injuries due to recurrent microtrauma. Pitchers may present with medial tendinitis, lateral impingement, posterior impingement, or ulnar nerve compression.[73]

Ruptures of the biceps tendon at its insertion into the radial tuberosity account for 3% to 10% of biceps tendon injuries.[56] Patients usually present with acute onset of pain in the antecubital region associated with lifting a heavy weight.[56,74]

Triceps rupture is rare (Fig. 10-30).[65] Anzel et al[56] reported eight triceps ruptures in 856 cases of upper extremity tendon

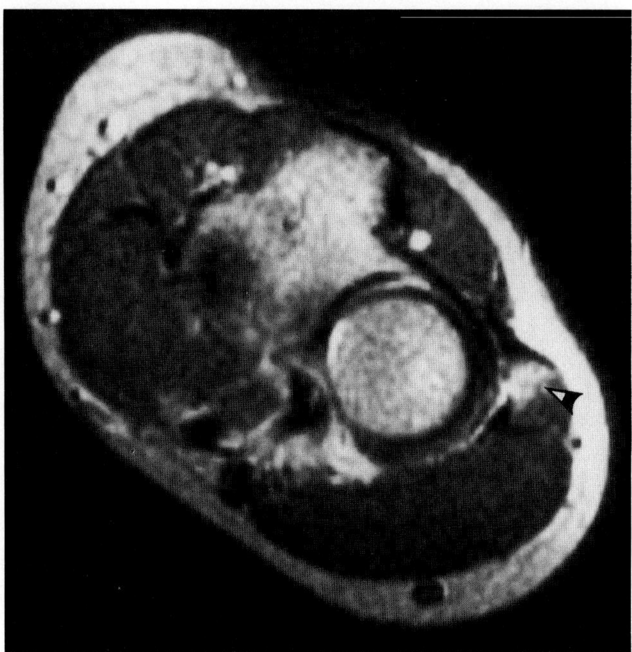

Fig. 10-31 Axial MR image of the elbow in a pitcher after several weeks of training. There is a first-degree muscle tear (arrowhead) seen as an area of high signal intensity near the annular ligament.

ruptures. Disruption of the distal tendon occurs with deceleration force to the arm while the triceps is contracted.

Snapping triceps tendon is an uncommon disorder. The condition occurs most commonly in young athletes. Snapping typically occurs medially and posteriorly. The sensation of snapping may be due to anomalous triceps insertions or subluxation of the ulnar nerve. Most frequently, the snapping is due to subluxation of the medial head of the triceps over the medial epicondyle.[63]

Muscle tears are uncommon, but when they occur typically the biceps or triceps is involved. These injuries occur in weight lifters and offensive linemen (triceps); in the latter they are due to the push-off used in blocking. Minor muscle tears may occur medially or laterally in pitchers (Fig. 10-31).

Imaging of the elbow may not be necessary for minor tendinitis. Nevertheless, radiography and MRI are often useful in clarifying the site and degree of injury. Routine radiographs may reveal avulsion fractures of the medial epicondyle in pitchers.[73] Soft tissue calcification may be noted in 25% of athletes with tendinitis. Bony exostosis on the ulna or epicondyles may also be evident.[69]

It is of special interest that characteristic radiographic features have been described for both biceps[61] and triceps[62] avulsion. The most commonly recognized tendon injury about the elbow is avulsion of the biceps tendon from the radial tuberosity.[62,67] Radiographically the radial tuberosity will often reveal hypertrophic changes or irregularity. This is best demonstrated on the lateral radiograph with the forearm in neutral rotation (Fig. 10-32).[61] Davis and Jassine[61] state that

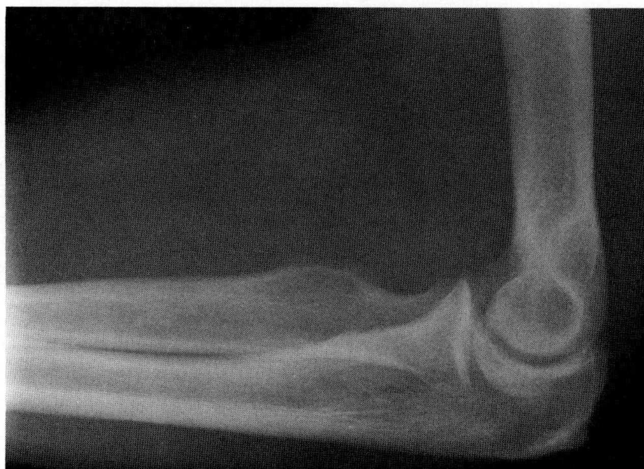

Fig. 10-32 Lateral view of the elbow demonstrating irregularity of the radial tuberosity due to chronic biceps avulsion. *Source:* Reprinted from *The Elbow and Its Disorders* by BF Morrey, 1985, WB Saunders, © Mayo Foundation.

this finding implicates a degenerative process as the etiology of the disruption. Up to 80% of patients have avulsion fractures detectable on lateral radiographs after triceps avulsion.[64,71]

MRI is rarely indicated for acute tendinitis but may be of value in patients who do not respond to conservative therapy. Injuries are most easily detected on T2-weighted axial and either coronal or sagittal images to determine the site and extent of injury (Fig. 10-33). Gradient-echo T2* images are

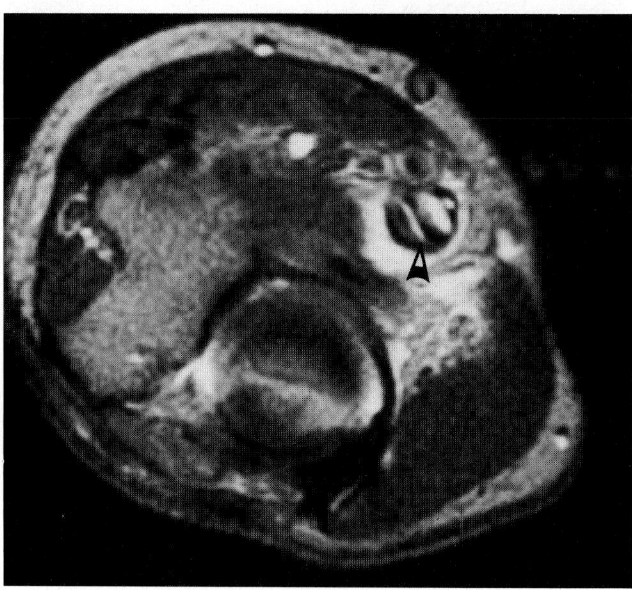

Fig. 10-33 Axial T2-weighted MR image (SE 2000/60) demonstrating high signal intensity in the biceps tendon (arrowhead) due to a second-degree strain. *Source:* Reprinted from *Magnetic Resonance Imaging of the Musculoskeletal System* by TH Berquist, 1990, Raven Press, © Mayo Foundation.

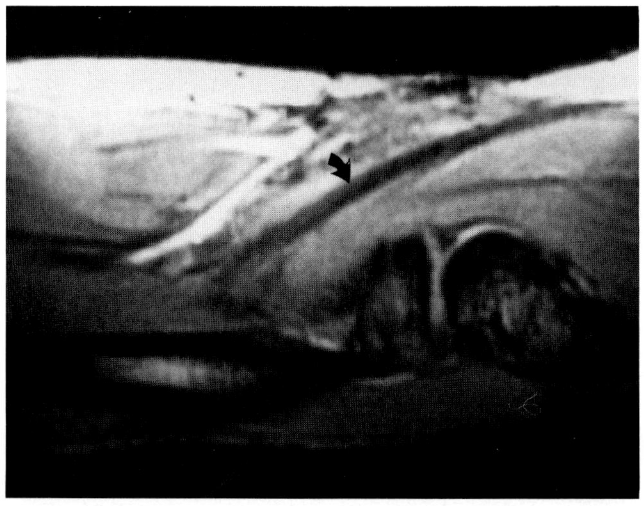

A

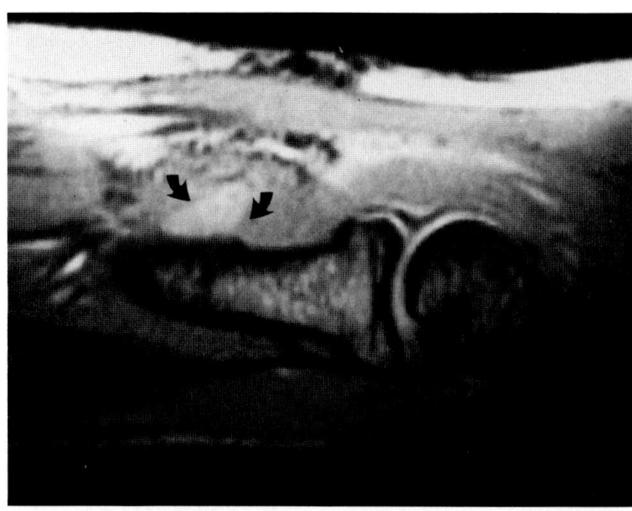

B

Fig. 10-34 Sagittal gradient-echo images of the elbow in various degrees of supination. (**A**) The tendon (arrow) is in the plane of section. (**B**) With slight supination the ganglion (arrows), which was causing the pain and snapping, can be identified. *Source:* Reprinted from *Magnetic Resonance Imaging of the Musculoskeletal System* by TH Berquist, 1990, Raven Press, © Mayo Foundation.

useful when motion studies, specifically pronation and supination, are important (Fig. 10-34). T2-Weighted images provide the best contrast between edema or hemorrhage and the low intensity of muscle and tendon units. Short T1 inversion-recovery sequences and fat-supressed T2-weighted images are also useful for similar reasons.[60]

MRI is also useful in assessment of healing. Signal intensity will return to normal if healing is complete. Scar tissue will have low signal intensity on both T1- and T2-weighted sequences (Fig. 10-35). Reinjury will result in new region of increased signal intensity at the site of recurrence.[60]

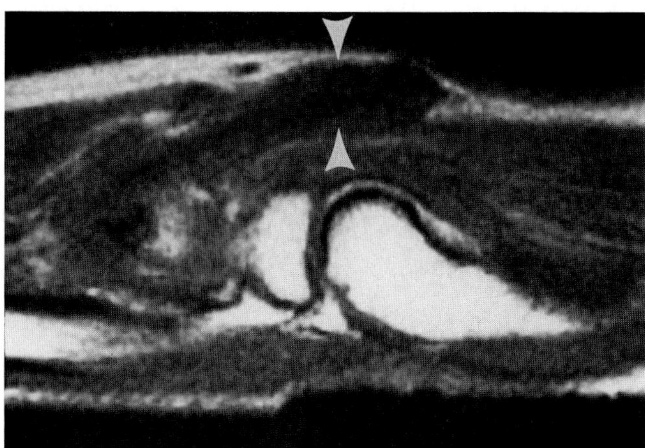

Fig. 10-35 Sagittal T2-weighted MR image of an old biceps tendon injury with thickening (arrowheads) but no increased signal intensity. This is an old injury with scarring.

Nerve Injury

Nerve injury about the elbow may be related to direct trauma, traction, recurrent subluxation, or fracture-dislocation. In athletes neural symptoms are often related to stretching and chronic friction or entrapment.[66,81,82,84]

It is important to appreciate the neuroanatomy to understand the location of a neural injury. The radial nerve and its posterior interosseous and superficial branches are susceptible to injury in several areas. Compression can occur from the lateral margin of the triceps to the distal forearm. The most common site of compression of the posterior interosseous branch is at the upper margin of or in the supinator.[81,82] Motor paralysis of the extensor muscles is common with compression of this branch of the radial nerve. Some patients present with minor symptoms similar to those of tennis elbow.[81] Compression of the superficial branch typically occurs in the proximal forearm or elbow region (Fig. 10-6).[81,82]

The ulnar nerve passes posterior to the medial epicondyle (Fig. 10-36) and enters the anterior compartment of the forearm several centimeters distal to the elbow. These areas are the most common sites of ulnar nerve compression. Compression more distally in the forearm is unusual.[81] Compression at the elbow may be due to bone or soft tissue abnormalities. Bony abnormalities in the medial epicondyle or an anomalous anconeus muscle (anconeus epitrochlaris) may compress the nerve. The nerve may also be compressed between hypertrophied ulnar and humeral heads of the flexor carpi ulnaris. Patients generally present with paresthesias in the fourth and fifth fingers. Later, sensory loss or flexion deformities due to motor loss can occur.[81,82,85] Recurrent ulnar nerve subluxation has been noted in up to 16% of athletes involved in throwing sports.[85]

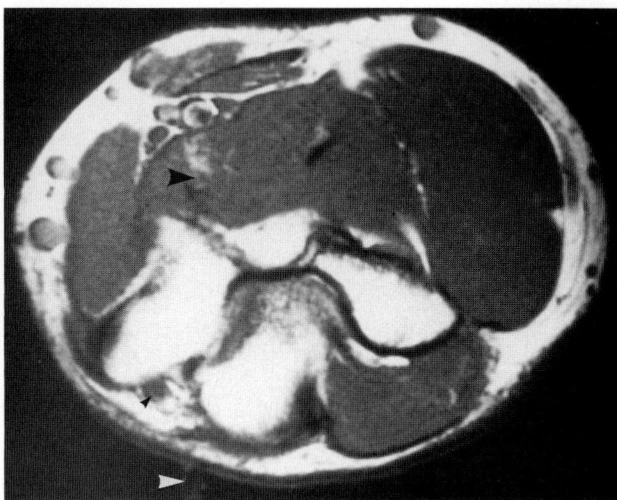

Fig. 10-36 Axial MR image demonstrating the ulnar nerve (small arrowhead). Note the flow artifact (large arrowheads).

The median nerve lies on the brachialis muscle near the brachial artery and biceps tendon in the medial aspect of the distal arm. At the elbow it passes along the humeral head of the pronator teres and then beneath it to lie between the flexor digitorum profundus and superficialis in the forearm. Compression typically occurs near the supracondylar process or near the origin of the pronator teres (Fig. 10-6).[81,82] Pronator teres syndrome is related to repetitive exertion or lifting. Patients present with vague discomfort and numbness in the median nerve distribution of the hand.[70] Therefore, carpal tunnel syndrome must be considered in the differential diagnosis.[60]

Imaging of patients with suspected nerve injury is best accomplished with MRI. The course of the nerves and their size dictate use of 5-mm thick axial images to follow these structures as they course about the elbow and into the forearm. Again, T2-weighted images are best because inflammatory changes in or around the nerves are more conspicuous. When ulnar nerve subluxation is considered, it may be best to select MPGR images with motion to define more clearly the position of the nerve.[60]

Bursitis

There are numerous superficial and deep bursae about the elbow. Superficially, the olecranon bursa lies in the posterior subcutaneous region (Fig. 10-37A). There may also be intratendinous and subtendinous bursae posteriorly. Medial and lateral superficial bursae (medial epicondylar and lateral epi-

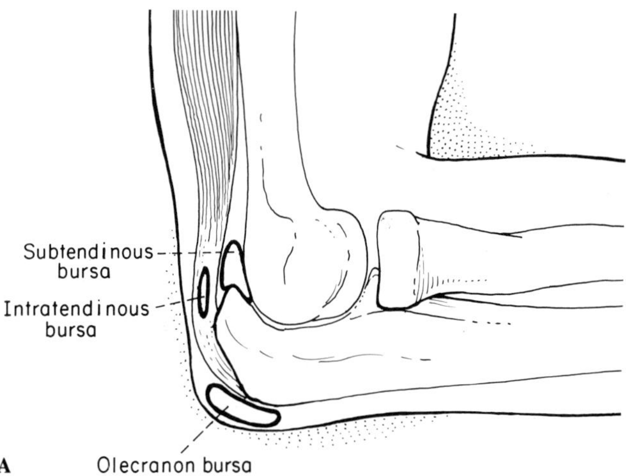

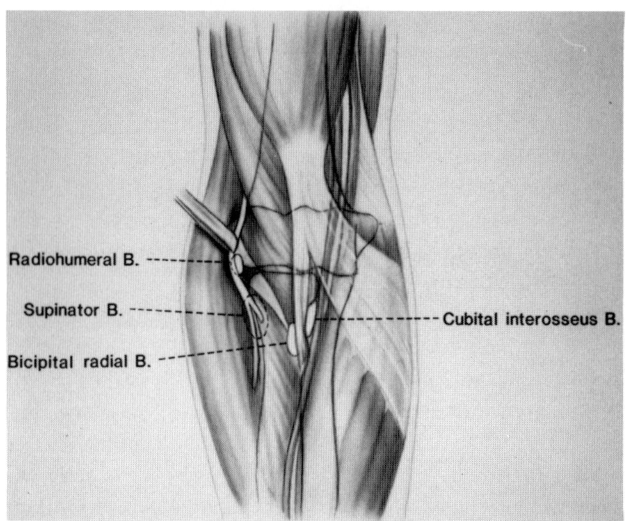

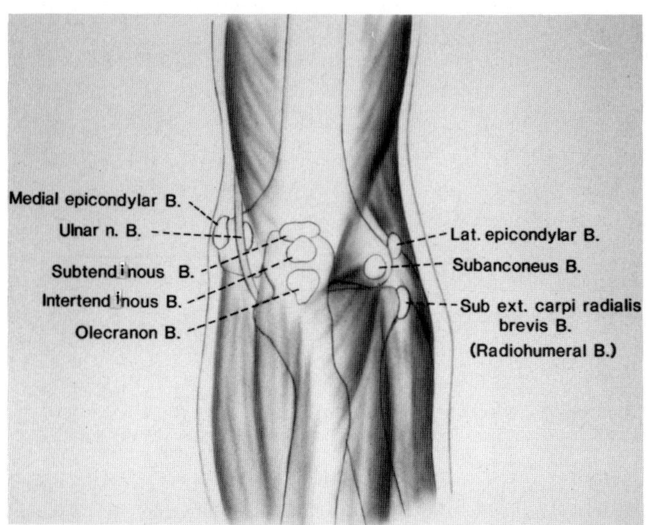

Fig. 10-37 Elbow bursae seen from lateral (**A**), anterior (**B**), and posterior (**C**) projections. Note their relationships to the neural structures. *Source:* Reprinted from *The Elbow and Its Disorders* by BF Morrey, 1985, WB Saunders, © Mayo Foundation.

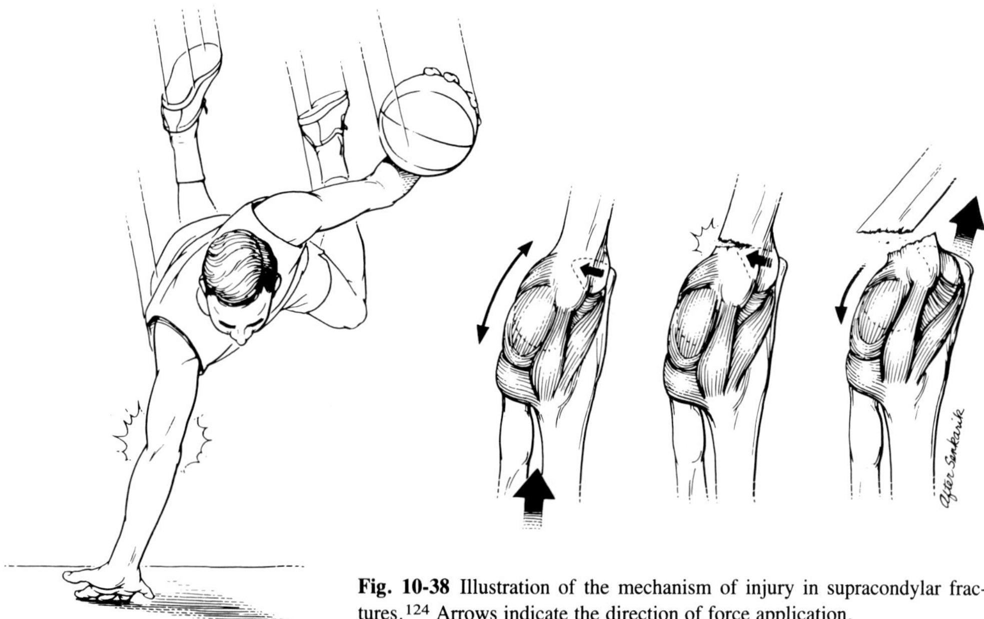

Fig. 10-38 Illustration of the mechanism of injury in supracondylar fractures.[124] Arrows indicate the direction of force application.

condylar) are also present and should not be confused with muscle tears on MR images.[60,74] Fig. 10-37, B and C demonstrates the other bursae of the elbow and their relationship to key neural structures.[74]

Any of these bursae may become inflamed and fluid filled. The olecranon bursa is most often affected because of its vulnerable location.[85] Although uncommon, the radiohumeral bursa (Fig. 10-37B) may be involved in tennis elbow.[74] Knowledge of the location of these bursae is important so that they may be identified correctly on T2-weighted MR images. In addition, aspiration and injection (bupivacaine and betamethasone) may be needed, which require a knowledge of the anatomy.[60,74]

FRACTURES AND OSSEOUS INJURIES

Supracondylar and Transcondylar Fractures

Approximately 80% of distal humeral fractures occur in children.[116,124] Fifteen percent of physeal injuries in children involve the distal humerus.[111,112,117] The usual mechanism of injury for the most common type of fracture is a fall on the outstretched hand causing extension at the elbow joint and a shearing fracture of the distal humerus (Fig. 10-38). The flexion fracture occurs from a direct blow to the posterior aspect of the flexed elbow and is much less common.[94,100,116]

Physical examination usually demonstrates variable amounts of swelling in the distal humeral region. The important bony landmarks retain their nominal relationships. With the elbow flexed, the medial and lateral epicondyles form the base of a triangle with the olecranon at the tip. The deforming force from the muscle causes displacement but does not alter the relationship. A careful neurologic and vascular examination is of paramount importance in the patient with a supracondylar fracture because the brachial artery as well as the median and ulnar nerves can be injured by the distal humeral fracture fragment (Fig. 10-39).[113] Injury to the brachial artery can

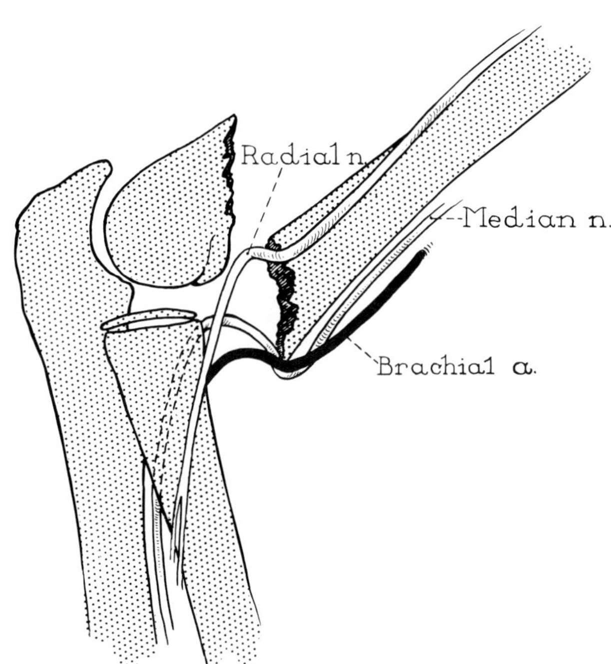

Fig. 10-39 Illustration of neurovascular injury in supracondylar fractures. *Source:* Reprinted with permission from Lipscomb PR and Burleson RJ, Vascular and neural complications in supracondylar fractures of the humerus in children, *Journal of Bone and Joint Surgery* (1955;37A:487–492), Copyright © 1955, Journal of Bone and Joint Surgery.

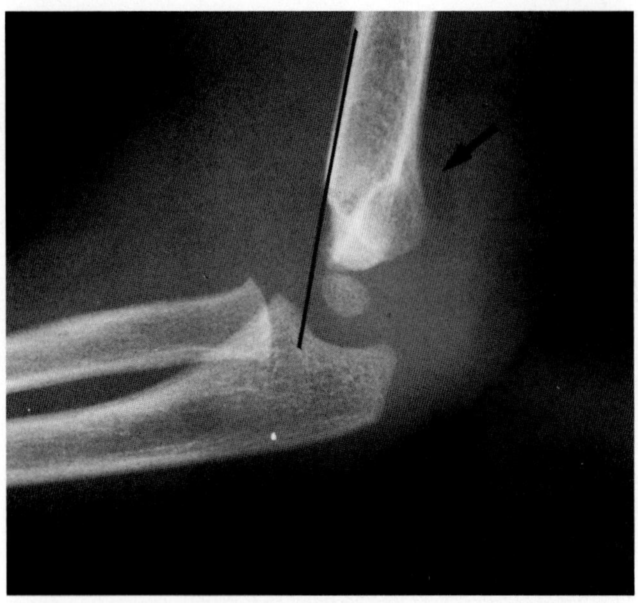

A

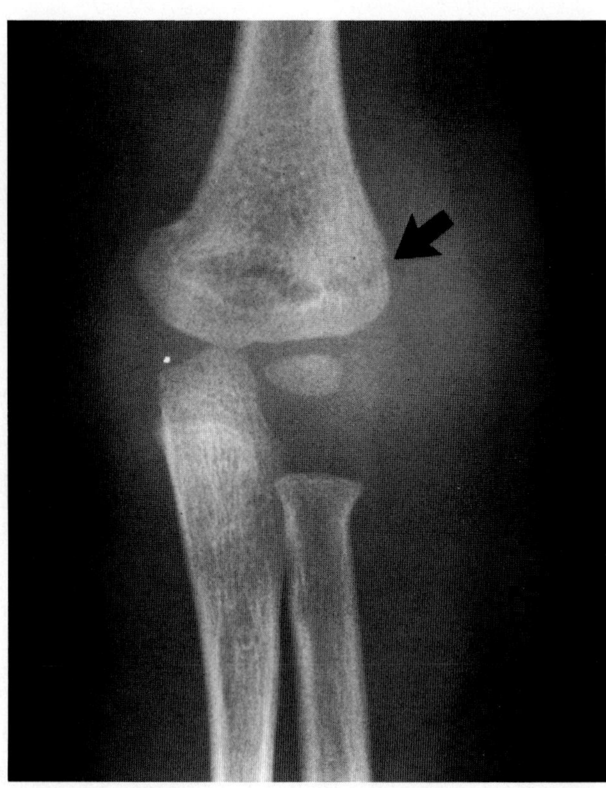

B

Fig. 10-40 (**A**) Lateral and (**B**) AP views of a subtle supracondylar fracture in a child. Note the posterior fat pad (arrow) and posterior capitellar displacement (behind the humeral line) in **A**. The fracture line is noted laterally (arrow) in **B**.

result in muscle and nerve ischemia of the extremity in the severe form known as Volkmann's ischemic contracture.[101,116]

Routine radiography in the AP and lateral projections is usually adequate for diagnosis of supracondylar fractures.[92] The lateral radiograph is particularly important. Appreciating displacement of the fat pads and, in children, the anterior humeral line is important in detecting subtle supracondylar fractures (Fig. 10-40).[92,97,108] With age, injuries are often more easily detected (Figs. 10-41 and 10-42).[91]

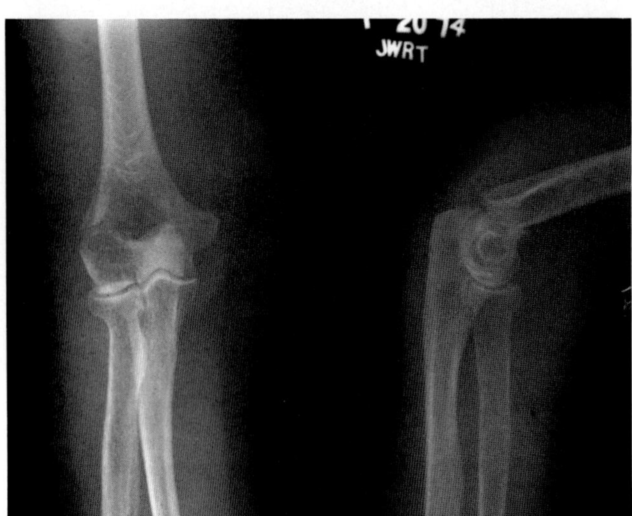

Fig. 10-41 AP and lateral views of the elbow in an adult demonstrating a displaced supracondylar fracture.

Epicondylar Fractures

Throwing, specifically in baseball pitchers, distributes significant stress to the wrist, elbow, and shoulder. The elbow moves from flexion to full extension with associated pronation or supination depending on the type of pitch. Throwing curve balls places extra stress on the medial epicondyle. The medial epicondyle is particularly vulnerable between ages 9 and 14, when organized baseball becomes more serious to participants and coaches.[86,96,112]

Chronic overuse may lead to soft tissue injury, separation, fragmentation (50% of adolescent pitchers), or accelerated growth (95% of adolescent pitchers) of the medial epicondyle (Fig. 10-43).[86] Osteochondral injuries to the radial head and capitellum occur less frequently (8%).[86,93]

Avulsion fractures of the epicondyle are uncommon in the adult because the physis has closed. This injury is more common in young pitchers (Fig. 10-44). Varus or valgus stresses that ordinarily cause an avulsion fracture of the epicondyle in the child result in a complex injury or fracture in the adult.[116] The mechanism of the medial epicondyle fracture is

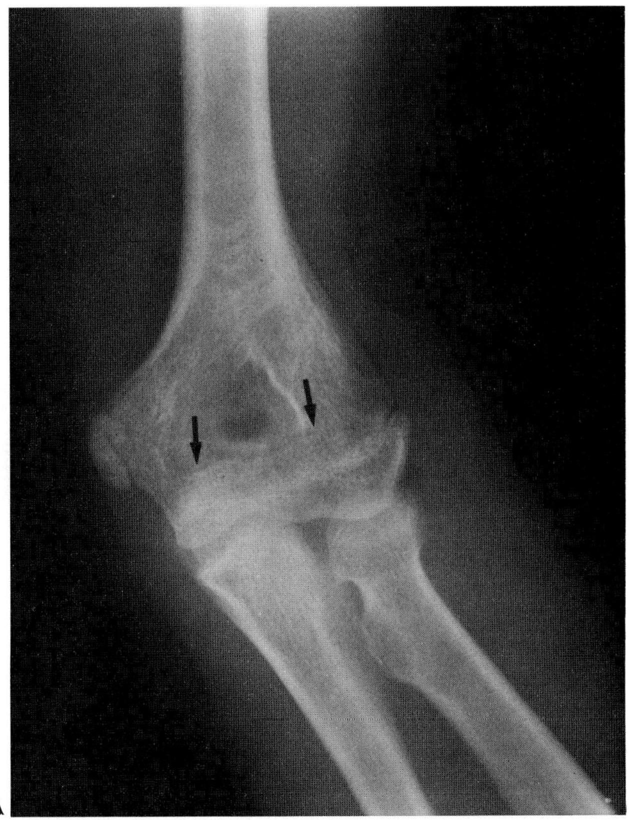

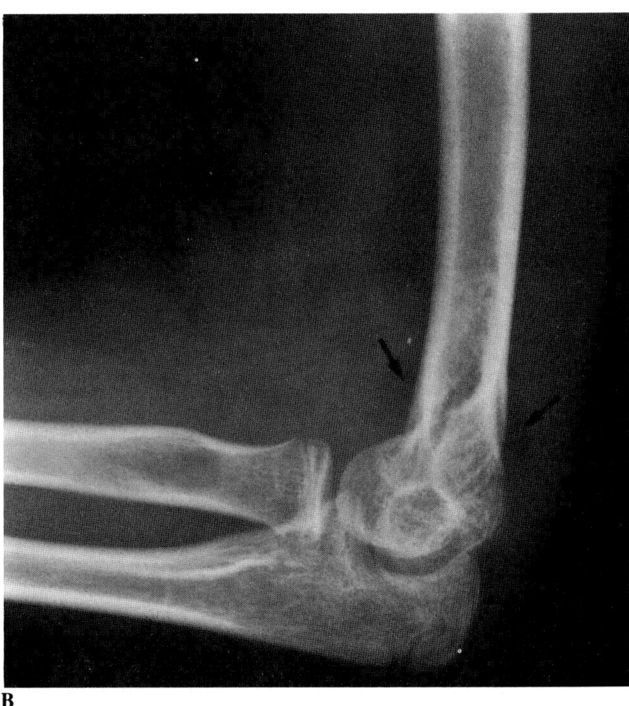

Fig. 10-42 (A) AP and (B) lateral views of the elbow in a teenager demonstrating a supercondylar fracture (arrows in A). Note the displaced fat pads (arrows in B).

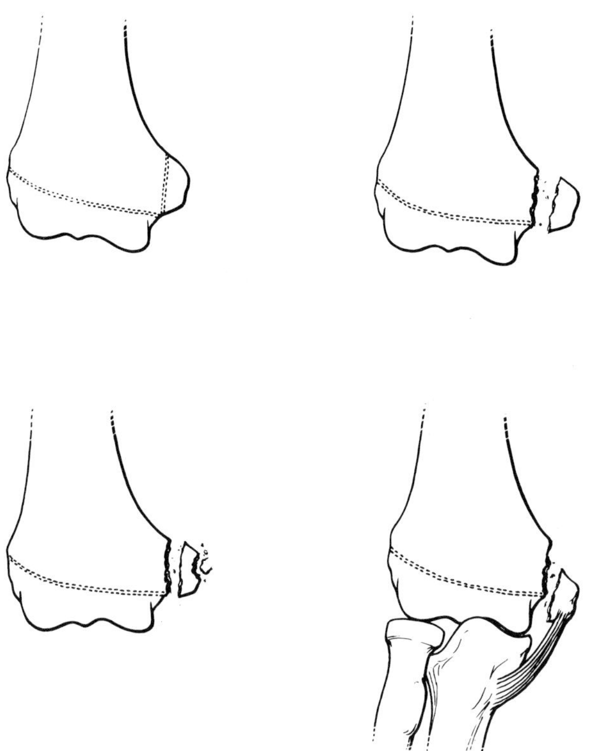

Fig. 10-43 Illustrations of injuries of the medial epicondyle due to pitching. (A) Normal, (B) separation and/or overgrowth, (C) fragmentation, (D) avulsion.

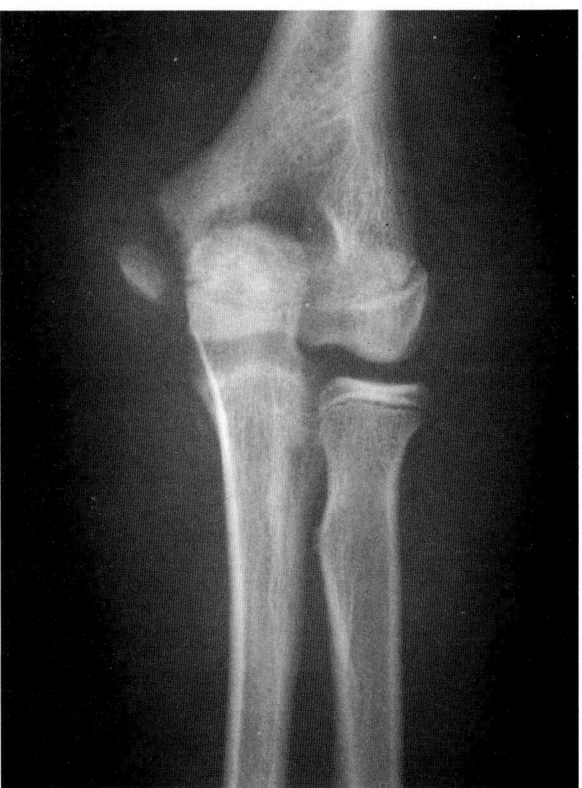

Fig. 10-44 AP view of the elbow demonstrating an avulsion fracture of the medial epicondyle.

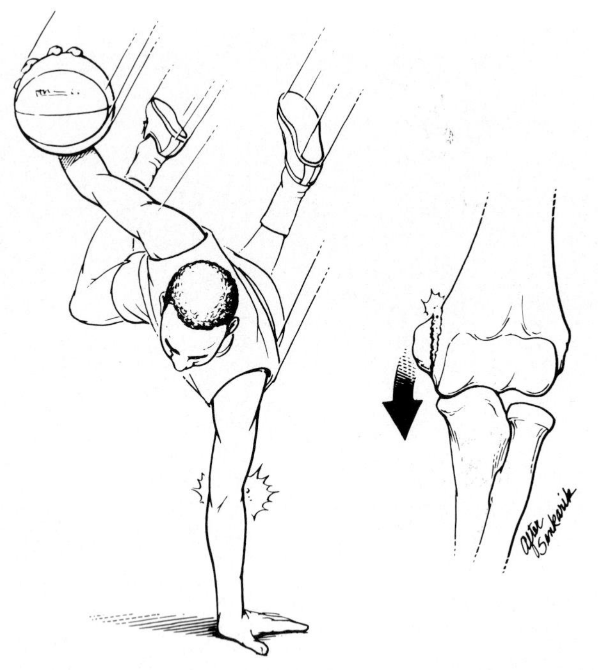

Fig. 10-45 Illustration of the mechanism of injury for medial epicondyle avulsion fractures.

an avulsion force that is transmitted across the medial collateral ligament from a valgus stress to the extended elbow (Fig. 10-45). The lateral epicondylar fracture is extremely rare.[116] It probably occurs with a mechanism of injury similar but opposite in direction to that involved in fractures of the medial epicondyle (Figs. 10-46 and 10-47). The elbow is forced into varus with avulsion forces applied by the extensor muscles and lateral ligament complex. The lateral epicondyle may be treated in a closed fashion if the displacement is less than 2 to 3 mm (Fig. 10-48). An accurate reduction of the medial epicondyle, however, is more crucial because the ligamentous integrity of the joint depends upon the position of the medial epicondyle.[116]

Occasionally, severe displacement of the medial epicondyle associated with elbow dislocation can result in entrapment of the fracture fragment in the joint after reduction (Fig. 10-49). This entrapment is often difficult to diagnose on the lateral view but is suggested by medial joint widening or visualization of the loose body on the radiograph. When this occurs, closed reductions are unsuccessful; open reduction with anatomic pinning must be undertaken.[116]

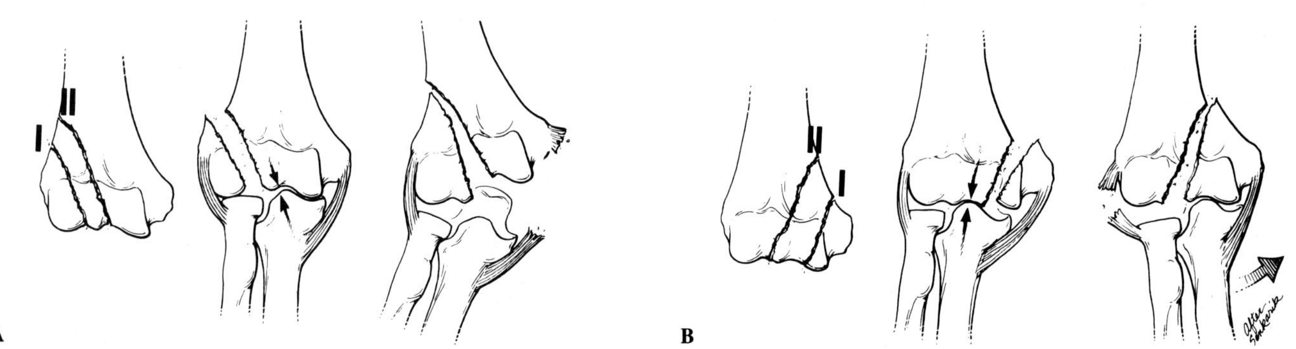

Fig. 10-46 Illustrations of lateral (**A**) and medial (**B**) epicondyle fractures. (**A**) Type I fractures spare the lateral trochlear ridge. Type II fractures involve the lateral trochlear ridge, which may lead to dislocation. (**B**) In type I fractures the lateral trochlear ridge is intact. In type II fractures the lateral trochlear ridge is involved, which may lead to medial dislocation.[100,116]

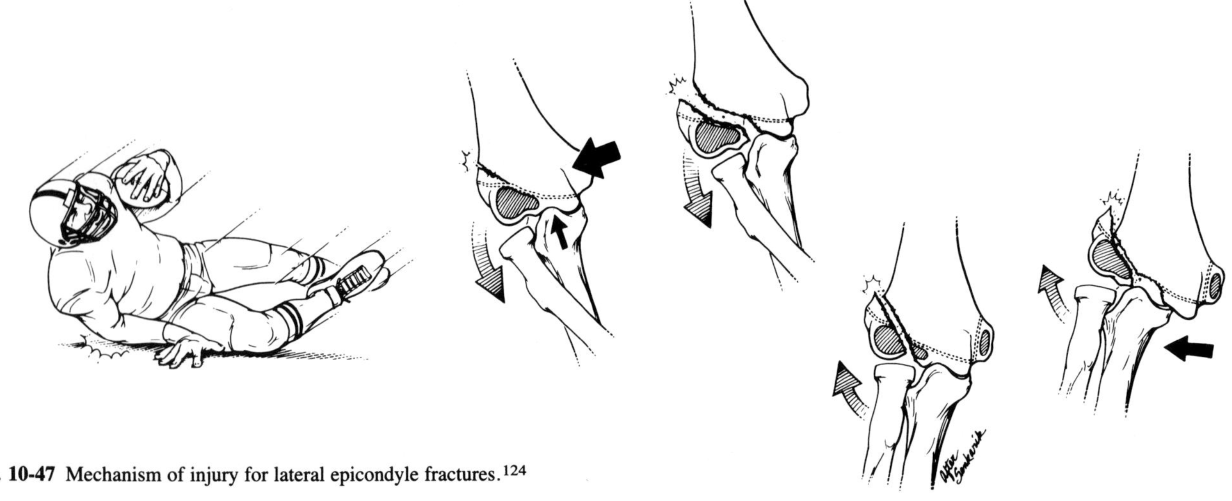

Fig. 10-47 Mechanism of injury for lateral epicondyle fractures.[124]

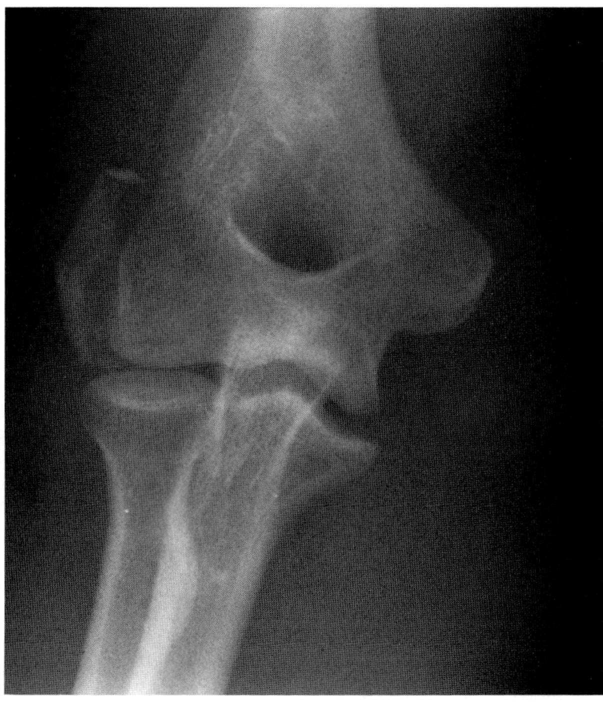

Fig. 10-48 Vertical fracture of the lateral epicondyle with lateral displacement.

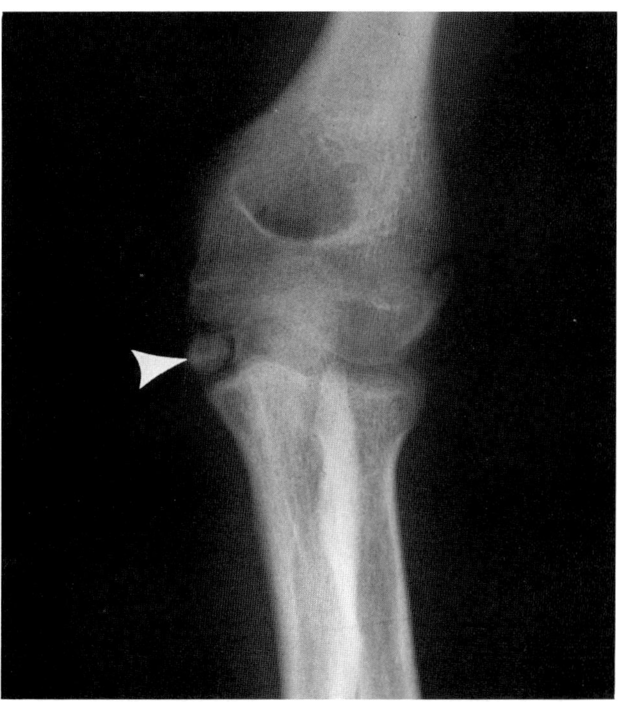

Fig. 10-49 AP view of the elbow demonstrating displacement of the medial epicondyle (arrowhead) into the joint.

T and Y Condylar Fractures

These fractures result from a direct blow to the proximal ulna, usually with the elbow in flexion. The fracture line is initiated in the central groove of the trochlea and extends across the olecranon and coronoid fossa, emerging across the medial and lateral supracondylar bony columns (Fig. 10-50).[94,98,100]

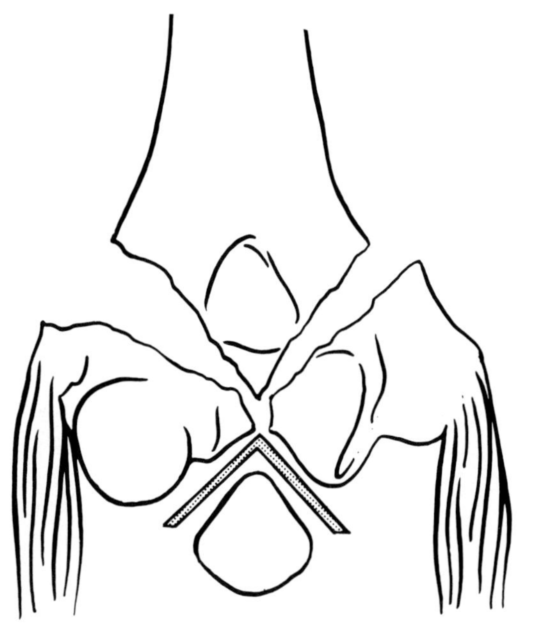

Fig. 10-50 Illustration of the mechanism of T and Y condylar fractures. The flexor and extensor muscles can cause significant displacement and rotation of the fragment. *Source:* Reprinted from *The Elbow and Its Disorders* by BF Morrey, 1985, WB Saunders, © Mayo Foundation.

Riseborough and Radin[121] distinguished four types of fracture. Type I fractures consist of undisplaced T or Y condylar fractures. The type II injury is one in which the condyles are displaced but not rotated. Type III fractures are those in which the medial and lateral condylar compartments are rotated. This rotation is caused by the action of the flexor and extensor muscle masses and results in the so-called inverted-V sign (Fig. 10-50). The type IV fracture is one with marked comminution.

In the T and Y supracondylar fracture there is usually massive swelling, and flexion-extension of the elbow is not possible. Routine radiographs clearly demonstrate the fracture (Fig. 10-51). No special techniques or views are required for the diagnosis, but the severity and degree of comminution are often more extensive than can be appreciated on the simple AP and lateral views. Oblique views are sometimes helpful in appreciating fully the precise nature of the fracture. Conventional tomography or CT may also be useful in complex cases. Three-dimensional CT evaluation may be needed for surgical planning.[92,107,109]

Complications of this fracture include improper reduction and the development of exuberant callus that can fill the olecranon fossa and thus limit motion.[95] Internal fixation devices can likewise limit motion if the fossae are crossed by screws or pins. These features of treatment can be detected

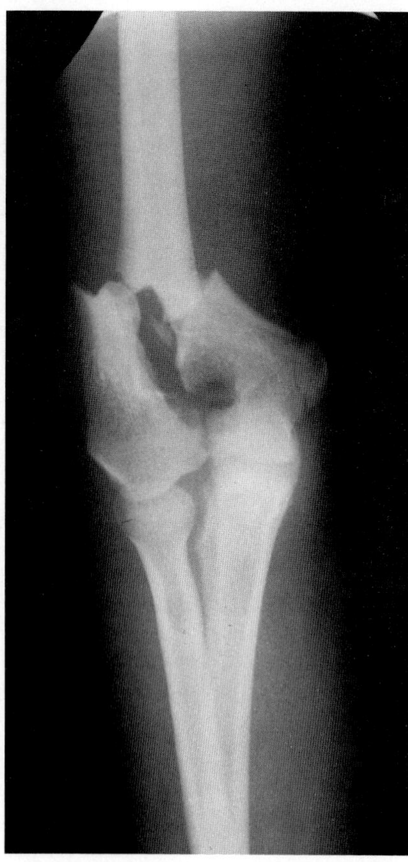

Fig. 10-51 AP view of the elbow demonstrating a type IV Y condylar fracture. Internal fixation is required in this setting.

radiographically with routine views, but occasionally tomography or flexion-extension views will be helpful. Nonunion occurs in about 2% to 5% of cases and is usually associated with inadequate surgical procedure.[100,116] Most nonunions occur with type III and IV injuries (Fig. 10-51).

Capitellar Fractures

These fractures are among the most difficult to diagnose accurately by the radiograph. The incidence is reported to be only 1% of all elbow injuries.[100,104,106] The mechanism of injury is either a direct blow or a fall on the outstretched hand.

Three types of capitellar fractures have been described. The type I fracture involves the entire capitellum or a major portion of it, often including a small portion of the trochlea. This fracture is difficult to detect on the AP radiograph but is easily identified on the lateral view (Fig. 10-52). Type II injury consists of a shearing fracture. Often there is little or no cancellous bone on the cartilage; as a result, this fracture is easily overlooked.[100,116] The fat pad sign is helpful in detecting an injury, and aspiration showing fat globules and a hemarthrosis should also raise one's suspicion of the likelihood of this fracture.[97] The type III injury is a comminuted fracture of the capitellum often associated with fracture of the radial head.[116] Associated rupture of the ulnar collateral ligament may occur in up to 13% of cases.[100] The mechanism of injury is a fall on the outstretched hand, causing a compression injury.

A

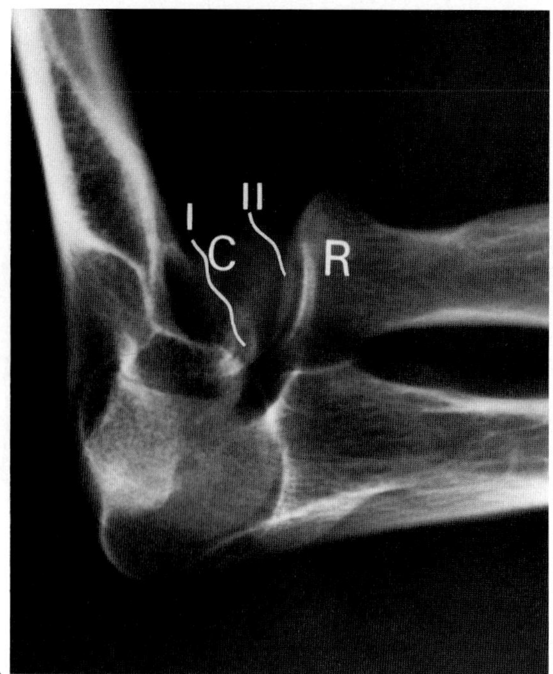

B

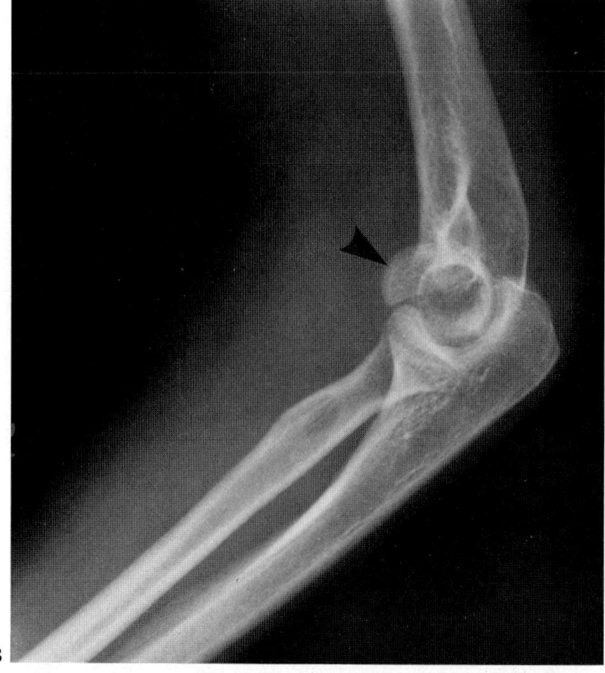

Fig. 10-52 **(A)** Lateral radiograph of the elbow demonstrating the fragment size of type I and II capitellar fractures. C, Capitellum; R, radius. **(B)** Lateral radiograph demonstrating a type I fracture (arrowhead).

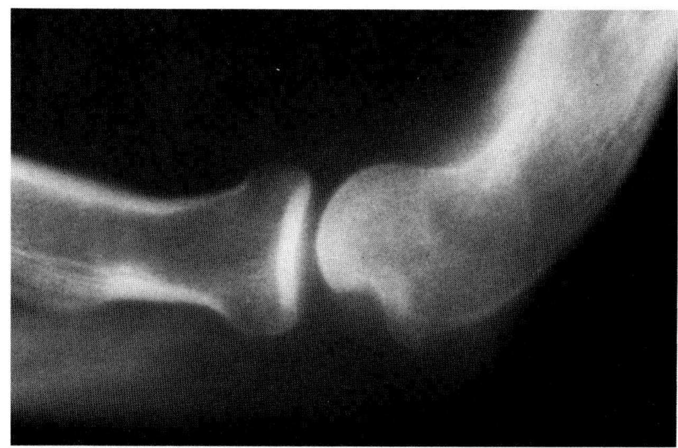

Fig. 10-53 Lateral tomogram of the elbow demonstrating an impacted osteochondral capitellar fracture.

The AP view is usually unrewarding for detection of all three types of fractures. The lateral view is sufficient for type I fractures, but oblique views of the elbow joint may be needed for detection of type II fractures. Lateral tomograms or CT scans may be needed for type II and III fractures (Fig. 10-53). The differential diagnosis for type II fracture includes fracture of the radial head. An important point of distinction is that the displacement of the capitellar fracture fragment is commonly superior to the capitellum (Fig. 10-52B), whereas the displacement of the radial head fracture fragments is not. For type II fractures, the sheared cartilage may have little or no osseous component (Fig. 10-54).

Fracture of the Humeral Condyles

Fracture of a humeral condyle is uncommon but may be seen to involve either the medial or the lateral structure.

An isolated fracture of the condyle can occur from one of two mechanisms. Both essentially involve an avulsion or a shearing type of fracture. A fall on the outstretched hand with the forearm in valgus can produce an axial load that, depending upon the distribution of the forces, may result in a shearing type of lateral condylar fracture or an avulsion type of medial condylar fracture. Conversely, a fall on the outstretched hand with an axial load and a varus angular component may produce a shearing type of medial condylar fracture and an avulsion type of lateral condylar fracture. Thus, four possible mechanisms obtain: shearing or avulsion of the medial condyle and shearing or avulsion of the lateral condyle.

This fracture has been classified into two types.[115,116] The type I lateral fracture involves only the capitellum and lateral epicondyle; the type I medial fracture includes the medial lip of the trochlea and the medial epicondyle. The type I lateral fracture includes none or only a small part of the lateral trochlea (Fig. 10-46). The type II lateral fracture involves the lateral half of the trochlea (Fig. 10-55); the type II medial fracture involves the entire trochlea. This classification is of major significance because the type II fracture, usually lateral, is associated with marked elbow instability. If this fracture is not appropriately treated with surgery, permanent and significant residual impairment can result.[110,115,116]

The diagnosis of an articular fracture of some type is suspected as a result of physical examination, which demonstrates that the posterior triangular relationship has been altered. In the adult, routine radiography readily demonstrates the nature of the injury. Because the distal humerus is primarily cartilaginous in children, however, this fracture, representing a Salter-Harris type IV, can be difficult to diagnose correctly (Figs. 10-56 and 10-57).

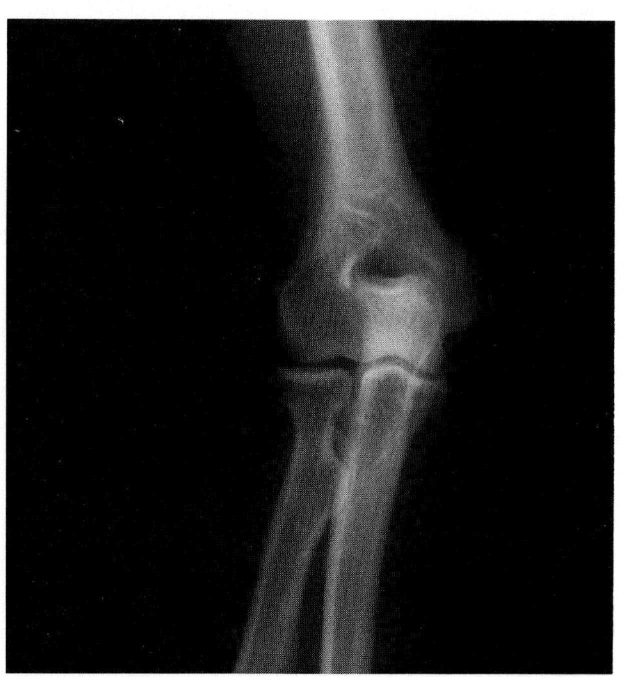

A

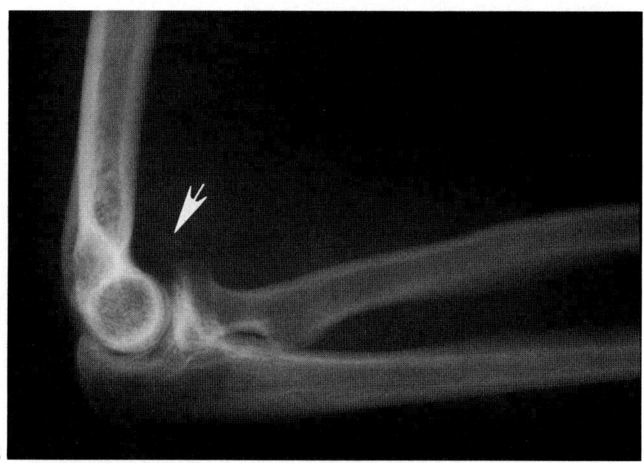

B

Fig. 10-54 (**A**) AP and (**B**) lateral views of the elbow. A tiny avulsed capitellar fragment (arrow) is seen only on the lateral view (arrow in **B**).

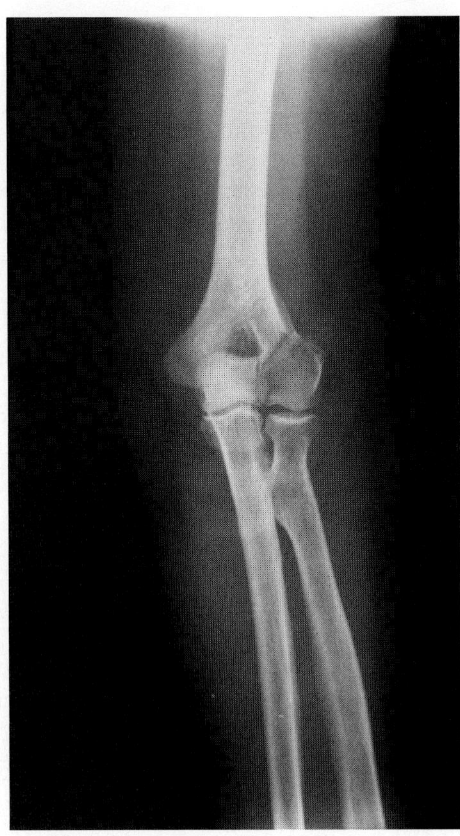

Fig. 10-55 AP view of the elbow demonstrating a type II lateral condyle fracture.

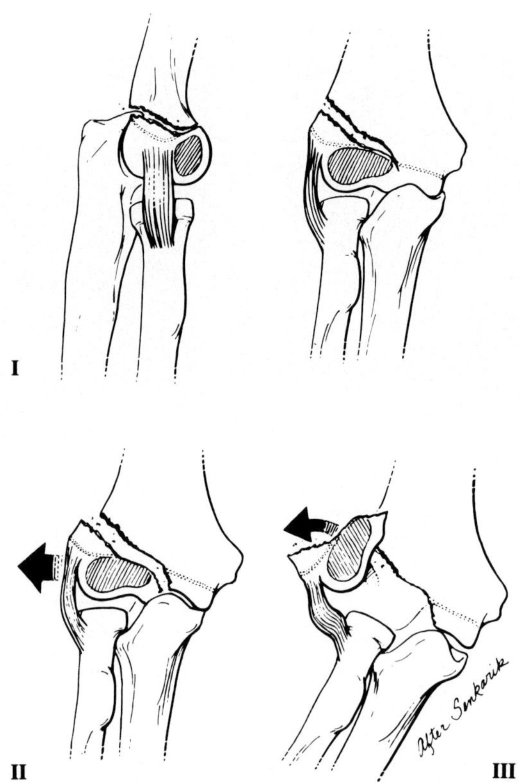

Fig. 10-56 Illustrations of Salter-Harris IV lateral condyle fracture with various degrees of displacement. Arrows indicate direction of force application. Stage I, undisplaced; stage II, slightly displaced; stage III, complete displacement.

Complications of this fracture include neurovascular compromise because the proximal fragment may impinge on or impale the neurovascular bundle.[113] The more common types of complications, however, involve inadequate reduction and the subsequent loss of proper position, motion, and stability owing to an incongruous joint.

Proximal Radial Fractures

Fractures of the head and neck of the radius are common injuries, accounting for approximately one-third of all elbow fractures.[88,90,102,116] These fractures result from a fall on the outstretched hand with the elbow partially flexed and pronated (Fig. 10-58). Because the neck of the radius makes an angle of about 15° with the shaft of the bone, in the pronated position the anterolateral margin comes into contact with the capitellum. Thus the proximal radius is vulnerable to a shearing type of fracture. Increasing amounts of force with this orientation result in a more extensive injury.[100,116]

Radial head and neck fractures may be undisplaced or minimally displaced (<2 mm, type I; Fig. 10-59). A type II fracture involves approximately one-third of the radial head with greater than 2 mm of displacement or 20° to 30° of angulation. The type III fracture involves comminution of the radial head (Fig. 10-60). The type IV fracture is any fracture of the radial head with dislocation of the ulnohumeral joint.[114,116] In the pediatric age group, most fractures involve the radial neck with various degrees of angulation and displacement (Fig. 10-61). If the fracture is of the radial neck, angulation of less than 20° to 30° is considered a type I fracture, angulation of greater than 20° to 30° is considered a type II fracture, and angulation of greater than 60° or dislocation is considered a type III fracture.[114,116,118]

A history of trauma is invariably present. On examination, marked local tenderness of the radiohumeral joint with extreme pain on pronation-supination is demonstrated.

Routine AP and lateral radiographs are usually sufficient to demonstrate this fracture (Figs. 10-59 and 10-60). A single view will often not reveal the fracture line, however, and oblique or radial head views are sometimes required before the true extent of the fracture is appreciated. A fat pad sign with the features on physical examination discussed earlier may be the only indication, but this should allow diagnosis even of minimally displaced type I fractures.[99] Distinguishing between a type II capitellar and a type I radial head fracture may be difficult. Additional views should be taken when there is doubt. Occasionally tomograms may be necessary to resolve the issue.[92,116]

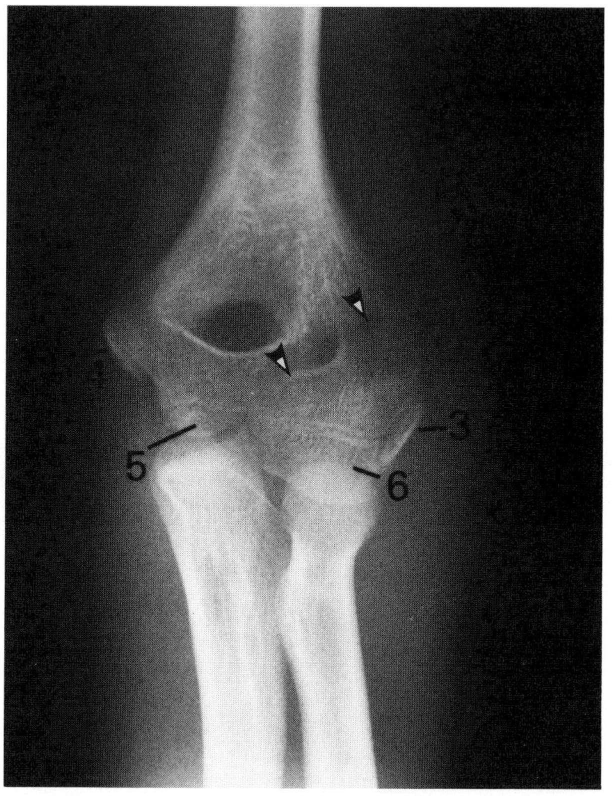

A

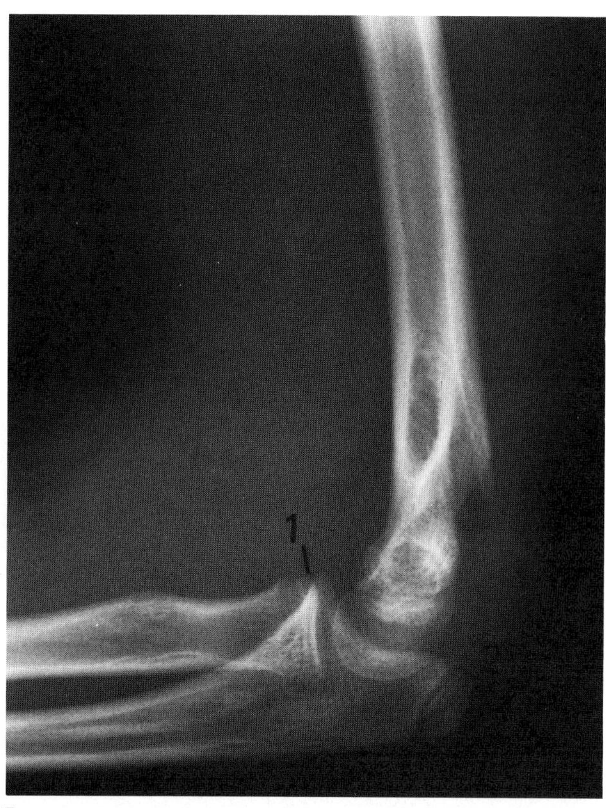

B

Fig. 10-57 (**A**) AP and (**B**) lateral views of the elbow demonstrating a Salter-Harris IV condylar fracture (arrowheads in **A**). 1, Radial epiphysis; 2, olecranon; 3, lateral epicondyle; 4, medial epicondyle; 5, trochlea; 6, capitellum.

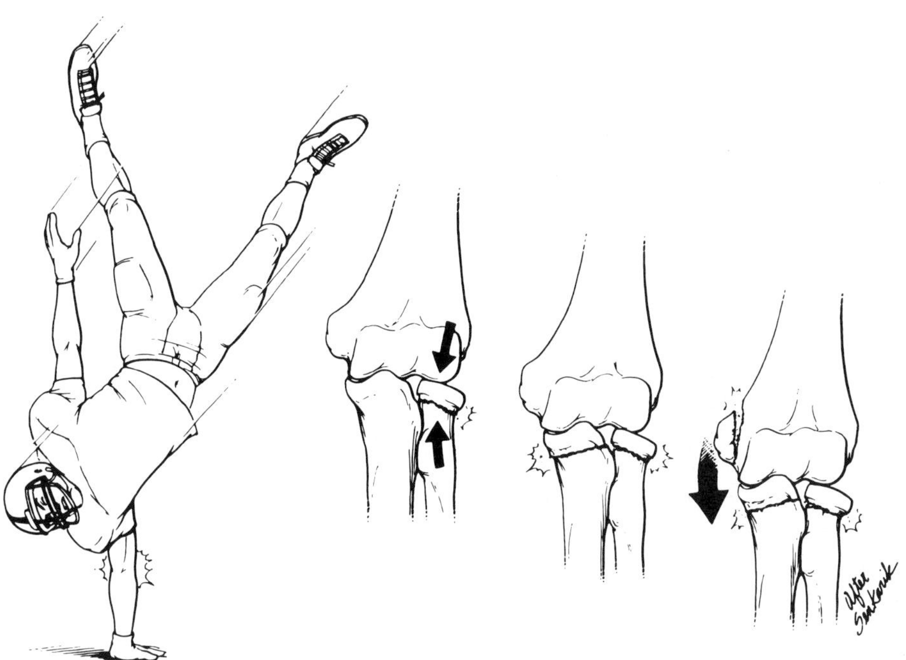

Fig. 10-58 Mechanism of radial head fracture (fall on the outstretched arm). Progressive force may result in fracture of the ulna and medial epicondyle.

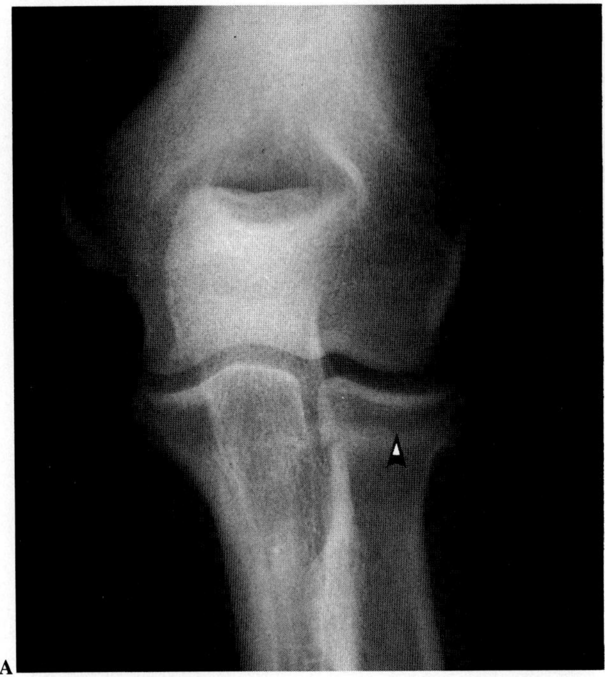

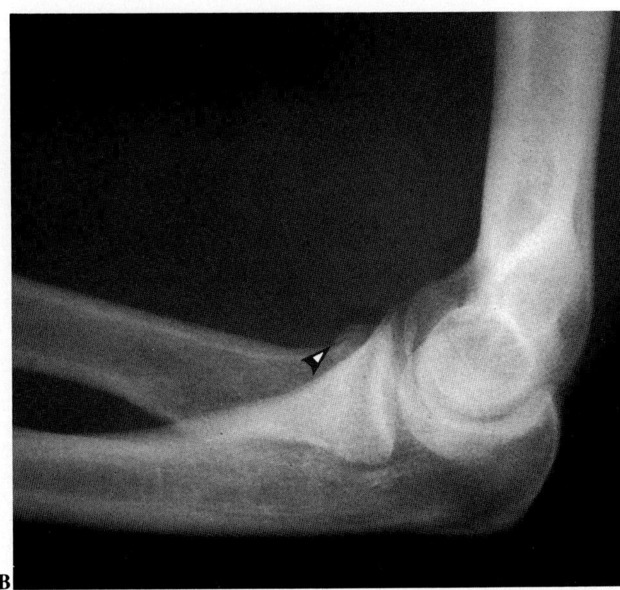

Fig. 10-59 (**A**) AP and (**B**) lateral views of an impacted type I radial neck fracture (arrowheads).

Proximal Ulnar Fractures

The olecranon is superficial and, therefore, particularly susceptible to trauma. Most fractures are intraarticular, which potentially affects stability and articular function. If the triceps with its fascial expansions has been disrupted, the fracture becomes even more displaced. Without this feature, the displacement is usually minimal.[116]

Fractures of the olecranon are usually the result of a direct blow, typically from a fall on the flexed elbow (Fig. 10-62A) or, less commonly, as a result of a hyperextension injury (Fig. 10-62B). The hyperextension injury is usually associated with other injury, for example elbow dislocation or radial head fracture. Greater comminution is observed in the older and younger age groups. A clean transverse line is often observed.

The AP radiograph of the elbow is not particularly helpful in defining the severity of the injury unless there is either medial or lateral displacement.[92] The lateral view is most useful because it not only demonstrates the precise orientation, displacement, and comminution of the fracture but also is helpful in revealing any associated fracture of the radial head or displacement of the distal fragment (Fig. 10-63). Failure to obtain a true lateral view before treatment is probably the most common error in the initial radiographic assessment of this type of injury.[116]

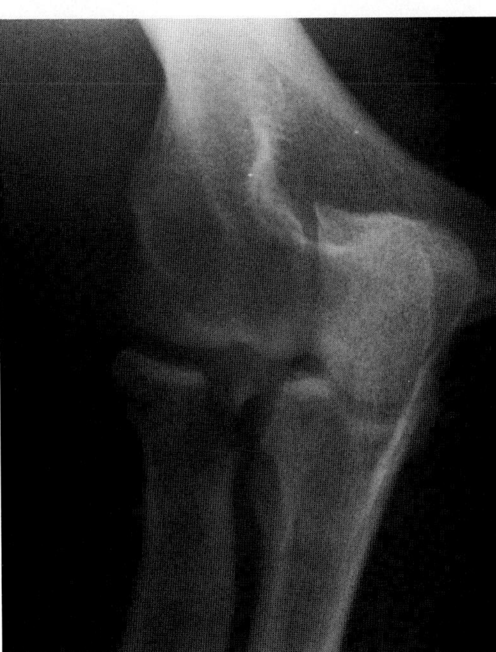

Fig. 10-60 Oblique view of the elbow in a patient with a single displaced radial head fracture.

Coronoid Fractures

Isolated coronoid fractures are uncommon. When present, they are most often associated with posterior dislocations of the elbow. In this setting, the incidence is 2% to 10%. Recurrent dislocation is associated with this injury.[120]

Most displaced coronoid fractures can be detected with routine radiography. Nevertheless, tomography or in some cases CT may be required to evaluate the injury fully. The coronoid is frequently partially obscured on routine radiographs.[92]

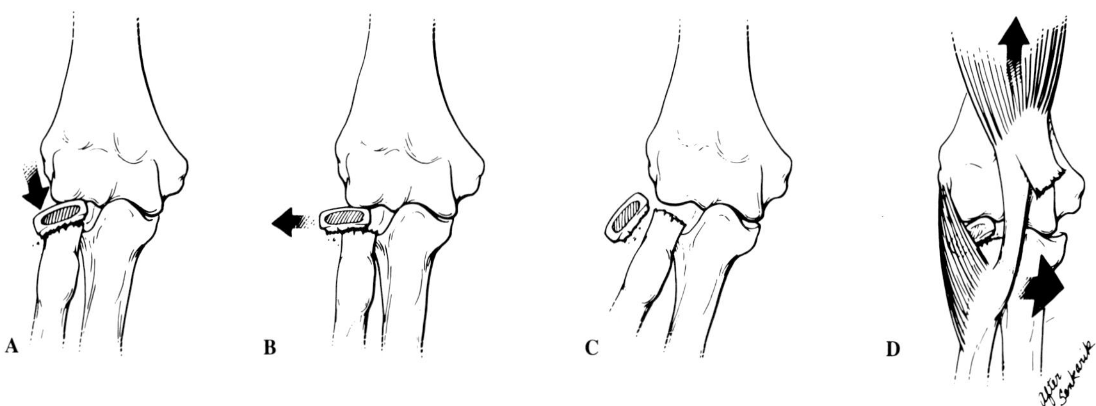

Fig. 10-61 Radial neck fractures with angulation (**A**), translocation (**B**), and total displacement (**C**). Biceps and superator muscles displace the distal fragment toward the ulna and upward (**D**).[124]

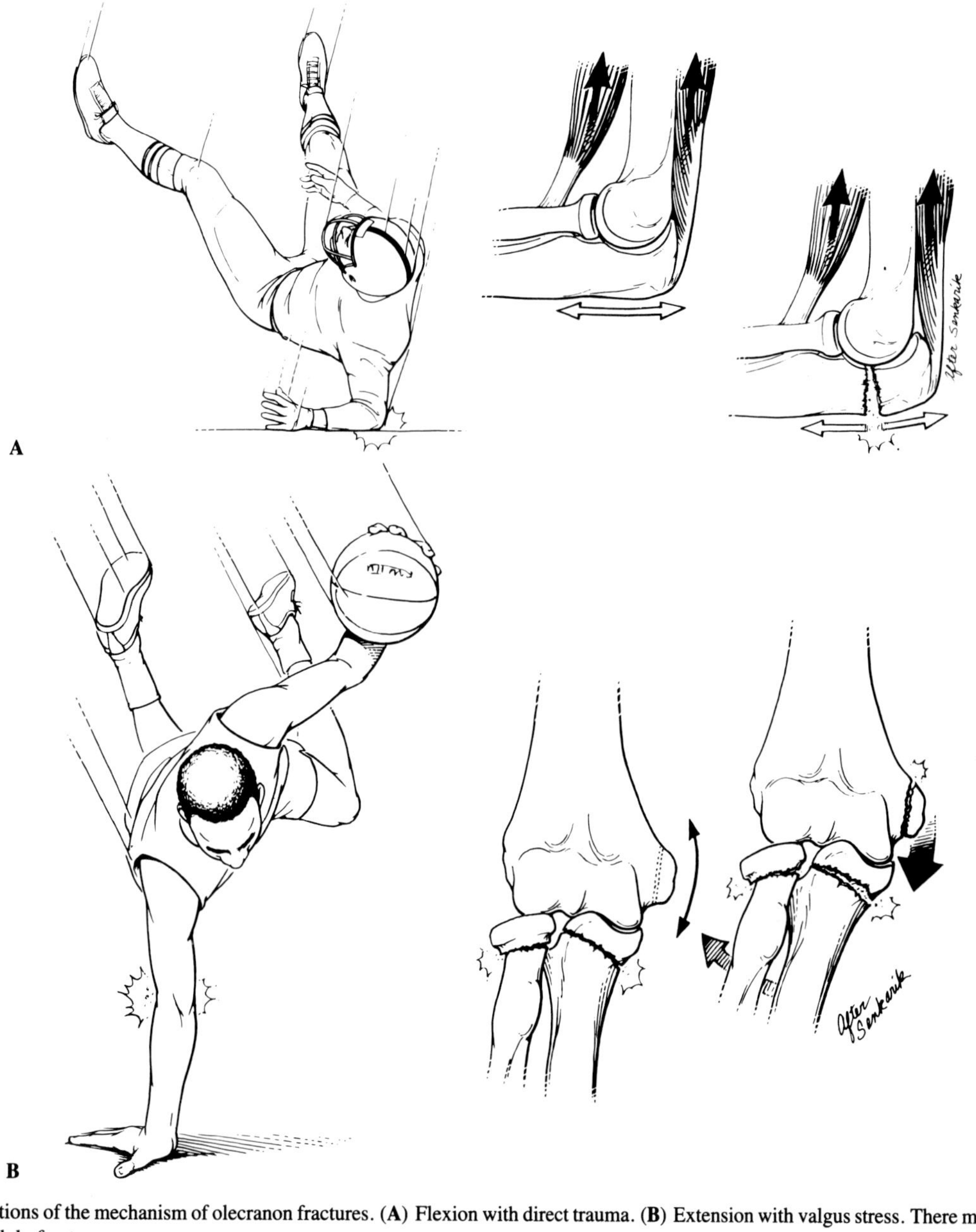

Fig. 10-62 Illustrations of the mechanism of olecranon fractures. (**A**) Flexion with direct trauma. (**B**) Extension with valgus stress. There may be associated radial and medial epicondyle fractures.

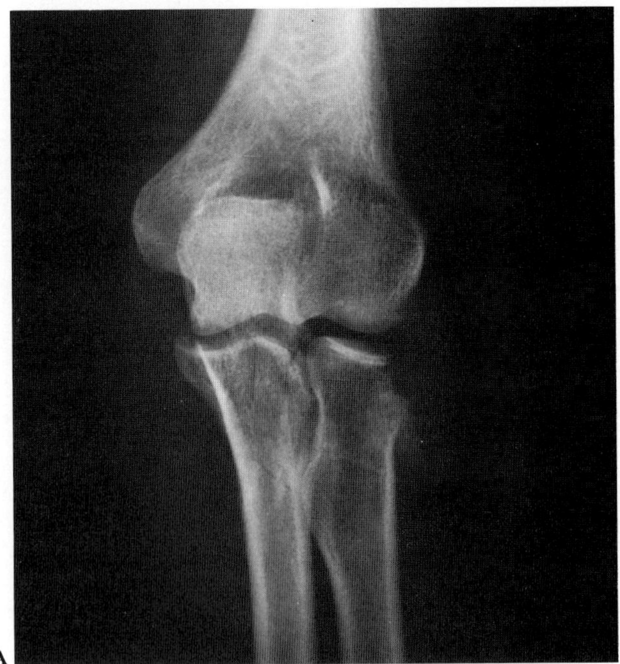

A

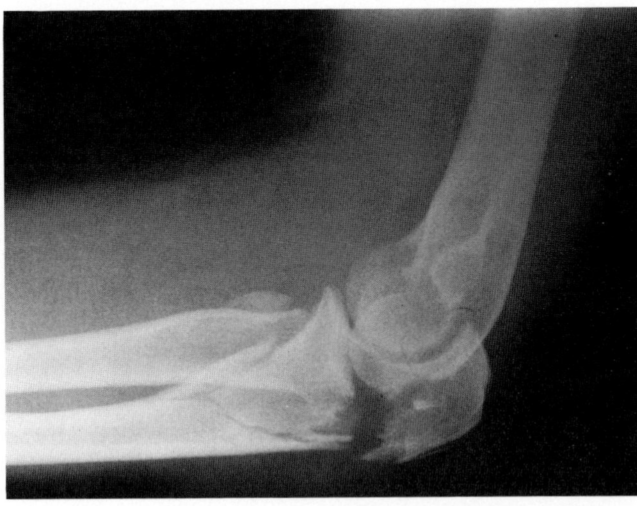

B

Fig. 10-63 (**A**) AP and (**B**) lateral views of the elbow in a patient with a comminuted olecranon fracture and radial head fracture.

Monteggia Fractures

The Monteggia fracture is a fracture of the proximal ulna with dislocation of the radial head.[91,100] Described in 1814 by Monteggia of Milan, this fracture was termed the Monteggia lesion by Bado.[89] These fractures are not common and represent about 7% of all ulnar fractures and thus about 0.7% of all elbow injuries.[92,116] A relatively simple classification of this fracture was proposed by Bado[89] and consists of the following types:

- *Type I*: fracture of the ulna with anterior dislocation of the radial head. This is the most common fracture, occurring in 50% to 75% of cases. It is a common type of fracture in children (Fig. 10-64).[89,116]
- *Type II*: fracture of the proximal ulna with a posterior or posterolateral dislocation of the radial head and a posterior angulation of the ulnar fracture. This is usually a more proximal fracture. It occurs most often in adults and represents about 10% to 15% of the Monteggia lesions.
- *Type III*: fracture of the ulna with a lateral and anterolateral dislocation of the radial head. This is a common type of fracture in children, representing 6% to 20% of Monteggia type lesions.
- *Type IV*: anterior dislocation of the radial head with fracture of the proximal third of the radius and ulna. This is the rarest of the Monteggia lesions and represents about 5% of cases.[89,119]

Three mechanisms have been proposed for this injury, and probably all three can give rise to one or another of the types. These include a direct blow to the posterior aspect of the ulna, a fall on the outstretched hand with the elbow flexed on impact, and hyperextension. Probably all three mechanisms are implicated in this type of fracture.[116]

Adequate radiographs in two or more planes are particularly important in this injury because the dislocation of the radial head may be missed in a single view. Certainly in severe cases the diagnosis is not difficult (Fig. 10-64). If the dislocation becomes inadvertently reduced at the time of positioning for radiography, the severity of the injury may be underestimated. This may occur in about 20% of cases.[116,119]

In the child the fracture usually can be reduced and hence treated by nonoperative modalities. For the adult, however, surgical intervention is the treatment of choice.[110,116]

Forearm Fractures

The radius and ulna are essentially parallel through the forearm with complex muscle groups, which can cause significant fracture deformity and rotation.[87,92,105]

Forearm fractures may occur with a direct blow, especially to the ulna, or they may be due to a fall on the outstretched hand.[92] Seventy-five percent of fractures involve both bones, 15% involve the ulna, and 10% involve the radius.[122] Fig. 10-65 illustrates the location of radial and ulnar fractures.[97]

Fractures may be undisplaced, but rotation and angulation are common as a result of muscle forces.[92,105] Even with proper reduction, complications such as cross-union can occur (Fig. 10-66).[103,122,123]

Routine AP and lateral radiographs are adequate for diagnosis. Both the elbow and the wrist should be included on the films to avoid overlooking subluxation or dislocation of these

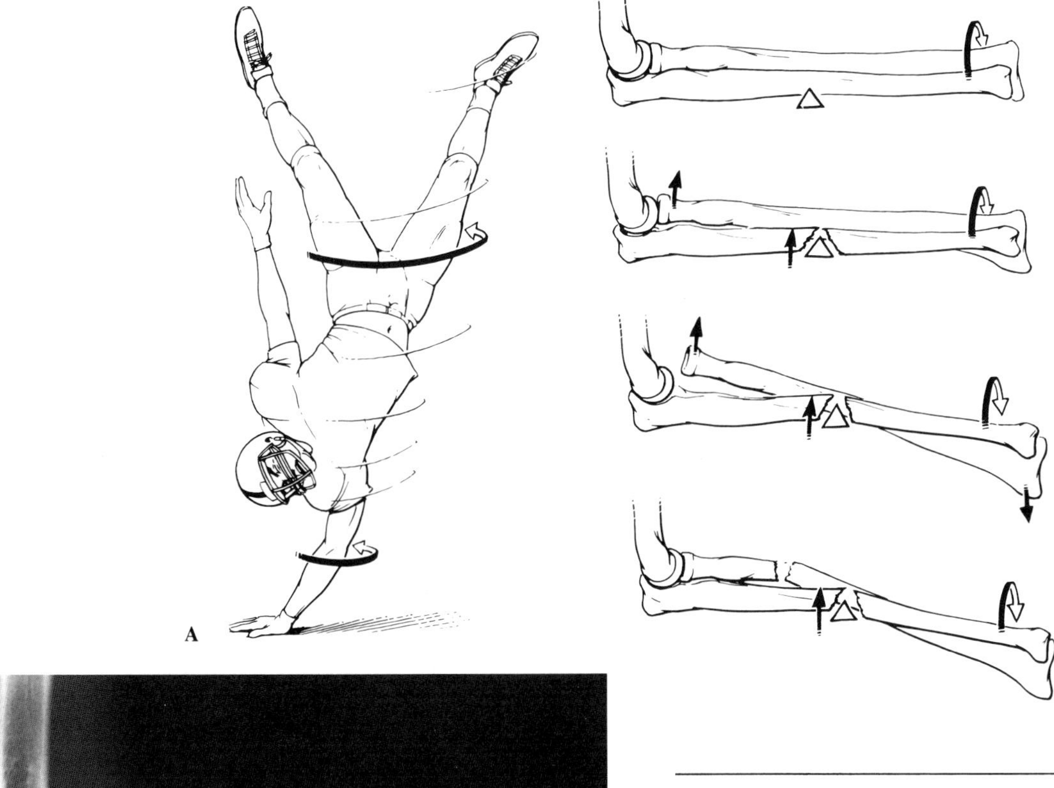

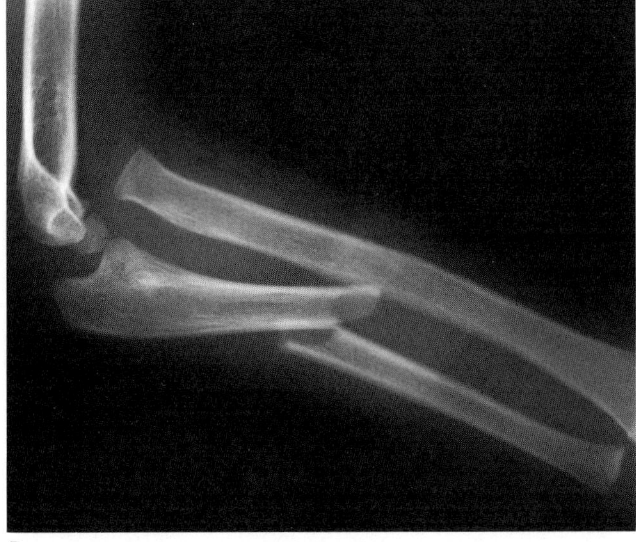

Fig. 10-64 **(A)** Illustration of the mechanism of Monteggia injury (fall on the outstretched arm with forearm pronated and trunk rotated). The pronation forces cause the ulna to fracture (top). The proximal ulnar fragment acts as a fulcrum, dislocating the radial head.[100,116] **(B)** Monteggia fracture in a child. The radial head is dislocated anteriorly.

articulations. This is particularly important when only one of the bones is fractured.[92]

Osteochondritis Dissecans

Chronic elbow pain, especially in adolescent athletes involved in throwing sports, is not unusual. In this setting, osteochondritis dissecans must be considered along with the other overuse injuries described earlier in this chapter. Patients generally present with dull aching pain in the throwing arm.

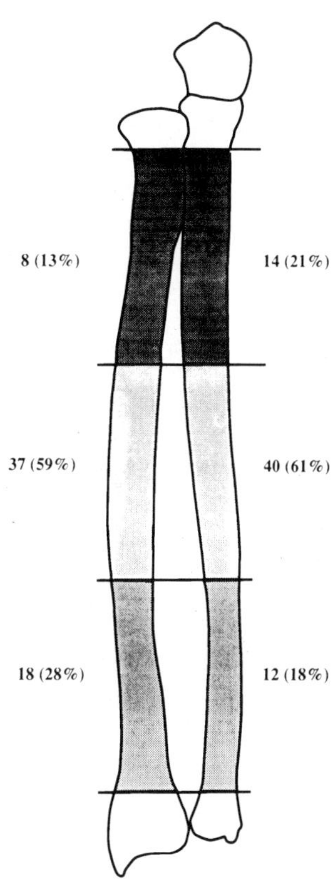

Fig. 10-65 Illustration of fracture locations in the radius and ulna. *Source:* Reprinted with permission from Chapman MW, Gordon JE, and Zissimos AG, Compression plate fixation of acute forearm fractures of the diaphysis of the radius and ulna, *Journal of Bone and Joint Surgery* (1989;71A:159–169), Copyright © 1989, Journal of Bone and Joint Surgery.

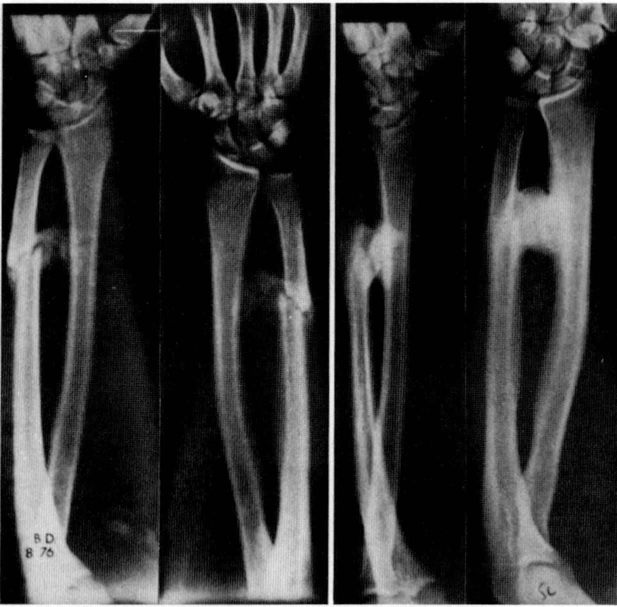

Fig. 10-66 Radiographs of the forearm demonstrating progressive cross-union. *Source:* Reprinted with permission from Vince KG and Miller JE, Cross union complicating fracture of the forearm, part I: adults, *Journal of Bone and Joint Surgery* (1987;69A:640–660), Copyright © 1987, Journal of Bone and Joint Surgery.

Swelling and limited motion are not uncommon. Rest typically relieves the pain.[93]

Staging of lesions is important radiographically. Type I lesions are intact with no fragment displacement. Type II lesions may be slightly displaced, but the articular surface will have a definite fissure or fracture. Type III lesions are detached.[93] Surgical intervention is often indicated in types II and III.

Conventional radiography is often of little value in the staging process. Radiographs are usually normal in the early stages. In children, comparison radiographs are useful because of the normal irregularity of the epiphysis. Tomography, CT, and arthrotomography are useful. MRI is noninvasive, however, and offers several advantages. Articular cartilage and bone can be evaluated in multiple planes (Fig. 10-67). In addition, other bone and soft tissue injuries that may mimic osteochondritis dissecans can be detected easily. Therefore, after routine radiographs clinicians frequently use MRI to evaluate athletes with subtle osseous or soft tissue injury.

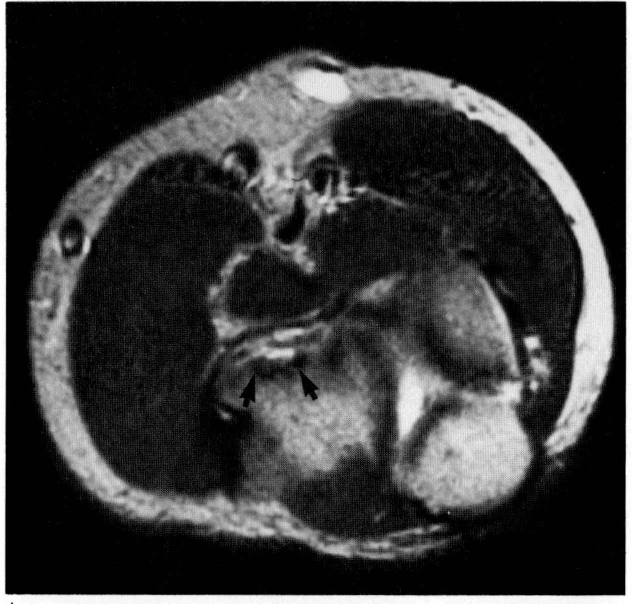

A

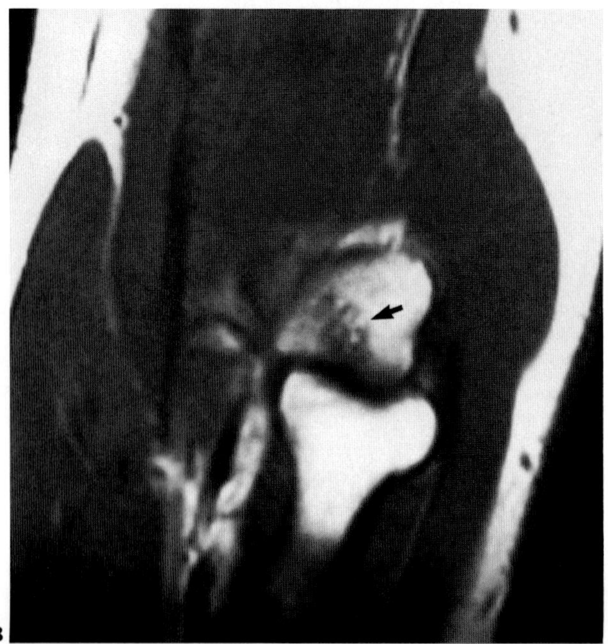

B

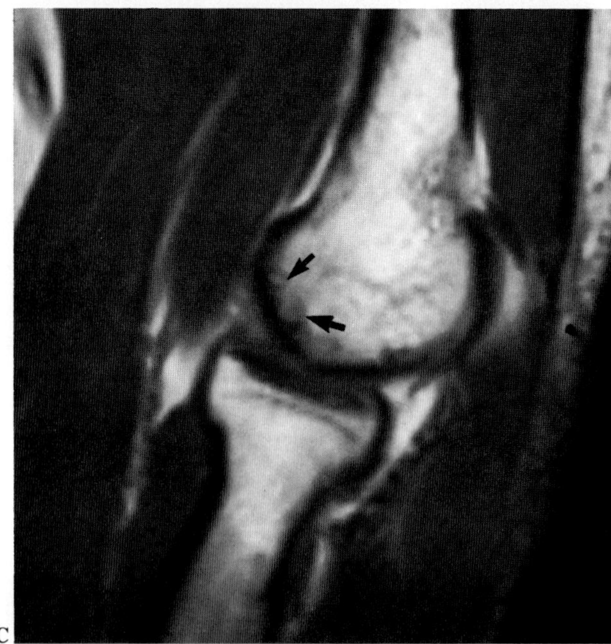

C

Fig. 10-67 MRI in osteochondritis dissecans. (**A**) Axial (SE 2000/60), (**B**) coronal, and (**C**) sagittal (SE 500/20) images demonstrate a type I lesion (arrows).

REFERENCES

Introduction

1. Axe MJ. Evaluation and treatment of common throwing injuries of the shoulder and elbow. *Del Med J*. 1987;59:593–598.

2. Leach RE, Miller JK. Lateral and medial epicondylitis of the elbow. *Clin Sports Med*. 1987;6:259–272.

3. Micheli LJ, Smith AD. Sports injuries in children. *Curr Probl Pediatr*. 1982:3–54.

4. Morrey BF. *The Elbow and its Disorders*. Philadelphia: Saunders; 1985.

5. Nirschl RP. Prevention and treatment of elbow and shoulder injuries in the tennis player. *Clin Sports Med*. 1988;7:289–308.

6. Wojtys EM, Smith PA, Hankin FM. A cause of ulnar neuropathy in a baseball pitcher. *Am J Sports Med*. 1986;14:422–424.

7. Yocum LA. The diagnosis and nonoperative treatment of elbow problems in the athlete. *Clin Sports Med*. 1989;8:439–451.

Anatomy

8. An KN, Hui FC, Morrey BF, Linscheid RL, Chao EY. Muscles across the elbow joint: a biomechanical analysis. *J Biomech*. 1981; 14:659–669.

9. Beals RK. The normal carrying angle of the elbow. *Clin Orthop Relat Res*. 1976;119:194–196.

10. Evans EM. Rotational deformity in the treatment of fractures of both bones of the forearm. *J Bone Joint Surg*. 1945;27:373–379.

11. Gay JR, Love JG. Diagnosis and treatment of tardy paralysis of the ulnar nerve. *J Bone Joint Surg*. 1947;29:1087–1097.

12. Guttierez LF. A contribution to the study of the limiting factors of elbow fixation. *Acta Anat*. 1964;56:146–156.

13. Hollinshead HW. The back and limbs. In: Hollinshead HW, ed. *Anatomy for Surgeons*. New York: Harper & Row; 1982;3.

14. Johansson O. Capsular and ligament injuries of the elbow joint. *Acta Chir Scand*. 1962;287(suppl).

15. Loomis LK. Reduction and after-treatment of posterior dislocation of the elbow: with special attention to the brachialis muscle and myositis ossificans. *Am J Surg*. 1944;63:56.

16. Morrey BF. *The Elbow and its Disorders*. Philadelphia: Saunders; 1985.

17. Morrey BF, Berquist TH. The elbow. In: Berquist TH, ed. *Imaging of Orthopedic Trauma*. 2nd ed. New York: Raven; 1991:675–730.

18. Morrey BF, Chao EY. Passive motion of the elbow joint. A biomechanical analysis. *J Bone Joint Surg Am*. 1976;58:501–508.

19. Simon WH, Friedenberg S, Richardson S. Joint congruence. *J Bone Joint Surg Am*. 1973;55:1614–1620.

Imaging Techniques

20. Arger PH, Oberkircher PE, Miller WT. Lipohemarthrosis. *Am J Roentgenol Radium Ther Nucl Med*. 1974;121:97–100.

21. Ballinger PW. *Merrill's Atlas of Roentgenographic Positions and Standard Radiologic Procedures*. 5th ed. St Louis, MO: Mosby; 1982.

22. Barr LL, Babcock DS. Sonography of the normal elbow. *AJR*. 1991;157:793–798.

23. Bassett LW, Mirra JM, Forrester DM, Gold RH, Berstein ML, Rollins JS. Post-traumatic osteochondral "loose body" of the olecranon fossa. *Radiology*. 1981;141:635–638.

24. Bernau A, Berquist TH. *Positioning Techniques in Orthopedic Radiology*. Baltimore: Urban & Schwarzenberg; 1983.

25. Berquist TH. *Imaging of Orthopedic Trauma*. 2nd ed. New York: Raven; 1991.

26. Berquist TH. *Magnetic Resonance Imaging of the Musculoskeletal System*. New York: Raven; 1990.

27. Berquist TH. The elbow and wrist. *Top Magn Resonance Imaging*. 1989;1:15–27.

28. Bledsoe RC, Izenstark JL. Displacement of fat pads in disease and injury of the elbow. A new radiographic sign. *Radiology*. 1959;73:717–724.

29. Bohrer SP. The fat pad sign following elbow trauma. *Clin Radiol*. 1970;21:90–94.

30. Brown R, Blazina ME, Kerlan RK. Osteochondritis of the capitellum. *J Sports Med*. 1974;2:27.

31. Eto RT, Anderson PW, Harley JD. Elbow arthrography with the application of tomography. *Radiology*. 1975;115:283–288.

32. Godfroy D, Pallardy G, Chevrot A, Zenny JC. Arthrography of the elbow: anatomical and radiological consideration and technical considerations. *J Radiol*. 1981;62:441–447.

33. Greenspan A, Norman A. Radial-head–capitellar view: an expanded imaging approach to elbow injury. *Radiology*. 1987;164:272–274.

34. Greenspan A, Norman A. The radial head, capitellar view. Another example of its usefulness. *AJR*. 1982;139:193.

35. Greenspan A, Norman A. The radial head, capitellar view. Useful technique in elbow trauma. *AJR*. 1982;138:1186–1188.

36. Greenspan A, Norman A, Rosen H. Radial head–capitellum view in elbow trauma: clinical application and radiographic anatomic correlation. *AJR*. 1984;143:355–359.

37. Hall-Craggs MA, Shorvon PJ, Chapman M. Assessment of the radial head–capitellum view and the dorsal fat pad sign in acute elbow trauma. *AJR*. 1985;145:607–609.

38. Hindman BW, Schreiber RR, Wiss DA, Ghilarducci MJ, Avolio RE. Supracondylar fractures of the humerus: Prediction of the cubitus varus deformity with CT. *Radiology*. 1988;168:513–515.

39. Hoffman AD. Radiography of the pediatric elbow. In: Morrey BF, ed. *The Elbow and its Disorders*. Philadelphia: Saunders; 1985:153–160.

40. Jasefsson PO, Andren L, Gentz CF, Johnell O. Arthrography of the distal elbow joint. *Acta Radiol Diagn*. 1984;25:143–145.

41. Kohn AM. Soft tissue alterations in elbow trauma. *Am J Roentgenol Radium Ther Nucl Med*. 1959;82:867–874.

42. London JT. Kinematics of the elbow. *J Bone Joint Surg Am*. 1981;63:529–535.

43. Mink JH, Eckhardt JJ, Grant TT. Arthrography in recurrent dislocation of the elbow. *AJR*. 1981;136:1242–1244.

44. Murry WA, Siegel MJ. Elbow fat pads with new signs and extended differential diagnosis. *Radiology*. 1977;124:659–665.

45. Norell HG. Roentgenologic visualization of the extracapsular fat. Its importance in the diagnosis of traumatic injuries to the elbow. *Acta Radiol*. 1954;42:205–210.

46. Obermann WR, Loose HWC. The os supratrochleare dorsale: a normal variant that may cause symptoms. *AJR*. 1983;141:123–127.

47. Page AC. Critical evaluation of the radial head–capitellum view in elbow trauma. *AJR*. 1986;146:81–82.

48. Pavlov H, Ghelman B, Warren RF. Double-contrast arthrography of the elbow. *Radiology*. 1979;130:87–95.

49. Roback DL. Elbow arthrography: brief technical considerations. *Clin Radiol*. 1979;30:311–312.

50. Rogers SL, MacEwan DW. Changes due to trauma in the fat plane overlying the supinator muscle: a radiographic sign. *Radiology*. 1969;92:954.

51. Smith DN, Lee JR. The radiological diagnosis of post-traumatic effusion of the elbow joint and its clinical significance: the displaced fat pad sign. *Injury*. 1978;10:115–119.

52. Surgson RD, Feldman F, Rosenberg ZS. Elbow joint: assessment with double-contrast CT arthrography. *Radiology*. 1986;160:167–173.

53. Teng MM, Murphy WA, Gilula LD, et al. Elbow arthrography: a reassessment of technique. *Radiology*. 1984;153:611–613.

54. Weston WJ. *Arthrography*. New York: Springer-Verlag; 1980.

55. Yousefzadeh DK, Jackson JH. Lipohemarthrosis of the elbow joint. *Radiology*. 1978;128:643–645.

Soft Tissue Injuries

56. Anzel SH, Covey KW, Weiner AD, Lipscomb DR. Disruption of muscles and tendons: analysis of 1,014 cases. *Surgery*. 1989;45:406–414.

57. Baker BE. Current concepts in the diagnosis and treatment of musculotendinous injuries. *Med Sci Sports Exerc*. 1984;16:323–327.

58. Barnes DA, Tullos HS. An analysis of 100 symptomatic baseball players. *Am J Sports Med*. 1978;6:62–67.

59. Bell SN, Morrey BF, Bianco AJ. Chronic posterior subluxation and dislocation of the radial head. *J Bone Joint Surg Am*. 1991;73:392–396.

60. Berquist TH. *Magnetic Resonance Imaging of the Musculoskeletal System*. 2nd ed. New York: Raven; 1990.

61. Davis WM, Jassine Z. An etiologic factor in the tear of the distal tendon of the biceps brachii. *J Bone Joint Surg Am*. 1956;38:1365–1368.

62. DeLee JC, Green DP, Wilkins KE. Fractures and dislocations of the elbow. In: Rockwood CA, Green DP, eds. *Fractures in Adults*. 2nd ed. Philadelphia: Lippincott; 1984;1:559–652.

63. Dreyfuss U. Snapping elbow due to dislocation of the medial head of the triceps. *J Bone Joint Surg Br*. 1978;60:56–57.

64. Farrar EL III, Lippert FG III. Avulsion of the triceps tendon. *Clin Orthop*. 1981;161:242–246.

65. Herrick RT, Herrick S. Ruptured triceps in a powerlifter presenting as a cubital tunnel syndrome. *Am J Sports Med*. 1987;15:514–516.

66. Jobe FW, Fanton GS. Nerve injuries. In: Morrey BF, ed. *The Elbow and its Disorders*. Philadelphia: Saunders; 1985:497–501.

67. Jorgensen U, Hinge K, Rye B. Rupture of the distal biceps brachii tendon. *J Trauma*. 1986;26:1061–1062.

68. Josefsson O, Gentz C, Johnell O, Wendenberg B. Surgical versus non-surgical treatment of ligamentous injuries following dislocation of the elbow joint. *J Bone Joint Surg Am*. 1987;69:605–608.

69. King JW, Brelsford HJ, Tullos HS. Analysis of the pitching arm of the professional baseball player. *Clin Orthop*. 1969;67:116–123.

70. Kopell HP, Thompson WAL. The pronator syndrome. *N Engl J Med*. 1958;259:713–715.

71. Levy M, Fischel RE, Stern GM. Triceps tendon avulsion with or without fracture of the radial head—a rare injury? *J Trauma*. 1978;18:677–680.

72. Linscheid RL, Wheeler DK. Elbow dislocations. *JAMA*. 1965;194:1171–1176.

73. Micheli LJ, Smith AD. Sports injuries in children. *Curr Probl Pediatr*. 1982:3–54.

74. Morrey BF. *The Elbow and its Disorders*. Philadelphia: Saunders; 1985.

75. Morrey BF, Askew LJ, An KN, Dobyns JH. Rupture of the distal biceps tendon: biomechanical assessment of different treatment options. *J Bone Joint Surg Am*. 1985;67:418–421.

76. Nirschl RP. Muscle and tendon trauma: tennis elbow. In: Morrey BF, ed. *The Elbow and its Disorders*. Philadelphia: Saunders; 1985:481–496.

77. Nirschl RP. Prevention and treatment of elbow and shoulder injuries in the tennis player. *Clin Sports Med*. 1988;7:289–308.

78. Norwood LA, Shook JA, Andrews JR. Acute medial elbow ruptures. *Am J Sports Med*. 1981;9:16–19.

79. Osborne G, Cotterill P. Recurrent dislocation of the elbow. *J Bone Joint Surg Br*. 1966;48:340–346.

80. Schwab GH, Bennett JB, Woods GW, Tullos HS. Biomechanics of elbow instability: the role of the medial collateral ligament. *Clin Orthop*. 1980;146:42–52.

81. Spinner M, Linscheid RL. Nerve entrapment syndromes. In: Morrey BF, ed. *The Elbow and its Disorders*. Philadelphia: Saunders; 1985:691–712.

82. Sutherland S. *Nerves and Nerve Injuries*. Baltimore: Williams & Wilkins; 1978.

83. Wadsworth TG. *The Elbow*. Edinburgh: Churchill Livingstone; 1982.

84. Wojtys EM, Smith PA, Hankin FM. A cause of ulnar neuropathy in a baseball pitcher. *Am J Sports Med*. 1986;14:422–424.

85. Yocum LA. Diagnosis and nonoperative treatment of elbow problems in the athlete. *Clin Sports Med*. 1989;8:439–451.

Fractures and Osseous Injuries

86. Adams JE. Injury to the throwing arm. *Calif Med*. 1965;102:127–132.

87. Anderson LD. Fractures of the shafts of the radius and ulna. In: Rockwood CA, Green DP, eds. *Fractures in Adults*. Philadelphia: Lippincott; 1984;1:511–558.

88. Arner O, Ekengren K, Von Schreeh T. Fractures of the head and neck of the radius. A clinical and roentgenographic study of 310 cases. *Acta Chir Scand*. 1957;112:115–134.

89. Bado JL. The Monteggio lesion. *Clin Orthop*. 1967;50:71–86.

90. Bakali MG. Fractures of the radial head and their treatment. *Orthop Scand*. 1970;41:320–331.

91. Beck C, Dabezies EJ. Monteggio fracture-dislocation. *Orthopedics*. 1984;7:329–331.

92. Berquist TH. *Imaging of Orthopedic Trauma*. 2nd ed. New York: Raven; 1991.

93. Bianco AJ. Osteochondritis dissecans. In: Morrey BF, ed. *The Elbow and its Disorders*. Philadelphia: Saunders; 1985:254–259.

94. Bryan RS, Bickel WH. T-Condylar fractures of the distal humerus. *J Trauma*. 1971;11:830–836.

95. Buxton JD. Ossification in ligaments of the elbow joints. *J Bone Joint Surg Am*. 1938;20:709–714.

96. Byron BG, Crow NE. Little Leaguer's elbow. *Am J Roentgenol Radium Ther Nucl Med*. 1960;83:671–675.

97. Chapman MW, Gordon JE, Zissimos AG. Compression plate fixation of acute forearm fractures of the diaphysis of the radius and ulna. *J Bone Joint Surg Am*. 1989;71:159–169.

98. Conn J, Wade P. Injuries of the elbow. A 10 year review. *J Trauma*. 1961;1:248–268.

99. Corbett RH. Displaced fat pads in trauma to the elbow. *Injury*. 1978;9:297–298.

100. DeLee JC, Green DP, Wilkins KE. Fractures and dislocations of the elbow. In: Rockwood CA, Green DP, eds. *Fractures in Adults*. 2nd ed. Philadelphia: Lippincott; 1984;1:559–652.

101. Edman P, Lohr G. Supracondylar fractures of the humerus treated wiht olecranon traction. *Acta Chir Scand*. 1963;126:505–516.

102. Essex-Lopresti P. Fractures of the radial head with distal ulnar dislocation. *J Bone Joint Surg Br*. 1951;33:244–247.

103. Failla JM, Amadio PC, Morrey BF. Post-traumatic proximal radioulnar synostosis. *J Bone Joint Surg Am*. 1989;71:1208–1213.

104. Fowles JV, Karsab MJ. Fracture of the capitellum humeri. *J Bone Joint Surg Am*. 1974;56:794–798.

105. Grace TG, Eversman WW. Forearm fractures. *J Bone Joint Surg Am*. 1980;62:433–438.

106. Grantham SA, Norris TR, Bush DC. Isolated fracture of the humeral capitellum. *Clin Orthop*. 1981;161:262–269.

107. Hindman BW, Schreiber RR, Wiss DA, Ghilarducci MJ, Avolio RE. Supracondylar fracture of the humerus: Prediction of cubitus varus deformity with CT. *Radiology*. 1988;168:513–515.

108. Hoffman AD. Radiography of the pediatric elbow. In: Morrey BF, ed. *The Elbow and its Disorders*. Philadelphia: Saunders; 1985:153–160.

109. Horne G. Supracondylar fracture of the humerus in adults. *J Trauma*. 1980;20:71–74.

110. Jessing P. Monteggia lesions and their complicating nerve damage. *Acta Orthop Scand*. 1975;46:601–609.

111. Klassen RA. Supracondylar fractures of the elbow in children. In: Morrey BF, ed. *The Elbow and its Disorders*. Philadelphia: Saunders; 1985:182–221.

112. Larson RL. Epiphyseal injuries in the adolescent athlete. *Orthop Clin North Am.* 1973;4:839–851.

113. Lipscomb PR, Burleson RJ. Vascular and neural complications in supracondylar fractures of the humerus in children. *J Bone Joint Surg Am.* 1955;37:487–492.

114. Mason MB. Some observations on fractures of the head of the radius with a review of one hundred cases. *Br J Surg.* 1954;42:123–132.

115. Milch H. Unusual fracture of the capitellum humeri and capitellum radii. *J Bone Joint Surg Am.* 1931;13:882–886.

116. Morrey BF. *The Elbow and its Disorders.* Philadelphia: Saunders; 1985.

117. Peterson HA. Physeal fractures. In: Morrey BF, ed. *The Elbow and its Disorders.* Philadelphia: Saunders; 1985:222–236.

118. Raden EL, Riseborough EJ. Fractures of the radial head. *J Bone Joint Surg Am.* 1966;48:1055–1061.

119. Reckling FW. Unstable fracture dislocation of the forearm (Monteggia and Galeazzi lesions). *J Bone Joint Surg Am.* 1982;64:857–863.

120. Regan W, Morrey BF. Fractures of the coronoid process of the ulna. *J Bone Joint Surg Am.* 1989;71:1348–1354.

121. Riseborough EJ, Raden EL. Intercondylar T-fractures of the humerus in the adult. *J Bone Joint Surg Am.* 1969;51:130–141.

122. Smith H, Sage FP. Medullary fixation of forearm fractures. *J Bone Joint Surg Am.* 1957;39:91–98.

123. Vince KG, Miller JE. Cross union complicating fracture of the forearm. Part I: adults. *J Bone Joint Surg Am.* 1987;69:640–660.

124. Wilkins KE. Fractures and dislocations of the elbow region. In: Rockwood CA, Wilkins KE, Kurg RE, eds. *Fractures in Children.* Philadelphia: JB Lippincott; 1984:363–576.

Chapter 11

Hand and Wrist

INTRODUCTION

Sports injuries to the lower extremities are more likely to result in reduced participation and prolonged rehabilitation than injuries to the hand and wrist. In some cases, even significant hand injuries (ie, fractures) do not prevent participation in sports.[3,12]

Injuries to the hand and wrist represent 25% to 30% of athletic injuries.[2,6,11,13] Direct trauma, such as a fall, and chronic overuse are commonly implicated. Direct trauma is common in contact sports. In order of decreasing frequency, the injury may result in a sprain, contusion, phalangeal fracture, or metacarpal fracture.[3] In children injuries occur most frequently in football, basketball, and gymnastics.[1,4,5,13] Skiing and martial arts also commonly result in hand and wrist injury. The hand and wrist are rarely injured in soccer and swimming.[2,6,8–10,13] In adults, other sports such as tennis, golf, racquetball, and bowling are implicated.[7,12]

ANATOMY

A thorough understanding of the complex bone and soft tissue anatomy of the hand and wrist is essential for optimizing the imaging approach to athletes with suspected injury. This chapter summarizes the pertinent normal and abnormal anatomic features related to traumatic conditions in the hand and wrist.

Osseous Anatomy

The wrist includes the distal metaphysis of the radius and ulna and the entire carpus. There are multiple articulations in the wrist. From the functional aspect, these fall into three main articular groups: the distal radioulnar joint, the radiocarpal articulation, and the so-called midcarpal articulation.[33]

The distal radial metaphysis and epiphysis are largely composed of cancellous bone with a relatively thin cortex, which explains the high frequency of fractures in this area. The extreme radial aspect is elongated distally as a styloid process. The distal articular surface of the radius has two fossae for the scaphoid and lunate, respectively. These are separated by a variably defined vertical ridge. This surface of the radius is inclined 14° toward the ulna in the frontal plane (Fig. 11-1A) and 12° toward the palmar surface in the lateral plane (Fig. 11-1B).[15] On the ulnar aspect of the distal radius is a separate concave joint surface called the sigmoid notch for articulation with the distal ulna. There are series of sulci and ridges on the dorsal radius that define the floor of the first through fourth dorsal tendinous compartments of the wrist. The most readily palpable protuberance of this surface is Lister's tubercle, which lies between the compartment of the radial wrist extensor tendons (second) and that of the extensor pollicis longus tendon (third). The first (most radial) dorsal compartment contains the abductor pollicis longus and extensor pollicis brevis tendons, and the fourth compartment contains the extensor digitorum communis tendons to all fingers as well as the proprius tendon of the index digit (Fig. 11-2).[20,33]

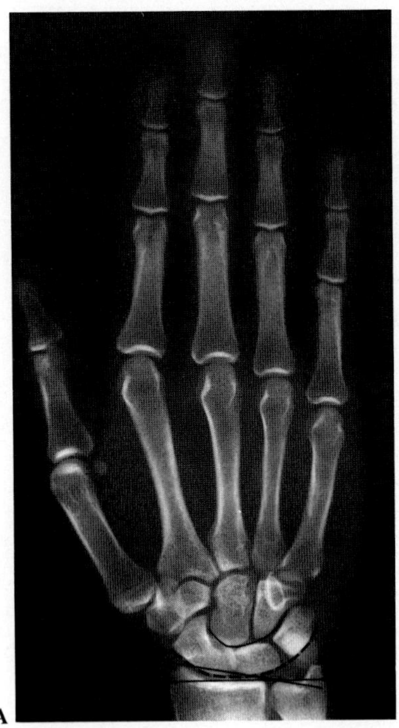

A

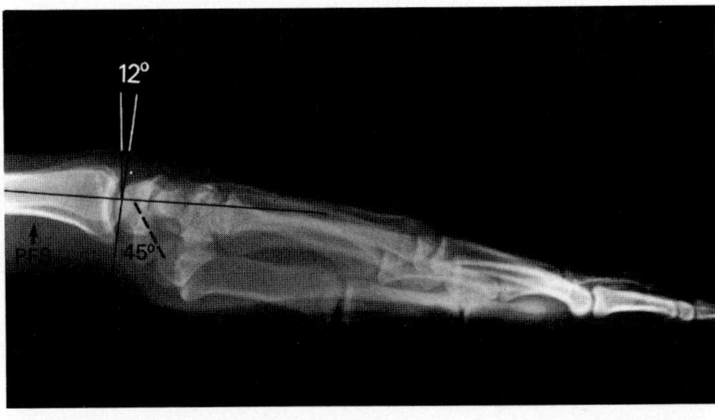

B

Fig. 11-1 (**A**) Posteroanterior (PA) and (**B**) lateral views of the right hand and wrist demonstrating the normal smooth arch formed by the carpal bones (dotted line in **A**), the distal radial angle (**B**), and the scapholunate angle (45°). PFS, Pronator fat stripe.

The distal ulna is also predominantly composed of cancellous bone but with a reasonably thick cortex. It has a spikelike, well-defined styloid process. Fracture of this process not infrequently accompanies a fracture of the distal radius. The ulnar head articulates with the distal radius, lunate, and triquetrum. It is usually separated from the latter two bones by an articular disc, which is a portion of the triangular fibrocartilage complex. The dorsal surface of the ulna has sulci for the fifth and sixth dorsal compartments of the wrist, which house the extensor digiti quinti and extensor carpi ulnaris tendons, respectively (Fig. 11-2). The position of the distal articular surface of the ulna relative to that of the radius may have significance in certain clinical situations and is defined by the term *ulnar variance*.[17] In most patients the ulna is either equal to (neutral) or 1 mm shorter than the radius. Ulnar variance is positive if the ulnar articular surface is more distal than that of the radius. Conversely, it is negative if the ulnar articular surface lies more proximally (Fig. 11-3). The distal radioulnar joint in conjunction with the proximal radioulnar joint at the elbow permits rotation of the radius about the ulna in the process of forearm pronation and supination. Normally an arc of 160° to 180° of rotation is possible.[15,33]

The carpus is composed of three anatomic groups (Fig. 11-4).[33] The proximal row (first anatomic group) consists of the scaphoid, lunate, triquetrum, and overlapping pisiform. The scaphoid and triquetrum are firmly bound to the lunate by strong interosseous ligaments. The stability of these articulations is essential for normal wrist mechanics.[32] The proximal articular surfaces of these three bones should define a smooth, unbroken arc in the frontal plane (Fig. 11-1A). In this same projection the scaphoid tubercle will present a ringlike appearance in the distal half of the bone, and the lunate should appear trapezoidal. The distance between the scaphoid and lunate or between the lunate and triquetrum should be relatively constant in all positions of the wrist. Normally this distance should not exceed 2 mm.[16] The position of the scaphoid and lunate should be congruous with the scaphoid and lunate fossae of the distal radius. Ulnar translation of the carpus relative to the radius may be seen in conditions of chronic wrist synovitis and in disruption of the radiocarpal ligament complex, particularly if accompanied by dorsal subluxation of the distal ulna. This instability pattern is characterized by the presence of an apparently widened joint space between the lateral radial articular surface and the scaphoid. In the lateral plane with the wrist in neutral, the lunate should generally be colinear with the radius and should appear symmetric within the lunate fossa. The scaphoid outline may be

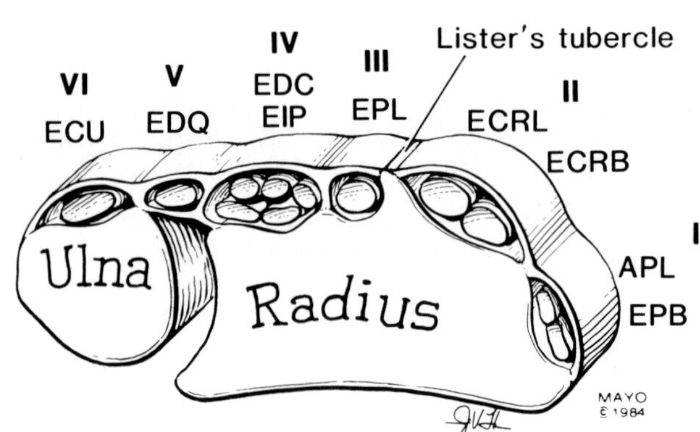

Fig. 11-2 Illustration of the distal radius demonstrating the six dorsal compartments. I, Abductor pollicis longus (APL) and extensor pollicis brevis (EPB); II, extensor carpi radialis longus (ECRL) and extensor carpi radialis brevis (ECRB); III, extensor pollicis longus (EPL); IV, extensor digitorum communis (EDC) and extensor indicis proprius (EIP); V, extensor digiti quinti (EDQ); VI, extensor carpi ulnaris (ECU). *Source:* Reprinted from *Imaging of Orthopedic Trauma* ed 2 by TH Berquist, 1991, Raven Press, © Mayo Foundation.

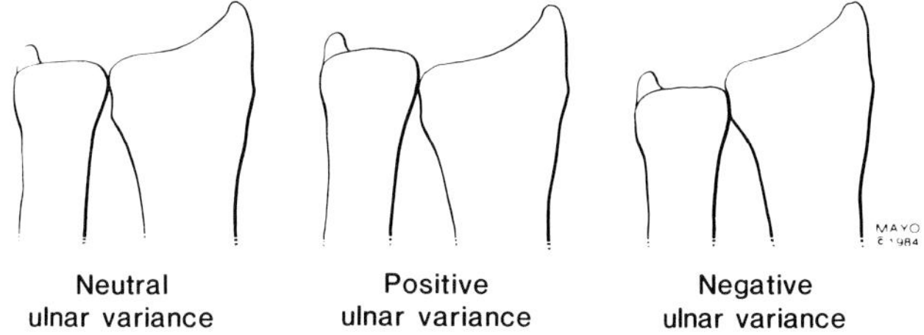

Fig. 11-3 Illustrations of neutral, positive, and negative ulnar variance. *Source:* Reprinted from *Imaging of Orthopedic Trauma* ed 2 by TH Berquist, 1991, Raven Press, © Mayo Foundation.

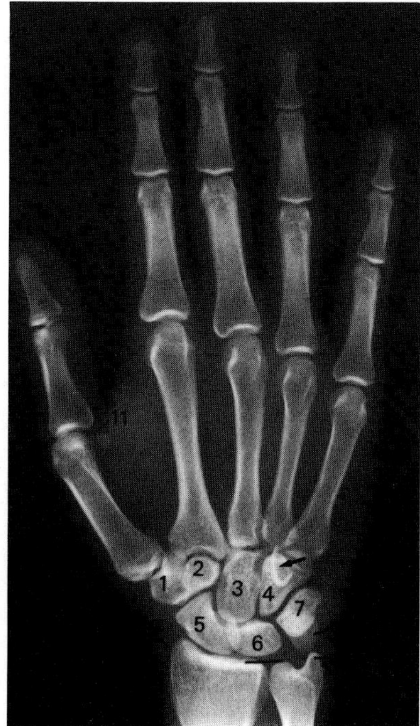

Fig. 11-4 PA view of the wrist demonstrating the carpal bones. 1, Trapezium; 2, trapezoid; 3, capitate; 4, hamate; 5, scaphoid; 6, lunate; 7, triquetrum; 8, pisiform and radial (9) and ulnar (10) styloid processes; 11, sesamoids of the thumb. The arrow indicates the hook of the hamate.

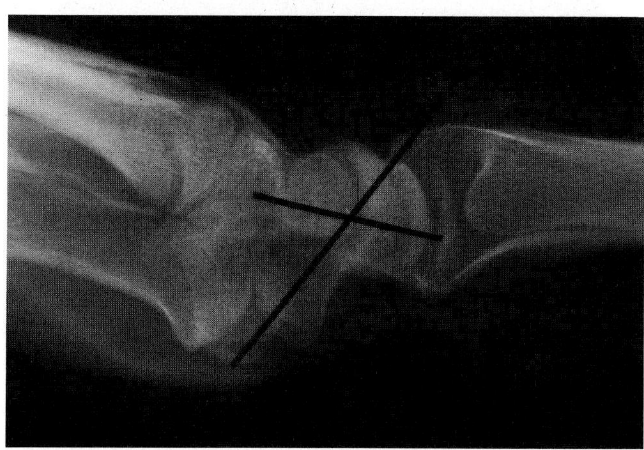

Fig. 11-5 Lateral view of the wrist demonstrating the normal position of the lunate and scaphoid and the scapholunate angle.

difficult to visualize owing to bony overlap. With the wrist in a neutral position, however, it should point obliquely in a palmar direction. A line drawn through its long axis should form an angle of 30° to 60° (mean, 47°) with a line drawn through the axis of the lunate (Fig. 11-5).[15,16] This angle is called the scapholunate angle and may be abnormal in certain collapse deformities of the wrist. The position of the scaphoid relative to the lunate, however, will vary with ulnar or radial deviation of the wrist.[22,30] This should be borne in mind when assessing the scapholunate angle. As the wrist moves from complete ulnar deviation to complete radial deviation, the scaphoid will subtend in an arc of 40° (Fig. 11-6). The pisiform is a true sesamoid bone, lying within the flexor carpi ulnaris tendon. It forms a synovial articulation with the triquetrum.[20,33–35]

The second anatomic group, the distal carpal row, consists of the trapezoid, capitate, and hamate, which are tightly bound by strong interosseous ligaments. The hook (hamulus) of the hamate will present an overlying ringlike appearance in the frontal projection (Figs. 11-1A and 11-4). On the lateral view the capitate should articulate congruently with the lunate; with the wrist in a neutral position, these two bones along with the radius should be colinear (Figs. 11-5 and 11-6).[23] This relationship may be lost in collapse deformities of the wrist.[25,33]

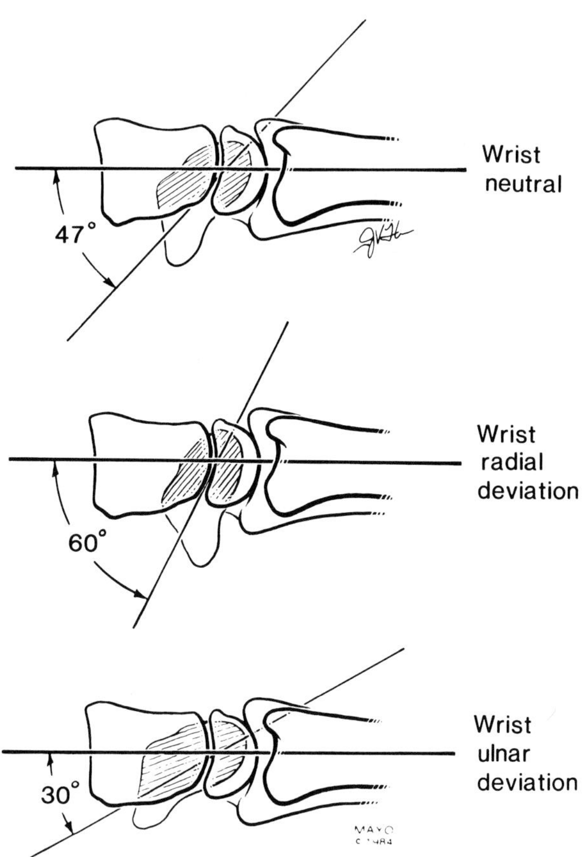

Fig. 11-6 Illustrations showing changes in the scapholunate angle with the wrist in neutral and in radial and ulnar deviation. *Source:* Reprinted from *Imaging of Orthopedic Trauma* ed 2 by TH Berquist, 1991, Raven Press, © Mayo Foundation.

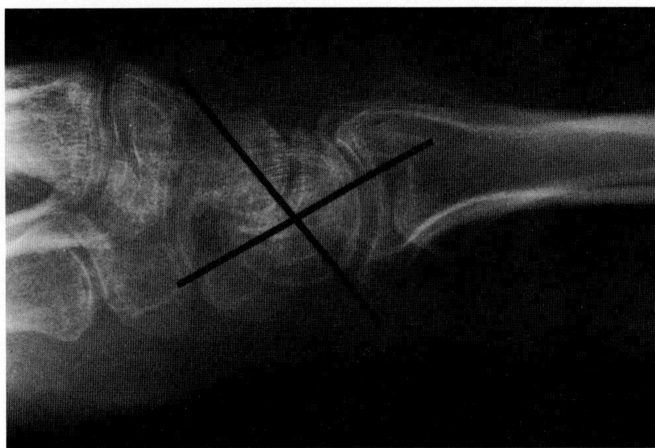

Fig. 11-7 Lateral view of the wrist demonstrating the dorsal intercalated segment instability collapse pattern (DISI). The scapholunate angle is increased, and the lunate is directed dorsally.

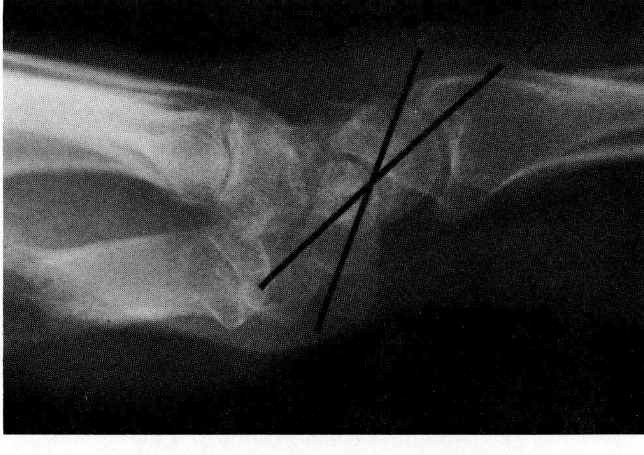

Fig. 11-8 Lateral view of the wrist demonstrating the volar intercalated segment instability collapse pattern (VISI). The scapholunate angle is decreased, and the lunate faces volarly.

Two basic patterns of collapse deformity are recognized and are defined by the direction of the lunate relative to the capitate.[25] The first and most common is a dorsal intercalated segment instability (DISI) pattern. This is characterized on the lateral projection by the lunate appearing to be dorsiflexed on the radius and the capitate palmar flexed on the lunate (Fig. 11-7). DISI is most commonly associated with fractures of the scaphoid and complete disruption of the scapholunate interosseous ligament.[18,25] In such cases, therefore, an additional radiographic finding will be an exaggeration of the scapholunate angle.[33]

The second major category of collapse deformity is referred to as a volar intercalated segment instability (VISI) pattern. This type is characterized by the lunate assuming a palmar flexed position relative to the radius with the capitate dorsiflexed relative to the lunate (Fig. 11-8).[24,25] It is most commonly associated with lunotriquetral ligament rupture or midcarpal sprains.[33] With VISI a reduction of the scapholunate angle is frequently seen.

It is important to emphasize that the diagnosis of either of these two collapse patterns can be made only on the basis of a true lateral radiograph with the wrist in a neutral position. The diagnosis is further supported by the apparent persistence of the collapse pattern on true lateral radiographs obtained with the wrist in a fully extended and fully flexed position.[25,33]

There are five metacarpals. The first (thumb) metacarpal lies outside the plane of the others in an oblique palmar direction. Each metacarpal is flared proximally and distally and is composed chiefly of cancellous bone and a narrow diaphysis of cortical bone (Fig. 11-1). The joint space of the carpometacarpal articulations, especially the second and third, may be poorly visualized on routine radiographs because of bony overlap. These joints have minimal motion. The fourth and fifth carpometacarpal joints, however, usually do have a well-defined joint space, which is best visualized on anteroposterior (AP) and oblique projections (Fig. 11-9), and also have a range of motion between 15° and 40°.[19] Adjacent metacarpals are stabilized with respect to each other by strong proximal interosseous ligaments and by the transverse metacarpal ligaments distally. The metacarpal head is eccentric in shape, its palmar aspect being broader than its dorsum. This configuration allows relaxation of the collateral ligaments with lateral motion for abduction of the fingers with the metacarpophalangeal joint in a position of extension. Conversely, flexion of the joint tightens the collateral ligaments and allows

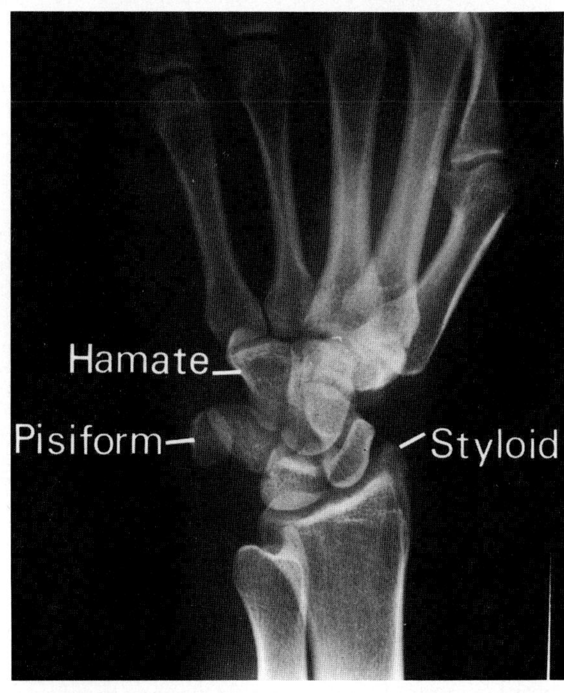

Fig. 11-9 Oblique view of the wrist demonstrating the bases of the fourth and fifth metacarpals.

for little lateral motion. In all positions of the metacarpophalangeal joint, however, the respective articular surfaces should appear congruent.[33]

The proximal and middle phalanges of the fingers are similar in structure, having flared proximal and distal ends composed chiefly of cancellous bone (Fig. 11-1). The diaphysis consists predominantly of cortical bone and is cylindric. The distal articular surface of the phalanges is bicondylar and is intimately congruent with the adjacent articulation on both frontal and lateral planes. The thumb lacks a middle phalanx and thus has only a single interphalangeal joint. The distal phalanx is foreshortened with its distal end flared in the shape of a blunt arrowhead on the frontal projection.[20,33]

Small, spheric sesamoid bones, although varying in position and number, are frequently seen in pairs volar to the metacarpophalangeal joints or in the interphalangeal joint of the thumb (Fig. 11-4). Moreover, occasionally accessory ossicles can be visualized about the hand and wrist. At least 16 accessory ossification centers have been reported.[28] The most significant of this group is probably the os centrale. If this ossification center fails to unite to the scaphoid, confusion with a so-called bipartite scaphoid may be possible. Another accessory ossicle described by some investigators is the so-called styloid bone, which lies in the region of the second and third carpometacarpal joint. Whether this represents a true accessory ossicle or a reactive process is debatable, but it may present as a symptomatic carpe bosseau. Other well-known accessory ossification centers are the lunula, which lies between the triquetrum and the ulnar styloid, and the os radiali externum at the distal end of the scaphoid. The order of ossification of the normal carpal bones is somewhat variable. In general, however, the center of ossification appears for the capitate at 6 months, for the hamate at 6 to 18 months, for the triquetrum at 2 years, for the lunate at 4 years, for the trapezium at 5 years, for the trapezoid at 6 years, for the scaphoid at 5 to 6 years, and for the pisiform at 10 years.[28,33]

Ligamentous Anatomy

The stability of the distal radioulnar joint and a major component of the ulnocarpal articulation depends on the integrity of the triangular fibrocartilage complex.[23,29,30] This complex consists of multiple components that blend together to form the triangular fibrocartilage proper (Fig. 11-10). The apex of the triangular fibrocartilage originates from the base of the ulnar styloid process and fans out to insert broadly along the ulnar margin of the distal radius. Perforations can occur centrally that may or may not be of clinical significance.[27,28,30] The dorsal and volar margins of the fibrocartilage are thickened, blending with the respective radioulnar ligaments, capsular ligaments of the wrist, and lunotriquetral interosseous ligaments. The ulnocarpal meniscus component arises near the insertion of the articular disc on the radius and courses distally, inserting into the triquetrum and hamate. Its extreme ulnar aspect blends with the ulnar collateral ligament

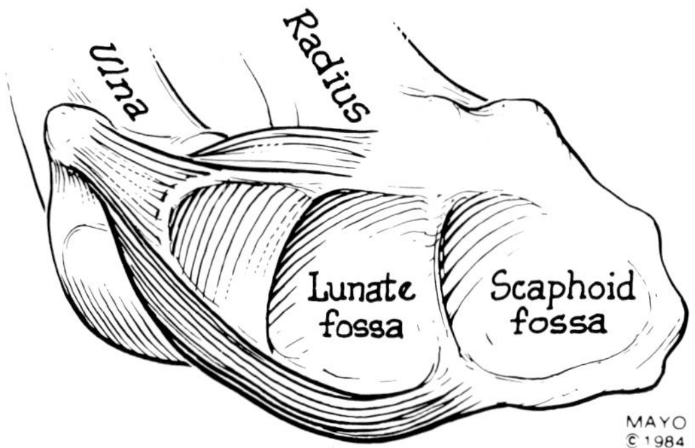

Fig. 11-10 Illustration of the triangular fibrocartilage complex. *Source:* Reprinted from *Imaging of Orthopedic Trauma* ed 2 by TH Berquist, 1991, Raven Press, © Mayo Foundation.

fibers. Other factors contributing to the stability of the distal radioulnar joint include the interosseous membrane of the radius and ulna, the extensor carpi ulnaris tendon and its retaining fibroosseous sheath, and finally the degree of concavity of the sigmoid notch of the radius.[20,33]

Both volar and dorsal ligaments contribute to the stability of the radiocarpal aspect of the wrist. The volar group is most significant clinically.[33] The palmar (volar) capsular ligaments are most obvious when viewed intracapsularly.[21,26,32] Basically they consist of two concentric arches originating from the volar lip of the radius and inserting into the triquetrum and triangular fibrocartilage complex (Fig. 11-11). The first arch is composed of the radiolunotriquetral ligament, which

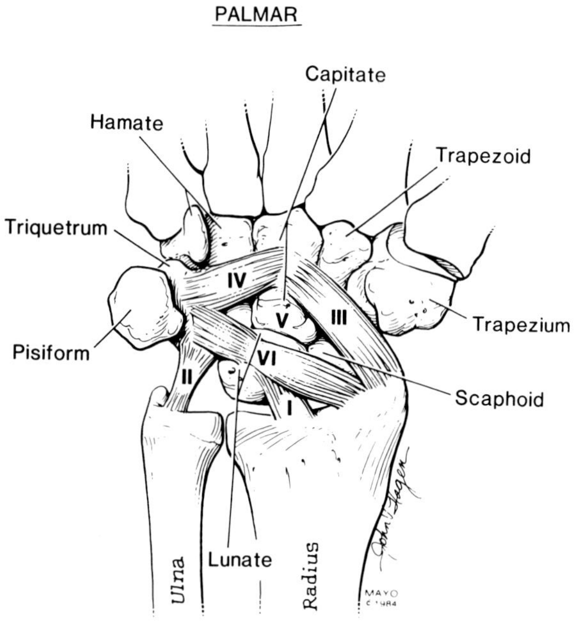

PALMAR
Capitate
Hamate
Trapezoid
Triquetrum
IV
V
III
Trapezium
Pisiform
VI
II
I
Scaphoid
Ulna
Lunate
Radius
MAYO

Fig. 11-11 Illustration of palmar ligaments of the wrist. I, Radiolunotriquetral; II, ulnotriquetral; III, radiocapitate; IV, capitotriquetral; V, space of Poirier; VI, radioscapholunate. *Source:* Reprinted from *Imaging of Orthopedic Trauma* ed 2 by TH Berquist, 1991, Raven Press, © Mayo Foundation.

courses from the radius across the volar surface of the lunate, inserts into the volar surface of the lunate, and then inserts firmly on the triquetrum. The ulnotriquetral ligament then completes the arch. The second arch is made up of the radiocapitate ligament, which originates more laterally on the radius, passes across the waist of the scaphoid, and inserts into the capitate. This arch is completed by the capitotriquetral ligament and the ulnotriquetral ligament. Between these two arches is a rather thinned area of the volar wrist capsule known as the space of Poirier. In addition to the double ligamentous arch of the palmar capsule there is a short but stout radioscapholunate ligament. This structure arises from the volar lip of the radius and courses obliquely distally and dorsally to insert on the volar and middle aspect of the scapholunate interosseous ligaments. The dorsal capsular ligaments of the wrist are relatively thin and of lesser significance than their palmar counterparts. The most important components are the radiolunotriquetral and ulnotriquetral ligaments (Fig. 11-12). Both dorsal and volar complexes are reinforced by a radial and ulnar collateral ligament complex.

In addition to the extrinsic capsular ligaments, intrinsic intercarpal ligaments contribute to the stability of the radiocarpal and intercarpal articulations. These include the scapholunate and lunotriquetral interosseous ligaments in the proximal carpal row and both dorsal and volar interosseous ligaments connecting the hamate, capitate, trapezoid, and trapezium. The preserved integrity of the extrinsic capsular and intrinsic intercarpal ligaments is essential for normal wrist stability and mechanisms.[16,21,22,24,31,33–35]

Ligamentous support of the carpometacarpal articulations is provided by longitudinally oriented dorsal and volar carpometacarpal ligaments. These vary in location, number, and strength according to the joint involved. The first carpometacarpal joint is relatively lax, allowing considerable motion in several degrees of freedom. Often its inherent instability is a source of clinical concern. The chief ligamentous support is provided by the palmar and dorsal oblique capsular ligaments. The former is strongest and most important. By contrast, the second and third carpometacarpal joints are extremely stable, having negligible motion. Strong, short capsular ligaments pass from the trapezoid to both radial and ulnar condyles of the second metacarpal on both volar and dorsal aspects of the joint. The third metacarpal base is stabilized by obliquely disposed dorsal ligaments passing from the trapezoid and capitate as well as by a volar ligament from the capitate and hamate. The fourth and fifth carpometacarpal joints have a moderate range of motion in the plane of flexion and extension and, therefore, are stabilized by less stout capsular ligaments. These arise on both dorsal and volar aspects from the capitate and hamate to the base of the fourth metacarpal and from the hamate along to the base of the fifth metacarpal. The carpometacarpal articulations are further stabilized by strong transverse intermetacarpal ligaments between the bases of the second through fifth metacarpals. Moreover, these same metacarpals are weakly stabilized distally by distal transverse intermetacarpal ligaments.[33]

Ligamentous support of the metacarpophalangeal joints is similar in all digits and depends primarily upon the collateral ligaments, the accessory collateral ligaments, and the fibrocartilaginous volar plate (Fig. 11-13). The collateral ligaments are well-defined capsular structures that arise from a dorsal position on either side of the metacarpal just proximal to its articular head. These structures then pass in a palmar and distal direction to insert onto the volar lateral aspect of the base of the proximal phalanx. The fibrocartilaginous volar plate arises from the base of the proximal phalanx and inserts into the volar aspect of the metacarpal just proximal to the articular surface. It is thick distally but becomes thin and compliant proximally. It is intimately associated with the distal intermetacarpal ligaments and proximal flexor tendon sheath pulley system. Between the collateral ligaments and the volar plate are the interconnecting fibers of the accessory collateral ligaments.

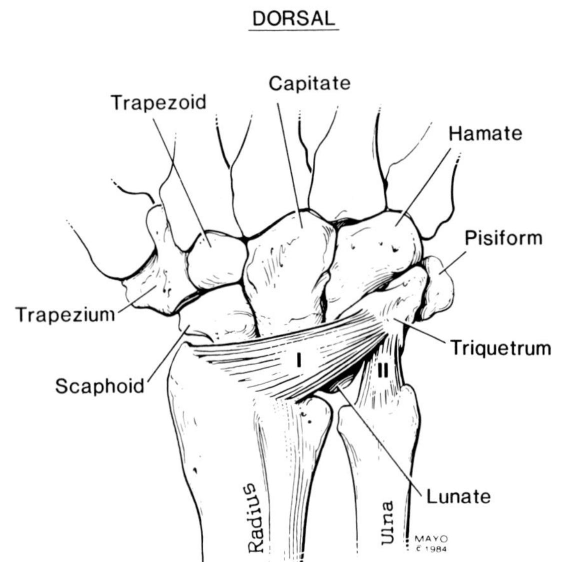

Fig. 11-12 Illustration of the dorsal ligaments of the wrist. I, Radiolunotriquetral; II, ulnotriquetral. *Source:* Reprinted from *Imaging of Orthopedic Trauma* ed 2 by TH Berquist, 1991, Raven Press, © Mayo Foundation.

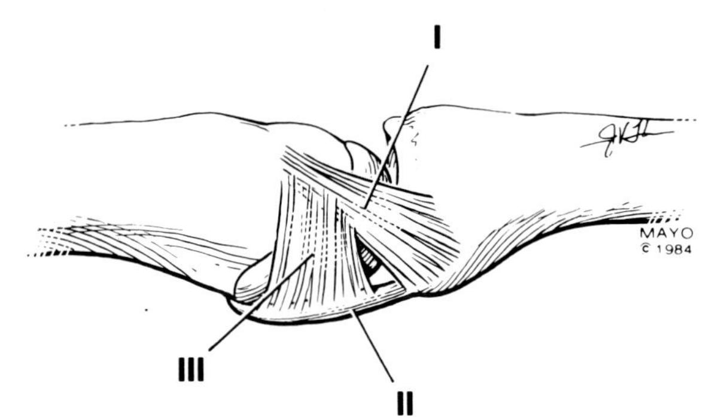

Fig. 11-13 Illustration of the metacarpophalangeal ligaments. I, Collateral ligaments; II, volar plate; III, accessory collateral ligaments. *Source:* Reprinted from *Imaging of Orthopedic Trauma* ed 2 by TH Berquist, 1991, Raven Press, © Mayo Foundation.

Dorsal to the collateral ligaments, the joint capsule is thin and closely associated with the extensor apparatus. As such, the dorsal capsule contributes relatively little stability to the joint. The metacarpophalangeal articulation allows considerable lateral motion, particularly in a position of extension, owing to the eccentricity and relatively spheric shape of the metacarpal head. Of particular clinical significance for collateral ligament injury is the metacarpophalangeal joint of the thumb. This joint is covered by a well-defined extensor aponeurosis, which may become interposed with complete ruptures of the ulnar collateral ligament.[23,33]

Ligamentous support of the interphalangeal joints is basically identical in all digits and is quite similar to the arrangement described earlier for the metacarpophalangeal joints.[23] The volar fibrocartilaginous plate of this joint, however, is thickened on its lateral extreme, where it is most firmly attached to the base of the middle (or distal) phalanges.[14] Proximally the laterally thickened portions are inserted into the proximal phalanx in close association with the flexor tendon sheath pulley system and form the so-called checkrein ligaments. In contrast to the metacarpophalangeal joints, the interphalangeal joints have little lateral motion. The collateral ligaments in the interphalangeal joint, therefore, are shorter and more rectangular in appearance. The dorsal capsule, although filmy, is reinforced at the base of the middle phalanx. In addition to the ligamentous structures discussed above and the inherent stability conferred by bony architecture, stability to all joints of the upper extremity is further augmented by musculotendinous structures crossing or inserting near the articulation.[23,33]

Muscular Anatomy

Many of the muscles and tendons that cross the wrist originate at the elbow or proximal forearm. These muscles of the forearm are largely responsible for flexion and extension of the wrist.[20,33] This section deals primarily with those muscles directly related to bones of the hand and wrist.

The chief flexors of the wrist are the flexor carpi radialis and the flexor carpi ulnaris. The palmaris longus is a minor flexor of the wrist.[20] Extension of the wrist is largely due to the extensor carpi radialis longus and brevis and the extensor carpi ulnaris. The primary muscles involved in radial deviation of the wrist are the abductor pollicis longus and the extensor pollicis brevis. Ulnar deviation of the wrist is accomplished primarily by the extensor carpi ulnaris.[19,20,33]

There are typically four lumbrical muscles that arise from the flexor digitorum profundus tendons and extend along the radial aspects of the second through fifth metacarpals to insert in the extensor aponeurosis of the proximal phalanx on the radial side. The flexor pollicis longus originates from the anterior aspect of the middle third of the radius. The tendon passes through the radial side of the carpal tunnel (Fig. 11-14) radial to the superficial and deep flexor tendons. A synovial sheath of the flexor pollicis longus tendon begins just proximal

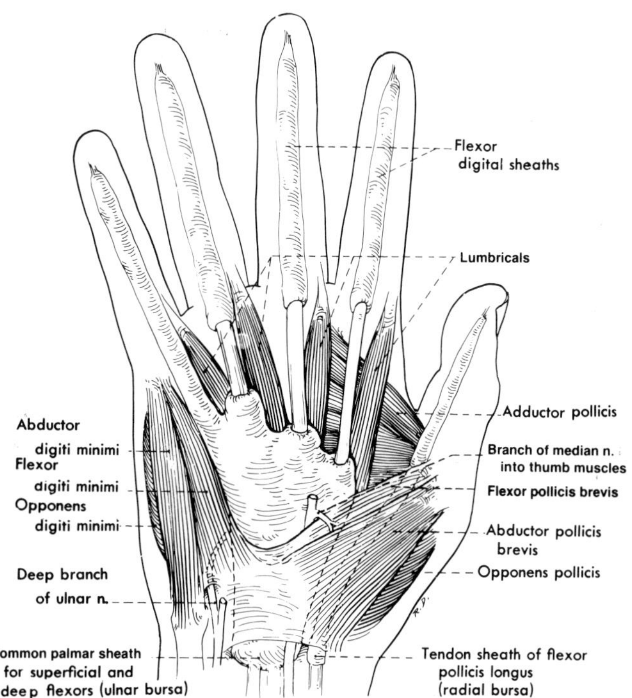

Fig. 11-14 Illustration of the muscles and flexor tendons of the hand and wrist. *Source:* Reprinted from *Anatomy for Surgeons, Vol 3, The Back and Limbs* ed 3 by HW Hollinshead, 1982, JB Lippincott.

to the flexor retinaculum and extends distally to the area of insertion of the tendon on the distal phalanx of the thumb.[20,33]

The interosseous muscles form the deepest layer of the muscles in the hand and are divided into palmar and dorsal groups. The palmar group consists of three muscles that take their origin on the radial aspect of the fifth and fourth metacarpals and the ulnar aspect of the second metacarpal. The muscles pass distally between the metacarpophalangeal joints to insert on the extensor aponeurosis. The four dorsal interossei originate from adjacent metacarpals, the first from the first and second metacarpal diaphyses, the second from the second and third, the third from the third and fourth, and the fourth from the fourth and fifth. The muscles pass dorsally and distally to insert with a palmar and dorsal slip into the bases of the proximal phalanges. The interosseous muscles, both palmar and dorsal, are innervated by the deep branch of the ulnar nerve and function in abduction and adduction of the fingers of the hand.[20]

The thenar eminence or muscle group comprises the abductor pollicis brevis and the superficial head of the flexor pollicis brevis, which overlie the opponens pollicis (Fig. 11-14). The abductor pollicis brevis arises from the flexor retinaculum and has deeper origins from the trapezium and trapezoid. This somewhat triangular muscle extends distally to insert in the radial aspect of the proximal phalanx of the thumb. It serves as the primary abductor of the thumb. The flexor pollicis brevis has two heads, one superficial and the other deep. The superficial head arises from the trapezium and flexor retinaculum, and the deep head arises from the trapezoid. The muscle extends distally to form a tendon that inserts on the radial flexor side of the base of the proximal phalanx of the thumb. Its primary function is flexion and rotation of the thumb. The opponens pollicis is partially covered by the abductors and flexors of the thumb and arises from the flexor retinaculum and trapezium to insert on the radial surface of the diaphysis of the first metacarpal. The adductor pollicis arises with both oblique and transverse heads. The transverse head arises from the ulnar surface of the third metacarpal diaphysis and the oblique head from the base of the third metacarpal and the flexor aspects of the trapezium, trapezoid, and capitate. The triangular muscle extends to insert at the base of the proximal phalanx of the thumb. This muscle serves to adduct the metacarpal and to flex the metacarpophalangeal joint of the thumb.[19,20]

The hypothenar muscle group consists of one superficial and three deep muscles (Fig. 11-14). The superficial muscle is the palmaris brevis, which arises from the ulnar side of the palmar aponeurosis and extends medially to attach into the skin along the medial border of the palm. This muscle is superficial to the ulnar nerve and artery.[20] The deep muscles include the abductor digiti minimi, flexor digiti minimi brevis, and opponens digiti minimi. The abductor digiti minimi is the most superficial of the three deep muscles. It arises from the distal surface of the pisiform and passes distally along the medial aspect of the hand to insert along the ulnar side of the base of the fifth proximal phalanx. This muscle abducts the little finger at the metacarpophalangeal joint. It acts along with the dorsal interosseous muscle in assisting in abduction or spreading of the fingers. The flexor digiti minimi brevis arises more distally than the abductor digiti minimi and takes its origin from the hook of the hamate and the flexor retinaculum. This muscle passes more obliquely and medially and inserts in the same position as the abductor. The main function of this muscle is to flex the fifth metacarpophalangeal joint. The third and final muscle of the deep hypothenar group is the opponens digiti minimi. This muscle is the deepest and arises deep to the abductor and flexor from the flexor retinaculum and distal hook of the hamate, taking an oblique course to insert along the ulnar aspect of the fifth metacarpal diaphysis. This muscle draws the fifth metacarpal anteriorly. All muscles of the hypothenar group are supplied by the deep branch of the ulnar nerve.[19,20]

Neurovascular Anatomy

The neurovascular anatomy of the hand and wrist is complex. Because there are numerous causes of nerve compression in this region, it is especially essential to understand the anatomy and relationship of these structures in the hand and wrist.[19,20,22] Evaluation of neurovascular anatomy is most easily accomplished by following the major nerve branches proximal to distal on axial magnetic resonance (MR) images. On the ulnar side of the distal forearm proximal to the carpal tunnel, the ulnar artery and nerve and their accompanying veins lie deep to the flexor carpi ulnaris (Fig. 11-15). The nerve is generally medial to the artery at this level. At the level of the pisiform, these structures pass along the lateral or radial side of the pisiform deep to the volar carpal ligament and then distally into the palm of the hand anterior to the flexor retinaculum but deep to the palmaris brevis muscle.[19,20] At the level of the pisiform, the ulnar nerve typically divides into superficial and deep branches. Also at the pisiform level the nerve and accompanying vascular structures lie between the volar carpal ligament and the flexor retinaculum in a space commonly known as Guyon's canal. Lesions proximal to or within the canal can produce both sensory and motor abnormalities in the ulnar nerve distribution.[20,22,33]

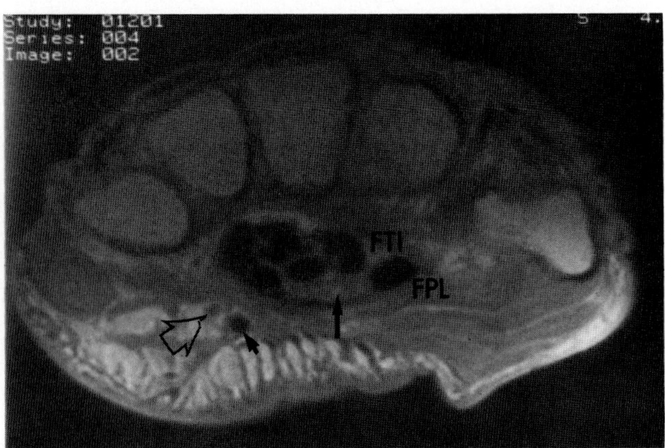

Fig. 11-15 Axial magnetic resonance (MR) image of the wrist demonstrating the median nerve (large black arrow), which lies superficial to the flexor tendons (FPL, flexor pollicis longus; FTI, flexor tendon to the index finger). The ulnar nerve (open arrow) and artery (small black arrow) are superficially located on the ulnar palmar surface.

The two flexor digitorum muscles (superficialis and profundus) are lateral to the ulnar nerve and vessels at the level of the wrist. The tendon of the palmaris longus lies superficially. The midline volar structures of the wrist, as they enter the carpal tunnel, tend to form three layers. The most superficial or anterior layer is formed by the flexor digitorum superficialis. The middle layer is formed by the superficial flexor of the index and middle fingers, and the most posterior or deepest layer is formed by the flexor digitorum profundus tendons. All tendons have a common sheath just before they pass under the flexor retinaculum. The palmaris longus tendon is the most superficial and midline structure at the wrist level.[19,22]

The median nerve lies deep to the flexor digitorum superficialis through much of the forearm (Fig. 11-15). Just proximal to the wrist, it emerges on the radial side of the superficial flexor and passes forward and medially to lie in front of the flexor tendons in the carpal tunnel. At the distal margin of the flexor retinaculum the median nerve divides into five or six branches.[20,22]

The complex vascular anatomy of the hand and wrist is illustrated in Fig. 11-16.[20]

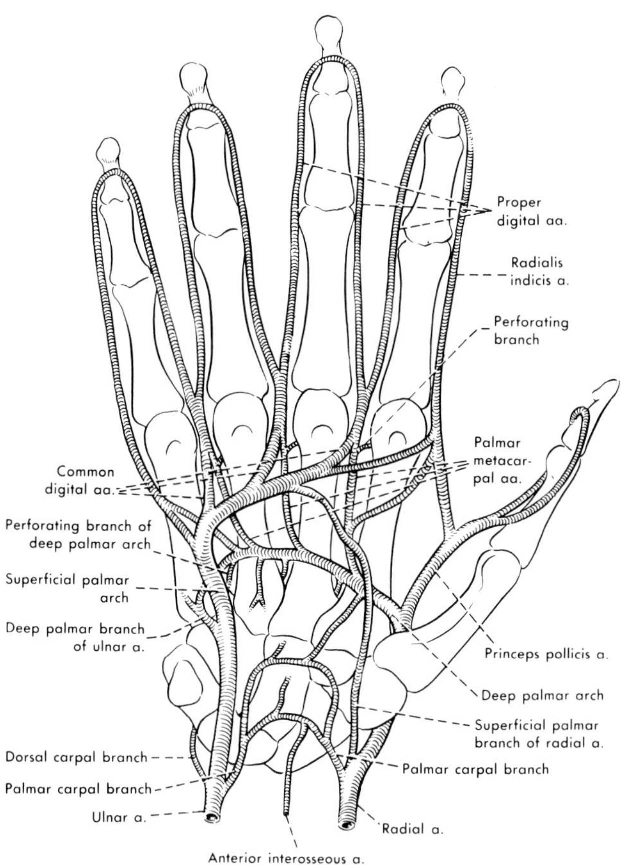

Fig. 11-16 Illustration of vascular anatomy. *Source:* Reprinted from *Anatomy for Surgeons, Vol 3, The Back and Limbs*, ed 3 by HW Hollinshead, 1982, JB Lippincott.

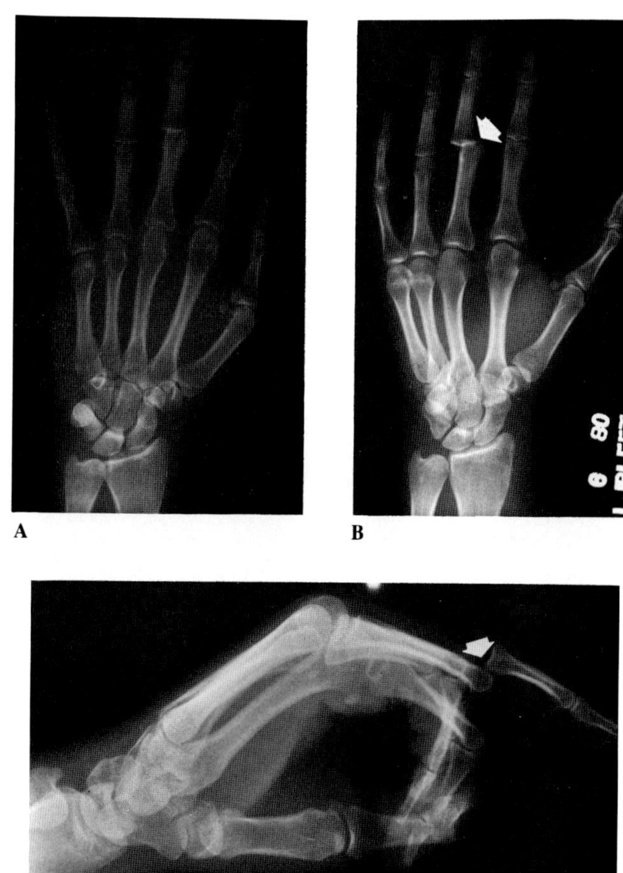

Fig. 11-17 (**A**) Anteroposterior (AP), (**B**) oblique, and (**C**) lateral views of the hand demonstrating a dorsal dislocation (arrows) of the third proximal interphalangeal joint. The isolated lateral view of the third finger with the uninvolved fingers flexed is the key to making the diagnosis.

IMAGING TECHNIQUES

Routine Radiography

There are numerous positioning techniques for evaluating the hand and wrist. Complex anatomy and subtle fractures often require multiple views or fluoroscopy for complete evaluation.[36–38,53]

Hand

Routine evaluation of the hand requires anteroposterior (AP), lateral, and oblique views (Fig. 11-17).[37,55]

The PA view is obtained with the patient sitting and the hand positioned on half an 8 × 10 inch cassette. The remainder of the cassette is shielded, allowing a second view to be obtained (Fig. 11-17, A and B). The fingers should be slightly spread and the palm laid flat against the cassette. The beam is perpendicular to the cassette and centered on the third metacarpophalangeal joint.[36–38] Careful radiographic analysis will demonstrate uniform cortical margins along the diaphyses of the phalanges and metacarpals. The proximal metaphysis expands just distal to the cortex of the joint space. Asymmetry in the metaphysis is common with torus fractures. The carpometacarpal joints should be parallel and uniform in width.[37,38,55]

The hand is rotated superiorly for the oblique view with the fingers slightly spread. A sponge can be used to maintain the proper position. The central beam is perpendicular to the cassette and centered on the metacarpophalangeal joints. The oblique view more clearly demonstrates the metacarpal heads (Fig. 11-17A) and the first and second carpometacarpal joints.

The lateral view is obtained with the ulnar side of the hand adjacent to the cassette and the thumb and fingers extended. The central beam is perpendicular to the cassette and centered on the metacarpophalangeal joints. This view is useful in evaluating dislocations (Fig. 11-17C) and fracture angulation.[37,55]

Fingers

Overlapping of the metacarpals and phalanges is common on the lateral and oblique views. Obtaining views of the digit in question provides better detail. In this way subtle injuries are more easily detected (Fig. 11-17C).

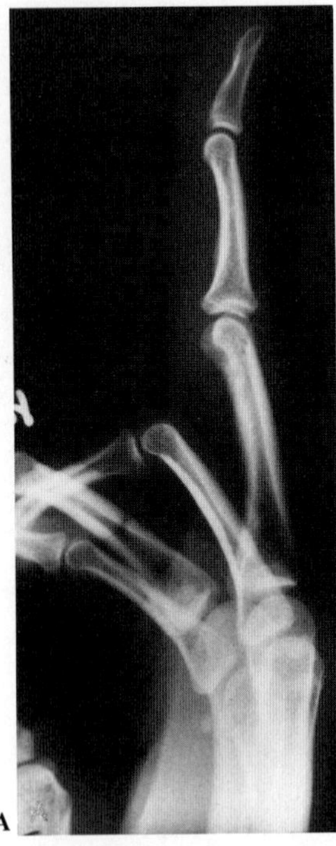
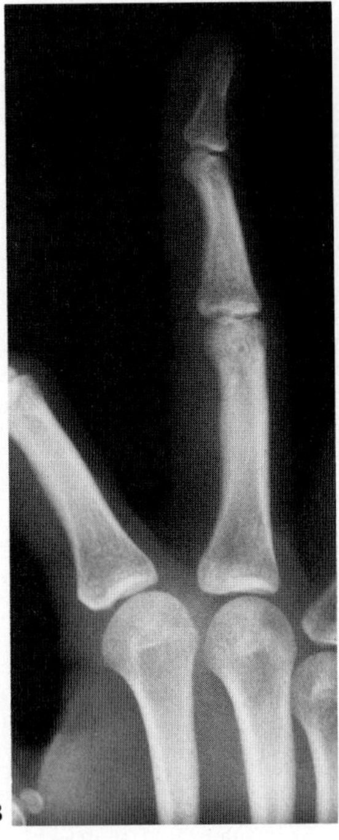
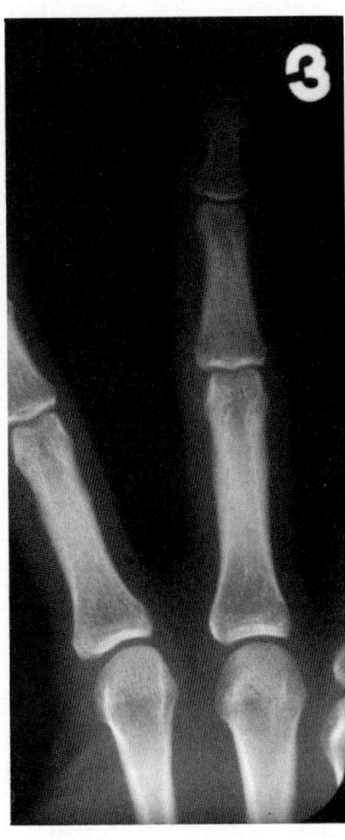

Fig. 11-18 (**A**) Lateral, (**B**) oblique, and (**C**) PA views of the third finger. *Source:* Reprinted from *Imaging of Orthopedic Trauma* ed 2 by TH Berquist, 1991, Raven Press, © Mayo Foundation.

Views of the individual fingers can be obtained with extremity cassettes or dental film. The finger being radiographed should be clearly marked on the film. The PA view is obtained with the finger flat on the cassette and the beam centered perpendicular to the proximal interphalangeal joint (Fig. 11-18C). The lateral view is essential in evaluating articular fractures (hyperextension volar plate fractures of the middle phalanx) and for determining the position and angulation of fractures.[37,38,76] This view is obtained with the ulnar side of the hand adjacent to the cassette and the finger separated by flexing the remaining digits (Figs. 11-17C and 11-18A). This may require taping or props to assist in positioning. Centering is the same as in the PA view. The oblique view (Fig. 11-18B) is obtained by rotating the hand as one would for the oblique view of the hand. The finger in question is isolated by flexing the remaining digits.[76]

Thumb

The PA view of the thumb is obtained with the thumb elevated from the film and the ulnar side of the hand adjacent to the cassette (Fig. 11-19). This results in some magnification. However, this position is much more easily maintained than the AP position, which requires that the hand be inverted with the dorsum of the thumb against the cassette.[37,38] The central beam is perpendicular to the cassette and centered on the metacarpophalangeal joint.

Stress views, especially of the first metacarpophalangeal joint, are frequently used to exclude ligament injury.[38,42,47,48] This study is more accurately performed fluoroscopically. Both thumbs should be in the PA position for comparison (Fig. 11-20A). Spot films are obtained in the neutral position and during radial and ulnar stress. Increase in the joint space on the stressed side (Fig. 11-20B) or subluxation indicates ligament injury. Swelling and pain may reduce accuracy in the acute setting. Intraarticular injection of 1% lidocaine (Xylocaine) allows more accurate assessment. If this

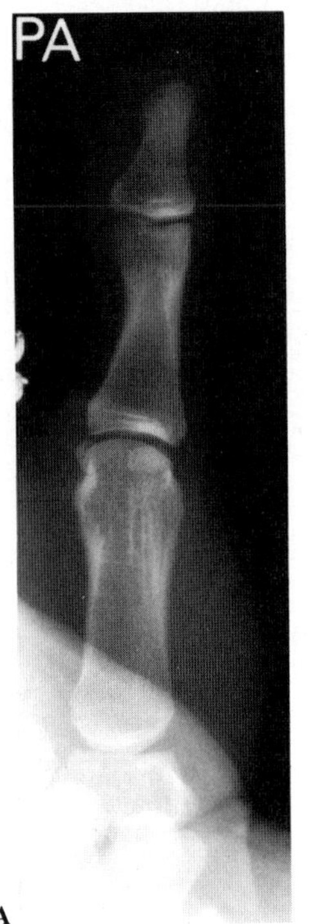

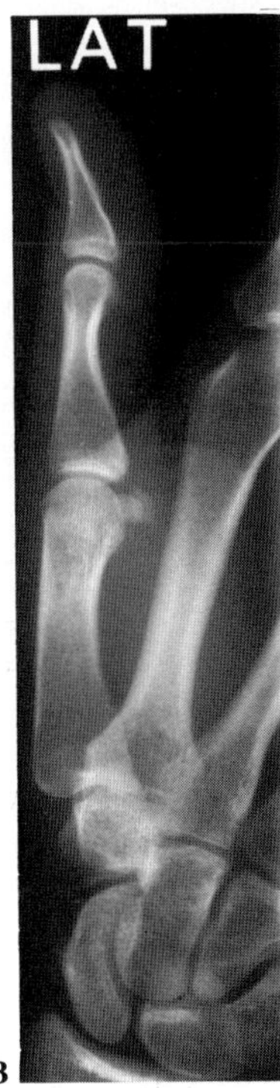

Fig. 11-19 (**A**) Normal PA and (**B**) lateral views of the thumb. *Source:* Reprinted from *Imaging of Orthopedic Trauma* ed 2 by TH Berquist, 1991, Raven Press, © Mayo Foundation.

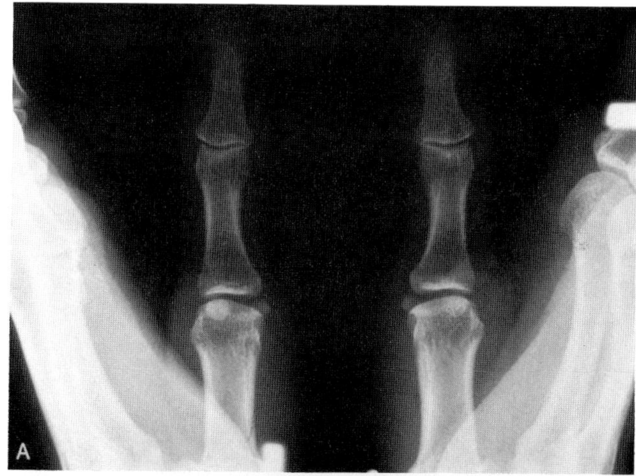

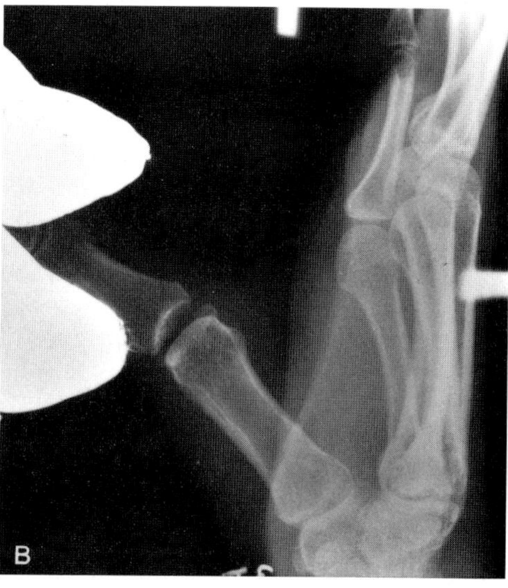

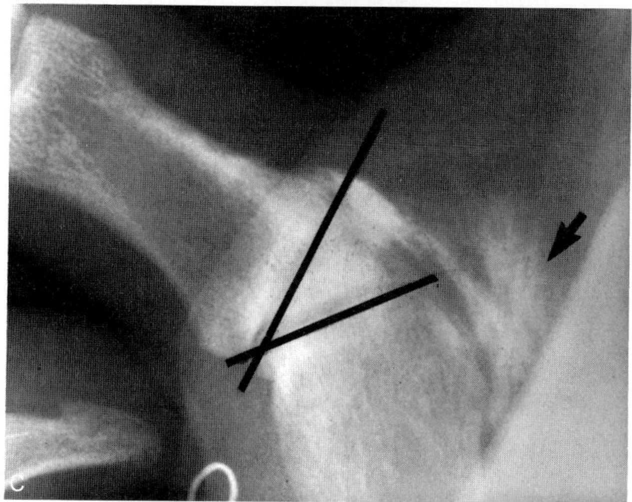

Fig. 11-20 (**A**) Neutral and (**B**) stress views of the right thumb. (**C**) The ulnar collateral ligament tear (arrow) is most obvious after injection of anesthetic and contrast material. Lines indicate angle of articular incongruency.

is needed, however, an arthrogram should be performed. The latter is more definitive (Fig. 11-20C).[76]

Wrist

PA, lateral, and oblique views are obtained after trauma. The position for the PA view of the wrist is similar to that used for the PA view of the hand except that the beam is centered on the wrist instead of the metacarpophalangeal joints.[56,76]

Careful examination of the PA view reveals significant bony and soft tissue anatomy. Subtle fractures on the radial side of the wrist, especially the scaphoid, are easily overlooked. The navicular fat stripe is a useful structure in this regard. This fat plane lies between the radial collateral ligament and the tendon sheaths of the abductor pollicis longus and extensor pollicis brevis (Fig. 11-21A). Although the fat plane is inconsistently seen in children, it is present in 96% of normal adults.[73] Terry and Ramin[73] noted absence or displacement of the fat stripe in 88% of fractures on the radial side of the wrist (Fig. 11-21B). These changes were noted in 87% of scaphoid fractures. Changes in the navicular fat stripe may be the only clue to a wrist fracture.[76]

The articular surfaces of the carpal bones should be parallel with 1- to 2-mm joint spaces.[37,38,51,58,76] Angling the tube 10° to the ulnar side of the wrist may optimize measurement of the scapholunate space.[58] Any change in the joint space or shape of the carpal bones may indicate subluxation or dislocation. Three arcs can be drawn on the normal PA view (Fig. 11-22). The first arc is formed by the proximal articular surfaces of the scaphoid, lunate, and triquetrum. The second arc is formed by the distal articular surfaces of these carpal bones. The third arc is formed by the proximal (convex) articular surfaces of the capitate and hamate. Any significant interruption of these arcs, other than where the trapezium, trapezoid, and pisiform are seen as overlapping structures on the PA view, suggests abnormality at the involved joint.

The distal radioulnar joint should also be demonstrated clearly on the PA view (see Fig. 11-22). This joint space normally measures about 2 mm. Ulnar variance should also be assessed on the PA view. The relationship of the distal radiocarpal and ulnocarpal joints is affected significantly by changes in wrist position. Supination increases, and pronation decreases, negative ulnar variance. Subtle positioning changes may also affect ulnar variance.[49]

Fluoroscopically positioned spot films are also useful to clarify suspected injuries. Alignment of the osseous structures is easily accomplished.[51,53,76]

Lateral view. Positioning for the lateral view of the wrist is similar to that for the hand except that the beam is centered on the wrist. On the lateral view the normal pronator fat stripe (Fig. 11-23) can be seen passing proximally from the ventral surface of the radius. This normally lies within 1 cm of the cortical surface of the distal radius. Subtle radial fractures will cause displacement or obliteration of the fat plane. This may

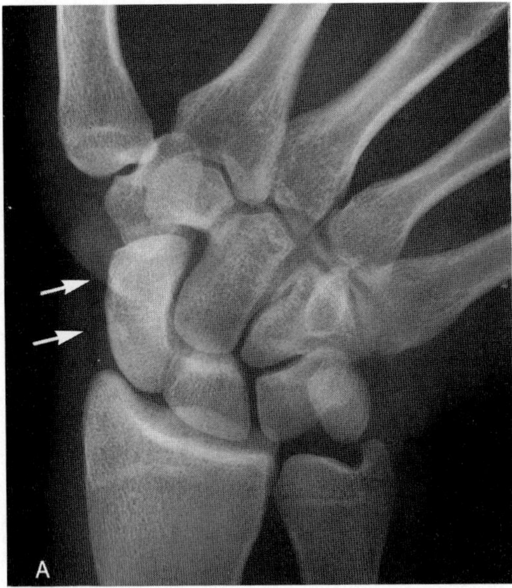

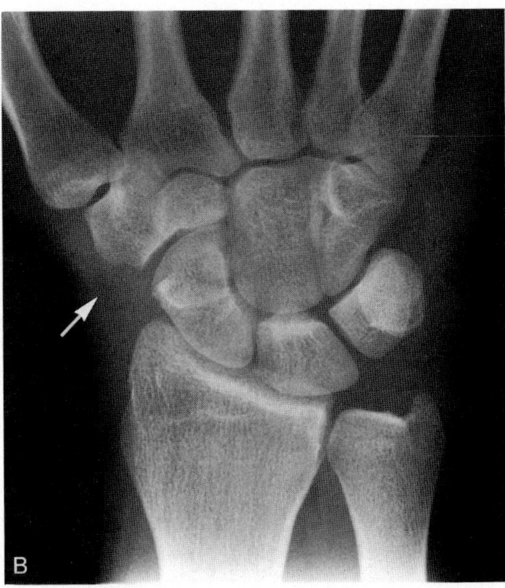

Fig. 11-21 (**A**) PA view (ulnar deviation) demonstrating the normal navicular fat stripe (arrows). (**B**) PA view of the wrist in a patient with a subtle scaphoid fracture showing obliteration of the fat stripe (arrow).

be the only indication of fracture. Dorsal swelling is also best seen on the lateral view.[76]

The relationship of the radius, lunate, capitate, and metacarpals is demonstrated clearly on the lateral view. The capitate is firmly attached to the third metacarpal. The convex proximal surface of the capitate articulates with the lunate, and the lunate articulates with the radius. A straight line can be drawn along the axes of the radius, lunate, capitate, and third metacarpal in the neutral position. Slight flexion or extension, however, will normally interrupt this line. The angle formed by the radius and scaphoid is normally about 136° (range, 121° to 153°; Fig. 11-23). The scapholunate angle is normally about 45°.[53,76]

Oblique views. Both oblique views may also be useful in acute wrist injuries (Fig. 11-24).[76] The internal oblique demonstrates the ulnar styloid and scaphoid tubercle. The external oblique demonstrates the pisiform more clearly. Subtle fractures of the radial and ulnar styloids are often only demonstrated on the oblique views.[76]

Scaphoid view. The scaphoid is the most frequently fractured carpal bone. These fractures are often subtle. Therefore, a scaphoid view should be obtained initially if a fracture is suspected. We routinely position the hand in ulnar deviation

Fig. 11-22 PA view of the wrist demonstrating the normal carpal arcs. Note the ring shadow (small arrow) formed by the hook of the hamate and the normal distal radioulnar joint (large arrow).

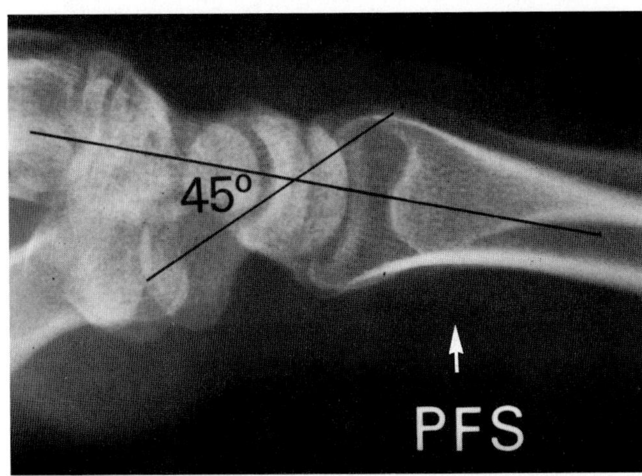

Fig. 11-23 Normal lateral view of the wrist demonstrating the normal scapholunate angle and pronator fat stripe (PFS).

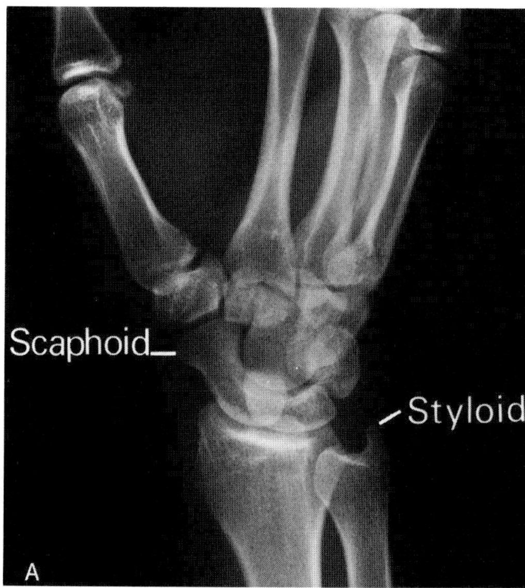

Fig. 11-24 (**A**) Normal internal and (**B**) external oblique views of the wrist.

with the palm down on the cassette (Fig. 11-25). The thumb is extended and in line with the radius. The beam is centered on the scaphoid and perpendicular to the cassette.[37,76] This clearly demonstrates the elongated scaphoid (Fig. 11-25).[76]

Carpal tunnel view. Several methods have been described for obtaining this view. A simple technique involves hyperextending the hand with the base of the wrist against the cassette. The hand can be positioned with the opposite hand used for support or with a strap to maintain the hyperextended position. The tube is angled toward the wrist at 40° from the horizontal (table top).[38,76]

The radiograph (Fig. 11-26) demonstrates the carpal tunnel and surrounding carpal structures. This is particularly useful in evaluating the hook of the hamate and soft tissues in the region of the carpal tunnel.[37,38,76]

Motion studies. Bending views of the wrist are useful to evaluate subtle bony or ligamentous injuries in patients with persistent pain. This series of radiographs includes the PA and lateral views. In addition, lateral views are obtained with maximal flexion and extension (Fig. 11-27, A and B), and PA views are obtained with radial and ulnar deviation (Fig. 11-27, C and D). Lateral and PA clenched fist views may also be included.[51,53] In certain cases fluoroscopy with vid-

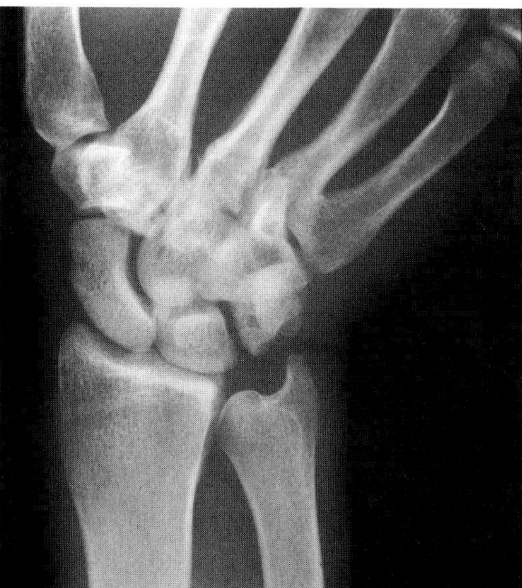

Fig. 11-25 Normal scaphoid view. Note the overlap of the carpometacarpal joints due to positioning.

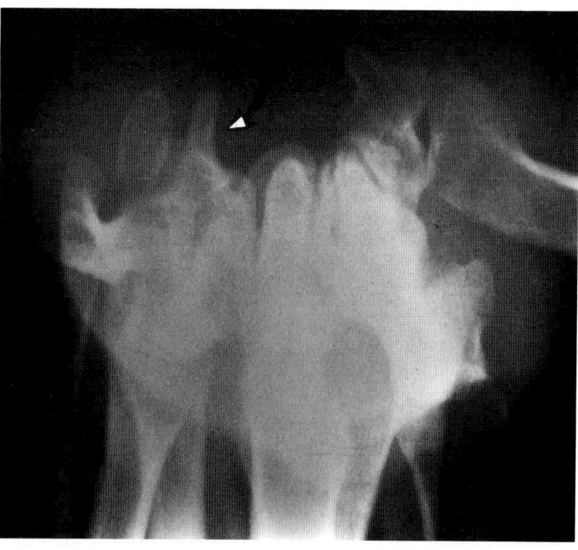

Fig. 11-26 Normal carpal tunnel view demonstrating the hook of the hamate (arrow).

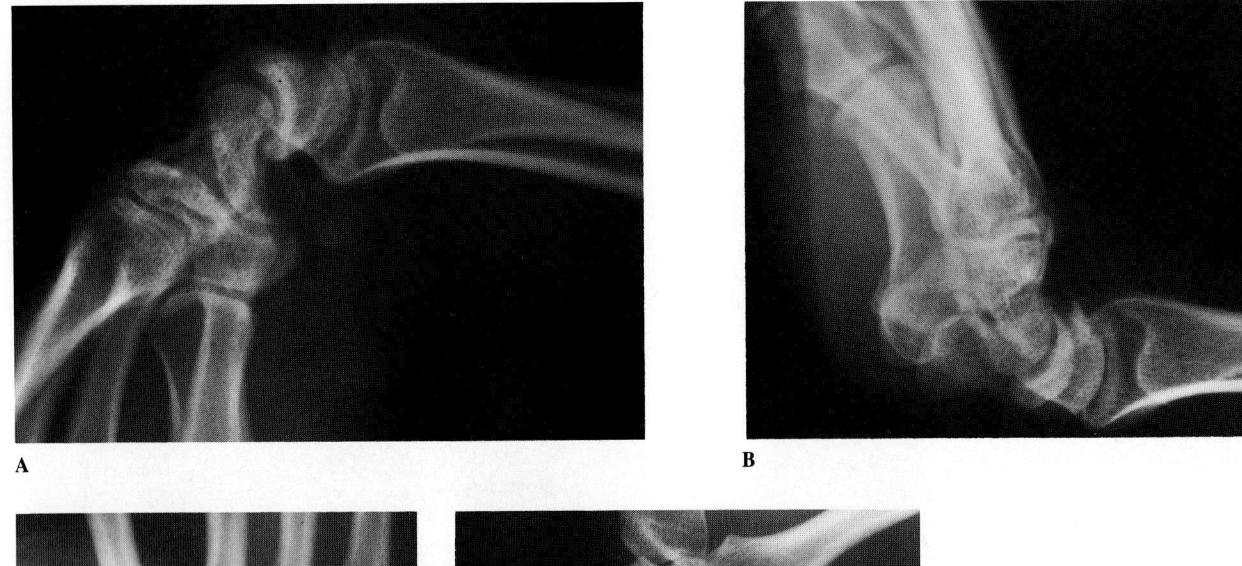

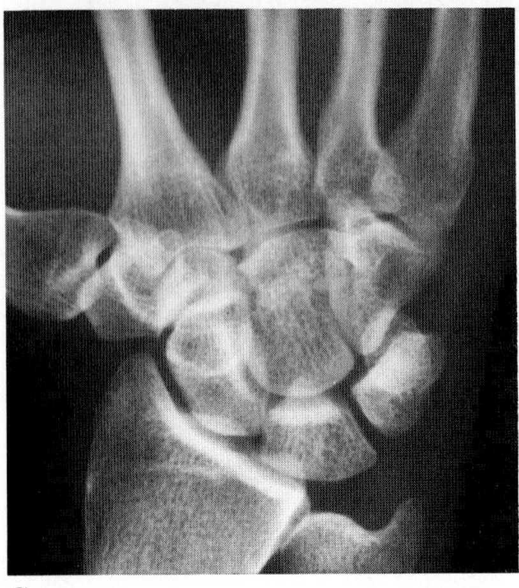

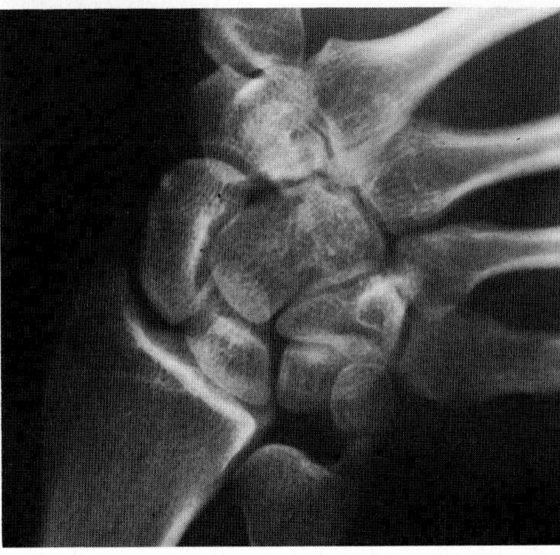

A B C D

Fig. 11-27 Radiographs of motion series. (**A**) Lateral flexion view. (**B**) Lateral extension view. (**C**) PA view in radial deviation. (**D**) PA view in ulnar deviation.

eotape or cineradiography may be helpful. These techniques allow review of the motion series for detection of more subtle abnormalities.[76]

The lateral dynamic views are obtained in the same manner as the views of the lateral wrist except that the wrist is flexed and extended. Dorsiflexion (hyperextension) and palmar flexion average 70° and 75°, respectively.[76]

With ulnar deviation (Fig. 11-27D) the scaphoid is elongated, and the lunate is more trapezoid in shape and articulates completely with the radius. During radial deviation (Fig. 11-27C) the lunate translates and only partially articulates with the radius. The scaphoid is foreshortened owing to palmar flexion. This provides a ringlike shadow distally that is similar to the ring sign seen with rotary subluxation. The scapholunate space (<2 mm) does not change with radial and ulnar deviation unless ligament injury is present.[76]

Tomography

Complex-motion, thin-section tomography (1- to 3-mm slices) is preferred for evaluating the hand and wrist.[53,71,76] Typically, tomograms are performed in the PA and lateral projections. Fluoroscopic positioning may be necessary, however, and flexion and extension tomograms may also be useful in certain situations.[72,76] Tomography after localizing radionuclide scans or in conjunction with arthrography is also useful in patients with chronic wrist pain or complex symptoms.[41,76]

Computed Tomography

In certain situations, computed tomography (CT) may provide additional information with regard to bone and soft tissue injuries.[44–46,53,61] In our practice, MRI has largely replaced CT for evaluating soft tissue injury and avascular necrosis.[39,40]

Technique is crucial. Routinely, 2- to 3-mm axial and direct coronal or sagittal images are obtained. The last are accomplished with the arm above the head, the elbow flexed, and the wrist in neutral position (coronal) or pronated (sagittal).[53,66] Acutely injured patients may not be able to tolerate the necessary positions for direct coronal and sagittal imaging. Recon-

Fig. 11-28 Illustrations of criteria for assessing radioulnar subluxation. **(A)** Supination. A perpendicular is drawn from the center of a line connecting the ulnar styloid and the central ulnar head. This should be in the center of the sigmoid notch. **(B)** Neutral. The ulnar head should lie between the marginal radial lines. **(C)** Pronation. A congruent arch is formed by the ulna and the synovial notch. **(D)** Use of all three criteria in a supinated wrist. RPL = radiopalmar line, RDL = radiodorsal line, C = arc of segmoid notch, C_1 = arc of ulnar head. *Source:* Reprinted with permission from Wechsler RJ, Wehbe MA, Rifkin MD, Edeiken J and Branch HM, Computed tomography diagnosis of distal radioulnar subluxation, *Skeletal Radiology* (1987;16:1–5), Copyright © 1987, Springer-Verlag. **(E)** Normal computed tomography arthrogram with marginal radioulnar lines marked.

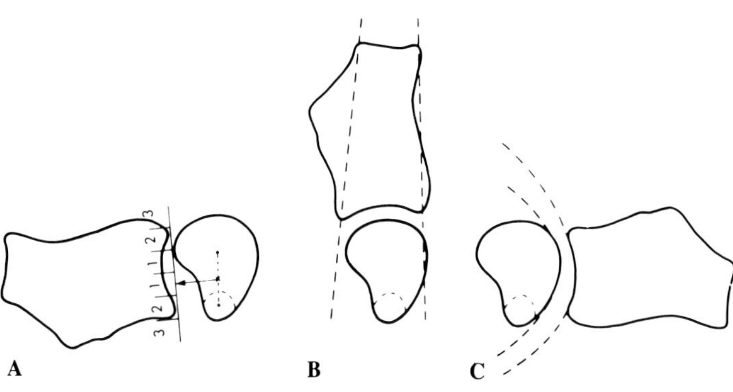

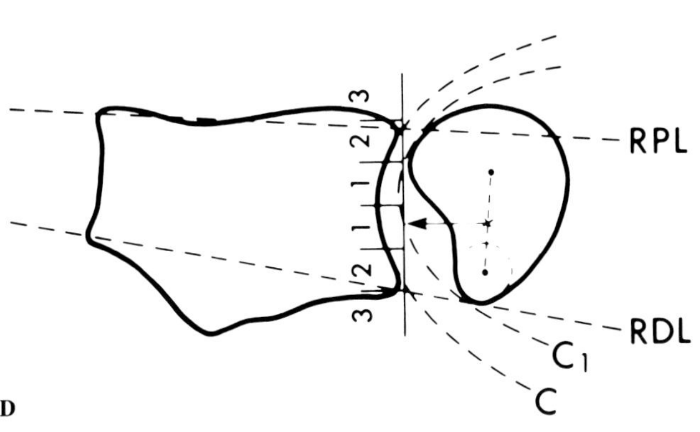

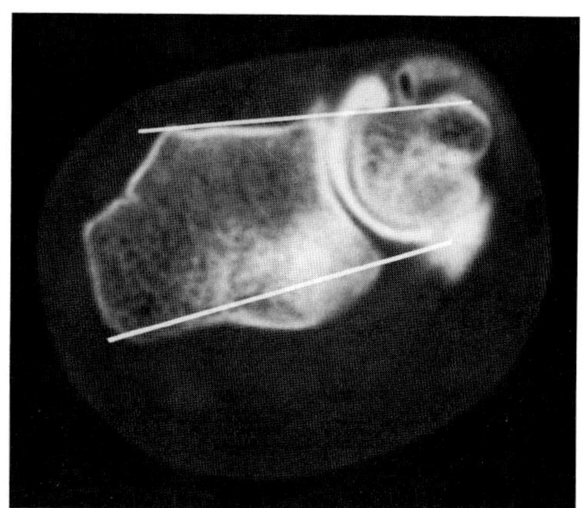

structed coronal and sagittal images can be obtained if the patient cannot tolerate positioning for direct coronal and sagittal images.[66,67]

CT is most frequently used to evaluate the distal radioulnar joint and subtle fractures or fracture healing.[65,67,75] Recently, postarthrographic CT has also been effective in evaluating subtle triangular fibrocartilage complex injuries.[66]

At the Mayo Clinic we use CT most frequently for evaluating subluxation and/or dislocation of the distal radioulnar joint. Axial images in the symptomatic position may be diagnostic. In some cases neutral, pronation, and supination images are required to detect subtle subluxation. The normal wrist is generally examined for comparison.[75] This can be done simultaneously, but positioning must be symmetric. This may be difficult to achieve in symptomatic patients. Figure 11-28 demonstrates the normal relationships of the distal radius and ulna.[75]

Complex injuries can also be evaluated with three-dimensional reconstruction. This is not commonly required in routine trauma series, however.[76]

Radionuclide Imaging

Three-phase radionuclide imaging of the hand and wrist is a useful technique for evaluating acute and chronic trauma-related disorders.[76] In this setting ^{99m}Tc coupled to phosphate compounds such as methylene diphosphonate (MDP) is most often used. Three-phase imaging provides additional advantage compared to the usual static delay (2- to 3-hour) bone images (phase III of a three phase study).[53,64] The first phase (rapid flow images) provides valuable flow information. This phase is obtained by means of rapid sequential imaging during the first 1 to 2 minutes after injection while the isotope is intravascular.[64] Soft tissue distribution is accomplished during phase II (5 to 10 minutes after injection), when the isotope is in the extracellular fluid space.[53,64] Abnormal uptake in diffuse regions is not unusual during the early phases (phases I and II) of soft tissue injuries. The lack of focal radionuclide uptake on delayed images (phase III) is useful in excluding osseous involvement (Fig. 11-29).[53,76]

The most common indication for radionuclide three-phase imaging in the hand and wrist is exclusion of the following: subtle osseous injury, reflex sympathetic dystrophy, bone ischemia, and early inflammation or infection.[50,53,54,57,64]

Magnetic Resonance Imaging

MRI has become increasingly useful in defining soft tissue abnormalities, subtle bone lesions, and ischemic changes in the hand and wrist. When properly performed, MRI may replace more conventional techniques in diagnosing certain disorders of the hand and wrist.[39,77]

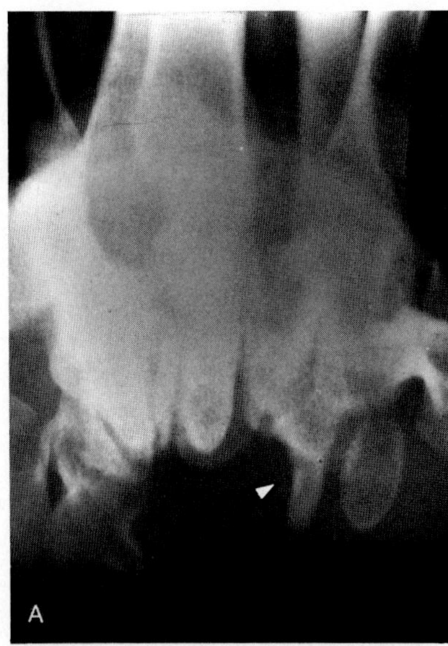

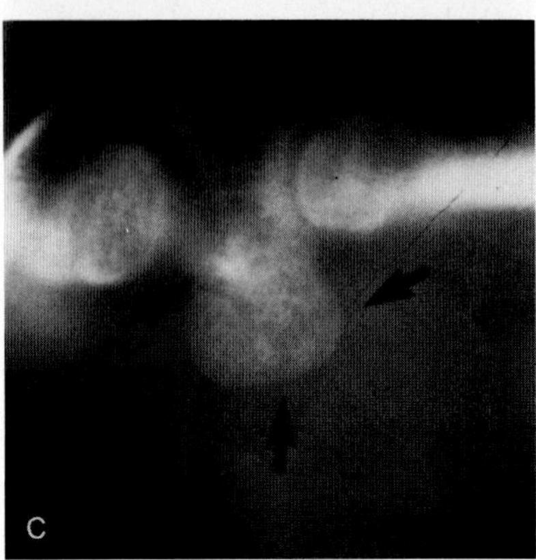

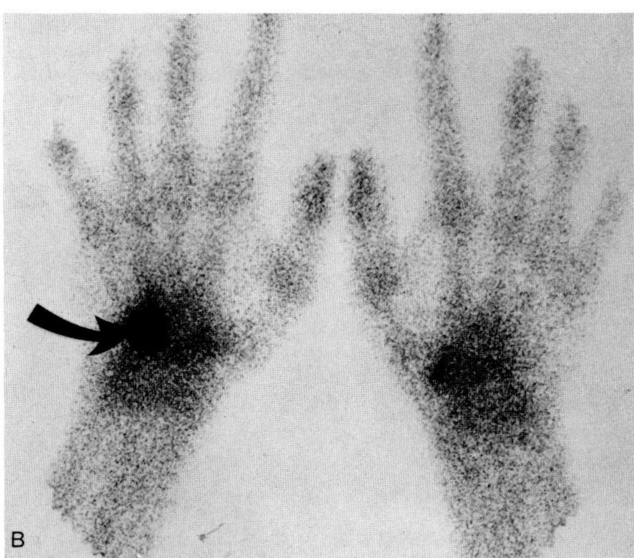

Fig. 11-29 Evaluation of a golfer with pain in the palm after a drive that was hit badly. (**A**) Carpal tunnel view shows a normal hamate hook (arrow). (**B**) Bone scan several days later shows focal tracer uptake in the hamate region (arrow). (**C**) Tomogram shows an undisplaced Y fracture (arrows). *Source:* Reprinted from *Imaging of Orthopedic Trauma* ed 2 by TH Berquist, 1991, Raven Press, © Mayo Foundation.

MR examinations of the hand and wrist can be difficult to perform because of limitations in positioning and coil selection. Patient comfort is an essential part of the examination. If the position is difficult to tolerate, one can expect significant problems with motion artifact. In an initial review of upper extremity MR studies performed at the Mayo Clinic, motion artifacts or incomplete studies due to patient discomfort were noted in 25% of cases.[39,40]

Positioning depends upon patient size, information required (ie, motion studies), software, and coil availability. Uniform signal intensity is most easily obtained with a wraparound, partial-volume, or Helmholtz coil system. The small flat coils (3 and 5 inches) are also adequate for hand and wrist imaging (Fig. 11-30). Flat coils allow more flexibility for positioning and motion studies. When patient size allows, it is best to position the arm at the side. Dual coils are now available that allow simultaneous evaluation of both hands and wrists. The wrist can also be positioned over the abdomen with the elbow flexed. The coil must be supported and separated from the abdominal wall, however, or motion artifact becomes a problem. Large patients may need to be rotated with the arm above the head. This position is difficult to tolerate because of shoulder discomfort (Fig. 11-31).[39,40]

Optimal quality in hand and wrist imaging requires a small field of view (FOV). We typically use an 8- to 12-cm FOV for examinations with both flat and partial-volume coils. Off-axis, small-FOV images are needed if the coil is positioned away from the central axis of the magnet (Fig. 11-30A). Therefore, if this software is not available one must position the patient's arm above the head to achieve the proper FOV (Fig. 11-31).[39]

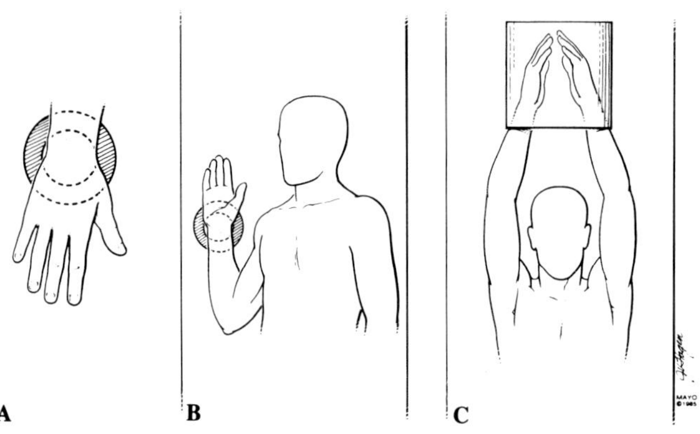

Fig. 11-30 Positioning options for the wrist. (**A**) Flat circular coil with the arm at the side. (**B**) Flat coil with the elbow flexed and the patient rotated. (**C**) Both wrists above the head in a head coil. Positioning is difficult with this technique.

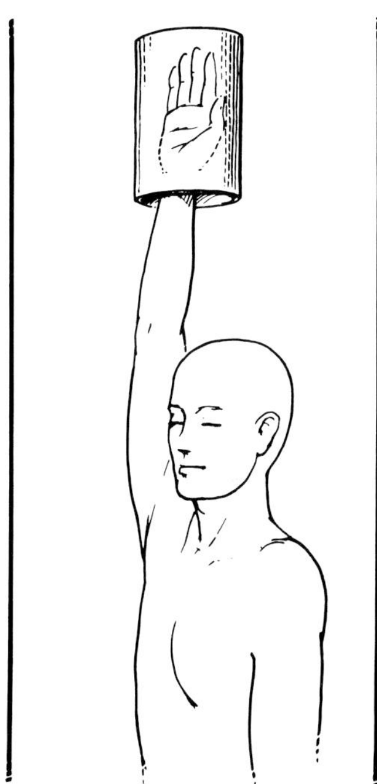

Fig. 11-31 Patient positioned with the arm above the head in a circumferential partial-volume coil.

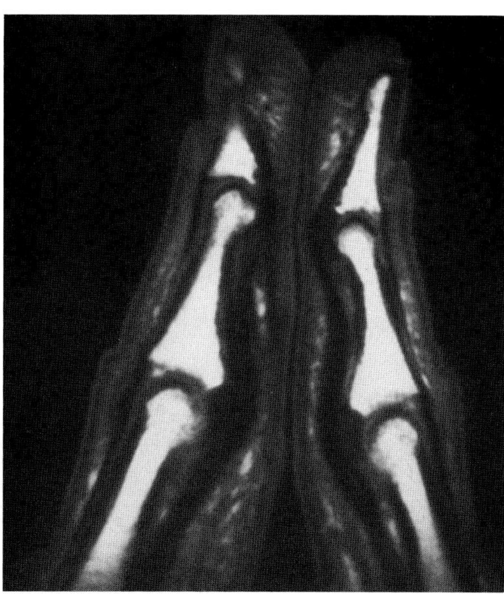

Fig. 11-32 Normal sagittal images of the index fingers demonstrating the flexor and extensor tendons.

Once the patient has been positioned, the proper pulse sequences and image planes must be selected to demonstrate the anatomy and pathology. An effective screening examination can be accomplished by beginning with either a coronal or a sagittal scout (SE 150–400/20). This should include the full area of the hand and wrist to be examined. We typically follow this sequence with an axial T2-weighted sequence (SE 2000/20–30, 60–80) with 5-mm thick slices, minimal interslice gap, a 256 × 256 matrix with one excitation (8 minutes 56 seconds) or a 256 × 192 matrix with two excitations (13 minutes). A small FOV (8 to 12 cm) with no phase, no frequency wrap, and presaturation techniques is used to reduce flow artifacts and to maximize image quality. The second sequence chosen varies depending on the findings of the first sequence or the clinical indication for the examination. A coronal T1-weighted sequence (SE 500/20) with 3- to 5-mm slices, no skip, and other setup data noted above is usually adequate as a second sequence to provide a good screening technique for bone and soft tissue pathology.[39,40,76]

Additional sequences may be indicated in specific clinical situations or when abnormalities are evident on the initial sequences that dictate further sequences to characterize the lesion. For example, if an abnormality is suspected in a specific phalangeal segment, sagittal T2-weighted (SE 2000/30,60) or gradient-echo sequences (echo time, 13 msec; repetition time, 100 to 400 msec; flip angle, 30° to 70°) will define the structures, including vasculature, to better advantage. The sagittal sequence should be performed with thin slices (3 mm) and aligned with the tendon or osseous structure of interest (Fig. 11-32).[39]

Specific anatomic areas can be examined with the 3-inch coil, an 8-cm FOV, and sequences that may differ from those described above for the screening examination. Specifically, the scaphoid is demonstrated most completely in the coronal and sagittal planes. T1- and T2-weighted sequences should be performed to evaluate fully the bone and articular anatomy. Evaluation of the distal radioulnar joint often requires pronation, supination, and neutral T2-weighted axial images. This allows functional anatomic analysis and evaluation of subtle soft tissue abnormalities. Cine motion studies can be performed quickly with gradient recalled acquisition in steady state (GRASS) or GRASS interleaved (GRIL) sequences. Soft tissue abnormalities in the carpal tunnel can be studied with axial (SE 2000/30,60 and SE 500/20) sequences. These images provide more than adequate evaluation of the median nerve and surrounding structures. Vascular anatomy is demonstrated most completely with GRASS or volume reconstruction techniques.[39,40]

MR techniques can be useful in acute and chronic musculoskeletal injuries of the hand and wrist (Table 11-1). Most acute skeletal injuries are adequately diagnosed with routine radiography. CT and isotope studies are valuable supplemental radiographic techniques.[39,40]

MRI is not frequently used for diagnosis of skeletal injuries in the hand and wrist. Nevertheless, it is not unusual to detect subtle injuries that may not be evident on routine radiographs or tomograms. Detection of stress fractures and osteochondral fractures with MRI has also been reported. Cortical bone appears black on MR images. Therefore, cortical fractures are most easily appreciated on T2-weighted images (SE 2000/60–80). Edema and hemorrhage in marrow will also have higher signal intensity than normal marrow with these

Table 11-1 Hand and Wrist Trauma

Anatomic Region/Indication	*Imaging Work-Up*
Osseous trauma	
Distal radius and ulna	Routine radiographs, tomography if needed
Carpal bones	Routine radiographs, radionuclide scans plus tomography if indicated
Metacarpals and phalanges	Routine radiographs
? Avascular necrosis	Routine radiographs, MRI if negative
Distal radioulnar joint (subluxation-dislocation)	CT with or without arthrography or MRI [gradient-echo technique with cine motion studies (neutral, pronation, supination)]
Ligament injuries	Arthrography
Capsules and ligaments of metacarpophalangeal and interphalangeal joints	Arthrography
Muscle and tendon injuries	MRI
Neural injury	MRI

Source: Reprinted from *Imaging of Orthopedic Trauma* ed 2 by TH Berquist, 1991, Raven Press, © Mayo Foundation.

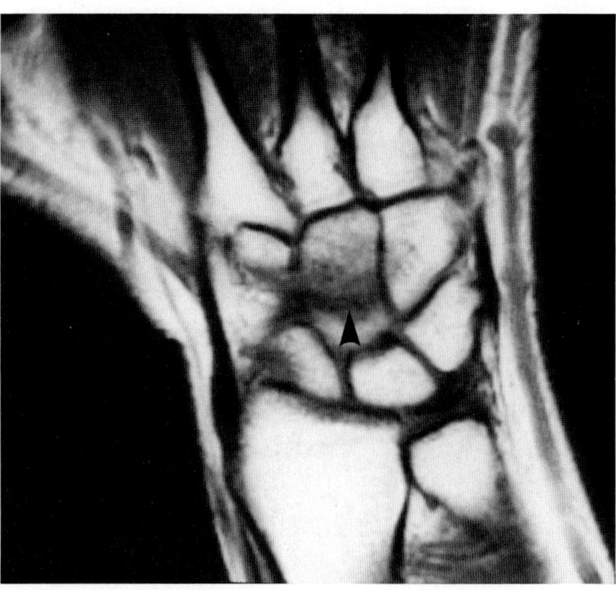

Fig. 11-33 Coronal (SE 500/20) MR image of the wrist demonstrating a capitate fracture (arrowhead).

parameters. Fracture lines and adjacent reactive changes have low signal intensity compared to normal marrow on T1-weighted (SE 500/20) sequences (Fig. 11-33). Compression injuries with trabecular condensation are seen as areas of low intensity on both T1- and T2-weighted sequences.[39,40]

Articular or joint-related injuries of the hand and wrist are usually evaluated with arthrography, motion studies, stress views, and, in certain cases, postinjection CT or conventional tomography (Table 11-1). Arthrography is still valuable for confirming suspected ligament injuries. In addition, diagnostic and therapeutic injections can be performed in conjunction with arthrography and tenography.[39,40,53,68,69]

MRI is most useful for evaluating soft tissue trauma, specifically muscle and tendon injuries, neural compression syndromes, and capsule disruptions (Table 11-1). Tears in the triangular fibrocartilage complex can be detected, especially if they occur near the thicker ulnar margin. Zlatkin et al[77] reported an accuracy of 95% for MR detection of these tears. MRI had a sensitivity of 100% and a specificity of 92% compared to 89% and 90% for arthrography.[77]

Evaluation of the intercarpal ligaments and distal radioulnar joint is usually accomplished with arthrography and CT.[76] Nevertheless, MRI has also demonstrated significant potential in these areas. Although experience is limited, Zlatkin et al[77] reported an accuracy of 90% for the scapholunate ligament and slightly less accurate results (80%) for the lunotriquetral ligament.

Technique is important. Dual coupled flat coils, a small FOV (8 to 12 cm), and T2-weighted sequences (SE 2000/20,60) or gradient-echo sequences (repetition time, 200 to 700 msec; echo time, 12 or 31 msec; flip angle, 25° to 30°) with T2* weighting are most useful. The coronal plane and thin (1- to 3-mm) slices are also best suited to evaluate the triangular fibrocartilage complex and ligaments.[39,77] At this time, arthrography is still useful for detection of interosseous ligament and triangular fibrocartilage complex injuries.[39,40,69]

Muscle and tendon tears are also most easily demonstrated with T2-weighted sequences. To define accurately the extent of injury, we usually use axial and either coronal or sagittal image planes. Subtle tendon abnormalities may be better demonstrated on gradient-echo motion studies. Axial images in neutral, pronation, and supination are also best for evaluating the distal radioulnar joint.

MRI is a proven technique for detection of avascular necrosis.[39,40] In the wrist, these changes are seen most commonly in the lunate and after scaphoid fractures (Fig. 11-34). Carpal bones are smaller, so that the MR features of osteonecrosis may be more difficult to interpret. Uniform loss of signal intensity on short echo time/repetition time sequences is the most reliable sign of avascular necrosis (Fig. 11-34), specifically in the lunate. Similar changes also can occur in the other carpal bones but are less common. Patchy or focal signal intensity changes have also been noted. When small focal areas of reduced signal intensity are noted in the carpal bones on a T1-weighted sequence, the diagnosis may be difficult (Fig. 11-35).[39,40] Comparison with T2-weighted images is somewhat useful. In the early stages the signal intensity will be increased. Later, when bone sclerosis occurs, the signal intensity will be reduced on both T1- and T2-weighted sequences.

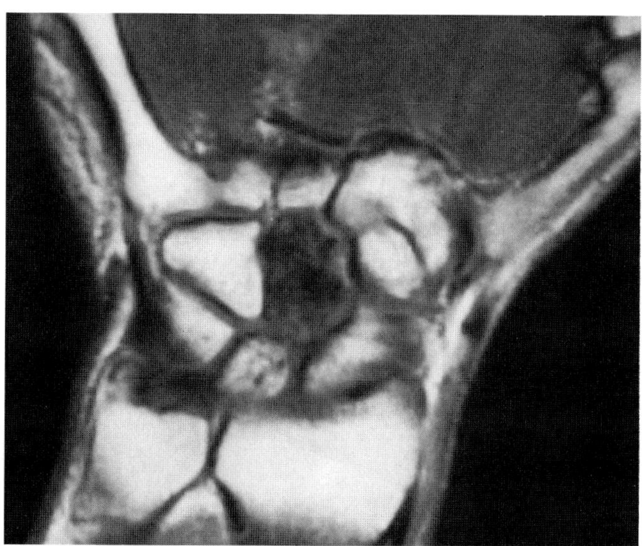

Fig. 11-34 Coronal (SE 500/20) MR image demonstrating low intensity in the capitate due to avascular necrosis.

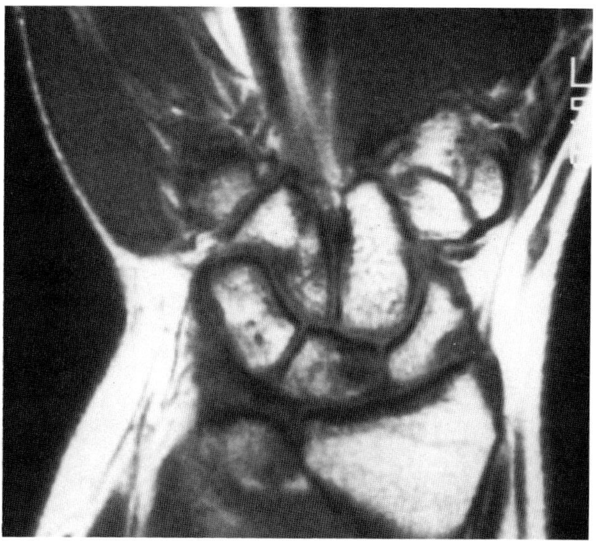

Fig. 11-35 Coronal (SE 500/20) MR image demonstrating a focal area of low signal intensity in the lunate due to a degenerative cyst.

In either setting, comparison with routine radiographs is important. Well-marginated lucent areas are usually degenerative and should not be confused with osteonecrosis. This appearance can also be seen with conditions such as ulnolunate abutment syndrome.[39,40]

MRI has been useful in detection and monitoring of the response of avascular necrosis to conservative therapy. In several cases, the signal intensity in an otherwise low-signal lunate has returned to normal with conservative therapy. This finding correlated with improvement in the patients' symptoms. Although isotope studies can also be used for identification of avascular necrosis, the MR findings are more informative, and the anatomy is demonstrated more clearly.[39,40]

Arthrography, Tenography, and Diagnostic Injections

Wrist Arthrography

Wrist arthrography allows evaluation of the articular cartilage and synovium. The integrity of the ligaments, triangular fibrocartilage complex, and joint compartments can also be assessed.[76]

Arthrography is most commonly used to evaluate patients with posttraumatic wrist pain. The number of injections and the initial injection site depend upon the clinical indication and suspected pathology. All routine radiographs should be reviewed. We also routinely examine the wrist with video fluoroscopy before injection to search for additional clues to the underlying injury.[76]

Technique. The examination may be performed with the patient seated next to the fluoroscopic table or supine with the arm extended and the hand resting palm down. The latter method allows easier access to the patient and decreases the concern for syncopal attacks. The dorsum of the wrist is prepared with the usual sterile technique.

The radiocarpal joint is entered with the wrist flexed over a cushion to open the dorsal radiocarpal joint (Fig. 11-36). The injection site is checked by positioning the needle tip just distal to the radius and on the radial side of the scapholunate joint (Fig. 11-36). Palpation of the dorsal joint space and distal radial tubercle will assist in proper needle site selection. A 0.5-inch, 25-gauge needle is used to inject a small amount of 1% lidocaine (Xylocaine) into the skin. In most patients the same needle will easily reach the joint space and can be used to perform the procedure. If cultures are required or if the soft tissues are thick, a 1.5-inch, 22-gauge needle may be required. Needle position and depth can be confirmed by gently rotating the wrist into the lateral position. The joint should be aspirated before the injection of contrast material. Fluid specimens for culture and synovial fluid analysis may be required in certain cases. Injection of a small test dose of contrast material (meglumine diatrizoate) should demonstrate free flow away from the needle tip. When the proper position has been obtained, 1.5 to 3.0 mL of contrast material is injected. This should be done slowly and observed fluoroscopically to confirm the site of any intercompartmental communication.[43,74,76]

After the injection the needle is removed, and the wrist is gently exercised under video fluoroscopic guidance. In addition, films are obtained in the PA, lateral, oblique, and bending (flexion, extension, and radial and ulnar deviation) positions. In certain situations repeat films may be required after the initial films have been studied.

Injection of the distal radioulnar joint or midcarpal joint (Fig. 11-36A) is performed with the hand palm down. When a previous injection has already been performed, 2 to 3 hours

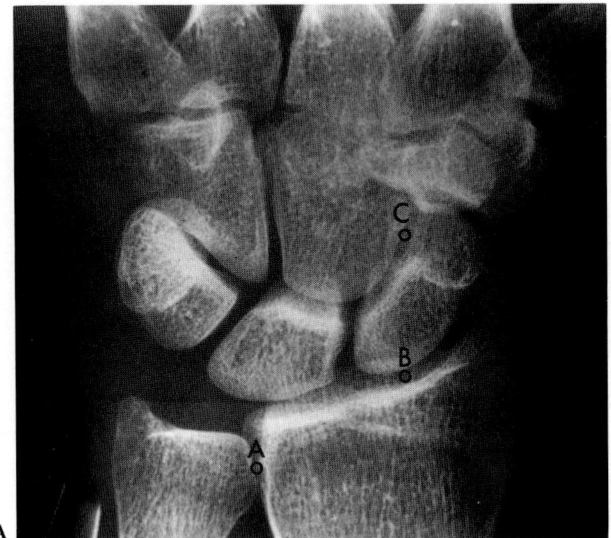

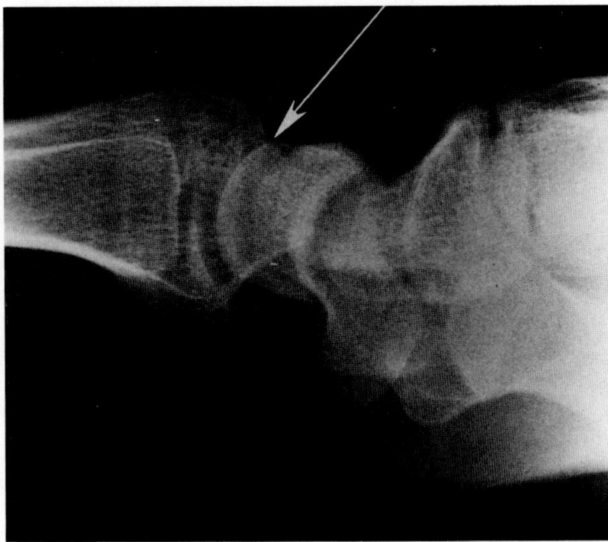

Fig. 11-36 Injection sites for wrist arthrography. (**A**) PA view of the wrist with injection sites for the distal radioulnar joint (A), radiocarpal joint (B), and midcarpal joint (C). (**B**) Lateral view demonstrating the angle of entry for the radiocarpal joint (arrow).

are required to allow the initial contrast medium to dissipate.[52,59,60]

There is some controversy as to how many compartments should be injected. Levinsohn et al[59,60] state that three injections (radiocarpal, midcarpal, and distal radioulnar joint) are required. Manaster[63] suggests that this may not be necessary in all cases if her technique is used. We also frequently use fewer than three injections (Fig. 11-37). Digital technique may be useful for detection of subtle abnormalities.[62] This technique is useful if it is used routinely and if equipment is readily available. We typically use videotape fluoroscopy, arthrography, and occasionally tenography, however. Diagnostic injection with lidocaine or bupivacaine may also be indicated for better localization of the symptomatic compartment.

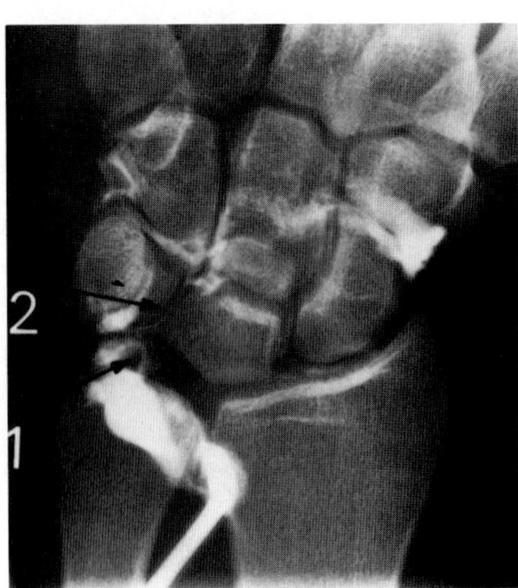

Fig. 11-37 Evaluation of a football center with chronic ulnar pain that reduced his ability to snap the ball for field goals and punts. Injection of the distal radioulnar joint shows a defect in the triangular fibrocartilage complex (1) and a lunotriquetral ligament tear (2). All three compartments are filled with a single injection.

Double-contrast technique is rarely used in wrist arthrography. Occasionally trispiral tomography or CT is used in conjunction with arthrography.[44,66,76]

Normal arthrographic anatomy. The anatomy of the hand and wrist was discussed earlier in this chapter. The compartments of the wrist should be reemphasized for proper arthrographic evaluation and selection of diagnostic injection sites.[76] These include the radiocarpal joint, distal radioulnar joint, intercarpal joint, carpometacarpal joints, first carpometacarpal joint, and pisotriquetral joint (Fig. 11-38).[43,59,76]

Communications between the compartments of the wrist in normal patients have been noted by numerous investigators (Fig. 11-39). The most common problem is differentiating communication of the radiocarpal and intercarpal compartments from a ligament tear in asymptomatic patients.

Injection of the radiocarpal joint will normally demonstrate no communication with the midcarpal or distal radioulnar joint. Communication with the pisotriquetral joint is commonly noted, radiocarpal-pisotriquetral communication occurring in 75% of cases.[52,76] Intracompartmental communications must be correlated with the clinical findings in each patient. Normal recesses are present in the prestyloid region and are volar to the distal radius. There is no communication with the tendon sheaths in the normal wrist.[43,74,76]

Abnormal arthrogram. Arthrography is most commonly performed to evaluate patients with posttraumatic wrist pain or instability. In assessment of ligament injuries the arthrogram

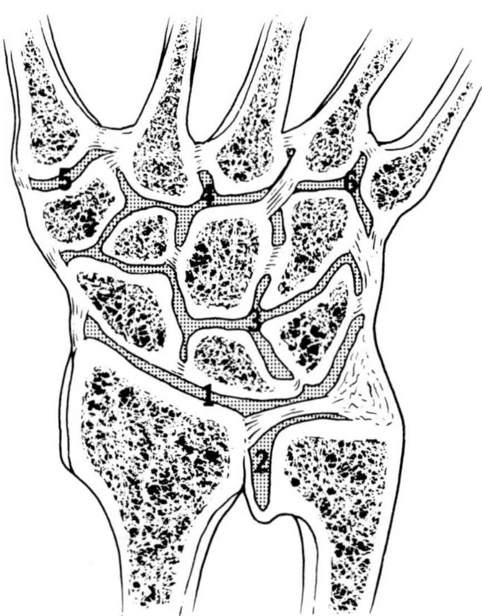

Fig. 11-38 Illustration of the normal compartments of the wrist. 1, Radiocarpal; 2, distal radioulnar; 3, midcarpal; 4, carpometacarpal; 5, first carpometacarpal; 6, outercarpal metacarpal.

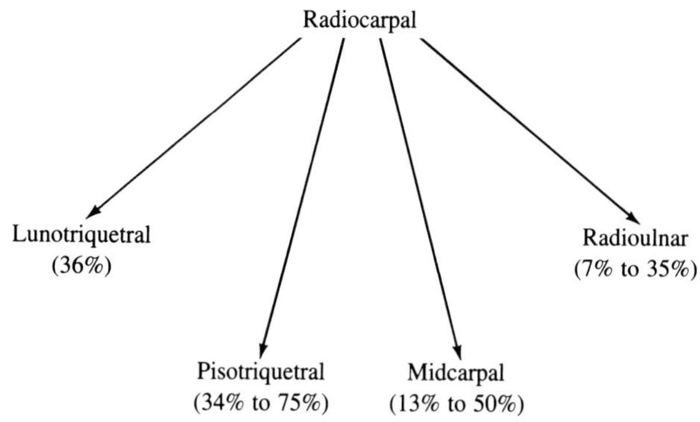

Fig. 11-39 Intercompartmental communications of the wrist. *Source:* Berquist TH, *Magnetic Resonance Imaging of the Musculoskeletal System*, 1990, Raven Press.

must be correlated with clinical findings, including the age of the patient. Patients with ligamentous disruption will demonstrate communication between the compartments of the wrist. The scapholunate ligament is commonly involved. This results in communication between the radiocarpal and midcarpal joints. To be significant, point tenderness or other local symptoms should correlate with the area of abnormality on the arthrogram. The bones may also be malaligned. This may present with widening or loss of the parallelism of the joint space (Fig. 11-40). In addition, a decrease in the radioscaphoid angle or the ring sign may be present. The latter is due to the vertical position of the scaphoid.

Lunotriquetral perforations are also common. This lesion was reported in 52% of cases in the series of Levinsohn et al.[60] This lesion is frequently associated with triangular fibrocartilage complex abnormalities (Fig. 11-37).[60,76] Up to 80% of these patients will also have positive ulnar variance. Both midcarpal and radiocarpal injections may be necessary to clarify isolated lunotriquetral injuries.[76]

Occasionally local synovial irregularity or tendon communication may be evident.[75] Levinsohn et al[60] noted capsular lesions in 31%, lymphatic filling in 12%, and tendon sheath communication in 10% of patients with chronic posttraumatic pain.

Arthrography is necessary to detect adhesive capsulitis. The volume is reduced, and recesses are obliterated.[63] Radiocarpal injection is most effective in this setting.[49]

Identification of periarticular ganglia may be difficult arthrographically. Frequently more contrast material (5 mL or more) and repeat exercise are necessary. Communication is more frequent with the midcarpal joint than with the radiocarpal joint. Therefore, the midcarpal joint should be injected when a ganglion is suspected. If injection of the wrist fails to demonstrate the mass, a direct injection of the ganglion may be useful. Currently, MRI is used more frequently to identify ganglia.[76]

Arthrography may be useful for evaluating other disease processes as well.[43,74,76] In the athlete, however, chronic and acute injuries are the most common indications.

Arthrography of the Hand

Arthrograms of the hand are most commonly obtained to evaluate ligament injury, instability, and cartilage abnormalities.[42,47,48,70,76] The technique is most often used to evaluate the first metacarpophalangeal joint of the thumb. Injury to the capsule and ulnar collateral ligament is common. This injury, formerly associated with gamekeepers, is commonly caused by skiing or other sporting injuries. The patient

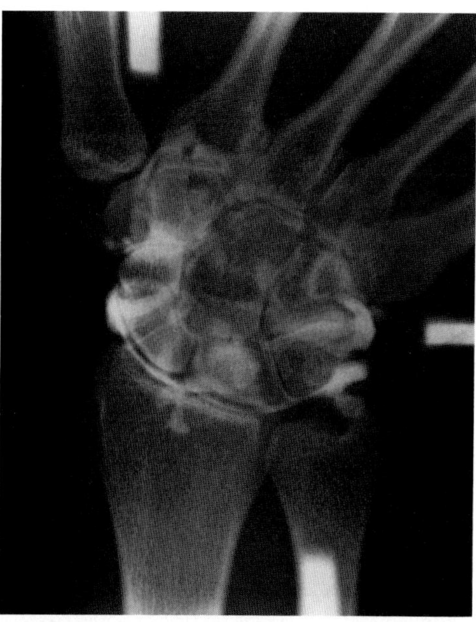

Fig. 11-40 Arthrogram after injection of the radiocarpal joint demonstrating filling of the midcarpal joint due to a scapholunate ligament tear.

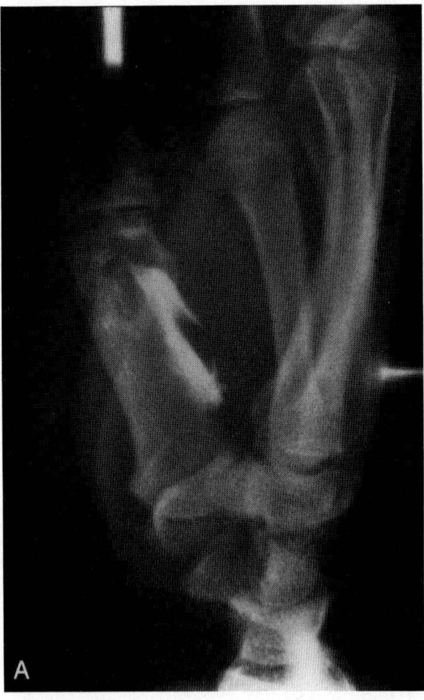

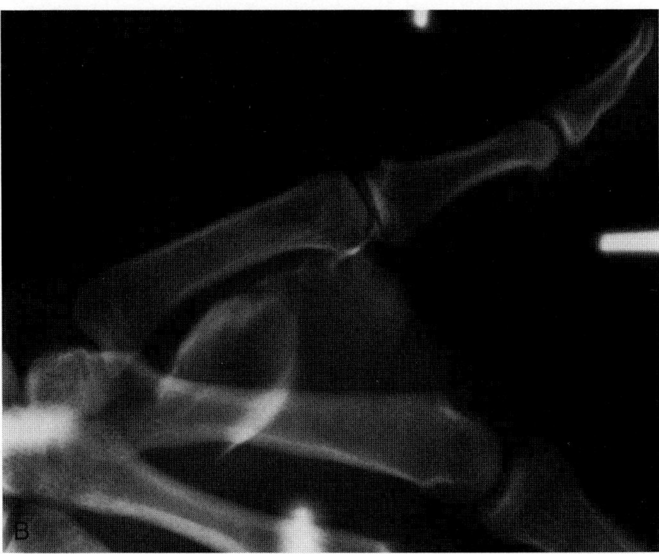

Fig. 11-41 (**A**) AP and (**B**) lateral arthrograms of the first metacarpophalangeal joint demonstrating ulnar extravasation of contrast agent with extension along the adductor pollicis longus due to ulnar collateral ligament tear with volar plate involvement. *Source:* Reprinted from *Imaging of Orthopedic Trauma* ed 2 by TH Berquist, 1991, Raven Press, © Mayo Foundation.

falls with the arm extended and the thumb forced into radial deviation. Subluxation or dislocation, resulting in weakness and decreased pinch strength, may occur.[42,76] Bowers and Hurst[42] described associated chip fractures of the distal metacarpal in 55 of 109 cases.

Examination of the second through fifth metacarpophalangeal joints and the proximal interphalangeal joints may also be required. Arthrography is effective, although less commonly requested, in evaluation of these articulations.

The examination is performed with the patient prone to avoid syncopal attack.[76] The joint is prepared with sterile technique. A 0.5-inch, 25-gauge needle is used for the injection of local anesthetic and the contrast material. The injection site should be dorsal and contralateral to the side of suspected injury. Most commonly single-contrast technique is used. Meglumine diatrizoate (1.0 to 1.5 mL) is injected. If ligament injury is not the primary concern, different techniques may be required. Study of the articular cartilage may be facilitated by double-contrast technique (0.1 to 0.3 mL of contrast material with 1 mL of air). Occasionally trispiral tomography or magnification technique may be useful.[76]

The injection and postinjection filming should be fluoroscopically monitored. Films are taken in AP and lateral projections and with ulnar and radial stress. Hyperextended lateral views are obtained if hyperextension injury is suspected.

Arthrograms are most accurate in the acute posttraumatic period. Extravasation of contrast material from the ulnar aspect of the capsule indicates capsular disruption with or without associated involvement of the ulnar collateral ligament (Fig. 11-41). If contrast material extends along the plane of the adductor pollicis muscle, a tear of the ulnar collateral ligament with involvement of the volar plate is likely (Fig. 11-41).[42,76]

In patients with chronic instability or old capsular tears the arthrogram will demonstrate irregularity, but extravasation of contrast material may not occur. Chronic tears may fill in with fibrous tissue.

Examination of the interphalangeal joints is performed as easily and as accurately as examination of the metacarpophalangeal joints. Ligament and capsule tears result in extravasation of contrast material. Associated periarticular fractures may occur (Fig. 11-42).[70,76]

Tenography

Tenography of the hand and wrist is rarely indicated after trauma. Resnick[68] has described this technique in evaluation of patients with rheumatoid arthritis. When arthrograms are negative, diagnostic tenograms (Fig. 11-43) are useful when combined with diagnostic injection to localize symptoms and to assist in selecting proper therapy.[76]

FRACTURES AND DISLOCATIONS

Distal Radial Fractures

Fractures of the distal radius account for a significant percentage of trauma about the wrist. They account for 17% of all fractures seen in emergency departments.[126] It is also the wrist fracture that most frequently requires manipulative reduction

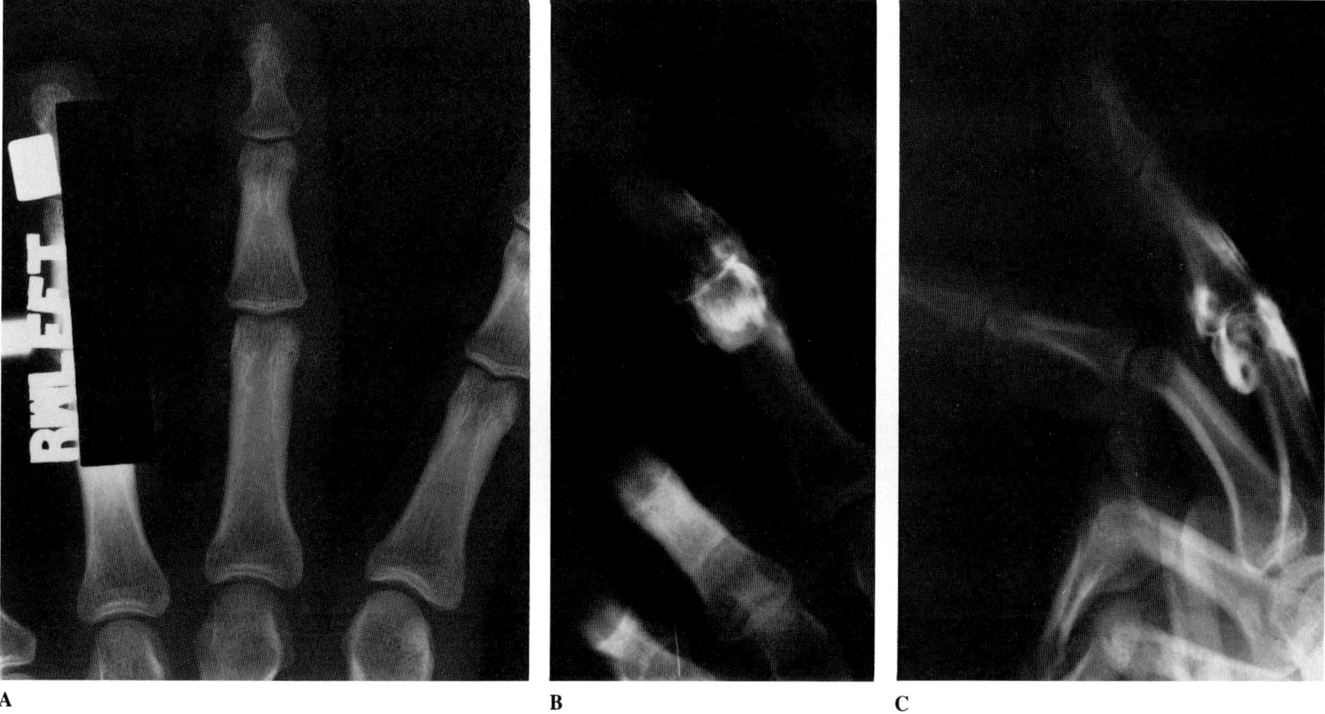

Fig. 11-42 Avulsion of the radial collateral ligament of the middle finger. (**A**) PA view shows soft tissue swelling with a small avulsion fracture. (**B**) PA arthrogram shows irregularity on the radial side of the joint. (**C**) The lateral view is less useful.

and hence careful sequential radiographic monitoring. Most fractures of the distal radius fall into one of five eponymic categories.[161]

Colles' Fracture

The Colles fracture, first described by Abraham Colles in 1813 before the discovery of the X ray, is the most common fracture of the distal radius.[126,161] This term is so well known that frequently, but incorrectly, it is applied to all bony injuries of the radius. The term *Colles' fracture*, however, should be restricted to those fractures of the distal radial metaphysis or epiphysis, with or without intraarticular involvement, that are either displaced and angulated or have the tendency to displace or angulate in the dorsal direction.[125,126,161] Most commonly there is dorsal cortical comminution, but this is not a necessary feature of the fracture. There may or may not be an associated fracture of the ulnar styloid. There should be no demonstrable radiocarpal subluxation.[161]

Radiographic evaluation can usually be adequately completed for this fracture with simple PA and lateral planar films (Fig. 11-44). Interpretation, both before and after reduction, should take into account the following characteristics of the fracture: direction of displacement or angulation, if present (which, by definition, should be dorsal); degree of comminution; presence or absence of intraarticular involvement of the radiocarpal or distal radioulnar joint; degree of apparent loss of radial length (or apparent positive ulnar variance); and degree of loss of the ulnar inclination of the radial articular surface (normally 14°) on the PA projection and loss of the volar tilt of the articular surface (normally 12°) on the lateral projection.[125,126]

The mechanism of injury in Colles' fracture is usually a fall onto the outstretched hand (Fig. 11-45). In an elderly patient

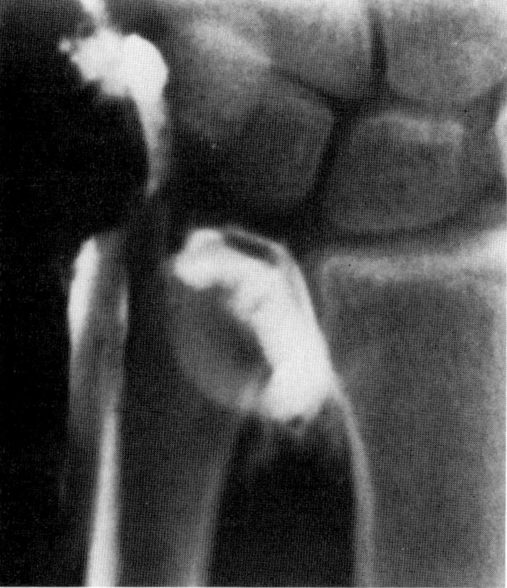

Fig. 11-43 Tenography in a tennis player with chronic ulnar pain. Injection of the distal radioulnar joint with contrast material and anesthetic had no effect on the patient's symptoms. Injection of the extensor carpi ulnaris tendon sheath relieved the symptoms and revealed an extrinsic deformity (arrow) near the ulnar styloid. This was released surgically.

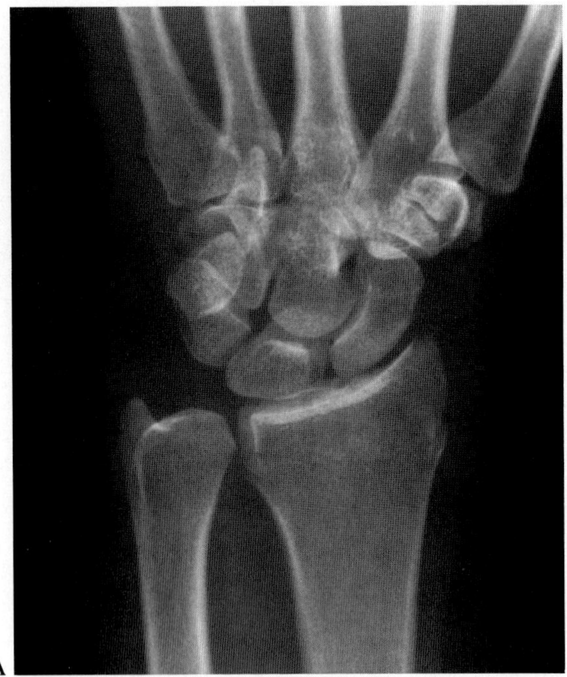

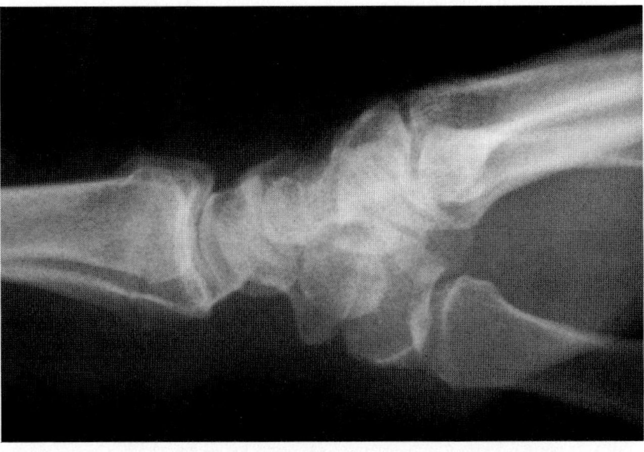

Fig. 11-44 Colles' fracture. (A) PA and (B) lateral radiographs demonstrate a fracture of the distal radius that enters the distal radioulnar joint (arrow). The distal radial angle is neutral on the lateral view (B) as a result of dorsal impaction. Note also the widening of the scapholunate space and the distal radioulnar joints due to ligament injury.

with considerable osteoporosis, this may represent a relatively trivial trauma. In a younger patient, however, a moderately violent force may be necessary to produce this fracture. In the latter instance, therefore, considerably more accompanying soft tissue injury can be anticipated, which may have implications in terms of the treatment options (Fig. 11-45).

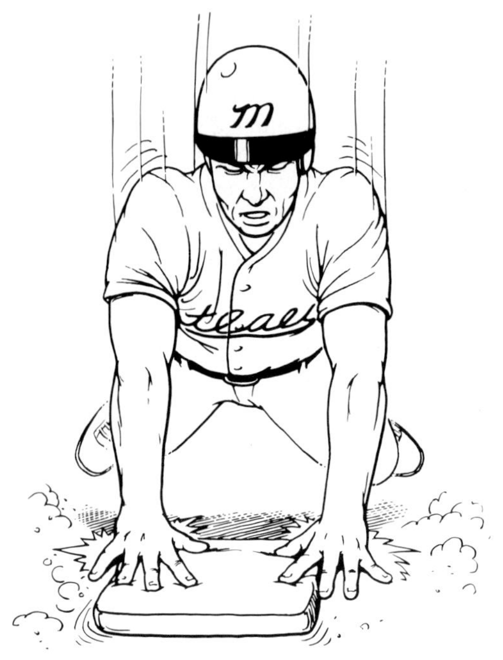

Fig. 11-45 Illustration of the mechanism of most wrist injuries: a fall or slide on the outstretched hand with the wrist dorsiflexed.

The goal of treatment with the Colles type fracture is bony union in as close to an anatomic position as possible and reasonable. Therefore, the minimally acceptable position will vary with the patient's age, the presence of other injuries, and other factors. In general, maintenance of radial length (neutral ulnar variance; Fig. 11-44), 0° to 10° of palmar tilt of the articular surface (lateral projection), 14° of ulnar inclination of the articular surface (PA projection), and articular congruity are the criteria for evaluating adequacy of reduction.[161] The stable fracture (nondisplaced, minimally displaced, or reduced with maintenance of position) is managed by cast immobilization in 75% to 80% of patients.[125]

Complications after Colles' fracture are relatively frequent, with a reported rate of 31%.[95] Eight major complications were described by Cooney et al[95]: compressive neuropathy (7% to 9%), arthrosis, malunion, tendon rupture, unrecognized associated injuries, fixation complications, Volkmann's ischemic contracture, and shoulder-hand syndrome. Median nerve injury is most easily identified on MRI. Similarly, injury to the tendons of the extensor pollicis longus or, less frequently, the flexor digitorum profundus or flexor pollicis longus may be evaluated with MRI. Tenography is less useful and more difficult to perform after acute injury.[83] Unrecognized injuries include scaphoid fractures, ligament injury, and radial head fracture (Fig. 11-44).[95]

The major problems are related to limited finger motion as a result of posttraumatic autonomic dysfunction syndrome (sympathetic dystrophy), median nerve compression, residual wrist pain and deformity, and wrist or forearm limitations in range of motion.[161] The first condition is often radiographically apparent by extreme bony rarefaction distal to the

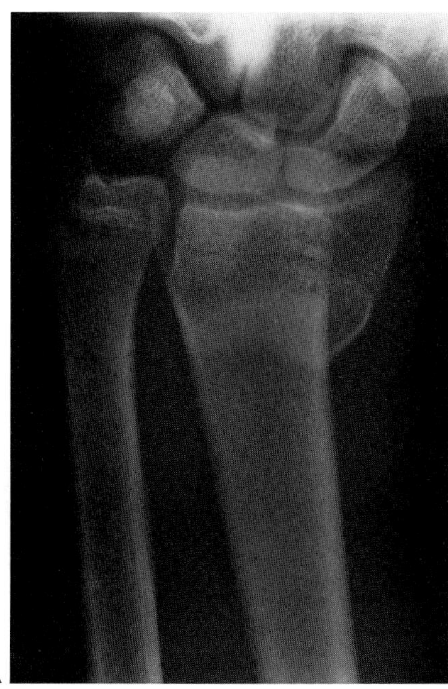
A

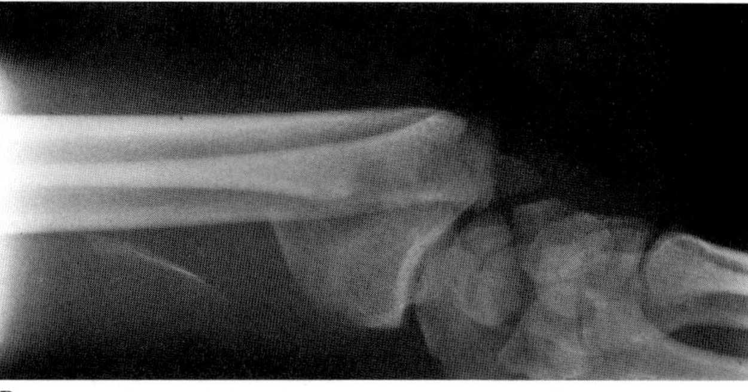
B

Fig. 11-46 Smith's fracture. (**A**) PA and (**B**) lateral views of a fracture of the distal radius and ulnar styloid with volar displacement. This particular injury occurred in a football player as a result of forced palmar flexion of the wrist during tackling.

wrist. The latter complications correlate fairly well with the adequacy of reduction. Nonunion of Colles' fracture is extremely rare.[95]

Smith's Fracture

The term *Smith's fracture* should be restricted to those fractures of the distal radial metaphysis or epiphysis, with or without articular involvement, that are displaced or angulated in the palmar direction (Fig. 11-46). There may or may not be an associated fracture of the ulnar styloid. There should be no radiocarpal subluxation.[161] In general, the Smith fracture can be adequately classified as extraarticular, juxtaarticular, or intraarticular with or without displacement or comminution.

The mechanism of injury as originally suggested by Smith was hyperflexion from a fall on the palmar-flexed wrist. Others suggest that a blow to the dorsum of the wrist and hand or a hypersupination type injury with a fall onto the extended wrist may reproduce this fracture type.[161]

The goals of treatment and the criteria for an acceptable reduction are basically identical to those for Colles' fracture. The complications of the Smith fracture are virtually identical to those of the Colles fracture. Residual subluxation of the distal radioulnar joint with pain or impaired grip strength is not uncommon.[161]

Barton's Fracture

The Barton fracture, by definition, represents a marginal rim fracture of the radius that displaces along with the carpus, in this way producing a fracture-subluxation (Fig. 11-47). The latter feature therefore distinguishes this fracture from an intraarticular Colles or Smith fracture.[102,161] In his original description, Barton described the injury as involving the dorsal or palmar lip of the radius. The palmar variety of this fracture is more commonly seen.[102,161] Considerable confusion is present in the literature regarding the terminology of Barton and reverse Barton fractures. The terms have been applied depending on whether the dorsal or palmar lip of the radius is fractured. A distinction in terminology between palmar and dorsal Barton type fractures will obviate any confusion in this regard.[161]

Adequate radiographic evaluation generally requires only PA and lateral radiographs (Fig. 11-47). It may be particularly important to obtain a high-quality true lateral projection to appreciate the degree of carpal subluxation accompanying the fracture fragment. At times, particularly when assessing the adequacy of reduction, lateral trispiral tomograms or CT scans in the coronal and sagittal planes may be helpful to evaluate the articular congruity of the distal radius.[161]

Adequate classification of the Barton fracture simply notes the location of the marginal fracture as palmar or dorsal with or without comminution. By definition, the fracture is always intraarticular, exhibits some displacement, and is accompanied by a subluxation of the carpus.

The palmar Barton fracture probably occurs by a mechanism similar to that described for Smith-type injuries with

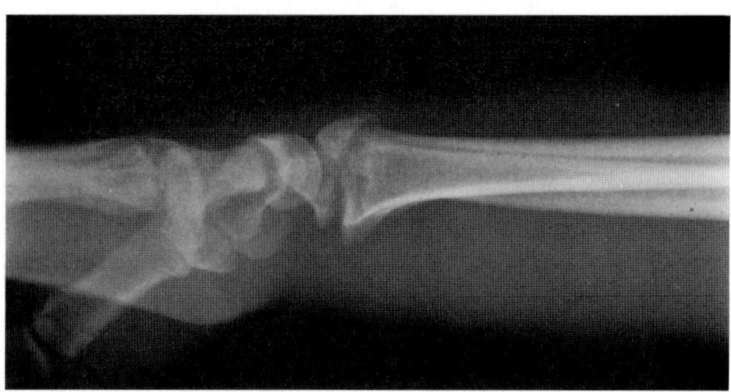

Fig. 11-47 Lateral view of the wrist demonstrating a dorsal Barton fracture.

perhaps an exaggerated degree of loading in compression across the wrist. The dorsal variety most often results from a fall that produces wrist extension and forearm pronation under compressive loading.

Reduction by simple longitudinal traction usually is readily achieved. Occasionally impaction of the fracture fragments may prevent adequate closed reduction. The major difficulty with this injury, however, is maintenance of a perfect reduction. The palmar Barton fracture should be immobilized in the opposite position compared to the dorsal fracture.[161] If an anatomic closed reduction is not achieved, or if the fracture conveys the impression of marked instability at the time of reduction, some means of internal fixation is advised.[161]

The same complications outlined for Colles' fracture may occur with this injury. The major late sequela of the Barton type fracture, however, is residual radiocarpal subluxation and articular incongruity leading to degenerative arthrosis of the wrist.[105] Evaluation of this injury is most easily accomplished with CT.[161]

Chauffeur's Fracture (Radial Styloid Fracture)

Chauffeur's fracture is an intraarticular fracture of the distal radius involving the radial styloid. The fracture line typically originates at the junction of the scaphoid and lunate fossae on the radial articular surface and courses laterally in a transverse or oblique direction. It is best appreciated radiographically on a PA projection (Fig. 11-48). The lateral projection may reveal few if any abnormalities.[161]

This fracture may be simple or comminuted, displaced or undisplaced. By definition it is intraarticular. There should be no evidence of radiocarpal subluxation.[161] The probable mechanism of this fracture is direct axial compression transmitted through the scaphoid.[161]

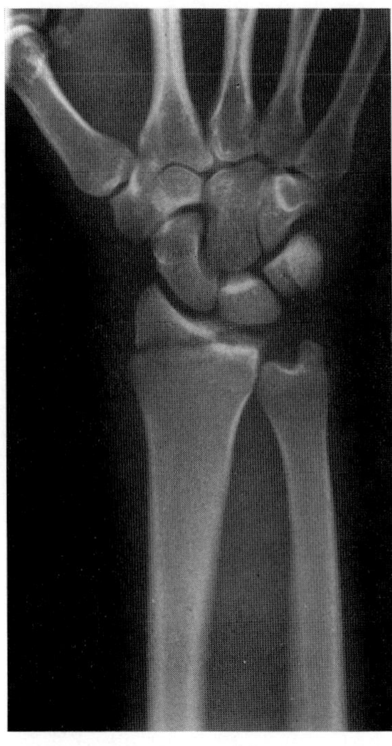

Fig. 11-48 PA view of the wrist demonstrating a typical Chauffeur fracture.

If the fracture is nondisplaced or only slightly displaced (<1 mm of articular depression), simple cast immobilization is sufficient. Because the brachioradialis tendon inserts on the radial styloid, an above-elbow cast with the elbow in 90° of flexion is advisable at least for the first 3 weeks. Usually 6 weeks is sufficient for complete bony union. Complications are similar to those discussed for other groups of distal radius fractures.

Galeazzi's Fracture

The Galeazzi fracture refers to a fracture of the radius that usually, but not always, involves the diaphysis at the junction of the middle and distal thirds with an associated subluxation of the distal radioulnar joint.[132] The latter feature may not always be apparent at the time of initial injury and may not become apparent until treatment is under way. Variants of the Galeazzi fracture include fractures involving the distal metaphysis or the more proximal diaphysis of the radius and cases involving fracture of the distal ulna in association with the radius injury. This injury is particularly important to recognize and differentiate from a Colles type fracture because its treatment is quite different. Routine PA and lateral projections of the forearm are usually adequate to make the diagnosis (Fig. 11-49). Localized views of the wrist in the AP and true lateral positions may be necessary, however, to evaluate the distal radioulnar joint.[161]

The fracture may be comminuted, but usually it is a simple oblique or transverse fracture of the distal radial diaphysis. It may be initially nondisplaced. Displacement characteristically involves the distal radial fragment, which shortens and angulates in a radial direction by the pull of the brachioradialis. Usually only the displaced variety will exhibit significant radioulnar subluxation radiographically.[161]

A fall onto the outstretched hand with hyperpronation of the forearm is the usual cause of this injury. Occasionally a direct

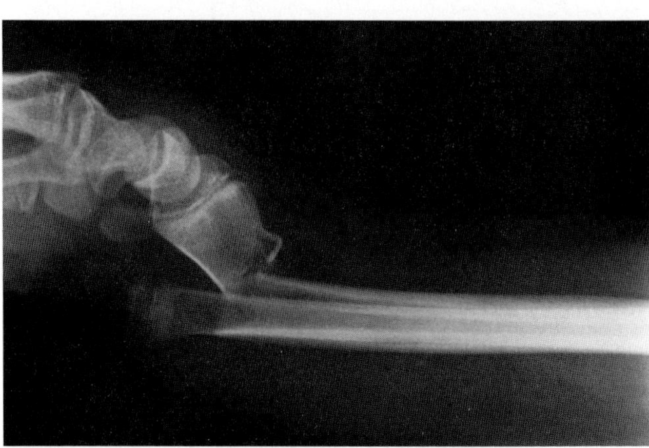

Fig. 11-49 Galeazzi's fracture. Lateral view of the wrist demonstrating a fracture of the distal radius with radioulnar dislocation.

blow on the dorsoradial aspect of the wrist may produce the fracture. Closed treatment is unsatisfactory in 92% of cases. Therefore, in nearly all cases this fracture should be managed by reduction and internal stabilization.

The most frequent complication of the Galeazzi fracture is malunion of the radius and residual subluxation of the distal radioulnar joint. This results most often from inadequate treatment, usually because of the physician's failure to recognize the differences between this fracture and either the Colles or the Smith variety. In contrast to the injuries mentioned above, delayed union or nonunion is not unusual with Galeazzi's fracture. If the fracture is seen late, chronic symptomatic subluxation of the distal radioulnar joint may require distal ulna excision.[161]

Other Fracture Types

In addition to the fracture groups mentioned above, variations of any of these involving an accompanying fracture of the distal ulna can be seen. Isolated fractures of the ulnar styloid do occur, but they are infrequent (Fig. 11-50). If the fracture is undisplaced, radionuclide studies may be indicated to identify bone involvement in patients with posttraumatic ulnar wrist pain.

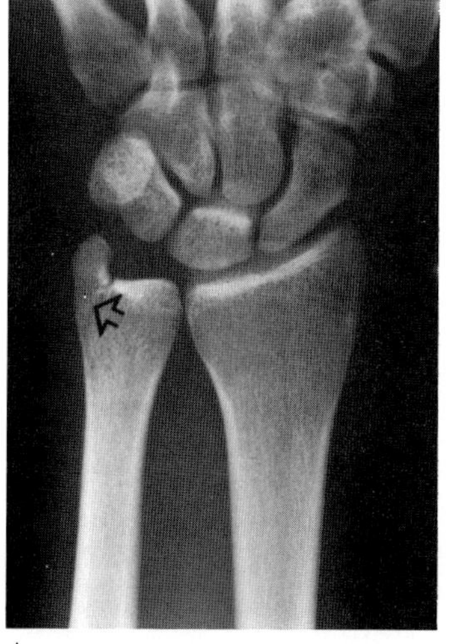

A

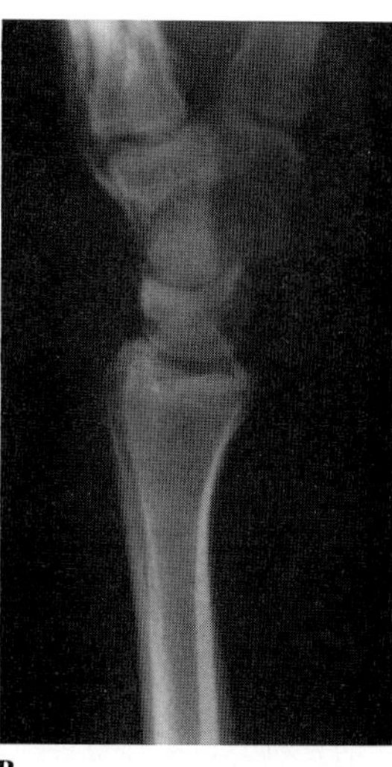

B

Fig. 11-50 (**A**) PA and (**B**) lateral views of the wrist in a soccer player with an isolated ulnar styloid fracture (arrow).

Injury to the Immature Radius and Ulna

Similar mechanisms result in fractures of the distal radius and ulna in children and adolescents. Because the capsule and ligaments are two to five times stronger than the growth plate, the growth plate is more often involved in children.[92] Injuries may result from acute trauma or chronic overuse.[80,87,91,128]

Acute fractures typically involve the radial and ulnar physes; in younger children, torus fractures commonly occur (Fig. 11-51). Physeal fractures are usually Salter-Harris type II.[92] Overuse growth plate injuries tend to involve the distal radius and spare the ulnar physis. Chronic compressive loading, particularly in gymnasts, is believed to result in trauma to the growth plate that, if not treated, can lead to early closure and positive ulnar variance with dysfunction of the distal radioulnar joint.[80,87,91]

Patients usually present with distal radial pain. Radiographs (Fig. 11-52) may reveal irregularity, cystic change, and wid-

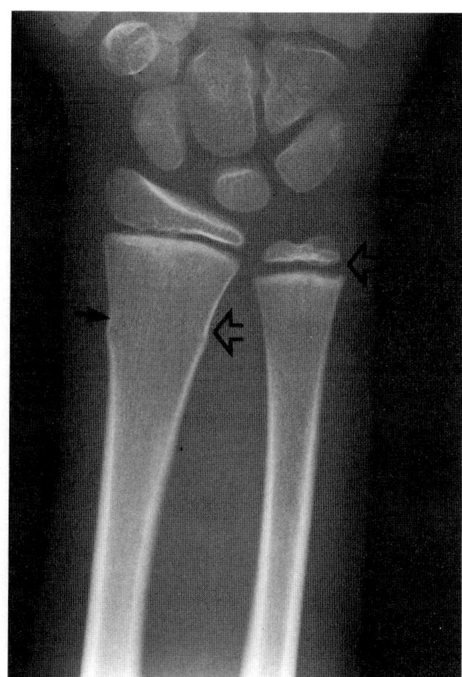

A

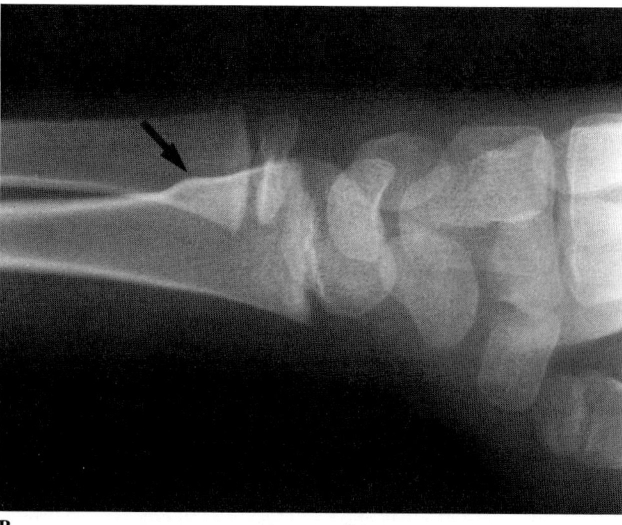

B

Fig. 11-51 (**A**) PA and (**B**) lateral views of the wrist in a young child demonstrating a torus fracture of the distal radius (arrows) and widening of the ulnar growth plate due to a Salter-Harris I injury.

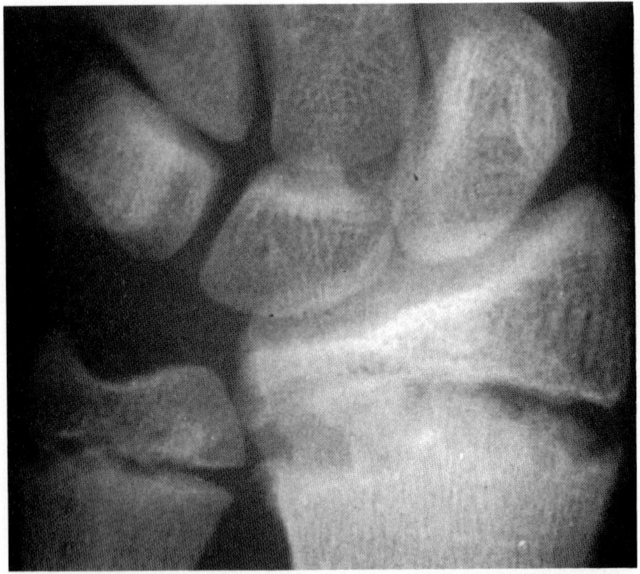
A

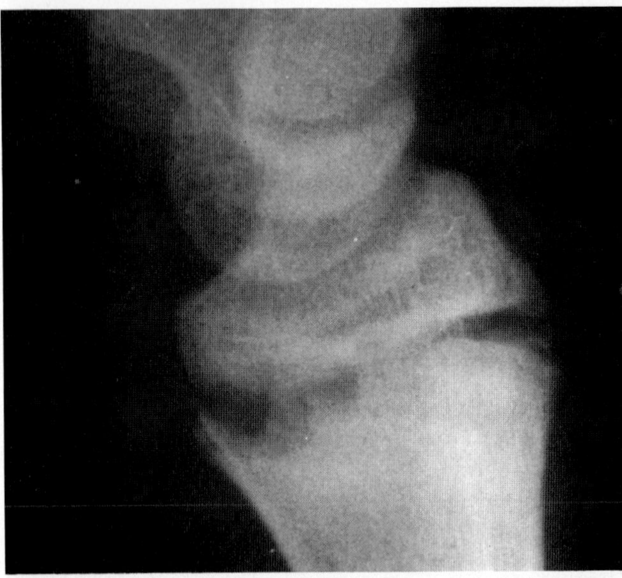
B

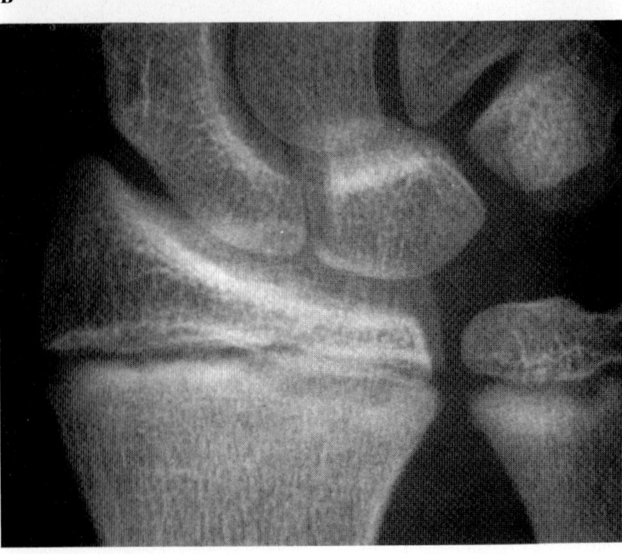
C

ening of the growth plate in the early stages. Premature closure may result later if the condition is not treated.

Diagnosis of both acute and chronic injuries is generally easily accomplished with PA and lateral radiographs. Follow-up studies typically show excellent response to rest (chronic) or cast immobilization (acute) of these injuries (Fig. 11-52).[93]

Dislocations About the Distal Radius

Dislocations of the distal radioulnar joint or, rarely, the radiocarpal joint may occur without an accompanying fracture.

Distal Radioulnar Joint, Dorsal Dislocation

This is the most common type of dislocation-subluxation of the distal ulna.[100,119,121] The usual cause is a hyperpronation injury to the wrist. Clinically the patient maintains the forearm in a position of moderate pronation and resists supination. The distal ulna is usually prominent dorsally.[136] Radiographic evaluation may reveal only subtle abnormalities. On a true lateral view of the wrist, the distal ulna should appear dorsally displaced. Minor degrees of forearm rotation may obscure this finding, however. Perhaps of greater significance is the PA

Fig. 11-52 (**A**) PA and (**B**) lateral radiographs of the wrist in a male gymnast with stress injury to the distal radial growth plate. Note the widening and irregularity. (**C** and **D**) Three months later, after the patient rested from athletic activity, the radiographs were nearly normal. *Source:* Reprinted with permission from Carter SR and Aldridge MJ, Stress injury of the distal radial growth plate, *Journal of Bone and Joint Surgery* (1988;70B:834–836), Copyright © 1988, Journal of Bone and Joint Surgery.

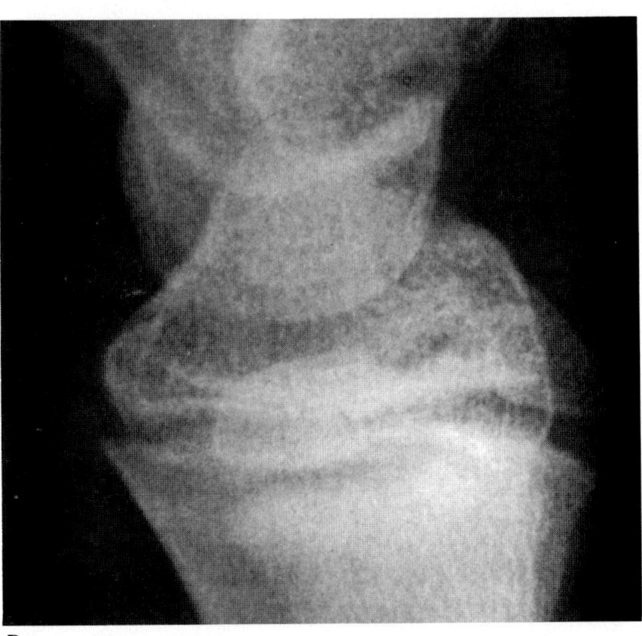
D

projection, which suggests overlap, widening, or incongruity of the distal radioulnar joint (Fig. 11-53).[156] Images in the axial plane (CT or MRI) may be useful in diagnosing these injuries.[161]

Distal Radioulnar Joint, Volar Dislocation

This injury results from a hypersupination stress to the forearm.[161] Clinically, the patient presents with the forearm maintained in supination. The wrist appears narrowed in the lateral plane, and there may be a prominence or fullness over the palmar ulnar aspect of the wrist. Radiographic evaluation should suggest palmar displacement of the distal ulna on the lateral view and overlap of the distal radius and ulna in the frontal plane. Reduction may be more difficult in this case than in the dorsal counterpart.

Radiocarpal Dislocation

In the absence of significant bony injury to the distal radius or as a variant of a perilunate dislocation, radiocarpal dislocation is extremely rare.[107] Displacement of the carpus in both palmar and dorsal directions has been more commonly reported with perilunate dislocation.[161]

Carpal Fractures

Fractures of the carpus frequently involve multiple bones or a single bone in association with significant ligamentous injury. The possibility of such combinations must be kept in mind when these injuries are imaged.

Scaphoid

The scaphoid is the most frequently fractured carpal bone.[96,104,122,155] Scaphoid fractures account for 55% to 70% of all carpal injuries.[120,161] Whether justified or not, the prognosis for these injuries is considered poor. Union rates ranging from 50% to 95% have been reported.[113] One must also exclude transcaphoid-perilunate dislocation (discussed later) when evaluating the fractured scaphoid. Failure to recognize significant concomitant soft tissue injury may lead to serious errors in management.[110] Although rare, associated injuries of the radial head have been reported. Too much attention to this more obvious area of symptoms can lead to overlooking of scaphoid fractures.[112]

If nondisplaced, fractures of the scaphoid may be difficult to detect on routine radiographs. The minimum requirements include PA, lateral, and scaphoid views. Changes in the navicular fat stripe, as mentioned earlier, may be noted (Fig. 11-54). If a high index of clinical suspicion persists despite negative initial films, repeat radiographic evaluation approximately 2 weeks after the injury may be indicated. Usually, but not always, a fracture line may be obvious at this stage. If there should still be some doubt as to the presence of a fracture after the second radiographic study, further evaluation with ^{99m}Tc-labeled MDP bone scans and trispiral tomography may be indicated. Generally in such cases a bone scan is used as a screening study, and trispiral tomography is used only if bone scan shows focal abnormality in the scaphoid region.

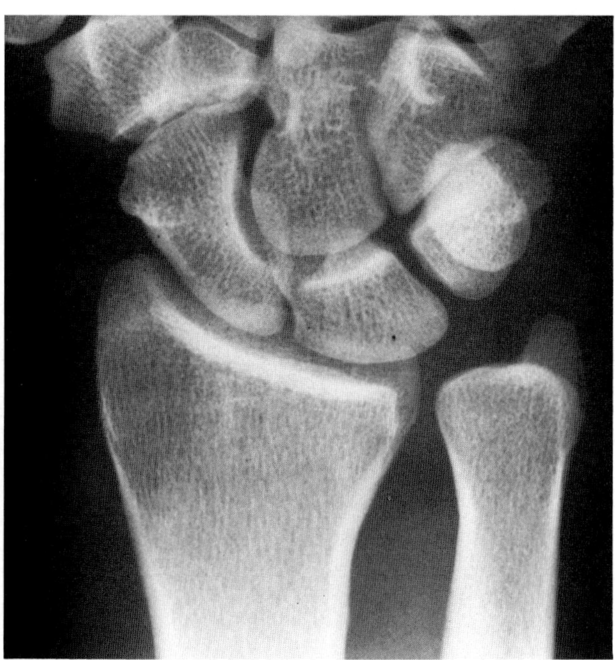

Fig. 11-53 PA view of the wrist demonstrating widening of the distal radioulnar joint (arrow) due to dorsal subluxation.

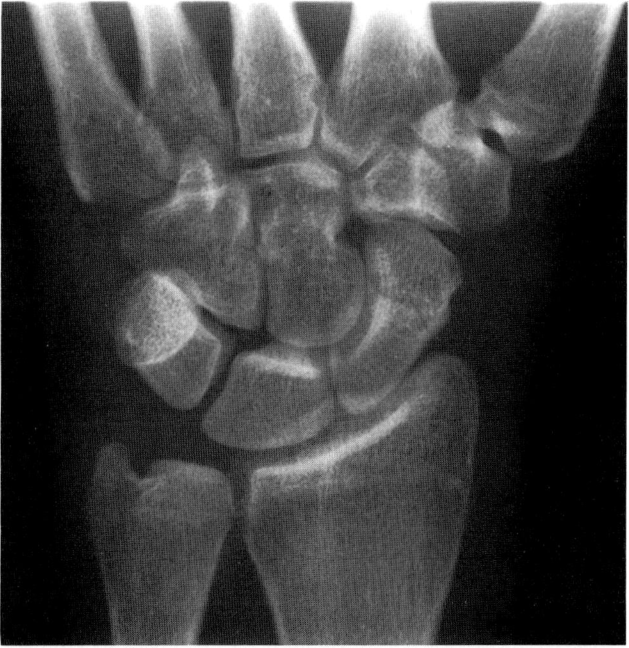

Fig. 11-54 PA view of the wrist in a patient with an undisplaced scaphoid fracture. There is swelling and obliteration of the fat stripe (arrow).

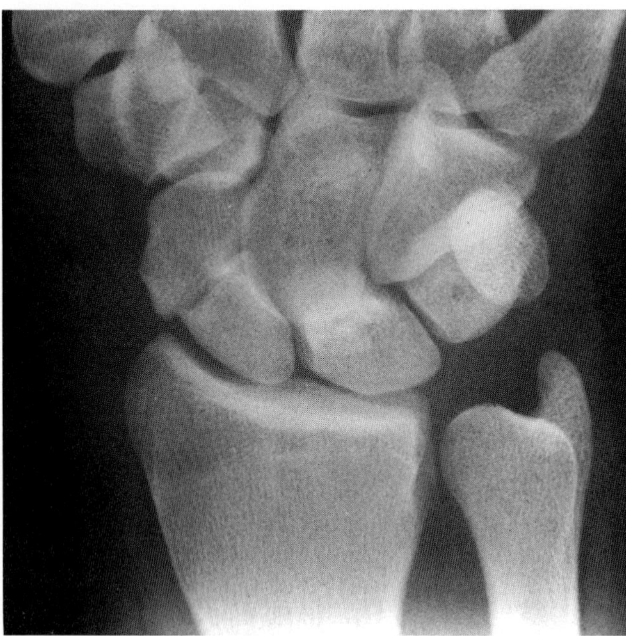

Fig. 11-55 PA view of the wrist demonstrating an obvious scaphoid fracture. Note the overlap of the intercarpal joint due to an associated perilunate dislocation.

Lack of an area of increased isotope uptake in the carpus effectively rules out a fracture.[138,161]

If the fracture is displaced, there is usually little difficulty in diagnosing the scaphoid fracture on routine radiographic views (Fig. 11-55). Trispiral tomography, however, particularly in the lateral plane, may be extremely helpful in assessing the degree of displacement or angulation of the fracture, the adequacy of an attempt at reduction, or the presence of any associated carpal instability patterns (Fig. 11-56). In general most displaced scaphoid fractures involving the waist (middle third) will tend to exhibit angulation of the distal fragment in a palmar direction (Fig. 11-56), with resultant foreshortening of the carpal height, and a dorsiflexion instability pattern of the proximal scaphoid fragment and accompanying lunate.[145,146,151,162]

The scaphoid fracture is most often classified by the location of the fracture line and its direction.[96,142] Both these factors have a bearing on the prognosis as well as on the approach to treatment. The fracture may be classified according to location (eg, proximal third, middle third, or distal third), or it may involve only the tuberosity.[161] The prognosis for union is worst, and the risk of ischemic necrosis of the proximal bony fragment highest, with fractures of the proximal third.[96] Those fracture lines involving the distal third of the bone and tuberosity have the best prognosis and the least risk of osteonecrosis (Fig. 11-57). Middle third fractures involving the waist of the scaphoid are intermediate in terms of prognosis.

The direction of the fracture line has been classified by Russe[142] into three types (Fig. 11-58). Type I is basically perpendicular to the long axis of the wrist and oblique to the long axis of the scaphoid (Fig. 11-58). Because the fracture line is perpendicular to the direction of the forces acting on it, most stresses acting on it are compressive with little shear. Thus the situation is most favorable for bony union. The type II fracture line is perpendicular to the long axis of the

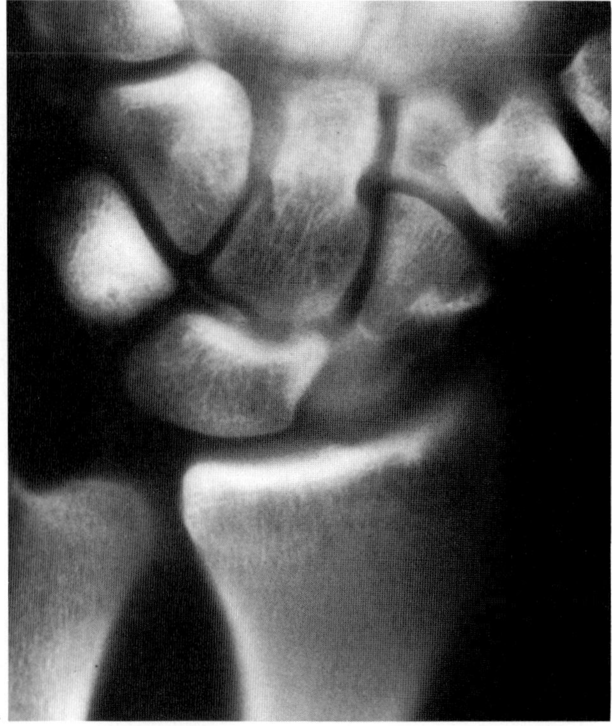

A

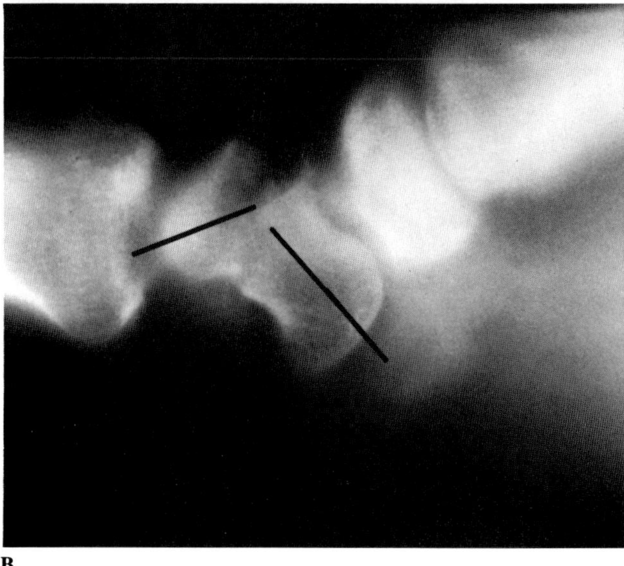

B

Fig. 11-56 (**A**) PA and (**B**) lateral thin-section complex-motion tomograms of the wrist demonstrating a scaphoid fracture with humpback deformity (lines in **B**) and an osteochondral capitate fracture.

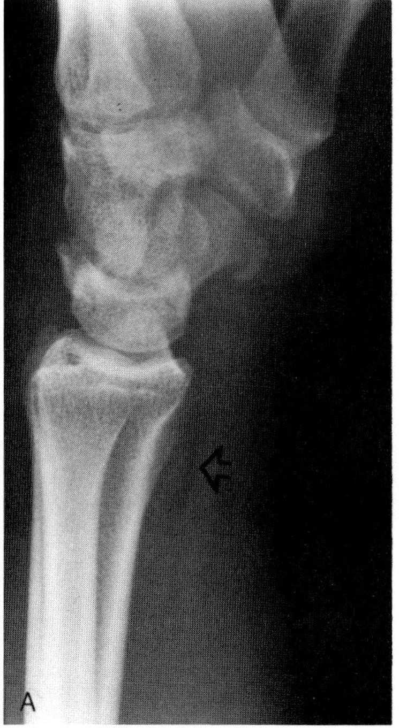

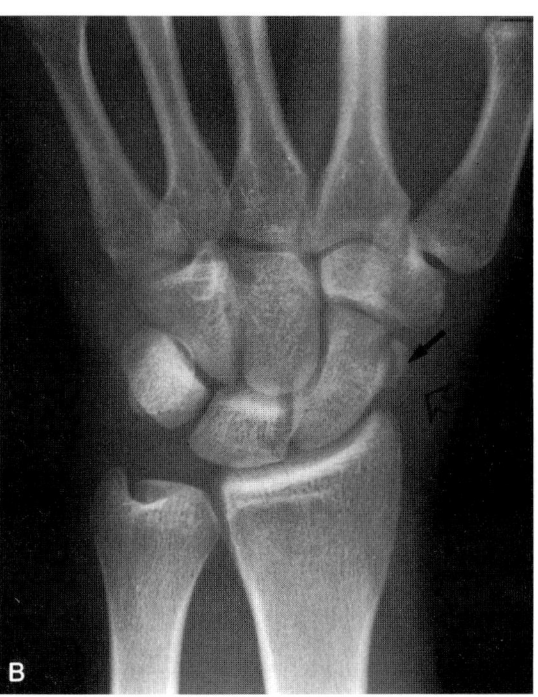

Fig. 11-57 Isolated fracture of the scaphoid tubercle seen on lateral (**A**) and PA (**B**) views. Note the displaced pronator and navicular fat stripes (open arrows). *Source:* Reprinted from *Imaging of Orthopedic Trauma* ed 2 by TH Berquist, 1991, Raven Press, © Mayo Foundation.

scaphoid (Fig. 11-58) and oblique to that of the wrist. A small shear vector acts on fractures of this sort, but most of the forces favor compression of the fragments. Type III has the least favorable prognosis, with the fracture line tending to parallel the long axis of the wrist (Fig. 11-58). Stresses acting across the fracture tend to produce shearing vectors rather than compression. As a result, fracture displacement and nonunion are highest with this type. Moreover, the type III fracture is most common with proximal third fractures. This further exacerbates the unfavorable prognosis.[142]

A fall onto the outstretched hand is the most common mechanism leading to a fracture of the scaphoid. In the laboratory, fracture of the scaphoid is most consistently produced by wrist hyperextension in a position of radial deviation. Applica-

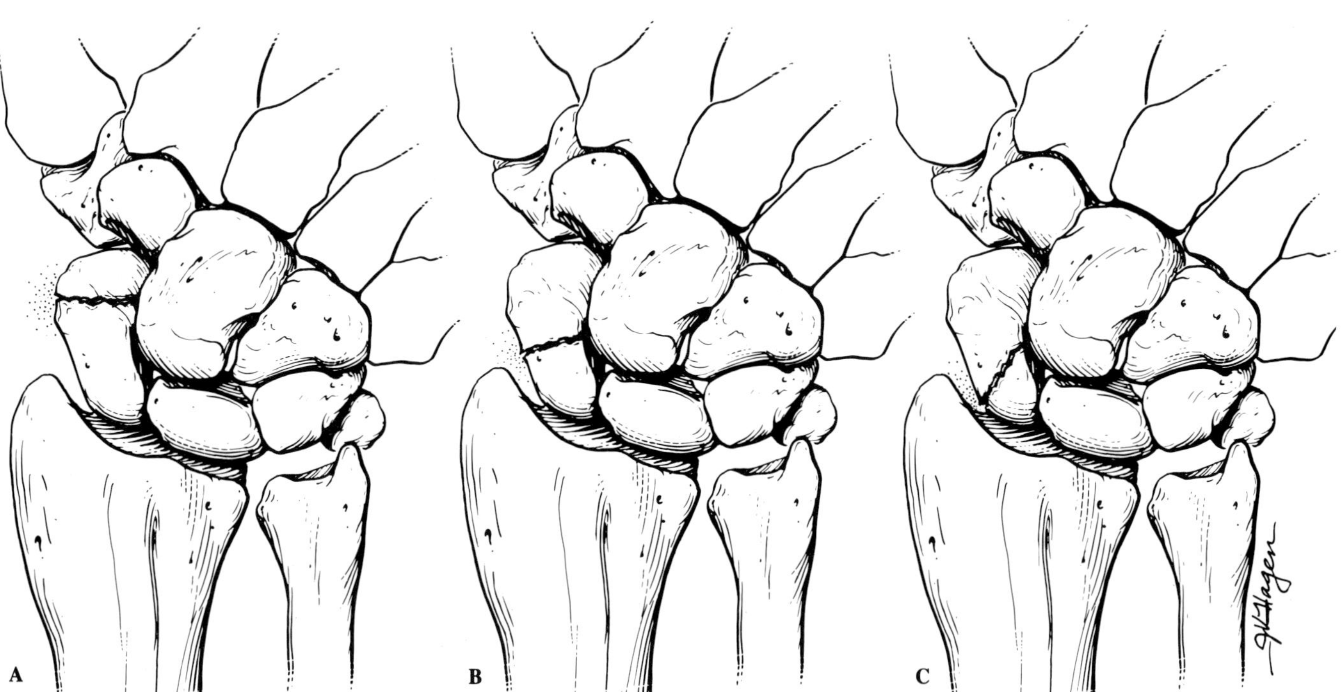

Fig. 11-58 Russe[142] classification of scaphoid fractures. (**A**) Type I, (**B**) type II, (**C**) type III.

tion of the deforming force more distally in the palm appears to produce a scaphoid fracture rather than a Colles-type fracture.[161]

Treatment considerations will vary with the location of the fracture within the scaphoid bone, the degree of displacement, and the degree of associated soft tissue injury. The latter two factors are often related. In general, it is wise to consider all displaced fractures inherently unstable; a high percentage of these actually represent spontaneous, partially reduced trans-scaphoid-perilunate dislocations.

Except under unusual circumstances, all nondisplaced scaphoid fractures should be treated by cast immobilization.[142,155] If adequate reduction is not possible by closed means, open reduction is indicated. Internal fixation and possibly repair of associated disrupted ligaments should be carried out.[161]

The scaphoid fracture is generally associated with numerous complications.[113,142,155,161] If the injury is recognized early, reduced adequately, and treated appropriately over a sufficient period, however, uneventful healing can be expected in more than 90% of cases.[110,161] Delayed union is perhaps the most common complication and is defined generally as failure of union within 3 months of the initiation of cast immobilization. It must be recognized, however, that a significant percentage of scaphoid fractures require 6 to 12 months of cast or splint immobilization to achieve union.[142,155]

Nonunion probably occurs in less than 10% of cases but is more prevalent in fractures of the middle or proximal third of the bone, in Russe type III fractures (vertical direction; Fig. 11-58), in comminuted fractures, and in fractures with unstable reductions. The most common preventable factors associated with nonunion include delay of diagnosis and inadequate treatment. PA and lateral tomograms or flexion-extension lateral tomograms are usually adequate for diagnosis.[145,146] MRI may be useful in this setting as well, however.[161]

Malunion most frequently results from failure to recognize an inadequate reduction. Usually it takes the form of palmar angulation of the distal fragment, producing the so-called humpback deformity (Fig. 11-56). This situation may then lead to foreshortening of the carpal height, which in turn leads to an exaggerated scapholunate angle and a dorsal carpal instability pattern.[142]

Avascular necrosis of the proximal scaphoid fragment is most prevalent with fractures involving the proximal third of the scaphoid.[103,142] It may also be seen, but less frequently, in middle third fractures. It is distinctly unusual with fractures involving the distal third of the bone. Radiographically this condition is characterized by increased radiopacity of the avascular portion. MRI is useful in early assessment of healing and avascular necrosis (Fig. 11-59).[83] When such radiopacity is present, delayed union or nonunion of the fracture is frequent. Revascularization occurs slowly over 1 to 2 years. Significant bony collapse of the avascular portion is unusual.[111,161]

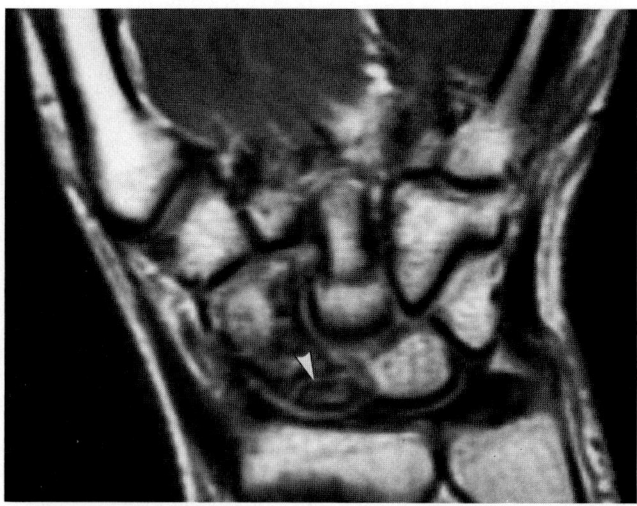

Fig. 11-59 MR image after a proximal third scaphoid fracture shows nonunion with high signal intensity (arrowhead) along the fracture due to fluid. There is normal signal intensity in the marrow of the proximal fragment, indicating no avascular necrosis.

The array of other complications common to all wrist injuries, including limited wrist or digit range of motion, autonomic dysfunction syndrome (sympathetic dystrophy), and carpal tunnel syndrome, may also be seen.

Triquetrum

The triquetrum is the second most commonly injured carpal bone.[95] Most often these are dorsal avulsion injuries, presumably at the site of the ulnotriquetral ligament insertion. More rarely, fractures of the body of the triquetrum are seen.[82] Usually these are nondisplaced, and often they are comminuted. The diagnosis is usually made by routine PA, lateral, and oblique wrist radiographs (Fig. 11-60). Trispiral tomograms may be useful, particularly to assess displacement of fractures involving the body.

Treatment of the dorsal avulsion fracture is symptomatic. A short-arm cast immobilizing the wrist in slight extension for 4 to 6 weeks is usually adequate. Fractures of the body that are nondisplaced are best treated by a long-arm cast for 4 to 6 weeks and then with a short-arm cast for 2 to 6 weeks more or until evidence of union is present. Significantly displaced fractures may be candidates for open reduction and internal fixation.[161]

Lunate

Considerable confusion and disagreement exist regarding fractures of the lunate and their relation to Kienböck's disease.[104,137] Some investigators hold that the etiology of Kienböck's disease is a fracture of the lunate, whereas others suggest that fracture and later fragmentation of the lunate are consequences rather than causes of Kienböck's disease. Acute traumatic fracture of the lunate can occur, however, and may or may not be followed by the typical radiographic findings of Kienböck's disease.

Fractures involving the body of the lunate may be extremely difficult to diagnose on routine radiographs. If a high index of clinical suspicion exists in spite of normal-appearing radiographs, further evaluation by trispiral tomography or bone scan may be warranted.[114] The fracture line usually occurs in the coronal plane (Fig. 11-61).

The mechanism of injury of the lunate fracture is usually hyperextension. Direct axial compression has also been suggested. Nondisplaced fractures should be treated at least initially by long-arm cast immobilization. These fractures require careful vigilance to ensure that displacement does not occur from compressive loads within the cast. Because of the position of the lunate, compressive deforming forces as a result of finger motion are difficult to avoid. Displaced fractures of the lunate are probably best managed by open reduction and internal fixation with Kirschner wires or miniature screws.[161]

Pisiform

Fractures of the pisiform usually result from a direct blow. This occurs when the base of the hypothenar eminence is struck directly in a fall or when the hand strikes a hard object such as a helmet. The fracture may be comminuted or simple. Displacement is usually not marked because this bone is enveloped in the tendon of the flexor carpi ulnaris.[154] Although routine radiographs may reveal a fracture line, the fracture is best visualized on a lateral projection with the wrist in a position of 30° supination (pisiform view; Fig. 11-62). Closed symptomatic treatment in a short-arm cast is recommended.[101] The major late complication is arthrosis of the pisotriquetral joint, which may require excision of the pisiform.[88,161]

Hamate

Fractures of the hamate may involve the body, the dorsal aspect,[114] the distal articular surface as a component of a carpometacarpal fracture-dislocation, or the hook (hamulus).[84,139,149] Fractures of the body are usually nondisplaced and can be diagnosed on routine PA, lateral, and oblique radiographs. These are stable injuries and can generally be managed adequately by short-arm cast immobilization for 4 to 8 weeks. Complications are unusual.

Fractures involving the distal articular surface as a component of a carpometacarpal dislocation are suggested on routine wrist radiographs. Detection of the fracture may require trispiral tomography (Fig. 11-63). These are unstable injuries and hence usually require internal fixation after closed or open reduction. The major late complication is degenerative arthrosis of the carpometacarpal articulation, particularly if the fracture heals with residual articular incongruity or joint subluxation.

Fracture of the hook (hamulus) is the most common injury to the hamate.[88,90,93,139,147,148] This is generally believed to be an avulsion fracture, presumably caused by the pull of the transverse carpal ligament that inserts on the hook of the hamate. The majority of fractures occur at the base of the hook.[148] These seem to be particularly prevalent in association with a dubbed golf swing and bad hits in racquet sports.[148,153]

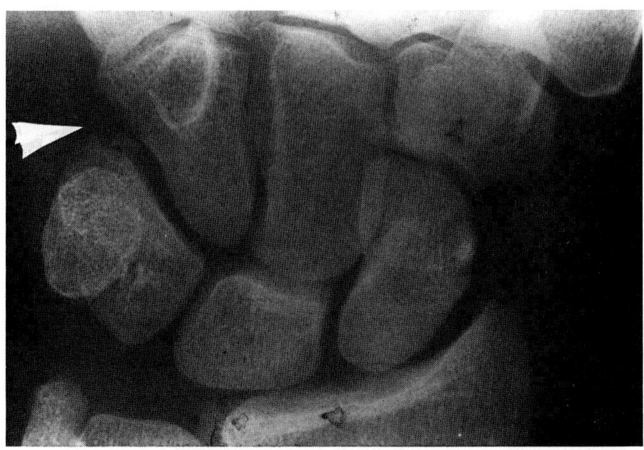

A

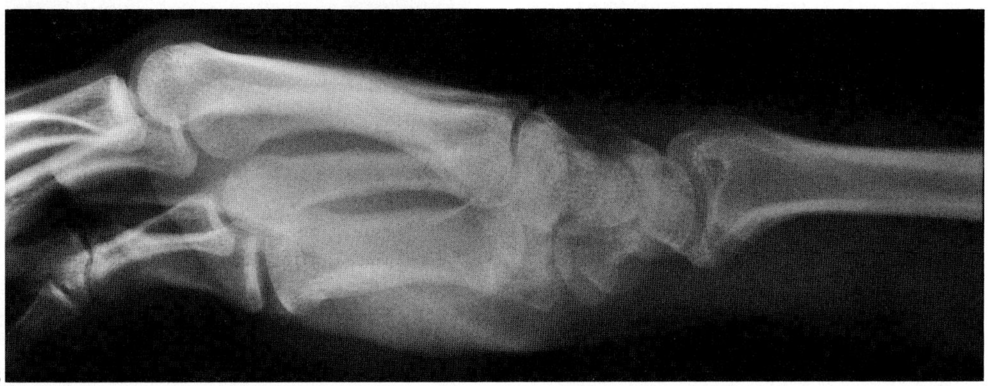

B

Fig. 11-60 **(A)** PA view of the wrist demonstrating a small triquetral fracture (arrow). **(B)** Most dorsal fractures are best seen on the lateral view.

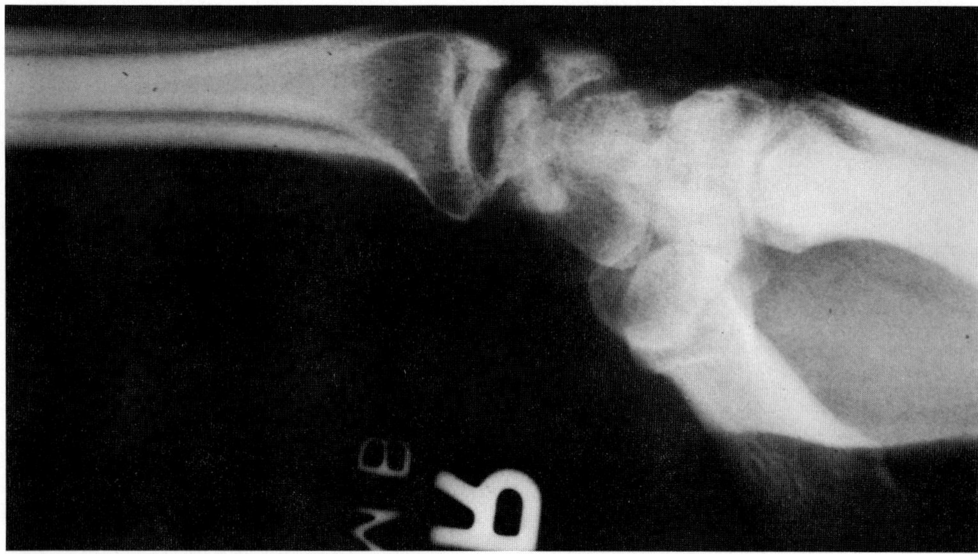

Fig. 11-61 Lateral view of the wrist demonstrating a lunate fracture. There is also avascular necrosis causing sclerosis and compression of the lunate.

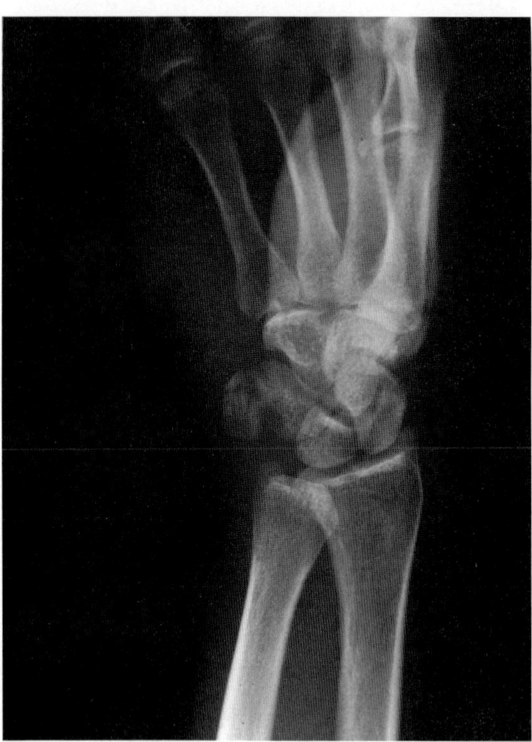

Fig. 11-62 Pisiform oblique view demonstrating an undisplaced fracture of the pisiform.

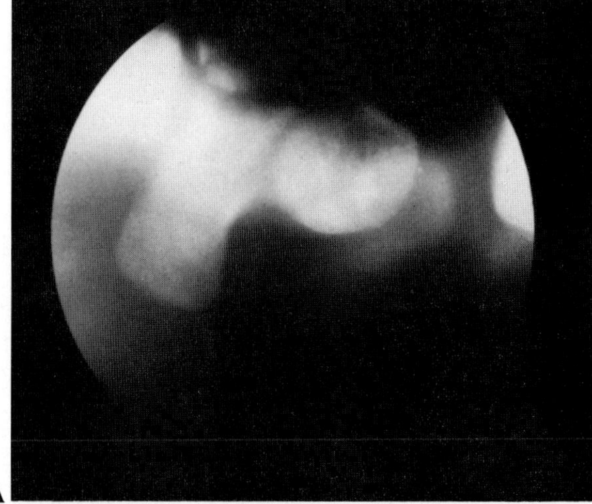

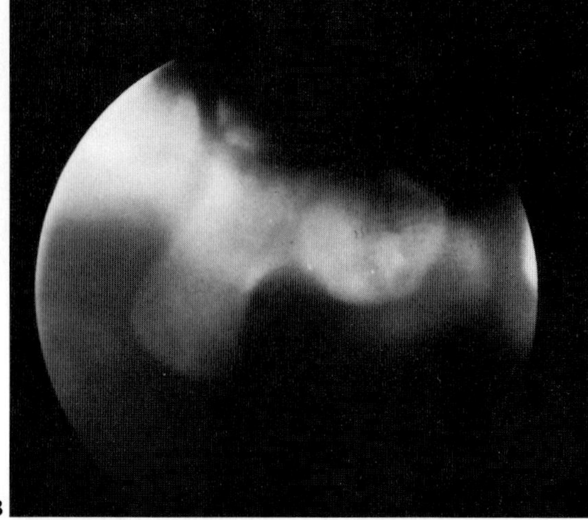

Fig. 11-63 Lateral tomograms of a dorsal articular fracture of the hamate.

The diagnosis is difficult to make on routine radiographs, but there are three useful radiographic signs that may be useful on the PA view: absence of the hook, sclerosis in the region of the hook, or lack of the normal cortical ring.[139] A carpal tunnel view may be helpful (Fig. 11-29). Trispiral tomography is diagnostic in most instances, but a localized bone scan may be useful in localizing the pathology before tomograms are obtained. CT may be useful in certain cases.[148]

Closed treatment by cast immobilization is unreliable for healing. Most clinicians recommend excision of the fractured fragment, although some suggest open reduction and internal fixation. Most complications of this injury result from failure to make the correct diagnosis. These include persistent pain, ulnar neuropathy, and attritional flexor tendon rupture.[99,161]

Capitate

Capitate fractures may involve the body, the distal articular surface as a component of a carpometacarpal fracture-dislocation, or the proximal pole (Fig. 11-64).[88,161] Fractures involving the body occur most commonly through the middle third and are transverse. They are usually the result of a hyperextension injury.[106] A direct blow over the dorsum of the capitate may also be responsible. Comminution may be present. Routine PA and lateral radiographs are usually sufficient to arrive at a diagnosis. If the fracture is nondisplaced, short-arm cast immobilization for 6 to 8 weeks is usually adequate. If displaced, the fracture is likely to be unstable. Internal fixation, usually with Kirschner wires, may be necessary in this setting.[161] Complications include nonunion, delayed union, and avascular necrosis of the proximal fragment. Fractures involving the distal articular surface are similar to those described for the same location in the hamate as part of the carpometacarpal dislocation.

Trapezoid

Fractures of the trapezoid are uncommon, and isolated dislocations are rare.[88,122,124,125] They may be seen as a component of a carpometacarpal fracture-dislocation. In such instances, the comments directed to this same injury in the capitate apply. Detection on routine radiographs is difficult. Trispiral tomography or CT is usually indicated.[115] It is not unusual to detect these subtle injuries when performing MR examinations to identify the cause of chronic wrist pain.[83] The major goal of treatment is stability of the trapezoid–second metacarpal articulation. This may require arthrodesis.

Trapezium

Fractures of the trapezium involve the body, the margin, or the ridge.[88,97,122] Those through the body are usually vertical and may result from direct axial compression on the thumb, hyperextension of the first metacarpal, or a blow to the adducted thumb. Comminution and displacement may be present. In addition to routine PA, lateral, and oblique radiographs, X-ray evaluation should include a true PA view of the first carpometacarpal joint and possibly trispiral tomograms. If the fracture is nondisplaced, short-arm cast immobilization with the thumb in moderate palmar abduction is usually adequate. If it is displaced, open reduction and internal fixation may be required. The chief complication of this fracture is degenerative arthrosis of the basilar thumb joints.[161]

Marginal fractures are not uncommon. Provided that they are not displaced, they are comparable in terms of treatment and prognosis to scaphoid tuberosity fractures (Fig. 11-65). If there is any displacement, careful radiographic scrutiny for evidence of subluxation of the joint should be carried out.[161]

Fractures of the ridge of the trapezium are generally believed to be avulsion fractures at the site of the transverse carpal ligament insertion. These may be difficult to visualize

Fig. 11-64 PA view of the wrist demonstrating a proximal capitate fracture (arrowhead).

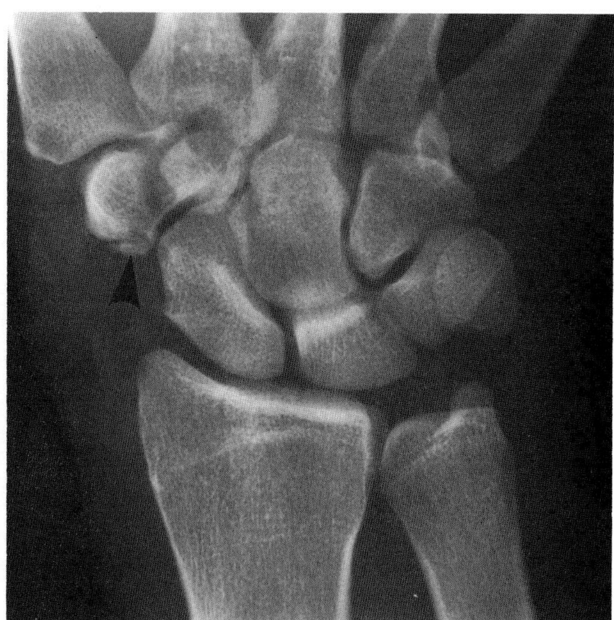

Fig. 11-65 PA view of the wrist demonstrating a margin fracture of the trapezium (arrowhead).

on routine radiographic views but can usually be seen on carpal tunnel views or trispiral tomograms. In terms of prognosis and treatment, they may be similar to fractures of the hook of the hamate. If the fracture is displaced or seen late, excision of the fracture fragment may be indicated.

Dislocations of the trapezium are rare and usually associated with other hand and wrist injuries.[150]

Carpal Dislocations

Dislocations of the carpus are uncommon and most frequently are associated with a perilunate injury or a variant of this injury.[109,118,129,131,143]

Dorsal Perilunate Dislocations and Variants

These injuries include a spectrum of findings that vary with the degree of associated trauma and the position of the force of impact on the wrist. Most are extreme hyperextension injuries resulting from a fall onto the dorsiflexed wrist (Fig. 11-45).[118,159,161]

Transscaphoid perilunate dislocation. This is the most common type of perilunate dislocation. Typically the lunate and proximal scaphoid fragment remain in articulation with the distal radius, and the remainder of the carpus and the distal scaphoid fracture are displaced in a dorsal direction (Fig. 11-66). Routine PA and lateral radiographs are usually adequate to suggest the injury. Oblique views or tomograms may be necessary to clarify the diagnosis, however, particularly with regard to associated carpal fractures. The incidence of scaphoid malunion or nonunion after this injury is significant. For this reason, unless a perfect and stable closed reduction is achieved, many clinicians advocate stable internal fixation with or without open repair of the disrupted or attenuated volar radiocarpal ligament complex.[161]

In addition to scaphoid nonunion or malunion, late complications and sequelae include carpal instability, limited range of motion of the wrist, median neuropathy, late degenerative arthritis, and occasionally avascular bony necrosis.[161]

Dorsal perilunate dislocation. This dislocation is essentially the same injury as the transscaphoid perilunate dislocation except that the scaphoid remains intact. The volar radiocarpal ligament complex is completely disrupted. The mechanism of injury and treatment principles are the same. The most significant late sequela is residual carpal instability (DISI).[143,161]

Anterior (volar) lunate dislocation. This injury is believed to represent a variant of the dorsal perilunate dislocation. It probably results from spontaneous reduction of the dorsally displaced carpus, which essentially settles on the lunate, displacing it in a palmar direction (Fig. 11-67). Closed reduction of this injury may be difficult and requires direct pressure over the displaced lunate in a dorsal direction in addition to longitudinal traction. The mechanism of injury and treatment principles are as outlined earlier.[161]

Volar Perilunate Dislocations and Variants

These injuries are extremely rare.[79,118,161] Most commonly they are associated with violent trauma that produces hyperflexion of the wrist. They can involve any combination of associated fractures or may lead to a posterior (dorsal) lunate dislocation by a mechanism similar to that described earlier. Complications after these injuries are frequent and include carpal instability, limited range of motion, avascular bony necrosis, and degenerative arthritis.

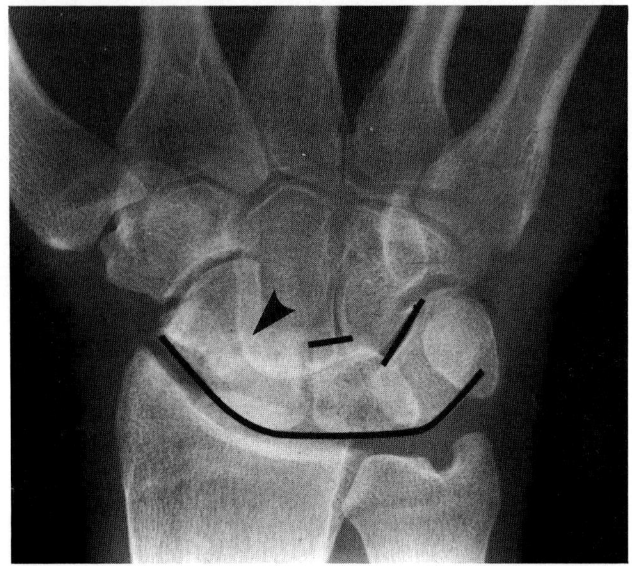

A

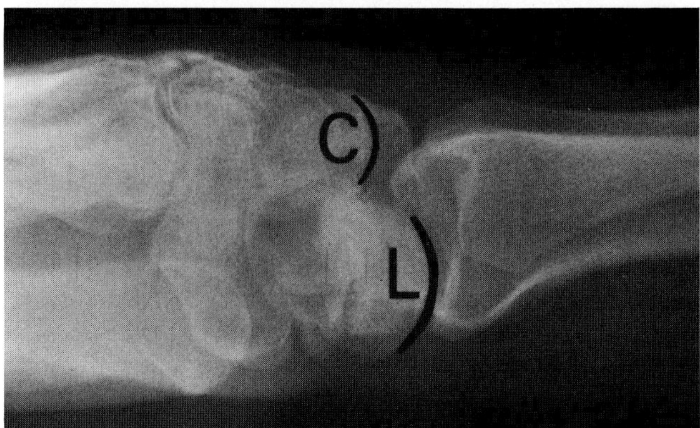

B

Fig. 11-66 Dorsal transscaphoid perilunate dislocation. (**A**) PA view shows interruption of the carpal arcs (lines) with a midscaphoid fracture (arrowhead). The lunate and proximal scaphoid maintain their relationship with the radius. (**B**) Lateral view shows dorsal displacement of the capitate (C) on the lunate (L).

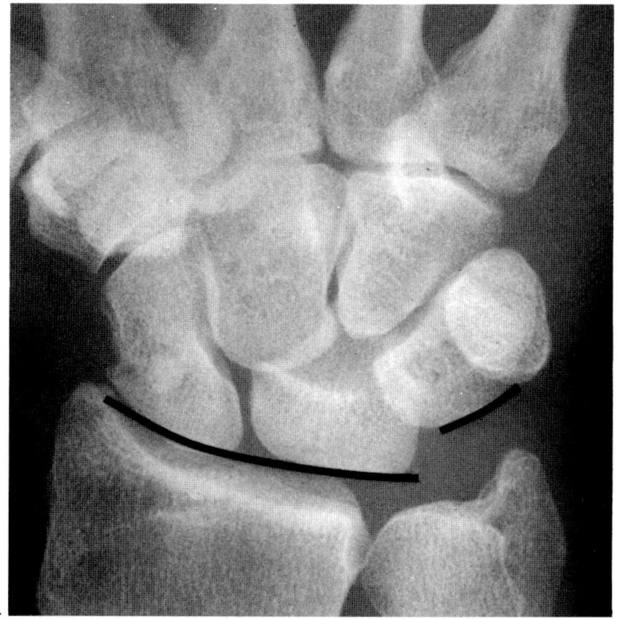

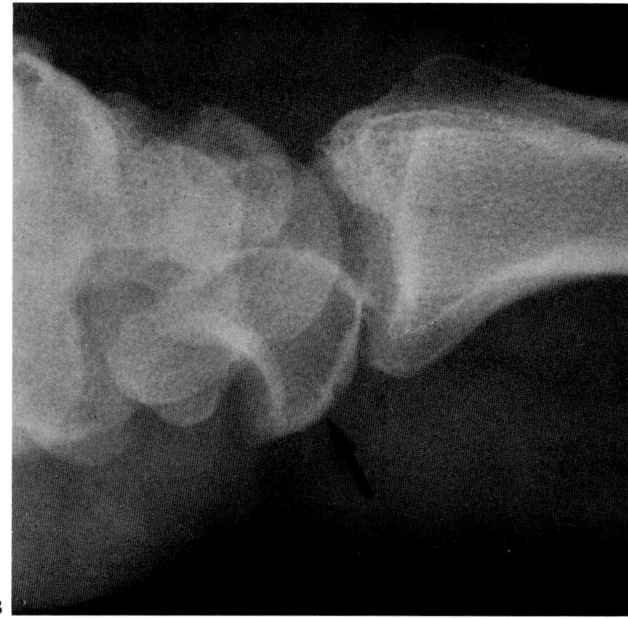

Fig. 11-67 Volar lunate dislocation. (**A**) PA view shows interruption of the arcs with elongation of the lunate. (**B**) Lateral view demonstrates volar displacement of the lunate (arrow).

Dislocations of the Carpus Other Than Perilunate

Although rare, dislocation of virtually every carpal bone has been described.[123,134,161] These occur either as isolated entities or in combination with other carpal dislocations or fractures. The most common nonperilunar carpal dislocations involve the trapezoid[117] and the trapezium.[116] Trapezoid dislocations occur most commonly in the dorsal direction, presumably from a hyperflexion stress to the second metacarpal. Palmar dislocations have also been described. Trapezial dislocations are most often associated with axial compression–adduction injuries. Associated marginal fracture is common.[161]

Diagnosis of subtle subluxation or dislocation may be difficult, especially when the typical scapholunate and lunate patterns described above are not present. Static instability (patterns seen on neutral routine radiographs) and dynamic instability (patterns seen only with motion) may both exist. The latter is more easily appreciated with video fluoroscopic studies.[85,152,161]

Carpometacarpal Dislocation

Carpometacarpal dislocation or subluxation is most often associated with an accompanying fracture of the distal carpal row or metacarpal base (Fig. 11-68).[108] These injuries may be difficult to define accurately on routine radiographs. Multiple oblique views, fluoroscopic spot views, or trispiral tomograms are often helpful. As an isolated injury without fracture, a carpometacarpal dislocation is rare (Fig. 11-69).[135,161] Most commonly they involve multiple rays or the border rays. The direction of displacement is usually dorsal, although volar dislocation has also been reported. These dislocations, particularly when they involve the first or fifth metacarpal, may be grossly unstable.[161] If the dislocations are reducible but unstable, percutaneous fixation is recommended. If they are irreducible, open reduction with internal fixation and possibly soft tissue repair is advisable.[161,162]

Metacarpal Fractures

Fractures of the metacarpals, particularly the fourth and fifth, are common.[141,161] The metacarpal involved, the type and location of the fracture line, the degree of displacement, the adequacy of rotatory alignment, and the presence of any associated soft tissue injury need to be identified radiographically for the purpose of treatment planning. In general, routine PA, lateral, and oblique radiographs are adequate for evaluation of these injuries. For discussion and treatment purposes, metacarpal fractures should be considered in three subgroups: thumb, stable rays (second and third metacarpals), and mobile rays (fourth and fifth metacarpals; Fig. 11-70). Within each of these groups, a similar fracture classification is applicable.

Thumb

The first metacarpal is highly mobile, and there is significant motion allowed at the carpometacarpal joint. Therefore, considerable tolerance exists for fracture angulation and rota-

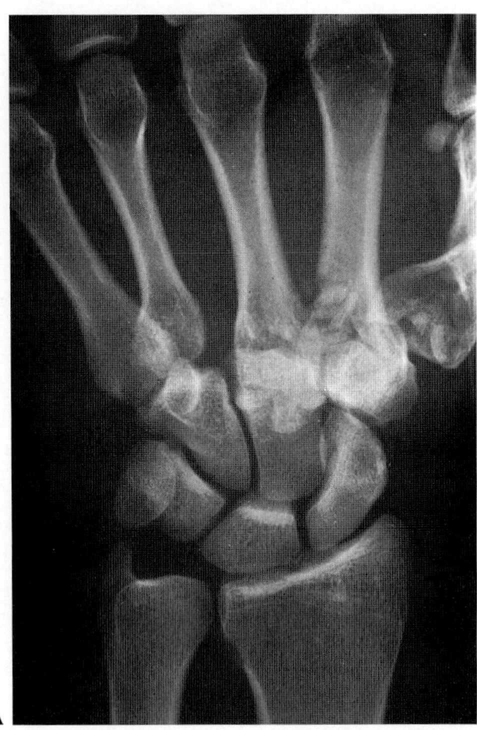

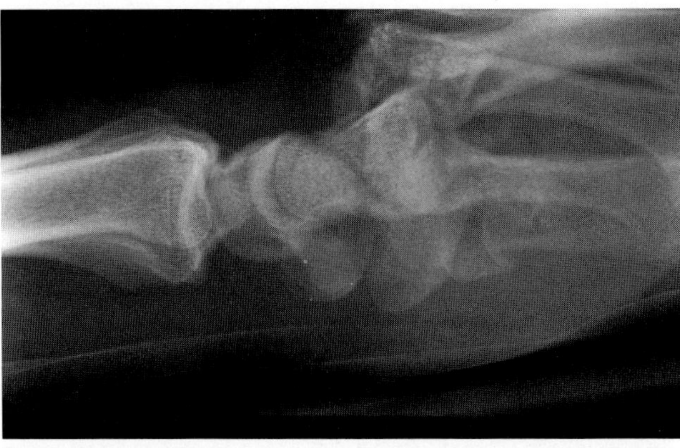

Fig. 11-68 (**A**) PA and (**B**) lateral radiographs demonstrating dorsal fracture-dislocations of the second and third metacarpals. The base of the thumb is also fractured.

tion. This same feature of high mobility of the basilar joint, however, is offset by the requirement that the thumb transmit a high magnitude of compressive load in pinch. This allows little tolerance for residual incongruity in the case of intraarticular fractures of the base.[161]

Extraarticular fractures of the metaphysis are relatively common (Fig. 11-71). They may be transverse or oblique and are usually angulated dorsally. Displacement may be present. Angulation of up to 20° in the adult and 40° in the child is acceptable. Fractures of the transverse plane are usually readily reduced by longitudinal traction. Maintenance of reduction is usually possible through a well-molded thumb spica cast that secures the thumb metacarpal in moderate palmar abduction and extension.[161]

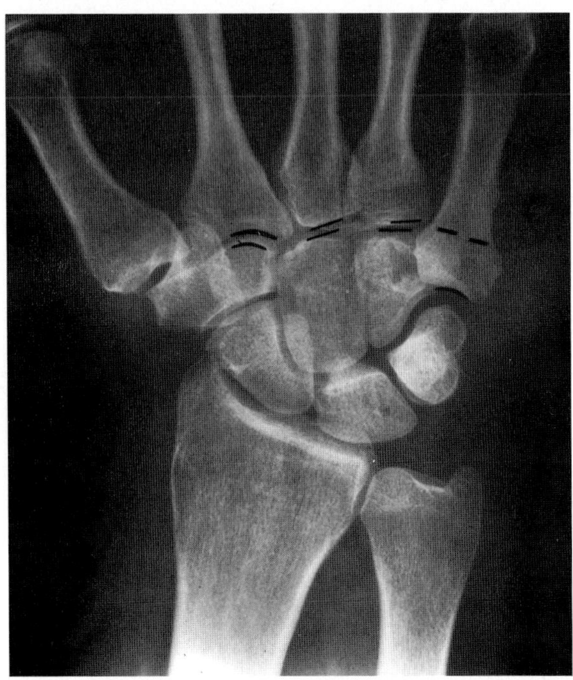

Fig. 11-69 PA view of the wrist demonstrating an isolated dislocation of the fifth metacarpal. The articular surfaces (lines) should be parallel at all levels.

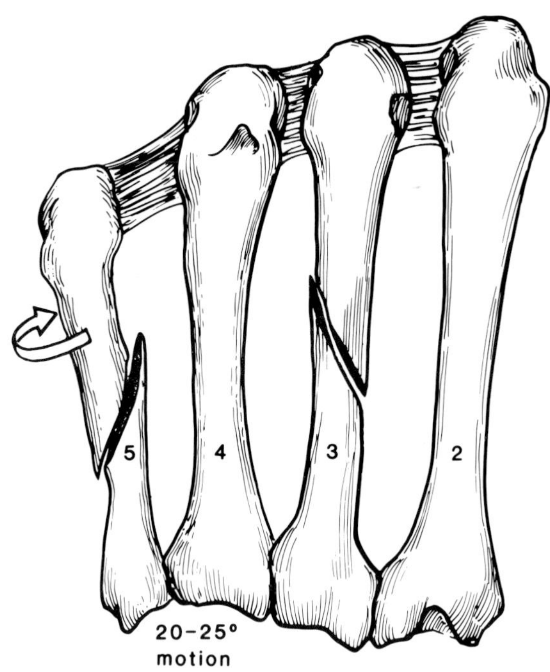

Fig. 11-70 Illustration of metacarpals two through five and the transverse metacarpal ligament. There is 20° to 25° of motion at the bases of the fourth and fifth metacarpals and increased laxity in the ligament, which allows greater rotation and shortening at the fracture site, especially with oblique fractures.

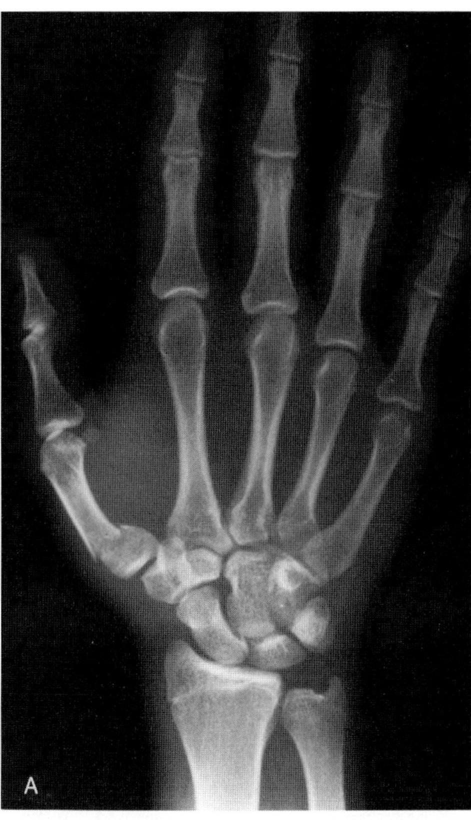

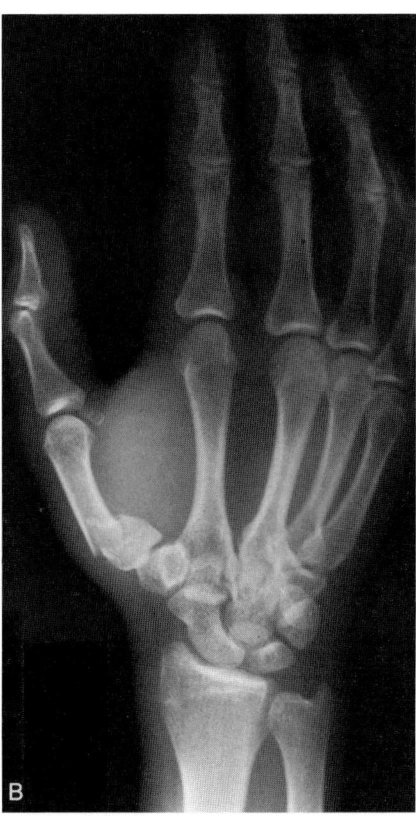

Fig. 11-71 (**A**) PA and (**B**) oblique views of a metaphyseal fracture of the thumb. *Source:* Reprinted from *Imaging of Orthopedic Trauma* ed 2 by TH Berquist, 1991, Raven Press, © Mayo Foundation.

Intraarticular basilar fractures are the most common fractures seen in the thumb.[141,161] They also are the most demanding in terms of treatment, there being little leeway for anything but anatomic reduction of the articular surface. Two basic fracture types, each with an attached eponym, are seen in this group.

The first, or Bennett's fracture (Fig. 11-72), is actually a fracture-subluxation of the first carpometacarpal joint. Characteristically the fracture line is oblique and divides a smaller proximal fragment, consisting of the volar (ulnar) lip of the first metacarpal base, from the remainder of the metacarpal, which becomes the distal fragment. The smaller proximal (volar or ulnar) fragment is anchored by the attached intermetacarpal and strong volar (ulnar) oblique ligaments. It therefore remains undisplaced relative to the trapezium. The larger distal fragment, however, consisting of essentially the entire first metacarpal, is characteristically unstable. It displaces proximally and falls into flexion. The proximal displacement is due primarily to the pull of the abductor pollicis longus and flexor pollicis longus tendons; the fall into flexion is due to the action of the strong adductor pollicis muscle.[161]

Reduction is usually possible by closed means and is accomplished by longitudinal traction on the thumb metacarpal accompanied by pronation. Maintenance of reduction by cast immobilization alone is difficult and unreliable. For this

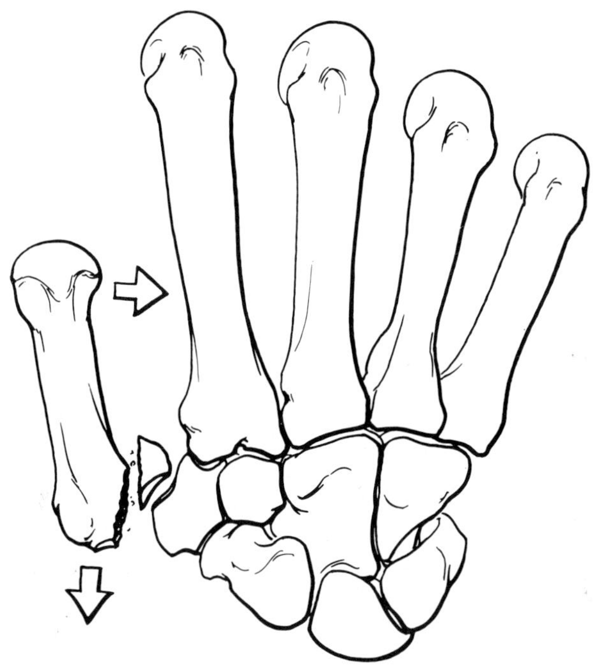

Fig. 11-72 Illustration of Bennett's fracture. The base of the metacarpal is pulled proximally by the abductor pollicis longus.

reason, internal fixation with percutaneously placed Kirschner wires is recommended.[161]

The second type of intraarticular basilar fracture of the first metacarpal is the Rolando fracture. This is by definition a comminuted injury, usually having a T or Y condylar component. The principles of management for the Rolando fracture are the same as for the Bennett type.[161]

In all intraarticular fractures of the base of the first metacarpal, the major late complication is degenerative arthrosis of the first carpometacarpal joint. The risk of this complication is increased by residual articular incongruity or joint subluxation and in highly comminuted injuries.[161]

Second through Fifth Metacarpals

The second and third metacarpals constitute the stable longitudinal axis of the hand (Fig. 11-70). Because there is essentially no motion at the carpometacarpal joints, angulation or rotational displacement is difficult to accept.

Neck fractures are common and usually result from axial compression or from a blow over the dorsum of the affected metacarpal. Displacement may be present. Characteristically the distal fragment falls into a position of palmar angulation as a result of the forces acting on the fracture from the intrinsic muscles and extrinsic flexor tendons (Fig. 11-73). Malrotation is often easily identified clinically. Malrotation is characterized chiefly by overlap of the fingers when the patient attempts to make a fist. In general, anatomic reduction of this fracture is required in the second and third metacarpals because of the lack of motion at their bases.[161]

Diaphyseal fractures are less common than fractures of the neck region. Nevertheless, they present the same array of problems regarding angulation or rotation. Spiral diaphyseal fractures are similar to transverse diaphyseal fractures but have a greater tendency toward shortening, instability, and malrotation (Fig. 11-74).[161]

Intraarticular basilar fractures are not common in the second and third metacarpals. With such injuries, however, stability of the carpometacarpal joint is the goal of treatment. Therefore, if the injury is unstable and comminuted, internal fixation, possibly with an attempt at primary arthrodesis of the carpometacarpal joint, may be necessary.

Mobility at the carpometacarpal joints of the fourth and especially the fifth rays allows a moderate degree of latitude for fracture angulation. For this reason anatomic reduction is less frequently necessary. Malrotation or excessive displacement and shortening are not acceptable, however.[161]

Neck fractures are the most common metacarpal fractures and are particularly likely to occur in the fifth ray. This injury is also known as the boxer's fracture (Fig. 11-75), which implies that the common mechanism of injury is a direct axial compression force over the ulnar side of a clenched fist. Displacement usually is not excessive, but characteristically there is palmar angulation of the distal fragment. The latter usually results from the deforming effects of the interosseous muscles and extrinsic digital flexors. Fracture angulation in the lateral plane of up to 40° in the fifth metacarpal and up to 25° in the fourth is compatible with minimal functional limitation.[161] Greater degrees of angulation may be accepted in children, who have significant growth potential, provided that no malrotation is present. The lateral view is essential in determining the degree of angulation (Figs. 11-73 and 11-75A).

Transverse diaphyseal fractures are less common but are associated with greater problems than injuries of the neck region (Fig. 11-76). Fracture union is less rapid, displacement and instability are more frequent, and angulation is less acceptable. Spiral diaphyseal fractures are more prone to shortening, instability, and malrotation than transverse frac-

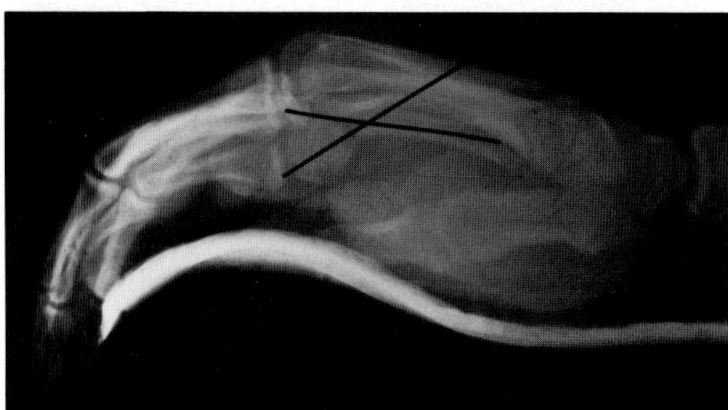

Fig. 11-73 Lateral view of the hand demonstrating volar (palmar) displacement of the distal metacarpal fragment.

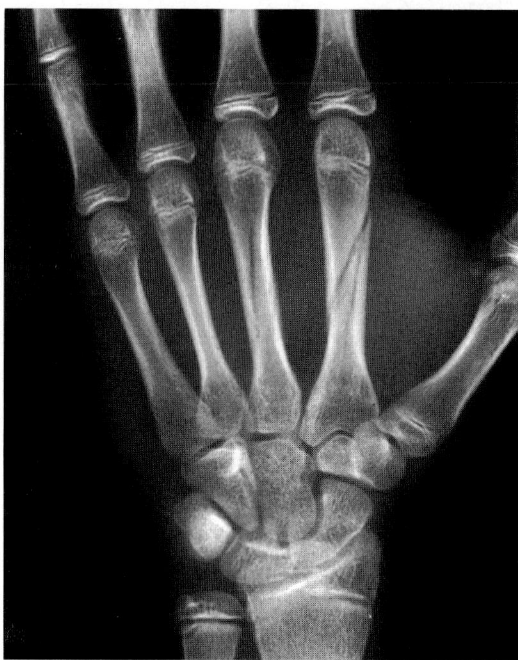

Fig. 11-74 PA view of the hand demonstrating spiral fractures of the second and third metacarpal diaphyses with slight shortening of the second.

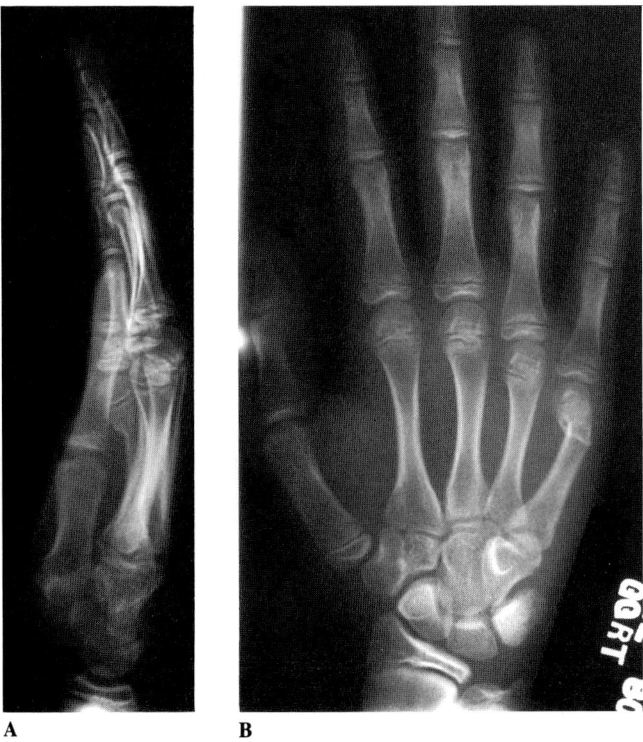

Fig. 11-75 (A) Lateral and (B) PA views demonstrating an angulated boxer's fracture.

tures of the middiaphysis (Fig. 11-70). It is not uncommon for multiple adjacent metacarpals to be affected. Internal fixation, either percutaneously or after open reduction, is frequently required.[98,161]

Extraarticular proximal metaphyseal fractures are not uncommon. They are usually impacted and stable. These fractures may be oblique or transverse. If there is no clinically apparent malrotation, reduction is rarely necessary. Because the interosseous muscles take their origin distal to the fracture, they do not represent a deforming force. Symptomatic treatment with a well-molded splint or short-arm cast that permits metacarpophalangeal joint range of motion is usually adequate.[161]

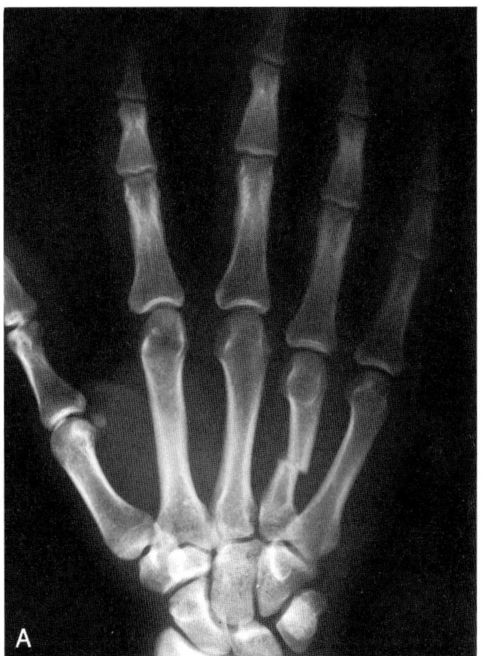

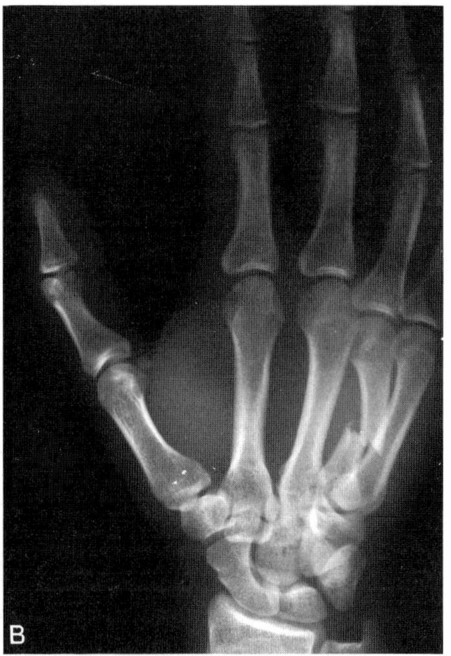

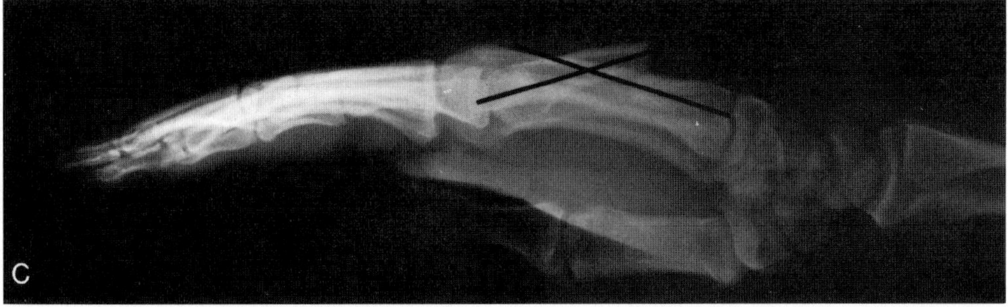

Fig. 11-76 (A) PA, (B) oblique, and (C) lateral views of a displaced, dorsally angulated (lines in C) transverse fracture of the fourth metacarpal. *Source:* Reprinted from *Imaging of Orthopedic Trauma* ed 2 by TH Berquist, 1991, Raven Press, © Mayo Foundation.

Intraarticular basilar fractures are particularly prevalent in the fifth metacarpal. In many respects this injury represents the fifth-ray counterpart of the Bennett fracture seen in the thumb. Instability, if present, usually results from the pull of the extensor carpi ulnaris tendon because it displaces the distal (metacarpal) fragment in a proximal direction.

Complications of Metacarpal Fractures

The chief complications of metacarpal fractures are limited range of motion, malunion, arthrosis, and nonunion. Limited joint range of motion is most commonly due to extension contractures of the metacarpophalangeal joints and flexion contractures of the proximal interphalangeal joints. These are often due to immobilization of the hand in an inappropriate position while awaiting fracture union. Occasionally these contractures can result from pericapsular fibrosis consequent to posttraumatic autonomic dysfunction (sympathetic dystrophy, Sudeck's atrophy). Furthermore, limited range of motion may be due to peritendinous adhesions of the extensor tendons. These may result from either associated soft tissue injury or adherence of the tendons to the fracture site.[161]

Metacarpophalangeal Joint Dislocations

Dislocations affecting the metacarpophalangeal joint are not frequent and usually are not accompanied by significant fracture. Occasionally small chip fractures at the site of collateral ligament or volar plate insertion or small shear fractures of the metacarpal head may be seen in association with this injury. Radiographically the lateral view of the involved joint is most useful. Usually the proximal phalanx is displaced dorsally relative to the metacarpal.[81,127,141] Displacement in the opposite direction has rarely been reported.[161]

Dorsal metacarpophalangeal joint dislocation usually results from hyperextension injuries.[127] It is most common in the thumb, where it may or may not be associated with an injury to the collateral ligaments (Fig. 11-77).[86,144,161] The dislocation may be simple or complex, the latter indicating an irreducible injury. Usually the volar fibrocartilaginous plate of the metacarpophalangeal joint is disrupted at its proximal attachment on the metacarpal and travels with the proximal fragment. This may prevent adequate reduction.

Dorsal metacarpophalangeal joint dislocations of the finger are most common in the index digit.[127,161] Unlike the situation in the thumb, a significant number of these injuries will not be amenable to closed reduction. Volar metacarpophalangeal dislocation is rare.

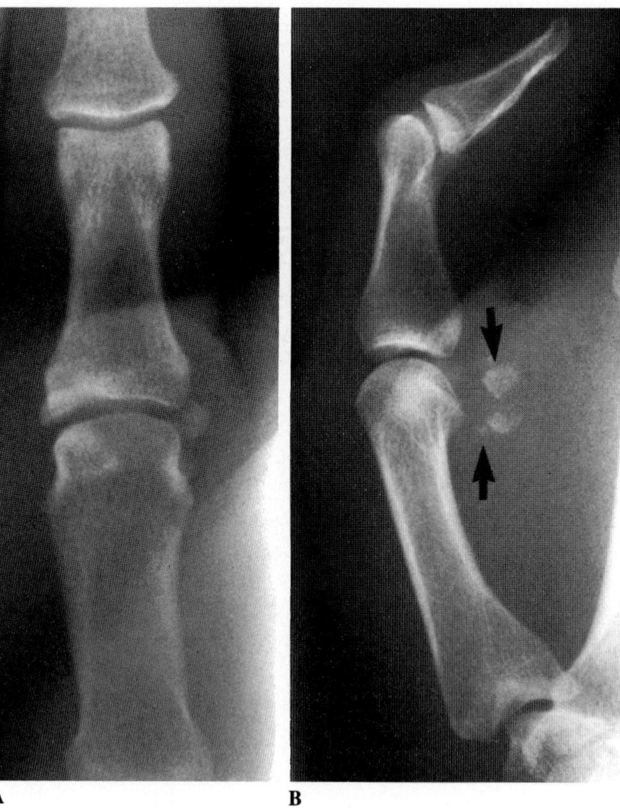

Fig. 11-77 (**A**) PA and (**B**) lateral views of a dorsal dislocation of the thumb that was reduced on the playing field. These views (taken after the game) show reduction but fractures of both sesamoids (arrows in **B**).

Phalangeal Fractures

As a group, fractures of the phalanges are the most common fractures in the hand.[89,141,150] Treatment varies with the particular phalanx fractured, the type and location of the fracture line, the degree of displacement or rotation, and the presence of associated soft tissue injury. Routine PA and lateral radiographs are usually adequate to evaluate these injuries. If possible, the involved finger should be separated from the other fingers to prevent overlap. Localized views of the injured phalanx with dental X-ray film may provide greater clarity.[161]

Proximal Phalanx

Fractures of the proximal phalanx are more common than those of the middle or distal phalanges. The adverse effects of malunion, shortening, and tendon adherence at the fracture site are more marked in the proximal phalanx than in distal fractures.[161]

Unicondylar and bicondylar fractures of the distal portion of the proximal phalanx (Fig. 11-78) are frequently unstable because of traction by the attached collateral ligament. Furthermore, in the bicondylar type, compressive forces acting across the proximal interphalangeal joint can spread the two condyles apart (Fig. 11-78). If nondisplaced, this fracture can often be adequately treated by splint protection. Careful radiographic monitoring of the fracture position during this time is advised. If the fracture is displaced, there is little allowance for deviation from the normal without adversely affecting joint function. In such cases open reduction and fixation with Kirschner wires or wire loop may be necessary.[161]

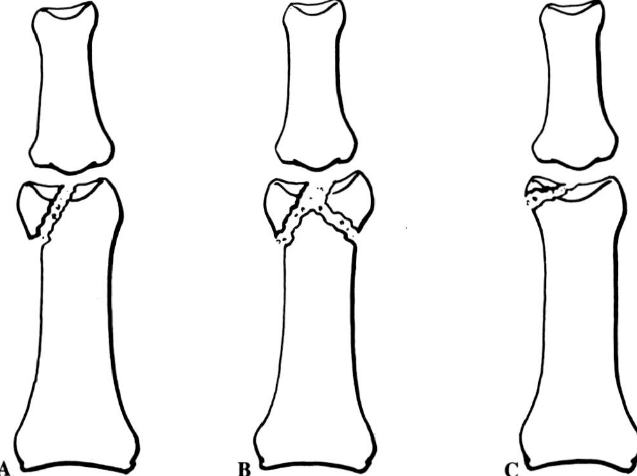

Fig. 11-78 Illustration of intraarticular fractures of the condyles of the proximal phalanx. (A) Unicondylar fracture, (B) bicondylar fracture, (C) osteochondral shear fracture.

Transverse fractures of the diaphysis are quite common. Angulation of the fracture, characteristically with the apex pointing in a palmar direction, is frequent (Fig. 11-79). This position results from the deforming forces of the intrinsic muscles, which act to flex the proximal fragment, and of the extrinsic extensor muscles, which act to extend the distal fragment. Angulation of more than 20° in the adult and 30° in the child should be corrected.[161]

Spiral or oblique fractures of the diaphysis are prone to shortening and/or malrotation. A long spiral fracture may extend into the epiphyseal region and impair joint motion by producing a bony block.

Transverse fractures of the proximal metaphysis are common, particularly in the fifth digit in children. Displacement is usual with angulation of the distal fragment dorsally and laterally and malrotation of the distal fragment in pronation. Closed reduction can usually be achieved.

Proximal condylar fractures are more easily managed than their distal counterparts. They are usually insignificantly displaced and are often impacted and stable. If so, simple protection by taping the involved digit to its neighbor on the side of the injury may be adequate treatment. If the fragment is displaced (Fig. 11-80), and particularly if it involves more than a third of the articular surface of the proximal phalanx, open reduction and internal fixation with Kirschner wires, a pullout suture, or a small bone screw may be necessary.[161]

Middle Phalanx

For the most part, fracture types seen in the middle phalanx are similar to those described for the proximal phalanx with the exception of fractures occurring about the base.

Volar lip fractures are the most common middle phalangeal fractures. This fracture characteristically is associated with a direct axial jamming or hyperextension injury. It may be

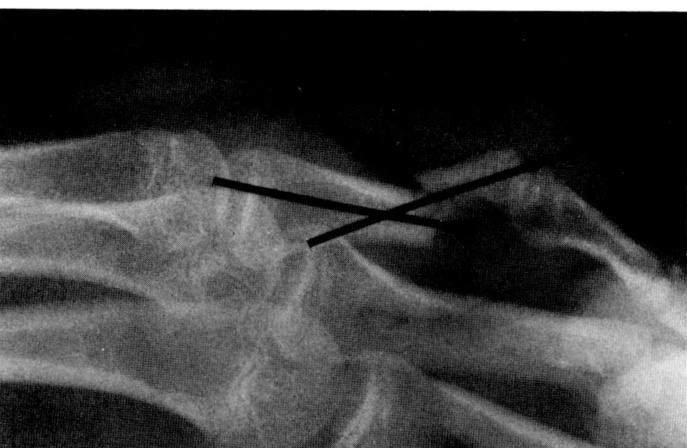

Fig. 11-79 Transverse fracture of the proximal phalanx in a wide receiver. The fracture is angulated in a volar (palmar) direction.

barely apparent radiographically (Fig. 11-81), or it may involve a sizeable portion of the proximal articular surface. If the latter is the case, when viewed laterally the fracture line characteristically courses obliquely in a dorsal and proximal direction.

The small chip fracture without dorsal subluxation or volar instability may be treated symptomatically with a monarticular finger splint to rest the proximal interphalangeal joint in 20° to 30° of flexion. Small chip fractures with either dorsal subluxa-

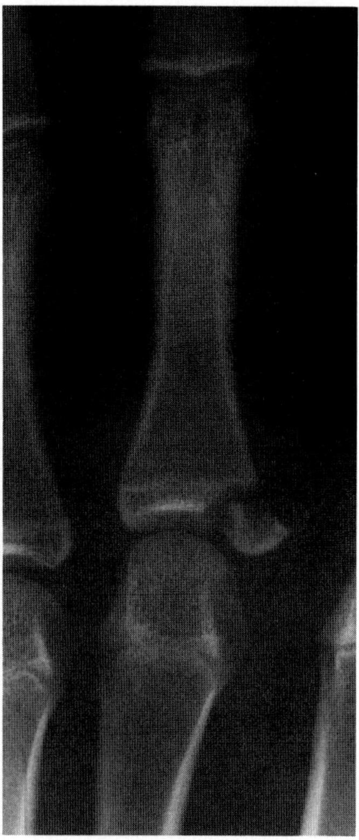

Fig. 11-80 Displaced proximal condylar fracture of the middle finger involving 25% of the articular surface.

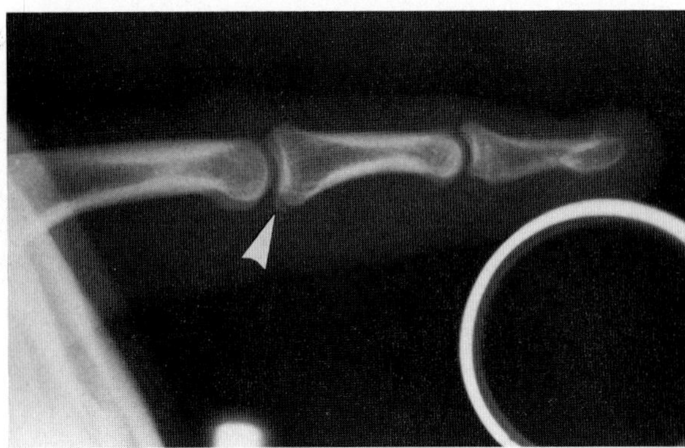

Fig. 11-81 Lateral view of the middle finger demonstrating a volar plate fracture (arrowhead) due to hyperextension injury during volleyball.

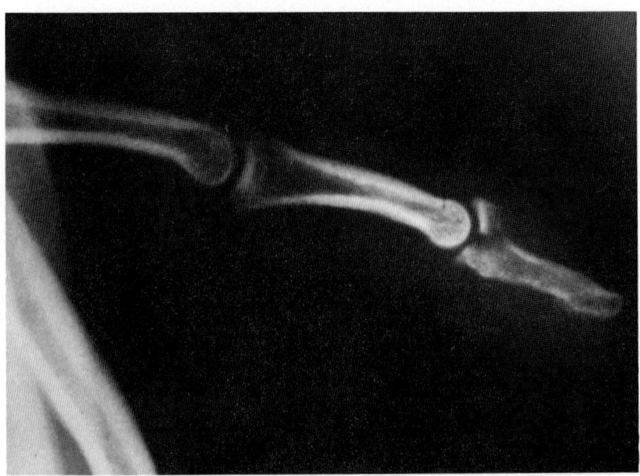

Fig. 11-82 Lateral view of the index finger demonstrating a displaced fracture of the dorsal base involving more than 50% of the articular surface.

tion or significant volar instability demand aggressive therapy. In these cases the most significant pathologic lesion involves the volar fibrocartilaginous plate, which is not radiographically obvious. This injury must be maintained in the minimum degree of flexion to prevent dorsal proximal interphalangeal joint subluxation.[161]

In general, displaced or undisplaced fractures involving less than one-third of the articular surface may be managed in a manner similar to that for the small chip fracture. Displaced fractures involving one-third or more of the articular surface, however, should be reduced with restoration of the articular congruity by either closed or open means.[160]

Dorsal plate fractures of the middle phalanx are uncommon.[161]

Distal Phalanx

Fractures of the distal phalanx are extremely common, but with few exceptions these require little in the way of treatment and are not associated with a high incidence of disabling sequelae.

Fractures are the most frequent injury to the distal phalanx. The true incidence of the fracture is unknown because it may not be accompanied by pain sufficient to warrant radiographic evaluation. Most often the mechanism of injury is a blunt crush to the fingertip. Frequently these fractures are accompanied by a nail bed laceration, a nail root avulsion, or a subungual hematoma that may obscure the underlying bone injury. Displacement may be present, particularly if there is a significant nail bed laceration. Most cases are minimally displaced and comminuted, however. They are often well stabilized by the overlying nail plate and the strong fibrous septa that characterize the fingertip tuft.[161]

Transverse fractures of the distal phalanx are distinguished from tuft fractures by the absence of distal comminution. The mechanism of injury, however, is similar. These fractures are also often associated with nail bed lacerations and nail root avulsion.

Like proximal base fractures of the middle phalanx, proximal base fractures of the distal phalanx are important. In contrast to the middle phalanx, however, the dorsal lip fracture of the distal phalanx is of greatest clinical significance. Fractures of the dorsal lip of the distal phalanx have also been termed mallet finger (Fig. 11-82).[157] The terminal portion of the extensor apparatus of the finger is inserted into the dorsal lip region. Consequently a displaced fracture will result in the inability to extend the distal phalanx completely. The mechanism of injury is most commonly a hyperflexion stress applied to the distal phalanx.[141,157] Presumably in such a situation avulsion of the dorsal lip of the distal phalanx results from the pull of the extensor tendon, or else rupture of the extensor tendon itself occurs.[130] Treatment of this injury depends primarily upon the size of the dorsal lip fragment and the presence or absence of volar joint subluxation.[130,133]

A small dorsal lip fragment constituting less than 30% of the articular surface of the distal phalanx can usually be managed with closed techniques. Dorsal lip fractures involving 30% or more of the articular surface should be reduced with restoration of articular congruity. Failure to achieve congruous articular reduction may be an indication for open reduction and fixation of the fracture.[157,161]

Volar lip fractures of the distal phalanx are unusual. They may or may not be associated with a large bony fragment and avulsion of the insertion of the flexor digitorum profundus tendon (Fig. 11-83).[140,158] If the latter occurs, dorsal subluxation of the distal interphalangeal joint may be present. Treatment usually depends on the presence or absence of associated flexor tendon injury. If there is associated flexor tendon injury, tenorrhaphy or open reduction of an attached bony fragment is indicated. Late complications may occur and are usually related to dysfunction of the flexor apparatus.[140,158]

Immature Phalanges

Phalangeal fractures in the immature skeleton typically involve the growth plate. Salter-Harris type II fractures are most common (Fig. 11-84A). Avulsion injuries may result in

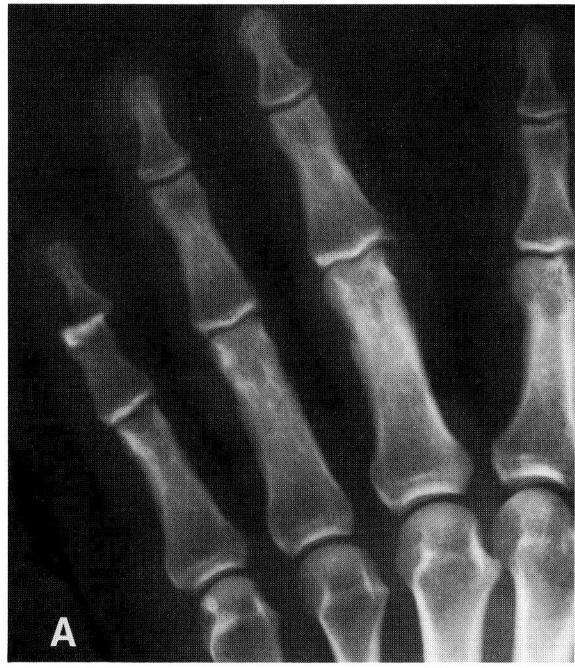

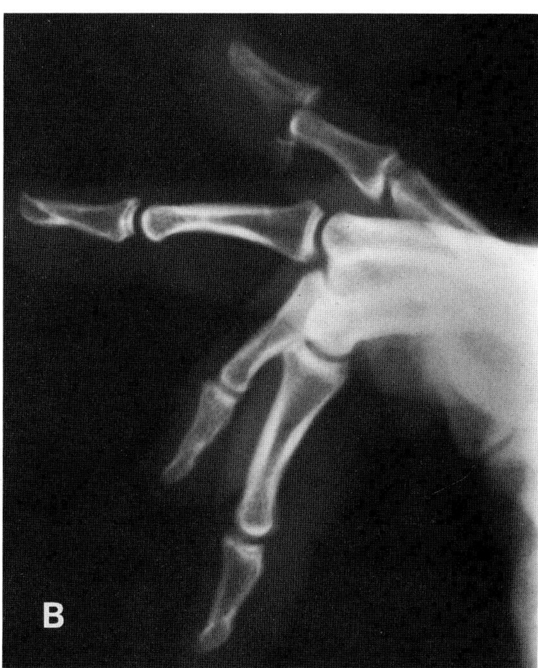

Fig. 11-83 (**A**) AP and (**B**) lateral views of the fifth finger demonstrating a large volar plate fracture with dorsal subluxation of the distal phalanx. *Source:* Reprinted from *Imaging of Orthopedic Trauma* ed 2 by TH Berquist, 1991, Raven Press, © Mayo Foundation.

type III fractures (Fig. 11-84, B and C). More complex fractures (Fig. 11-84D) are uncommon.

Dislocations of the Interphalangeal Joints

Dislocations affecting the proximal interphalangeal joint are common.[78,141,161] Less frequently this injury may occur in the distal interphalangeal joint. Often there may be accompanying bony injury, as in the dorsal or volar lip fractures of the middle phalanx discussed in the preceding sections. The dislocation almost always involves dorsal displacement of the middle phalanx on the proximal phalanx (Fig. 11-85).

Dorsal proximal interphalangeal dislocation usually results from an axial compression or hyperextension injury to the

Fig. 11-84 Illustrations of physeal injuries in children. (**A**) Salter-Harris type II fracture of the middle phalanx. (**B** and **C**) Salter-Harris type III avulsion injuries. (**D**) Salter-Harris type IV fracture of the middle phalanx.

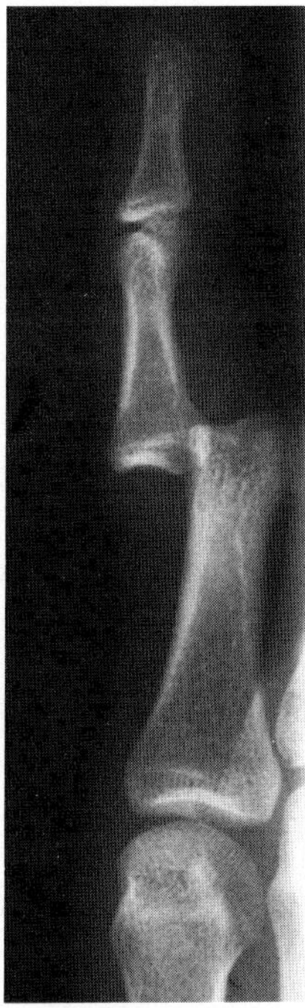

Fig. 11-85 Lateral view of the fifth finger demonstrating a dorsal dislocation of the interphalangeal joint.

fingertip (Fig. 11-85). In the absence of a displaced volar lip fracture there is disruption of the volar cartilaginous plate and variable degrees of collateral ligament injury.[161]

SOFT TISSUE AND MISCELLANEOUS INJURIES

There are numerous soft tissue and osseous overuse syndromes that may affect the hand and wrist. Tendinitis is common in athletes participating in racquet sports, rowing, and weight lifting.[167,171,173,178] Thumb injuries are particularly common in skiers.[167,169,172]

Diagnosis of these disorders is often based on the history and physical findings. Imaging and diagnostic or therapeutic injections are frequently required, however.[163,186]

Tendon Disorders

Tendon disorders, specifically tendinitis, may affect the flexor or extensor group.[167,186] De Quervain's tendinitis affects the tendons in the radial styloid region (Fig. 11-86). Inflammation is related to overuse due to pinch, grasp, or radial and ulnar deviation of the wrist.[167] The extensor pollicis brevis and abductor pollicis longus are affected in the region of the fibroosseous tunnel (Fig. 11-86). The condition is most common in racquet sports.[178] Patients typically present with pain in the anatomic snuff box with associated swelling.[167,168,178,187]

Intersection syndrome (squeaker's wrist) is an overuse syndrome that occurs slightly proximal to De Quervain's tendinitis (Fig. 11-86). There is a potential bursa located between the extensor carpi radialis longus and brevis and the abductor pollicis longus and extensor pollicis brevis. Irritation occurs with repetitive extension and radial deviation and is most frequently noted in rowers, weight lifters, and participants in racquet sports.[178] Patients present with pain, weak grasp, and crepitation (squeaker's wrist).[166,178]

Tendinitis may also involve the extensor carpi radialis longus and brevis. This condition is frequently associated with carpal boss. Carpe bosseau is not common. Patients present with a firm mass over the dorsum of the hand in the region of the second and third carpometacarpal joints. This may be tender and can be confused with a ganglion. This boss may be osteophytic or due to tendinitis at the extensor insertions. The former is obvious on routine radiographs.[94,186]

The extensor carpi ulnaris tendon may become inflamed in the region of the fibroosseous tunnel (Fig. 11-86). Chronic untreated inflammation can lead to recurrent subluxation.[165,178] The flexor carpi ulnaris and flexor carpi radialis are the most frequent flexor tendons affected. Less frequently the profundus tendon of the ring finger may be injured. Rupture of this tendon is particularly common in football players.[178]

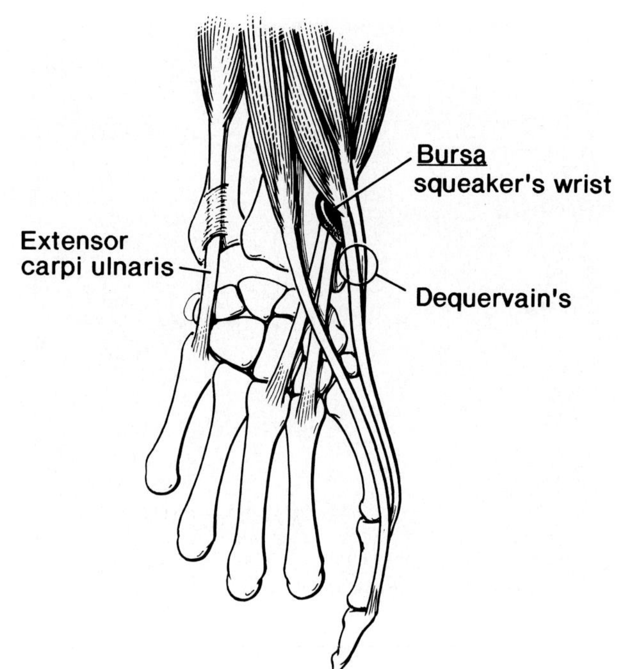

Fig. 11-86 Illustration of sites of De Quervain's tendinitis, squeaker's wrist, and extensor carpi ulnaris tendinitis or subluxation.

Although conservative therapy is usually adequate, it is not unusual for betamethasone-bupivacaine injections and on occasion surgery to be used to correct the above disorders. Imaging of these disorders may not be necessary, but definition of the exact etiology (ie, ganglion or boss, inflammation or rupture) and diagnostic or therapeutic injections often require imaging techniques.[163]

Routine radiographs provide important information in cases of tendon avulsion (Fig. 11-87), carpe bosseau, and calcific tendinitis.[161] Ultrasonography[170] may be useful in identifying tendon pathology, but MRI is more frequently employed in practice at the Mayo Clinic. Osseous and soft tissue (neural, vascular, tendon, or ligament) abnormalities can be evaluated (Figs. 11-88 and 11-89).[163,185] Contrast agent injections are useful to define tendon sheaths for purposes of diagnostic and therapeutic injection (Fig. 11-90). This ensures proper localization for injection. We typically use betamethasone and bupivacaine (the latter of which is longer acting than lidocaine) in a 1:1 ratio; 1 to 2 mL is injected depending on the site.

Ligament and Triangular Fibrocartilage Complex Injuries

Ligament injuries of the hand and wrist are usually due to acute trauma.[167,178,186] Skier's thumb, more commonly known as gamekeeper's thumb, is a common injury in downhill skiers but can also occur with cross-country skiing or other athletic activities where the thumb is forced into abduction or

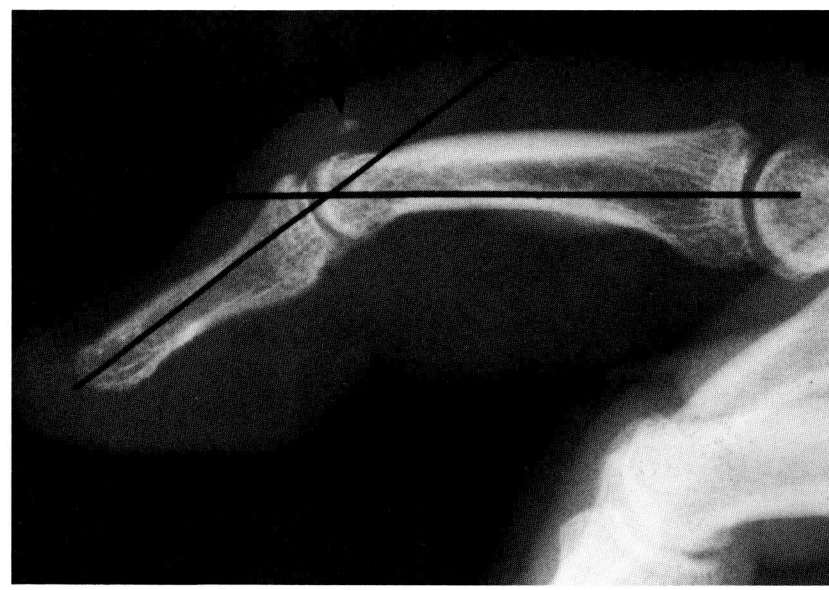

Fig. 11-87 Lateral radiograph of the index finger demonstrating a tiny avulsion fracture (arrow) with extensor tendon rupture and flexion deformity (lines) of the distal interphalangeal joint.

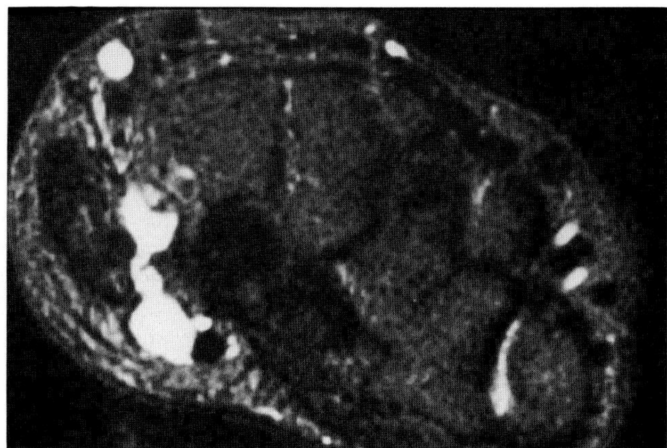

Fig. 11-88 Axial (SE 2000/50) MR image demonstrating a large dissecting ganglion compressing the ulnar nerve in a tennis player.

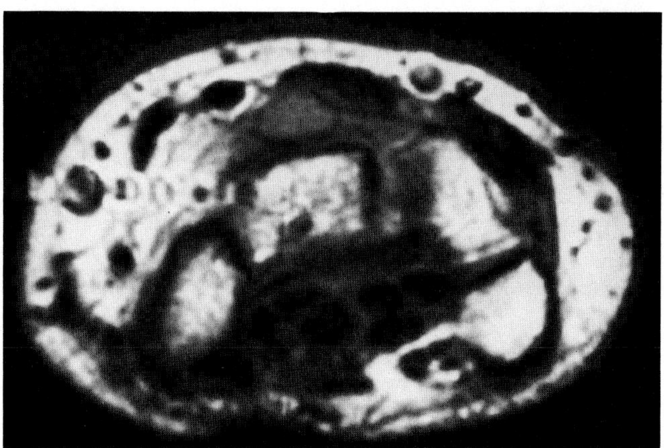

Fig. 11-89 Axial (SE 2000/60) MR image demonstrating inflammation around Guyon's canal and the ulnar nerve in a handball player.

hyperextension. The injury spectrum includes sprain or disruption of the ulnar collateral ligament or an avulsion.[166,169,172] This injury accounts for 15% to 20% of all ski injuries.[172] A rare variant is dislocation of the first carpometacarpal joint.[172]

Routine radiographs, including stress views, may be sufficient for diagnosis. Injection of anesthetic and contrast material into the metacarpophalangeal joint (Fig. 11-91) is most accurate, however.[186]

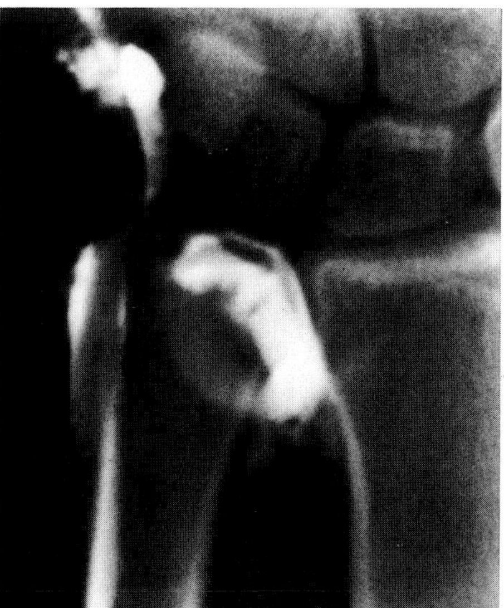

Fig. 11-90 Extensor carpi ulnaris tendon sheath and distal radioulnar joint injections used to evaluate and localize the site of symptoms. The distal radioulnar joint is normal, and injection of anesthetic had no effect. The extensor carpi ulnaris tendon sheath is constricted near the styloid. Anesthetic injection completely relieved the patient's symptoms.

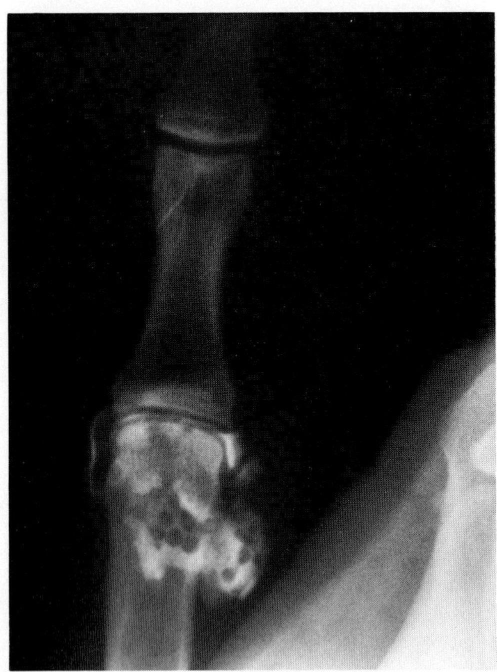

Fig. 11-91 PA arthrogram of the right thumb in a skier with ulnar collateral ligament rupture. Note the extravasation of contrast medium on the ulnar side.

Ligament injuries of the other digits also occur, primarily with dislocation. Ligament injuries and injuries of the triangular fibrocartilage complex are not uncommon in the wrist.[186]

Scapholunate ligament injury is often subtle and misdiagnosed.[186] The injury is usually the result of hyperextension with partial disruption of the volar radiocarpal ligament (Fig. 11-11). Routine radiographs may demonstrate widening (>2 mm) or proximal opening (Fig. 11-92A) of the scapholunate space on the PA view or dorsal collapse (DISI) pattern on the lateral view (Fig. 11-92B).[164] Arthrography or MRI can be used to confirm the diagnosis (Fig. 11-93).[174–184,186] Treatment is generally surgical.[186]

Lunotriquetral ligament injury may occur alone or in association with triangular fibrocartilage complex injuries.[174,186] Increase in the lunotriquetral space is not commonly seen, but VISI deformity may be evident on lateral views or motion studies. Arthrography (Fig. 11-94) or MRI confirms the diagnosis.[183,186]

Tears of the triangular fibrocartilage complex may occur with significant injuries such as dislocations or as a result of repetitive trauma. The latter is more common in athletes. Patients present with ulnar pain. There may be an associated click or crepitus. Arthrography (Fig. 11-94) or MRI is most effective for diagnosis.[174,186]

Ulnolunate Abutment Syndrome

Patients most frequently present with ulnar pain that may be confused with pain due to injury to the triangular fibrocartilage complex or other pathology. Usually, overuse or stress syndrome is responsible for this condition. Radionuclide scans demonstrate focal increased tracer uptake in the ulnar region. Tomography is most useful for demonstrating the characteristic features of positive ulnar variance with sclerosis, erosion, or cystic changes in the ulnar aspect of the proximal lunate (Fig. 11-95).[186] Surgery may be indicated if conservative therapy fails.

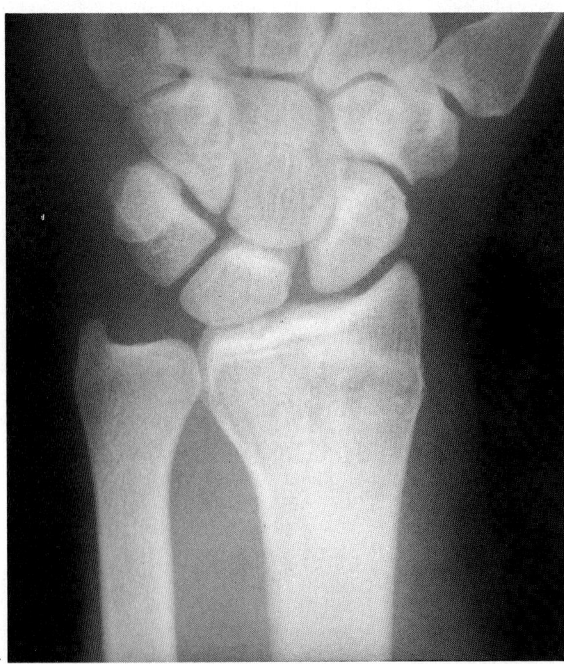

A

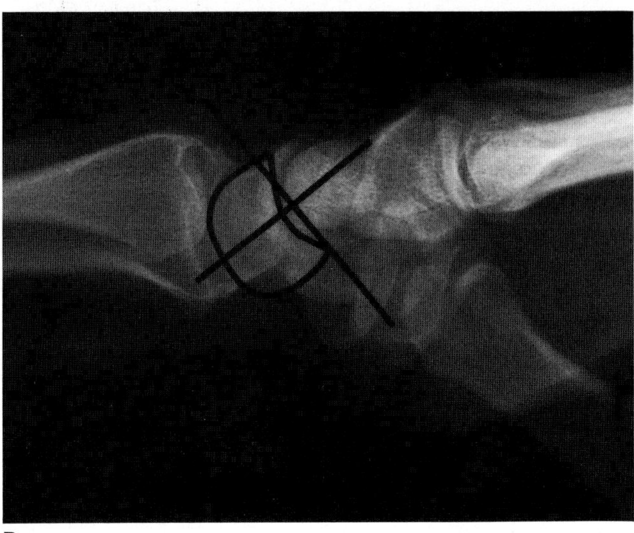

B

Fig. 11-92 Scapholunate ligament injury. There is widening of the scapholunate space on the PA view (**A**) and an increase in the scapholunate angle (lines) on the lateral view (**B**).

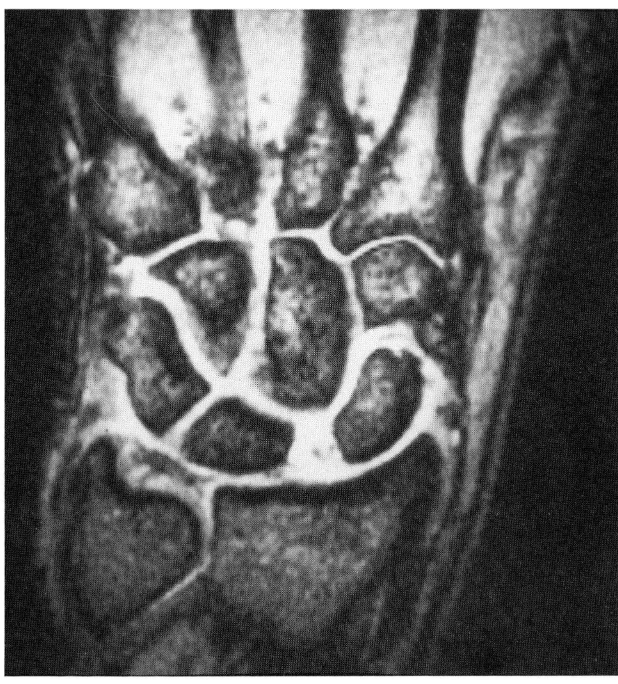

Fig. 11-93 Coronal gradient-echo image of the wrist demonstrating a scapholunate ligament tear.

Avascular Necrosis

Osteonecrosis most commonly involves the lunate, but the scaphoid and metacarpal heads may also be affected.[163,186]

Kienböck's disease (lunate avascular necrosis) is not an uncommon cause of vague wrist pain. It is most often associated with trauma (either a hyperextension injury or repetitive minor trauma). Routine radiographs are normal early. Therefore, diagnosis and exclusion of other causes of wrist pain are most easily accomplished with MRI. Diffuse decreased signal intensity (T1-weighted sequences) is the most diagnostic feature (Fig. 11-34). MRI is also useful in following patients undergoing conservative therapy. Signal intensity will return to normal with successful treatment.[163,189]

Avascular necrosis of the scaphoid or metacarpal heads is rare except after acute fracture. MRI is best suited for diagnosis of avascular necrosis in these areas as well.[163]

Neurovascular Injury

Injuries to neurovascular structures most commonly involve palmar or digital structures.[178,188] Vascular injury has been associated with racquet sports, handball, and bicycle touring. These sports primarily affect the ulnar artery near Guyon's canal. Thrombosis, dissection, and aneurysms have been reported.[178] Digital injuries have been reported in catchers and pitchers in baseball and in handball players. Repetitive trauma may also cause injury to the ulnar or median nerves.

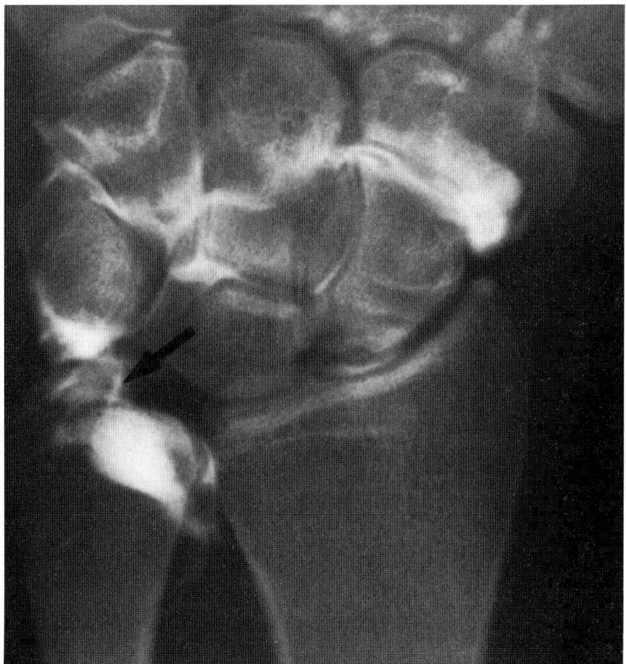

Fig. 11-94 Arthrography in a tennis player with ulnar wrist pain. Injection of the distal radioulnar joint demonstrates a triangular fibrocartilage complex tear (arrow) with communication with the midcarpal joint via a lunotriquetral ligament tear.

Angiography may be needed for diagnosis of vascular injury. New vascular software provides improved image quality for MR angiography, however. In addition, MRI is useful for detection of nerve or perineural pathology.[163]

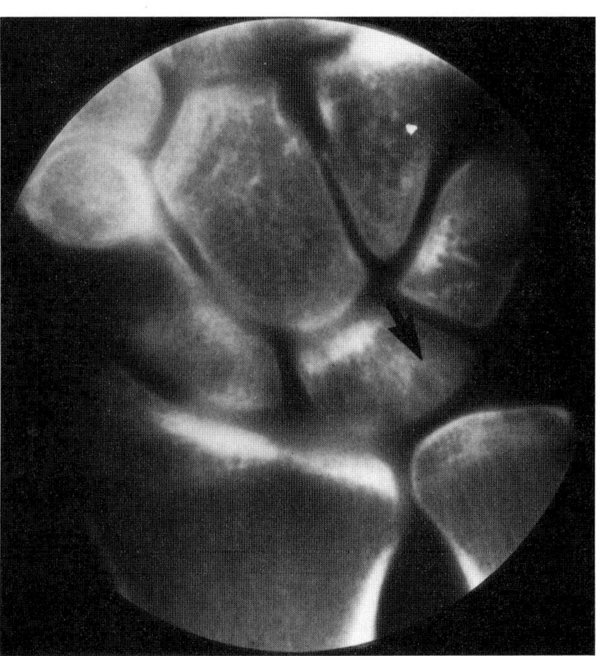

Fig. 11-95 Tomogram of the wrist demonstrating positive ulnar variance with a cystic area (arrow) in the lunate due to ulnolunate abutment syndrome.

REFERENCES

Introduction

1. Albanese SA, Palmer AK, Kerr DR, Carpenter CW, Lisi D, Levinsohn EM. Wrist pain and distal growth plate closure of the radius in gymnasts. *J Pediatr Orthop*. 1989;9:23–28.

2. Birrer RB, Halbrook SP. Martial arts injury: the results of a 5 year national survey. *Am J Sports Med*. 1988;16:408–410.

3. Brunet ME, Haddad RJ. Fractures and dislocations of the metacarpals and phalanges. *Clin Sports Med*. 1986;5:773–781.

4. Carter SR, Aldridge MJ. Stress injury of the distal radial growth plate. *J Bone Joint Surg Br*. 1988;70:834–836.

5. Carter SR, Aldridge MJ, Fitzgerald R, Davies AM. Stress changes of the wrist in adolescent gymnasts. *Br J Radiol*. 1988;61:109–112.

6. deLoes M, Goldie I. Incidence rate of injuries during sport activity and physical exercise in a rural Swedish municipality: incidence rates in 17 sports. *Int J Sports Med*. 1988;9:461–467.

7. Fakharzadeh FF. Stress fracture of the finger in a bowler. *J Hand Surg*. 1989;14A:241–243.

8. Hooper CJ. An unusual variety of skier's thumb. *J Hand Surg*. 1987; 12A:627–629.

9. Isani A, Melone CP. Ligamentous injuries of the hand in athletes. *Clin Sports Med*. 1986;5:757–772.

10. Johannsen HV, Noerregaard FOH. Prevention of injury in karate. *Br J Sports Med*. 1988;22:113–115.

11. Matter P, Ziegler WJ, Holzach P. Skiing accidents in the past 15 years. *J Sports Med*. 1987;5:319–326.

12. Osterman AL, Moskow L, Low DW. Soft-tissue injuries of the hand and wrist in racquet sports. *Clin Sports Med*. 1988;7:329–348.

13. Simmons BP, Lovallo JL. Hand and wrist injuries in children. *Clin Sports Med*. 1988;7:495–512.

Anatomy

14. Bowers WH, Wolf JW, Nehil JL. The proximal interphalangeal joint volar plate. I. An anatomical and biomechanical study. *J Hand Surg*. 1980;5: 79–88.

15. Dobyns JH, Linscheid RL. Fractures and dislocations of the wrist. In: Rockwood CA, Green DP, eds. *Fractures in Adults*. 2nd ed. Philadelphia: Lippincott; 1984:411–509.

16. Dobyns JH, Linscheid RL, Beckenbaugh RD, et al. Fractures of the hand and wrist. In: Flynn JE, ed. *Hand Surgery*. Baltimore: Williams & Wilkins; 1991:122–185.

17. Epner RA, Bowers WH, Guilford WB. Ulnar variance—the effect of wrist positioning and roentgen filming technique. *J Hand Surg*. 1982;7: 298–305.

18. Gilford WW, Bolton RH, Lambrinudi C. The mechanism of the wrist joint with special reference to fractures of the scaphoid. Guy's Hosp. Rep. 92: 52–59, 1943.

19. Green DP, Rowland SA. Fractures and dislocations in the hand. In: Rockwood CA, Green DP, eds. *Fractures in Adults*. 2nd ed. Philadelphia: Lippincott; 1984:313–409.

20. Hollinshead HW. *Anatomy for Surgeons*. New York: Harper & Row; 1982:3.

21. Kaplan EB. *Functional and Surgical Anatomy of the Hand*. 2nd ed. Philadelphia: Lippincott; 1965.

22. Kauer JMG. Functional anatomy of the wrist. *Clin Orthop*. 1980; 149:9–20.

23. Landsmeer JMF. The proximal interphalangeal joint. *Hand*. 1975;7: 30.

24. Lichtman DM, Schneider JR, Swafford AR, Mack GR. Ulnar midcarpal instability. Clinical and laboratory analysis. *J Hand Surg*. 1981;6: 515–523.

25. Linscheid RL, Dobyns JH, Beabout JW, Bryan RS. Traumatic instability of the wrist: diagnosis, classification, and pathomechanics. *J Bone Joint Surg Am*. 1972;54:1612–1632.

26. Mayfield J, Johnson R, Kilcoyne R. The ligaments of the human wrist and their functional significance. *Anat Rec*. 1976;185:417–428.

27. Mikic ZD. Age changes in the triangular fibrocartilage of the wrist joint. *J Anat*. 1978;126:307–384.

28. O'Rahilly R. A survey of carpal and tarsal anomalies. *J Bone Joint Surg Am*. 1953;35:626–642.

29. Palmer AK, Werner FW. The triangular fibrocartilage complex of the wrist—anatomy and function. *J Hand Surg*. 1981;6:153–162.

30. Seffafian S, Melamed JL, Goshgarian GM. Study of the wrist motion in flexion and extension. *Clin Orthop*. 1977;126:153–159.

31. Taleisnik J. The ligaments of the wrist. *J Hand Surg*. 1976;1: 110–118.

32. Volz RG, Lieb M, Benjamin J. Biomechanics of the wrist. *Clin Orthop*. 1980;149:112–117.

33. Wood MB, Berquist TH. The hand and wrist. In: Berquist TH, ed. *Imaging of Orthopedic Trauma*. 2nd ed. New York: Raven; 1991:749–870.

34. Youm Y, Flatt AE. Kinematics of the wrist. *Clin Orthop*. 1980;149: 21–32.

35. Youm Y, McMurthy RY, Flatt AE, Gillespie TE. Kinematics of the wrist. I. An experimental study of the radial-ulnar deviation and flexion-extension. *J Bone Joint Surg Am*. 1978;60:423–431.

Imaging Techniques

36. Abbitt PL, Riddervold HO. The carpal tunnel view: helpful adjuvant for unrecognized fractures of the carpus. *Skeletal Radiol*. 1987;16:45–47.

37. Ballinger PW. *Merrill's Atlas of Roentgenographic Positions and Standard Radiologic Procedures*. 5th ed. St Louis, MO: Mosby; 1982.

38. Bernau A, Berquist TH. *Orthopedic Positioning in Diagnostic Radiology*. Baltimore: Urban & Schwarzenberg; 1983.

39. Berquist TH. *Magnetic Resonance Imaging of the Musculoskeletal System*. 2nd ed. New York: Raven; 1990.

40. Berquist TH. The elbow and wrist. *Top Magn Resonance Imaging*. 1989;1:15–27.

41. Blair WF, Berger RA, El-Khoury GY. Arthrotomography of the wrist: an experimental and preliminary clinical study. *J Hand Surg*. 1985; 10A:350–359.

42. Bowers WH, Hurst LC. Gamekeeper's thumb. Evaluation by arthrography and stress roentgenography. *J Bone Joint Surg Am*. 1977;59: 519–524.

43. Braunstein EM, Louis DS, Greene TL, Hankin FM. Fluoroscopic and arthrographic evaluation of carpal instability. *AJR*. 1985;144: 1259–1262.

44. Bush CH, Gillespy T, Dell PC. High-resolution CT of the wrist: initial experience with scaphoid disorders and surgical fusions. *AJR*. 1987; 149:757–760.

45. Cone RO, Szabo R, Resnick D, Gelberman R, Taleisnick J, Gilula LA. Computed tomography of the normal radioulnar joints. *Invest Radiol*. 1983;18:541–545.

46. Cone RO, Szabo R, Resnick D, Gelberman R, Taleisnick J, Gilula LA. Computed tomography of the normal soft tissues of the wrist. *Invest Radiol*. 1983;18:546–551.

47. Curtis DJ, Downey EF. A simple first metacarpophalangeal stress test. *Radiology*. 1983;148:855.

48. Downey EF, Curtis DJ. Patient induced stress test of the first metacarpophalangeal joint: a radiographic assessment of collateral ligament injuries. *Radiology*. 1986;158:679–683.

49. Epner RA, Bowers WH, Guifford WB. Ulnar variance—the effect of wrist positioning and roentgen filming technique. *J Hand Surg*. 1982;7: 298–305.

50. Ganel A, Engel J, Oster Z, Farene I. Bone scanning in the assessment of fractures of the scaphoid. *J Hand Surg*. 1979;4:540–543.

51. Gilula LA. Carpal injuries: analytic approach and case exercises. *AJR*. 1979;133:503–517.

52. Gilula LA. Mid carpal wrist arthrography. *AJR*. 1986;146:645–646.

53. Gilula LA, Distouet JM, Weeks PM, Young LV, Wray RC. Roentgen diagnosis of the painful wrist. *Clin Orthop*. 1984;187:52–64.

54. Greyson ND, Tepperman PS. Three-phase bone studies in hemiplegia with reflex sympathetic dystrophy and the effect of disuse. *J Nucl Med*. 1984; 25:423–429.

55. Gruber L. Practical approaches to obtaining hand radiographs and special techniques in hand radiography. *Hand Clin*. 1991;7:1–20.

56. Hardy DC, Totty WG, Reinus WR, Gilula LA. Posteroanterior wrist radiography: importance of arm positioning. *J Hand Surg*. 1987;12A: 504–508.

57. Holder LE, Mackinnon SE. Reflex sympathetic dystrophy in the hands: clinical and scintigraphic criteria. *Radiology*. 1984;152:517–522.

58. Kindynis P, Resnick D, Kang HS, Haller J, Sartoris DJ. Demonstration of the scapholunate space with radiography. *Radiology*. 1990;175: 278–280.

59. Levinsohn ME, Palmer AK, Coren AB, Zinberg E. Wrist arthrography: the value of the three compartment injection technique. *Skeletal Radiol*. 1987;16:539–544.

60. Levinsohn ME, Rosen DI, Palmer AK. Wrist arthrography: value of the three-compartment injection method. *Radiology*. 1991;179:231–239.

61. Magid D, Thompson JS, Fishman EK. Computed tomography of the hand and wrist. *Hand Clin*. 1991;7:219–234.

62. Manaster BJ. Digital wrist arthrography: precision in determining the site of radiocarpal–mid carpal communication. *AJR*. 1986;147:563–566.

63. Manaster BJ. The clinical efficacy of the triple-injection wrist arthrography. *Radiology*. 1991;178:267–270.

64. Mauer AH. Nuclear medicine in evaluation of the hand and wrist. *Hand Clin*. 1991;7:183–200.

65. Mirro DE, Palmer AK, Levinsohn ME. Radiography and computerized tomography in the diagnosis of incongruity of the distal radioulnar joint. *J Bone Joint Surg Am*. 1985;67:247–252.

66. Quinn SF, Belsole RS, Green TL, Rayhack JM. Post-arthrography computed tomography of the wrist: evaluation of the triangular fibrocartilage complex. *Skeletal Radiol*. 1989;17:565–569.

67. Quinn SF, Murray W, Watkins T, Kloss J. CT for determining results of treatment of fractures of the wrist. *AJR*. 1987;149:109–111.

68. Resnick D. Roentgenographic anatomy of the tendon sheaths of the hand and wrist: tenography. *Am J Roentgenol Radium Ther Nucl Med*. 1975;124:44.

69. Resnick D, Dalinka MK. Arthrography and tenography of the wrist. In: Dalinka MK, ed. *Arthrography*. New York: Springer-Verlag; 1980: 165–175.

70. Rosenthal DI, Murray WT, Smith RJ. Finger arthrography. *Radiology*. 1980;137:647.

71. Smith DK, Linscheid RL, Amadio PC, Berquist TH, Cooney WP. Scaphoid anatomy: evaluation with complex motion tomography. *Radiology*. 1989;173:177–180.

72. Tehranzadeh J, Davenport J, Pas MJ. Scaphoid fracture: evaluation with flexion-extension tomography. *Radiology*. 1990;176:167–170.

73. Terry DW, Ramin JE. The navicular fat stripe. A useful roentgen feature for evaluating wrist trauma. *Am J Roentgenol Radium Ther Nucl Med*. 1975;124:25.

74. Tirman RM, Weber ER, Snyder LL, Koonce TW. Mid carpal wrist arthrography for detection of tears of the scapholunate and lunotriquetral ligaments. *AJR*. 1985;144:107–108.

75. Wechsler RJ, Wehbe MA, Rifkin MD, Edeiken J, Branch HM. Computed tomography diagnosis of distal radioulnar subluxation. *Skeletal Radiol*. 1987;16:1–5.

76. Wood MB, Berquist TH. The hand and wrist. In: Berquist TH, ed. *Imaging of Orthopedic Trauma*. 2nd ed. New York: Raven; 1991:749–870.

77. Zlatkin MB, Chis PC, Osterman AL, Schmoll MD, Dalinka MK, Kressel HY. Chronic wrist pain: evaluation with high-resolution MR imaging. *Radiology*. 1989;173:723–729.

Fractures and Dislocations

78. Agee JM. Unstable fracture-dislocations of the proximal interphalangeal joint of the fingers: a preliminary report of a new treatment technique. *J Hand Surg*. 1978;3:386–389.

79. Aitkin AP, Nalebuff EA. Volar transnavicular perilunar dislocations of the carpus. *J Bone Joint Surg Am*. 1960;42:1051–1057.

80. Albanese SA, Palmer AK, Kerr DR, Carpenter CW, Lisi D, Levinsohn EM. Wrist pain and distal growth plate closure of the radius in gymnasts. *J Pediatr Orthop*. 1989;9:23–28.

81. Baldwin LW, Miller DL, Lockhart LD, Evans EB. Metacarpophalangeal-joint dislocations of the fingers. *J Bone Joint Surg Am*. 1967; 49:1587–1590.

82. Bartone NF, Grieco RV. Fractures of the triquetrum. *J Bone Joint Surg Am*. 1956;38:353–356.

83. Berquist TH. *Magnetic Resonance Imaging of the Musculoskeletal System*. 2nd ed. New York: Raven; 1990.

84. Bowen TL. Injuries of the hamate bone. *Hand*. 1973;5:235–238.

85. Braunstein EM, Louis DS, Greene TL, Hankin FM. Fluoroscopic and arthrographic evaluation of carpal instability. *AJR*. 1985;144:1259–1262.

86. Browne EZ, Dunn HK, Snyder CC. Ski pole thumb injury. *Plast Reconstr Surg*. 1976;59:19–23.

87. Brunet ME, Haddad RJ. Fractures and dislocations of the metacarpals and phalanges. *Clin Sports Med*. 1986;5:773–781.

88. Bryan RS, Dobyns JH. Fractures of the carpal bones other than lunate and navicular. *Clin Orthop*. 1980;149:107–111.

89. Burton RJ. Fractures of the proximal phalanx of the finger. *Contemp Surg*. 1977;11:32–37.

90. Cameron HU, Hastings DE, Fournasier VL. Fracture of the hook of the hamate. A case report. *J Bone Joint Surg Am*. 1975;57:276–277.

91. Carter SR, Aldridge MJ. Stress injury of the distal radial growth plate. *J Bone Joint Surg Br*. 1988;70:834–836.

92. Carter SR, Aldridge MJ, Fitzgerald R, Davies AM. Stress changes of the wrist in adolescent gymnasts. *Br J Radiol*. 1988;61:109–112.

93. Carter SR, Eaton RG, Littler JW. Ununited fracture of the hook of the hamate. *J Bone Joint Surg Am*. 1977;59:583–588.

94. Conway WF, Destouet JM, Gilula LA, Bellinghausen HW, Weeks PM. The carpal boss: an overview of radiographic evaluation. *Radiology*. 1985;156:29–31.

95. Cooney WP, Dobyns JH, Linscheid RL. Complications of Colles fractures. *J Bone Joint Surg Am*. 1980;62:613–619.

96. Cooney WP, Dobyns JH, Linscheid RL. Fractures of the scaphoid: a rational approach to management. *Clin Orthop*. 1980;149:90–97.

97. Cordrey LJ, Ferrer-Torells M. Management of fractures of the greater multangular. *J Bone Joint Surg Am*. 1960;42:1111–1118.

98. Crawford GP. Screw fixation for certain fractures of the phalanges and metacarpals. *J Bone Joint Surg Am*. 1976;58:487–492.

99. Crosby EB, Linscheid RL. Rupture of the flexor profundus tendon of the ring finger secondary to ancient fracture of the hook of the hamate: review of the literature and report of two cases. *J Bone Joint Surg Am*. 1974;56: 1076–1078.

100. Dameron TB. Traumatic dislocation of the distal radioulnar joint. *Clin Orthop*. 1972;83:55–63.

101. Darrach W. Foreward dislocation at the inferior radioulnar joint with fractures of the lower third of the radius. *Ann Surg*. 1912;56:801.

102. De Oliveira JC. Barton's fractures. *J Bone Joint Surg Am*. 1973;55:586–594.

103. Desser TS, McCarthy S, Trumble T. Scaphoid fractures and Kienböck's disease of the lunate: MR imaging with histopathologic correlation. *Magn Resonance Imaging*. 1990;8:357–361.

104. Dunn AW. Fractures and dislocations of the carpus. *Surg Clin North Am*. 1972;52:1513.

105. Ellis J. Smith's and Barton's fracture—a method of treatment. *J Bone Joint Surg Br*. 1965;47:724–727.

106. Fenton RL. The naviculo-capitate fracture syndrome. *J Bone Joint Surg Am*. 1956;38:681–684.

107. Fernandez DL. Irreducible radiocarpal fracture-dislocation and radioulnar dissociation with entrapment of the ulnar nerve, artery, and flexor profundus II–V—case report. *J Hand Surg*. 1981;6:456–461.

108. Fisher MR, Rogers LF, Hendrix RW, Gilula LA. Carpometacarpal dislocation. *CRC Crit Rev Diagn Imaging*. 1984;22:95–126.

109. Fisk GR. An overview of injuries of the wrist. *Clin Orthop*. 1980;149:137–144.

110. Fisk GR. Carpal instability and the fractured scaphoid. *Ann R Coll Surg*. 1970;45:63–77.

111. Frykman G. Fractures of the distal radius including sequelae—shoulder-hand-finger syndrome, disturbance in the distal radioulnar joint, and impairment of nerve function. *Acta Orthop Scand*. 1967;108(suppl):1–55.

112. Funk DA, Wood MB. Concurrent fractures of the ipsilateral scaphoid and radial head. *J Bone Joint Surg Am*. 1988;70:134–136.

113. Gelberman RH, Welock BS, Siegel DB. Fractures and non-unions of the carpal scaphoid. *J Bone Joint Surg Am*. 1989;71:1560–1565.

114. Gillespy T III, Stork JJ, Dele PC. Dorsal fracture of the hamate: distinct radiographic appearance. *AJR*. 1988;151:351–353.

115. Gilula LA, Destouet JM, Weeks PM, Young LV, Wray RC. Roentgen diagnosis of the painful wrist. *Clin Orthop*. 1984;187:52–64.

116. Goldberg I, Amit S, Bahar A, Seelenfreeval M. Complete dislocation of the trapezium. *J Hand Surg*. 1981;6:193–195.

117. Goodman ML, Shankman GB. Update: palmar dislocation of the trapezoid—a case report. *J Hand Surg*. 1984;9:127–131.

118. Green DP, O'Brien ET. Classification and management of carpal dislocations. *Clin Orthop*. 1980;149:55–72.

119. Hamlin C. Traumatic disruption of the distal radioulnar joint. *Am J Sports Med*. 1977;5:93–96.

120. Hanks GA, Kolinak A, Bowman LS, Sebastianelli WJ. Stress fractures of the scaphoid. *J Bone Joint Surg Am*. 1989;71:938–941.

121. Heiple KG, Freehafer AA, Van't Hof A. Isolated traumatic dislocation of the distal end of the ulna and distal radioulnar joint. *J Bone Joint Surg Am*. 1962;44:1387–1394.

122. Hill NA. Fractures and dislocations of the carpus. *Orthop Clin North Am*. 1970;1:275–284.

123. Immermann EW. Dislocation of the pisiform. *J Bone Joint Surg Am*. 1948;30:489–492.

124. Inque G, Inagaki Y. Isolated palmar dislocation of the trapezoid associated with attritional rupture of the flexor tendon. *J Bone Joint Surg Am*. 1990;72:446–448.

125. Johnson RP. The acutely injured wrist and its residuals. *Clin Orthop*. 1980;149:33–44.

126. Jupiter JB. Fractures of the distal end of the radius. *J Bone Joint Surg Am*. 1991;73:461–469.

127. Kaplan EB. Dorsal dislocation of the metacarpophalangeal joint of the index finger. *J Bone Joint Surg Am*. 1957;39:1081–1086.

128. Knirk JL, Jupiter JB. Intra-articular fractures of the distal end of the radius in young adults. *J Bone Joint Surg Am*. 1986;68:647–659.

129. Lawlis JF, Gunther SF. Carpometacarpal dislocations. *J Bone Joint Surg Am*. 1991;73:52–58.

130. Leddy JP, Packer JW. Avulsion of the profundus tendon insertion in athletes. *J Hand Surg*. 1977;2:66–69.

131. Mayfield JK, Johnson RP, Kilcoyne RK. Carpal dislocations: pathomechanics and progressive perilunar instability. *J Hand Surg*. 1980;5:226–241.

132. Mikic ZD. Galeazzi fracture-dislocations. *J Bone Joint Surg Am*. 1975;57:1071–1080.

133. Mikio T, Yamamuro T, Kotoura Y, Tsuji T, Shimizu K, Itakura H. Rupture of the extensor tendons of the fingers. *J Bone Joint Surg Am*. 1986;68:610–614.

134. Minami M, Hamazaki J, Ishii S. Isolated dislocation of the pisiform: a case report and review of the literature. *J Hand Surg*. 1984;9:125–127.

135. Moore JR, Webb CA, Thompson RC. A complete dislocation of the thumb metacarpal. *J Hand Surg*. 1978;3:547–549.

136. Morrissy RT, Nalebuff EA. Dislocation of the distal radioulnar joint: anatomy and clues to prompt diagnosis. *Clin Orthop*. 1979;144:154–158.

137. Mouat TB, Wilkie J, Harding HE. Isolated fracture of the carpal semilunar and Kienböck's disease. *Br J Surg*. 1932;19:577–592.

138. Nielsen PT, Hederboe J, Thommesen P. Bone scintigraphy in the evaluation of fracture of the carpal scaphoid bone. *Acta Orthop Scand*. 1983;54:303–306.

139. Norman A, Nelson J, Green S. Fracture of the hook of the hamate: radiographic signs. *Radiology*. 1985;154:49–53.

140. Reef TC. Avulsion of the flexor digitorum profundus: an athletic injury. *Am J Sports Med*. 1977;5:281–285.

141. Ruby LK. Common hand injuries in the athlete. *Orthop Clin North Am*. 1980;11:819–839.

142. Russe O. Fracture of the carpal navicular. *J Bone Joint Surg Am*. 1960;42:759–768.

143. Russell TB. Intercarpal dislocations and fracture-dislocations. A review of 59 cases. *J Bone Joint Surg Br*. 1949;31:524–531.

144. Smith DK. Post-traumatic instability of the metacarpophalangeal joint of the thumb. *J Bone Joint Surg Am*. 1977;59:14–21.

145. Smith DK, Gilula LA, Amadio PC. Dorsal lunate tilt (DISI configuration): sign of scaphoid fracture displacement. *Radiology*. 1990;176:497–499.

146. Smith DK, Linscheid RL, Amadio PC, Berquist TH, Cooney WP. Scaphoid anatomy: evaluation with complex motion tomography. *Radiology*. 1989;173:177–180.

147. Stark HH, Chao E, Zemel NP, Rickard TA, Ashworth CR. Fracture of the hook of the hamate. *J Bone Joint Surg Am*. 1989;71:1202–1207.

148. Stark HH, Jobe FW, Boyes JH, Ashworth CR. Fracture of the hook of the hamate in athletes. *J Bone Joint Surg Am*. 1977;59:575–582.

149. Stein R, Siegel MW. Naviculo-capitate fracture syndrome. *J Bone Joint Surg Am*. 1969;51:391–395.

150. Swanson AB. Fractures involving the digits of the hand. *Orthop Clin North Am*. 1970;1:261–274.

151. Talersnik J. Carpal instability. *J Bone Joint Surg Am*. 1988;70: 1262–1268.

152. Tehranzadeh J, Davenport J, Pais MJ. Scaphoid fracture: evaluation with flexion-extension tomography. *Radiology*. 1990;176:167–170.

153. Torisu T. Fracture of the hook of the hamate by a golf-swing. *Clin Orthop*. 1972;83:91–94.

154. Vasilas A, Grieco RV, Bartone NF. Roentgen aspects of injuries to the pisiform bone and pisotriquetral injury. *J Bone Joint Surg Am*. 1960;42: 1317–1328.

155. Verdan C, Narakas A. Fracture and pseudoarthrosis of the scaphoid. *Surg Clin North Am*. 1968;48:1083–1095.

156. Vesley DG. The distal radioulnar joint. *Clin Orthop*. 1967;51:75–91.

157. Wehbe MA, Schneider LA. Mallet fractures. *J Bone Joint Surg Am*. 1984;66:658–669.

158. Wenger DR. Avulsion of the profundus tendon insertion in football players. *Arch Surg*. 1973;106:145–149.

159. Wesely MS, Barenfield PA. Trans-scaphoid, transcapitate, transtriquetral, perilunate fracture-dislocation of the wrist. *J Bone Joint Surg Am.* 1972;54:1073–1078.

160. Wilson JN, Rowland SA. Fracture-dislocation of the proximal interphalangeal joint of the finger. Treatment by open reduction and internal fixation. *J Bone Joint Surg Am.* 1966;48:493–505.

161. Wood MB, Berquist TH. The hand and wrist. In: Berquist TH, ed. *Imaging of Orthopedic Trauma.* 2nd ed. New York: Raven; 1991:749–870.

162. Yeager BA, Dalinka MK. Radiology of trauma of the wrist: dislocations, fracture dislocations, and instability patterns. *Skeletal Radiol.* 1985; 13:120–130.

Soft Tissue and Miscellaneous Injuries

163. Berquist TH. *Magnetic Resonance Imaging of the Musculoskeletal System.* 2nd ed. New York: Raven; 1990.

164. Braunstein EM, Louis DS, Green TL, Hankin FM. Fluoroscopic and arthrographic evaluation of carpal instability. *AJR.* 1985;144:1259–1262.

165. Burkhart SS, Wood MB, Linscheid RL. Post-traumatic recurrent subluxation of the extensor carpi ulnaris tendon. *J Hand Surg.* 1982;7:1–4.

166. Cooney WP III. Bursitis and tendinitis in the hand, wrist, and elbow: an approach to treatment. *Minn Med.* 1983;66:491–494.

167. Cooney WP III. Sports injuries to the upper extremity. *Postgrad Med.* 1984;76:45–50.

168. Dobyns JH, Sim FH, Linscheid RL. Sports stress syndromes of the hand and wrist. *Am J Sports Med.* 1978;6:236–254.

169. Engkvist O, Balkfors B, Lindsjo U. Thumb injuries in downhill skiing. *Int J Sports Med.* 1982;3:50–55.

170. Fomage BD, Schernberg FL, Rifkin MD. Ultrasound examination of the hand. *Radiology.* 1985;155:785–788.

171. Helal B. Chronic overuse injuries of the pisotriquetral joint in racquet game players. *Br J Sports Med.* 1979;12:195–205.

172. Hooper GJ. An unusual variety of skier's thumb. *J Hand Surg.* 1987;12A:627–629.

173. Johnson RK. Soft tissue injuries of the forearm and hand. *Clin Sports Med.* 1986;5:701–707.

174. Kong HS, Kurdynis P, Brahme SK, et al. Triangular fibrocartilage and intercarpal ligaments of the wrist: MR imaging. *Radiology.* 1991;181:401–404.

175. Levinsohn EM, Palmer AK, Coren AB, Zinberg EM. Wrist arthrography: the value of the 3-compartment injection technique. *Skeletal Radiol.* 1987;16:534–544.

176. Linscheid RL, Dobyns JH. Athletic injuries of the wrist. *Clin Orthop.* 1985;198:141–151.

177. Naso SJ. Compression of the digital nerve. A new entity in tennis players. *Orthop Rev.* 1984;13:506–508.

178. Osterman AL, Moskow L, Low DW. Soft tissue injuries to the hand and wrist in racquet sports. *Clin Sports Med.* 1988;7:329–348.

179. Palmer AR, Dobyns JH, Linscheid RL. Management of post traumatic instability of the wrist secondary to ligament rupture. *J Hand Surg.* 1978;3:507–532.

180. Pick RY. DeQuervain's disease: a clinical triad. *Clin Orthop.* 1977;143:165–166.

181. Posner MA. Injuries to the hand and wrist in athletes. *Orthop Clin North Am.* 1977;8:593–618.

182. Tapper EM. Ski injuries from 1939–1976. The Sun Valley experience. *Am J Sports Med.* 1978;6:114–121.

183. Tirman RM, Weber ER, Snyder LL, Koonce TW. Mid carpal wrist arthrography for detection of tears of the scapholunate and lunotriquetral ligament. *AJR.* 1985;144:107–108.

184. Wilson AJ, Gilula LA, Mann FA. Unidirectional joint communication in wrist arthrography: an evaluation of 250 cases. *AJR.* 1991;157: 105–109.

185. Wong EC, Jesmanowicz A, Hyde JS. High-resolution, short echo time MR imaging of the fingers and wrist with local gradient coil. *Radiology.* 1991;181:393–397.

186. Wood MB, Berquist TH. The hand and wrist. In: Berquist TH, ed. *Imaging of Orthopedic Trauma.* 2nd ed. New York: Raven; 1991:749–870.

187. Wood MB, Linscheid RL. Abductor pollicis longus bursitis. *Clin Orthop.* 1973;93:293–296.

188. Yasusuki H. Sports and peripheral nerve injury. *Am J Sports Med.* 1983;11:420–426.

189. Zlatkin MB, Chao PC, Osterman AL, Mitchell DS, Dalinka MK, Kressel HY. Chronic wrist pain: evaluation with high resolution MR imaging. *Radiology.* 1989;173:723–729.

Chapter 12

Stress Fractures

INTRODUCTION

The term *stress fracture* is commonly applied to a number of fractures resulting from repetitive stress that is of lesser magnitude than that required for an acute traumatic fracture. Daffner[12] states that a stress fracture results from muscular activity on bones rather than from direct trauma. Most stress fractures are fatigue fractures resulting from abnormal muscular tension on normal bone.[12,18] These usually occur in the lower extremity in association with significant changes in physical activity. Fatigue fractures are commonly reported in military personnel.[24,25,28,43] Insufficiency fractures occur when normal stress or muscle tension acts on bone with abnormal elastic resistance.[8–10,14,18,48]

Participants in unorganized sports frequently give a history of starting a new activity such as track, jogging, or fitness classes.[38] Usually several weeks after starting the activity the patient will note local pain. Symptoms are usually relieved by rest. If the activity is continued, the pain generally increases.[18]

Stress fractures occur in 10% of athletes. The incidence approaches 16% in runners.[35] Injuries are bilateral in 17% of cases. Stress fractures in athletes differ somewhat from the commonly reported findings in military recruits. This difference is probably related to the types of activity and the lower fitness level in military recruits at the time training is initiated. Table 12-1 summarizes the location of common stress fractures and the activities in which they often arise.

Physical examination may reveal local tenderness or swelling over the fracture.[4,18] These fractures may be evident in 66% and 25% of patients, respectively. This is especially true of stress fractures in the fibular and tarsal regions.[35] Children may have slight temperature elevation.[18] Clinically most stress fractures arise distal to the knee. The importance of this lies mainly in that differentiation from other entities may be difficult. For example, stress fractures of the proximal tibia may result in periosteal new bone formation, leading the physician to suspect a primary bone tumor. Similarly, if the metatarsal is involved there may be exuberant periosteal reaction suggesting either osteomyelitis or tumor.[32] In either case the history of repetitive stress is helpful in suggesting the diagnosis.[19,25]

RADIOGRAPHIC EVALUATION

There are multiple imaging techniques available for evaluating musculoskeletal conditions. Except with isotope studies, detection of stress fractures may be difficult in the early stages.[12,24,35] Early diagnosis is especially important with stress fractures of the femoral neck; displacement of these fractures can occur, resulting in a significant increase in morbidity.[4] Matheson et al[35] reported that an average of 13 weeks passed before the diagnosis of stress fractures could be established.

Routine radiographs are almost always normal initially. Blickenstaff and Morris[4] described the phases of stress fractures. During the first 5 to 14 days osteoclastic resorption leads to local osteoporosis. This is followed by periosteal or endosteal callus formation. Swelling and increased vascularity

Table 12-1 Common Stress Fractures

Location	Activity or Sport	References
Foot	Marching Running Basketball Ballet Jumping Cycling Skiing	12,18,22,24,41,43, 47,52
Tibia	Running Ballet	5,13,16,19,24,35, 40,41
Fibula	Running Jumping	2,20,24,40
Patella	Hurdling	12,17,18,24
Femur	Long distance running Ballet	12,26,34,35,40,44
Pelvis	Running Gymnastics Bowling	4,15,35,40,44
Spine	Weight lifting Football (blocking) Ballet	12,18,21,35,38
Ribs	Backpacking Orienteering Golf	12,25,37,45,52
Coracoid	Trap shooting	46
Humerus	Baseball	4,35
Ulna	Baseball Wheelchair racing	12,25
Hand	Golf Tennis Baseball Weight lifting Gymnastics	12,25,27,40,49

accompany these changes. Continued activity results in fracture. The fracture defect may be primarily cortical or trabecular. Greaney et al[24] reported isotopic findings in 250 military personnel. Twenty-three percent of fractures were considered cortical, and 77% were cancellous. Routine radiographs were positive in only 40% of cortical and 26% of trabecular stress fractures. Cortical fractures may present with endosteal or periosteal callus with or without a lucent cortical defect.[4,5] Tomography is often necessary to define a fracture line. Stress fractures in cancellous bone may appear as a hazy area of increased density or a sclerotic line due to trabecular compression.[4]

Metabolic activity around stress fractures may allow isotope detection as early as 24 hours after the injury.[24,35,36] The bone changes must progress to cause a 30% to 50% change in the bone density before radiographs will be positive. This usually takes 10 to 21 days.[24,42]

Classification of stress fractures may be useful in certain cases. Wilson and Katz[52] categorized fractures according to their radiographic appearance. Type I fractures present with a lucent line with no associated periosteal reaction, type II fractures reveal cancellous sclerosis and endosteal callus, type III fractures have external callus, and type IV fractures present with a mixture of types I to III.

Devas[18] divided stress fractures into compression and distraction categories. Compression fractures are equivalent to torus fractures. These most commonly occur in children and elderly patients and are usually located in the femoral neck and tibia. Distraction fractures are similar to greenstick fractures and may be transverse, oblique, or longitudinal. Transverse fractures are the most significant in that complete fracture and displacement may occur.

Stress fractures differ in their appearance depending upon their location. Therefore, early diagnosis and appearance are important mainly in determining which fractures are likely to displace.[12,44]

Early attempts at radiographic diagnosis of stress fractures with the use of magnification techniques, xeroradiography, thermography, conventional tomography, and computed tomography (CT) have been useful in certain cases.[1,24,35,41,51] Magnetic resonance imaging (MRI) may be useful in certain situations because of the strong signal obtained from medullary bone. Detection of cortical changes may be more difficult.[3]

Despite new imaging techniques, isotope studies with ^{99m}Tc remain most useful in early detection of stress fractures.[24,35] Greaney et al[24] noted normal radiographs in 50% of their patients with stress fractures even during follow-up. Radiographic techniques are still extremely important in determining the nature of isotope abnormalities. Differential diagnostic challenges may occur with osteogenic sarcoma, chronic osteomyelitis, and osteoid osteoma.[3,12,16,32] Problems in diagnosis and treatment of stress fractures vary depending upon location and fracture type.[35]

Foot

Military studies have provided a large controlled population for study of tarsal and metatarsal stress fractures. Wilson and Katz[52] studied 250 patients, and Greaney et al[24] studied 250 marine recruits. Although statistics vary somewhat, most investigators agree that stress fractures in the foot, at least in the military population, most commonly involve the metatarsals (Table 12-1).[24,52] March fractures are common in military recruits. Stress with marching is applied maximally to the second and third metatarsals (Fig. 12-1). Less commonly the fourth metatarsal is involved.[18,52] Initial radiographs are usually normal. Follow-up films in 10 to 14 days will often demonstrate a small, lucent cortical defect or early periosteal change. Metatarsal stress fractures most commonly involve the middle or distal shaft of the metatarsals.

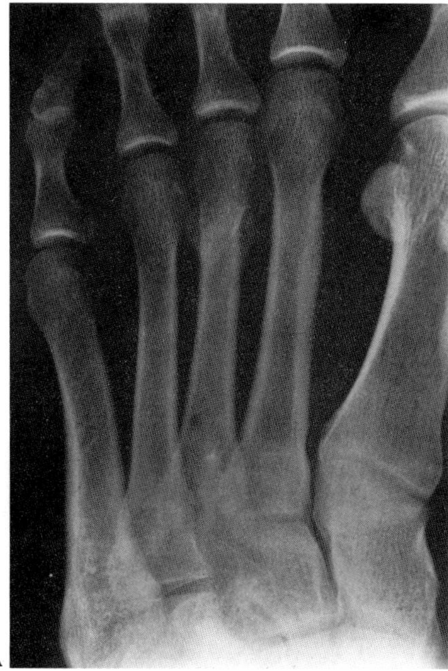

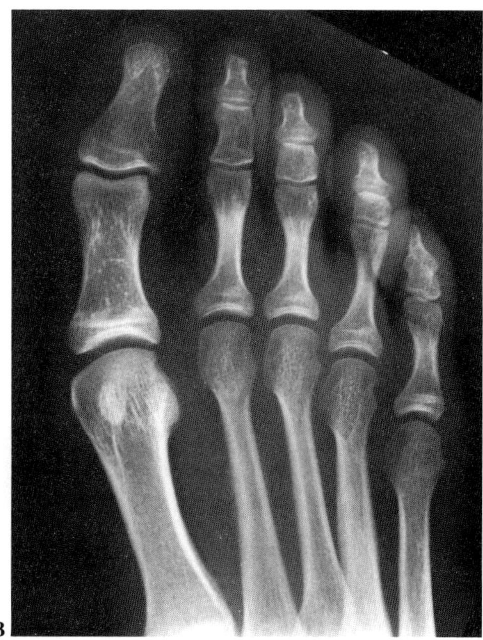

Fig. 12-1 Metatarsal stress fracture. (**A**) Healing stress fracture of the left third metatarsal neck. (**B**) More subtle early stress fracture of the second metatarsal diaphysis.

Metatarsal stress fractures are not uncommon in civilians and athletes.[18,40] Matheson et al[35] reported metatarsal stress fractures in 9% of 320 athletes studied. The finding is most common in runners and may relate to a change in training patterns or footwear (Tables 12-2 and 12-3). Pain with weight bearing may begin in the first few weeks after the change in activity. This pain is usually reproducible each time the activity is resumed. The pain is usually well localized.[12,18,40]

Wilson and Katz[52] noted calcaneal stress fractures nearly as frequently as metatarsal fractures. Calcaneal stress fractures were most common in the series of Greaney et al.[24] Associated stress fractures of the upper tibia medially were noted in 60%.[22,24]

Calcaneal stress fractures occur less frequently in civilians, but again there seems to be an association with footwear that increases heel stress. When asked to describe their pain, patients normally point to the medial and lateral sides of the heel rather than to the plantar surface. Physical examination often reveals pain on squeezing of the heel.

Radiographically a hazy or speckled appearance may be noted. This usually progresses to a sclerotic band if stress continues (Fig. 12-2).[24,52] Trabecular stress fractures rarely produce periosteal changes. Isotope scans will demonstrate a linear area of increased tracer uptake and may be positive within 24 hours but almost certainly will be positive in 72 hours.[24,36]

Table 12-2 Stress Fractures and Associated Sports Activities

Activity	*Incidence (%)*
Running	69
Fitness and aerobics classes	8
Racquet sports	5
Basketball	4
Soccer	2
Baseball	2
Other (skating, ice hockey, volleyball, gymnastics, etc)	10

Source: Matheson GO, Clement DB, McKenzie DC, Tauton JE, Lloyd-Smith DR, MacIntyre JE, *American Journal of Sports Medicine* (1987;15:46–58), American Orthopaedic Society for Sports Medicine.

Table 12-3 Stress Fractures in Athletes

Location	*Incidence (%)*
Tibia	49
Tarsal	25
Metatarsal	9
Femur	7
Fibula	7
Pelvis	2
Sesamoid	<1
Spine	<1

Source: Matheson GO, Clement DB, McKenzie DC, Tauton JE, Lloyd-Smith DR, MacIntyre JE, *American Journal of Sports Medicine* (1987;15:46–58), American Orthopaedic Society for Sports Medicine.

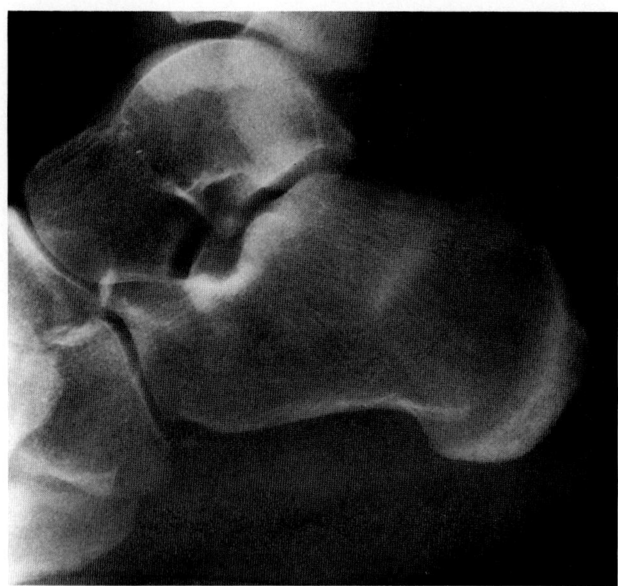

Fig. 12-2 Lateral view of the calcaneus demonstrating a linear zone of condensation of the midcalcaneus due to stress fracture.

Stress fractures involving the tarsal navicular, talus, phalanges, and sesamoids typically occur less frequently.[23,40,41,51] Tarsal stress fractures are second only to tibial fractures in athletes, however (Table 12-3). Matheson et al[35] reported tarsal stress fractures in 25% of 320 athletes compared to an incidence of 49% for the tibia. An acute traumatic event is usually recalled by athletes with tarsal stress fractures. Despite this clinical history, delay in diagnosis is more common than with stress fractures in other locations. Prognosis is also more guarded.[35,38] Pavlov et al[41] accomplished diagnosis of tarsal navicular fractures with isotope scans and tomography. Isotope scans (^{99m}Tc), especially the plantar view, were useful in localizing the abnormality and tomograms in defining the fracture.

Most navicular fractures are sagittal and involve the middle and medial thirds of the navicular.[41,51] In a series of patients reported by Torg et al,[51] treatment of navicular fractures was successful with non–weight bearing. Simple restrictions of activity led to nonunion in seven of nine patients, however.

Tibia

Tibial stress fractures are common in the military and athletic populations.[24,35,38,40,51] The incidence of tibial stress fractures in the series of Greaney et al[24] was 73%. Cortical involvement is much more common in the tibia. Matheson et al[35] found tibial stress fractures to be the most common fracture in athletes (49% of 320 cases; Tables 12-2 and 12-3).

Stress fractures may arise anywhere along the length of the tibia.[35,53] Classically, they occur on the posteromedial aspect or in the proximal tibia at the junction of the metaphysis and diaphysis (Fig. 12-3). Variations are not uncommon, however (Fig. 12-4). Miller et al[38] reported tibial stress fractures to be most common in the midtibia and then in the distal and

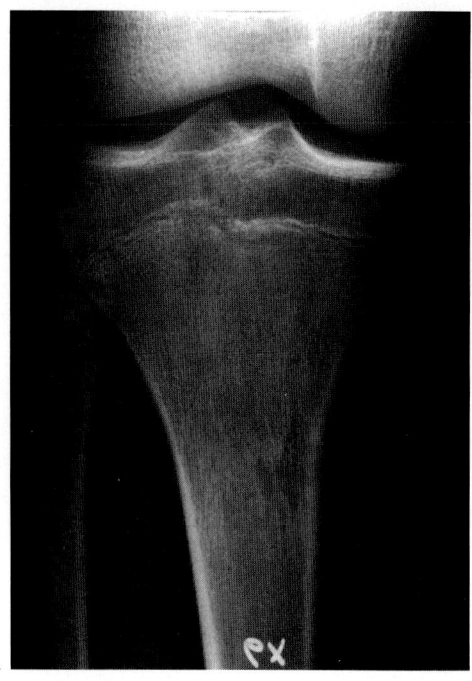

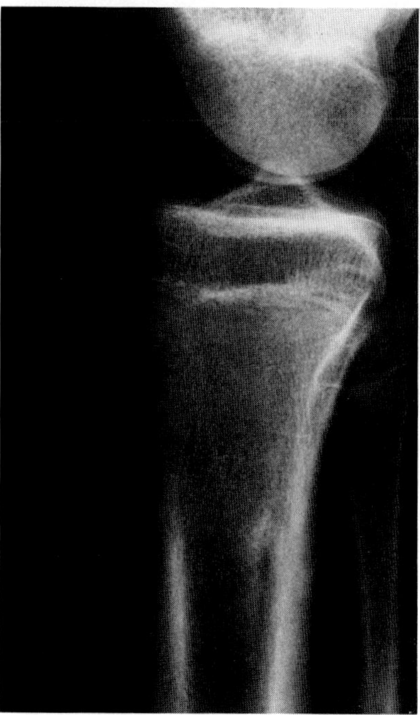

Fig. 12-3 Typical posteromedial stress fracture of the tibia demonstrated on (**A**) anteroposterior (AP) and (**B**) lateral views.

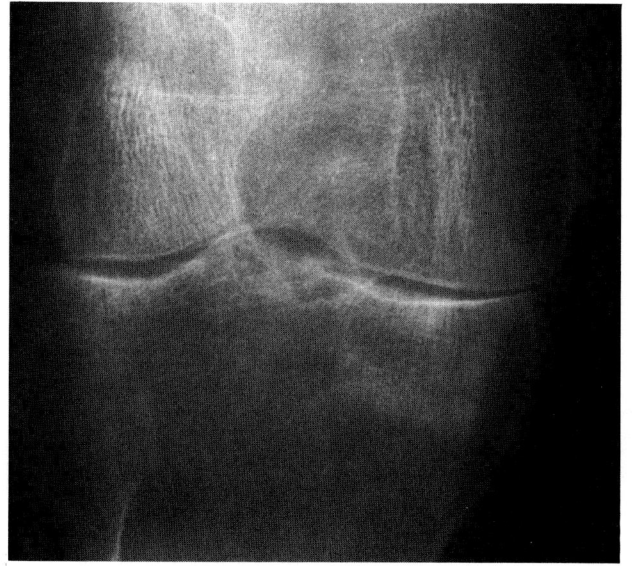

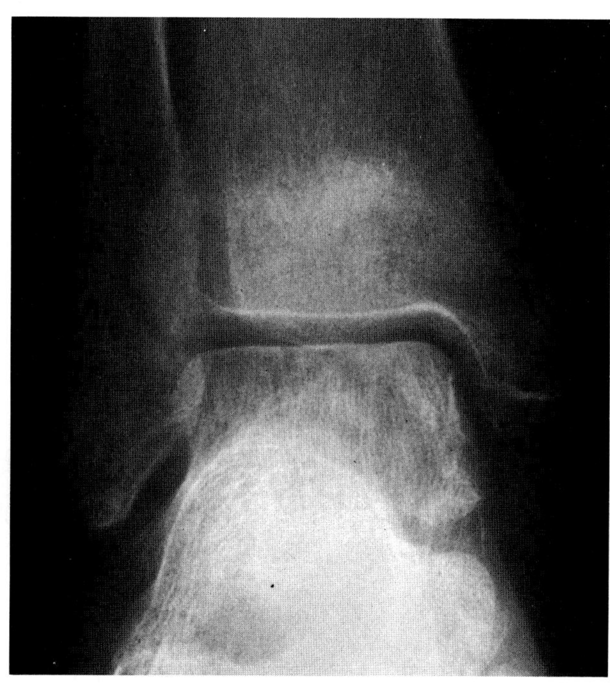

Fig. 12-4 Tibial stress fractures in marathon runners. **(A)** AP view of the knee demonstrates a linear zone of condensation medially due to a stress fracture. Note the marked joint space narrowing. **(B)** AP view of the ankle demonstrating a distal tibial stress fracture.

proximal segments. Ballet dancers often develop stress fractures in the midtibia.[5,6,16,39]

Almost any form of strenuous activity may precede stress fractures of the tibia; hence jogging, racquetball, and any form of running may be responsible. In the past when the athlete first started training for a sport, leg pain was called shin splints. It was recognized that this condition would not improve unless the activity was halted. Probably at least some of these cases were early stress fractures.

Isotope studies will be positive soon after symptoms begin if a stress fracture is present.[11,24,36,42] Radiographs may remain negative for 2 to 3 weeks.[24] The earliest finding may be subtle periosteal reaction. Tomograms will often demonstrate the fracture line and may assist in differentiating a stress fracture from a primary bone tumor (Fig. 12-5). The latter condition may be difficult to differentiate from a stress fracture if there is no clear-cut history of change in physical activity.[32]

Usually the pain present with stress fractures is sufficient to cause patients voluntarily to restrict their activities. This may be the only treatment necessary. Persistent pain with simple weight bearing may indicate the need for more aggressive therapy, however, such as crutches or even a long-leg cylinder cast. Radiographic changes may be helpful in this decision-making process. Hallel et al[26] described tibial fractures as grade I if periosteal reaction involved one cortex, grade II if changes were circumferential, and grade III if the fracture was displaced. Tibial stress fractures rarely displace. Grade II fractures, however, may require more aggressive therapy than the less extensive grade I fractures.

Fibula

Stress fractures involve the fibula less frequently than the tibia. Ovara et al[40] reported an incidence of 14.1% in 142 athletes with stress fractures. The incidence in other series is only about 7%.[50] The fibula is a non–weight-bearing bone. Therefore, the fractures are due to muscle stress.[18,52] This stress is most commonly applied with calf muscle contraction during running.[18]

Femoral Shaft

Stress fractures of the femoral shaft are not common. Ovara et al[40] reported an incidence of 2.8%. Femoral stress fractures occur in about 7% of athletes.[35] Midfemoral involvement is most common, and fractures of the distal femur and femoral neck are the next most common.[38] Femoral stress fractures are often associated with cavus foot.[35] Fractures are most frequent in long distance runners and occasionally in ballet dancers.[7,33,34,47] Highly motivated, well-conditioned athletes tend to be at risk for this type of fracture.[26,34] Luchini et al[34] reported femoral shaft fractures in long distance runners who were totally asymptomatic before the fracture. This was attributed to muscle fatigue resulting in transfer of stress to the femoral shaft. Early recognition of this fracture is important because displacement tends to occur (Fig. 12-6). Treatment of femoral shaft fractures may require open reduction and internal fixation if displacement occurs.

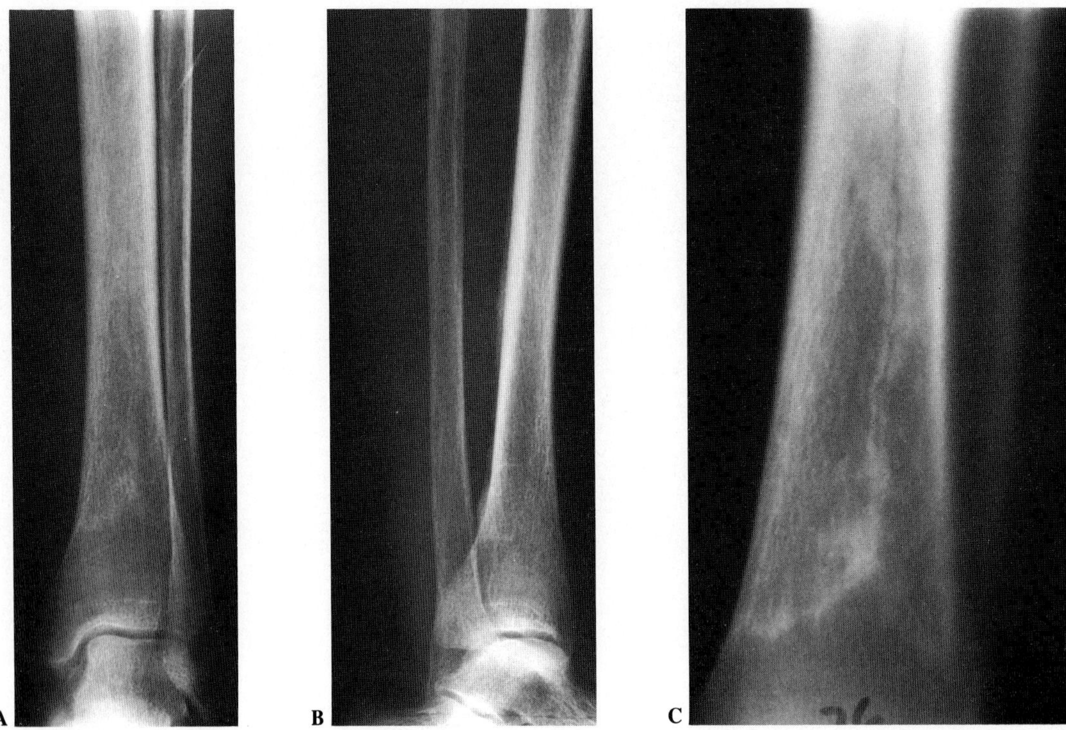

Fig. 12-5 Longitudinal tibial stress fracture. (**A**) AP view shows subtle condensation distally (arrows) with a longitudinal lucent line. (**B**) Lateral view shows periosteal new bone formation posteriorly. (**C**) AP tomogram clearly demonstrates the fracture.

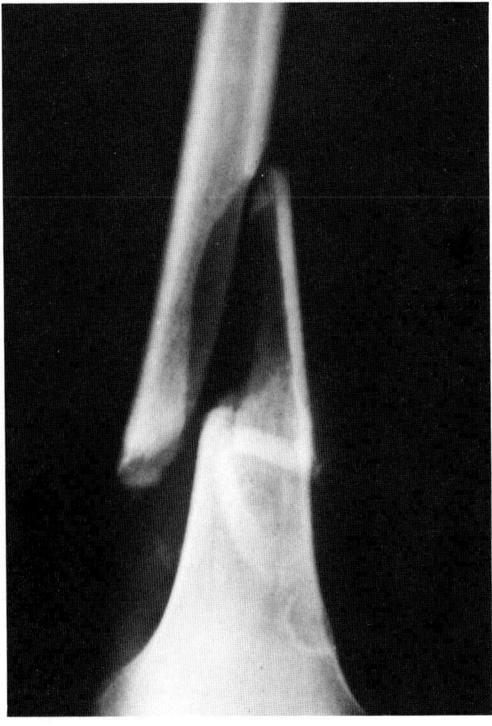

Fig. 12-6 AP view of the femur demonstrating a displaced, comminuted fracture in a long distance runner.

Femoral Neck

Stress fractures of the femoral neck were more common than diaphyseal stress fractures in the series by Ovara et al.[40] Detection may be difficult clinically (Fig. 12-7). The patient's pain will frequently be referred to the knee, and point tenderness may be difficult to elicit.[18,44] Early diagnosis and treatment are essential because progression of this type of fracture may lead to eventual displacement.[4,18,26] Classification of femoral neck fractures is useful in determining which fractures tend to displace.[4,18,36] Devas[15,18] classified fractures as transverse or compression. Compression fractures occur at the base of the femoral neck medially (calcar). They often present with localized osteoporosis, which progresses to periosteal callus formation. This type usually occurs in young patients. Osteoid osteoma should be considered in this location as well. History and tomography are useful in differentiating these two conditions. Compression stress fractures usually do not displace and can be treated with non–weight bearing. Transverse fractures occur in older patients. Initially a defect in the inferior cortex of the neck will be seen. This frequently progresses to a complete fracture and displacement. Devas[15,18] noted displacement in 11 of 18 transverse fractures (Fig. 12-7).

Blickenstaff and Morris[4] classified femoral neck fractures according to their radiographic appearance. A type I fracture

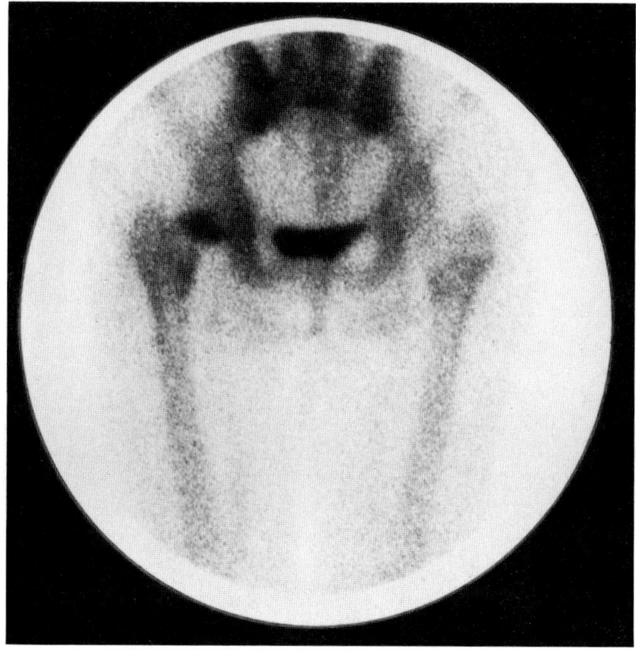

A

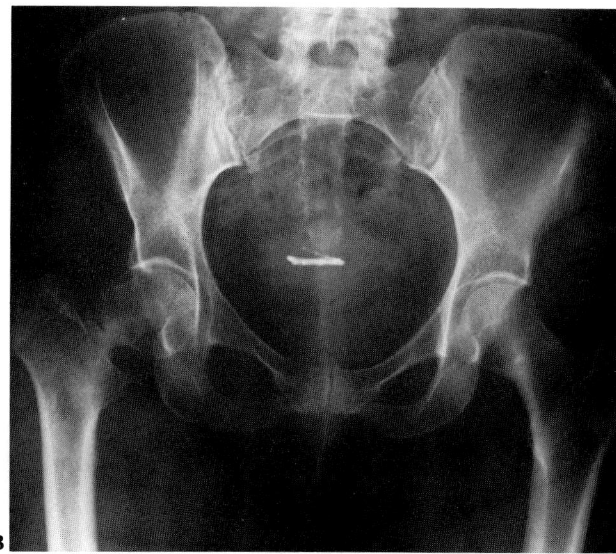

B

Fig. 12-7 Femoral neck stress fracture. (**A**) Radionuclide scan demonstrates increased tracer uptake in the right femoral neck due to a stress fracture. (**B**) Radiograph of the pelvis several weeks later demonstrates progression to a complete fracture.

demonstrates callus only, type II shows fine calcar fracture with or without extension across the femoral neck, and type III is displaced. These investigators indicated that, once a fracture line is visible, internal fixation is indicated. Patients with type I fractures were treated conservatively, requiring about 9.5 weeks of hospitalization. Displaced fractures only healed without complication 20% of the time. The average hospital stay was 59 weeks. Complications included malunion, non-union, and avascular necrosis.

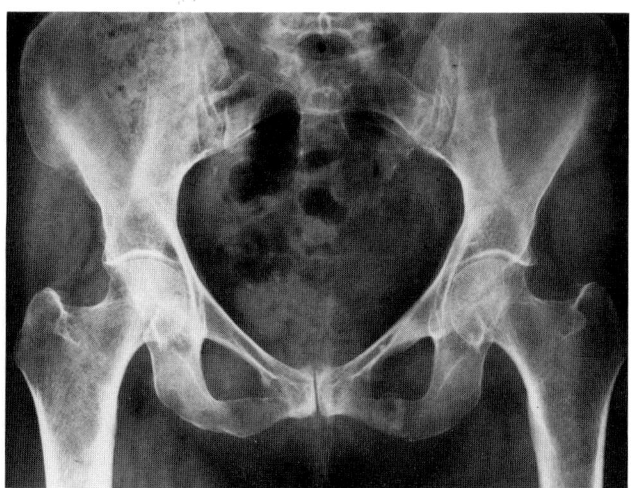

Fig. 12-8 AP view of the pelvis demonstrating a stress fracture of the left inferior pubic ramus. There is also condensation (arrow) in the superior pubic ramus due to a second fracture.

Pelvis

Stress fractures in the pelvis most frequently involve the pubic arch and sacrum.[8–10,12] They may be related to running, gymnastics, and bowling (Fig. 12-8).[12,18]

Insufficiency fractures in this region are becoming more common as the incidence of joint replacement procedures increases. Patients with severe rheumatoid arthritis are now able to walk and bear weight, which results in insufficiency fractures in the pubic arch and other locations.[8–10,14,48]

Pubic arch stress fractures tend to occur in older individuals. Patients frequently notice pain in the groin or hip with weight bearing. Treatment consists of activity restriction or partial weight bearing with crutches.

Other Locations

Stress fractures in the spine, upper extremities, and ribs are uncommon compared to the lower extremity.[27,29–31,45,46,49] Stress fractures may occur in the spinous processes and lumbar pars in weight lifters and football linemen who repeatedly lift heavy weights.[12,18,24,48,52] Evaluation of the pars may be accomplished with isotope studies and subsequent localized (1- to 3-mm thick) tomograms. On occasion, CT scanning may be used to evaluate the posterior elements (Fig. 12-9). This technique is especially helpful in excluding other bone and soft tissue abnormalities. MRI may provide even better sensitivity for detection of soft tissue abnormalities.[3]

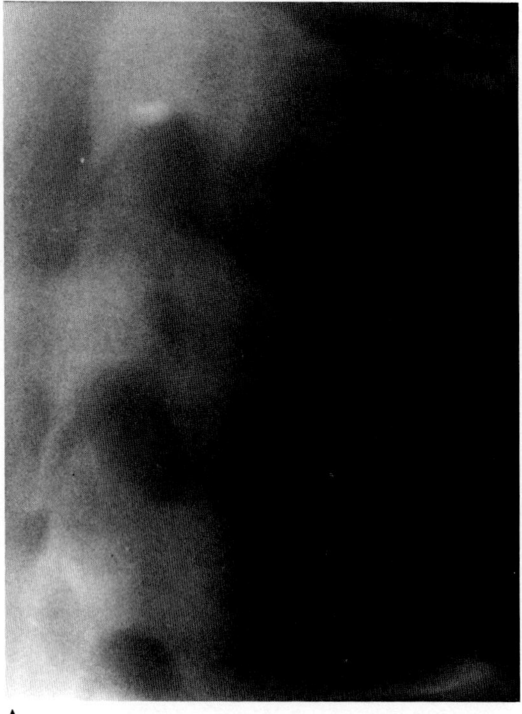

A

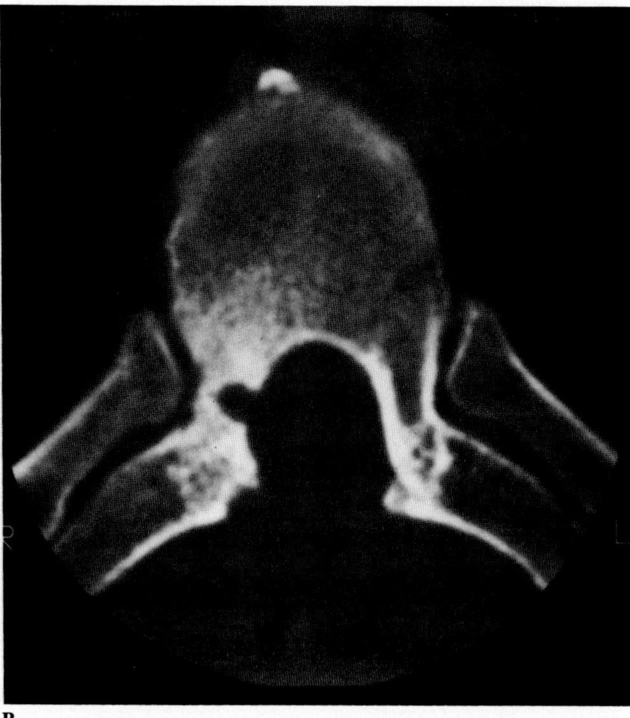

B

Fig. 12-9 **(A)** Lateral tomogram and **(B)** computed tomogram demonstrating a stress fracture of the pedicle. *Source:* Reprinted from *Imaging of Orthopedic Trauma* ed 2 by TH Berquist, 1991, Raven Press, © Mayo Foundation.

Upper extremity stress fractures have been described in baseball players, golfers, and trap shooters (Table 12-1).[12,27] Stress fractures of the ribs have been reported in golfers and orienteers.[37] Fractures of the first ribs can develop after prolonged use of heavy back packs.[12]

SUMMARY

The diagnosis of a stress fracture should be considered in patients presenting with pain after a change in activity, especially if the activity is strenuous and the pain is in the lower extremities. Because evidence of the stress fracture may not be apparent for weeks on routine radiographs, proper use of other imaging techniques will allow an earlier diagnosis. Prompt diagnosis is especially important in the femur, where displacement may occur.

REFERENCES

1. Allen JG. Longitudinal stress fractures of the tibia: diagnosis with CT. *Radiology*. 1988;167:799–801.

2. Bargren JH, Tilson DH Jr, Bridgefort OE. Prevention of displaced fatigue fractures of the femur. *J Bone Joint Surg Am*. 1971;53:1115–1117.

3. Berquist JH. *Imaging of Orthopedic Trauma*. 2nd ed. New York: Raven; 1991.

4. Blickenstaff LD, Morris JM. Fatigue fractures of the femoral neck. *J Bone Joint Surg Am*. 1966;48:1031–1047.

5. Burrows HJ. Fatigue fractures of the fibula. *J Bone Joint Surg Br*. 1948;30:266–279.

6. Burrows HJ. Fatigue fracture of the middle of the tibia in ballet dancers. *J Bone Joint Surg Br*. 1956;38:83–94.

7. Butler JE, Brown SL, McConnel BG. Subtrochanteric stress fractures in runners. *Am J Sports Med*. 1982;10:228–232.

8. Casey D, Mirra J, Staple TW. Parasymphyseal insufficiency fractures of the os pubis. *AJR*. 1984;142:581–586.

9. Cooper KL, Beabout JW, McLeod RA. Supraacetabular insufficiency fractures. *Radiology*. 1985;157:15–17.

10. Cooper KL, Beabout JW, Swee RG. Insufficiency fractures of the sacrum. *Radiology*. 1985;156:15–20.

11. Daffner RH. Anterior tibial striations. *AJR*. 1984;143:651–653.

12. Daffner RH. Stress fractures. *Skeletal Radiol*. 1978;2:221–229.

13. Darby RE. Stress fractures of the os calcis. *JAMA*. 1967;200: 1183–1184.

14. DeSmet AA, Neff JR. Pubic and sacral insufficiency fractures: clinical course and radiologic findings. *AJR*. 1985;145:601–606.

15. Devas MB. Longitudinal stress fractures. *J Bone Joint Surg Br*. 1960;42:508–514.

16. Devas MB. *Stress Fractures*. Edinburgh: Churchill Livingstone; 1975.

17. Devas MB. Stress fractures in children. *J Bone Joint Surg Br*. 1963; 45:528–541.

18. Devas MB. Stress fractures of the femoral neck. *J Bone Joint Surg Br*. 1965;47:728–738.

19. Devas MB. Stress fractures of the patella. *J Bone Joint Surg Br.* 1960;42:71–74.

20. Devas MB, Sweetnan R. Stress fractures of the fibula. *J Bone Joint Surg Br.* 1956;38:818–829.

21. Farquharson-Roberts MA, Fulford PC. Stress fractures of the radius. *J Bone Joint Surg Br.* 1980;62:194–195.

22. Gilbert RS, Johnson HA. Stress fractures in military recruits—a review of twelve years' experience. *Mil Med.* 1966;131:716–721.

23. Goergen TG, Venn-Watson EA, Rossman DJ, Resnick D, Gerler KH. Tarsal navicular stress fractures in runners. *AJR.* 1981;136:201–203.

24. Greaney RB, Gerber FH, Laughlan RL. Distribution and natural history of stress fractures in US Marine recruits. *Radiology.* 1983;146:339–346.

25. Grusd R. Pseudofractures and stress fractures. *Semin Roentgenol.* 1978;13:81–82.

26. Hallel T, Amit S, Segal D. Fatigue fractures of the tibial and femoral shaft in soldiers. *Clin Orthop.* 1976;118:35–43.

27. Hanks GA, Kalenak A, Bowman LS, Sebastianelli WJ. Stress fractures of the carpal scaphoid. *J Bone Joint Surg Am.* 1989;71:938–941.

28. Hartley JB. "Stress" or "fatigue" fractures in bone. *Br J Radiol.* 1943;16:255–262.

29. Kitchin ID. Fatigue fracture of the ulna. *J Bone Joint Surg Br.* 1948;30:622–623.

30. Kroening PM, Shelton ML. Stress fractures. *Am J Roentgenol Radium Ther Nucl Med.* 1963;89:1281–1286.

31. Laferty JF, Winter WG, Ganilaro SA. Fatigue characteristics of posterior elements of the vertebra. *J Bone Joint Surg Am.* 1977;59:154–158.

32. Levin DC, Blazena ME, Levina E. Fatigue fractures of the shaft of the femur: simulation of malignant tumor. *Radiology.* 1967;89:883–885.

33. Lombardo SJ, Benson DW. Stress fractures of the femur in runners. *Am J Sports Med.* 1982;10:219–227.

34. Luchini MA, Sarokhan AJ, Micheli LJ. Acute displaced femoral-shaft fractures in long distance runners. *J Bone Joint Surg Am.* 1983;65:689–691.

35. Matheson GO, Clement DB, McKenzie DC, Tauton JE. Lloyd-Smith DR, MacIntyre JE. Stress fractures in athletes. A study of 320 cases. *Am J Sports Med.* 1987;15:46–58.

36. Matin P. The appearance of bone scans following fractures, including immediate and long-term studies. *J Nucl Med.* 1979;20:1227–1231.

37. McKenzie DC. Stress fractures of the rib in an elite oarsman. *Int J Sports Med.* 1989;10:220–222.

38. Miller TW, Heck LL, Kight JL, McCarroll JR, Shelbourne KD, VanHove ED. A clinical and radiological review of stress fractures in competitive and noncompetitive athletes. *Indiana Med.* 1987;80:942–949.

39. Nussbaum AR, Treves ST, Micheli L. Bone stress lesions in ballet dancers: scintigraphic assessment. *AJR.* 1988;150:851–855.

40. Orava S, Puranen J, Ala-Ketola L. Stress fractures caused by physical exercise. *Acta Orthop Scand.* 1978;49:19–27.

41. Pavlov H, Tord JS, Freiberger RH. Tarsal navicular stress fractures: radiographic evaluation. *Radiology.* 1983;148:641–645.

42. Prather JL, Nusynowitz ML, Snowdy HA, Hughes AD, McCortney WH, Bragg RJ. Scintigraphic findings in stress fractures. *J Bone Joint Surg Am.* 1977;59:869–874.

43. Protzman RR, Griffis CG. Stress fractures in men and women undergoing military training. *J Bone Joint Surg Am.* 1977;59:825.

44. Provost RA, Morris JM. Fatigue fracture of the femoral shaft. *J Bone Joint Surg Am.* 1969;51:487–498.

45. Rasad S. Golfer's fracture of the ribs. Report of 3 cases. *Am J Roentgenol Radium Ther Nucl Med.* 1974;120:901–903.

46. Sandrock AR. Another sports fatigue fracture. Stress fracture of the coracoid process of the scapula. *Radiology.* 1975;117:274.

47. Schneider HJ, King AY, Brownson JL, Miller EH. Stress injuries and development changes of lower extremities in ballet dancers. *Radiology.* 1974;113:627–632.

48. Schneider R, Kaye JJ. Insufficiency fractures of the long bones occurring in patients with rheumatoid arthritis. *Radiology.* 1975;116:595–599.

49. Stark HH, Jobe FW, Boyes JH, Ashworth CR. Fracture of the hook of the hamate in athletes. *J Bone Joint Surg Am.* 1977;59:575–582.

50. Symeonides PP. High stress fractures of the fibula. *J Bone Joint Surg Br.* 1980;62:192–193.

51. Torg JS, Pavlov H, Cooley LH, et al. Stress fractures of the tarsal navicular. *J Bone Joint Surg Am.* 1982;64:700–712.

52. Wilson ES, Katz FN. Stress fractures. An analysis of 250 consecutive cases. *Radiology.* 1969;92:481–486.

53. Zlatkin MB, Bjorkengren A, Sartoris DJ, Resnick D. Stress fractures of the distal tibia and calcaneus subsequent to acute fractures of the tibia and fibula. *AJR.* 1987;149:329–332.

Index

A

Abduction, 176
Accessory ligament, 36, 37
Accessory navicular, 172, 173
Acetabular fracture, 74, 87–89
  complex, 88
  complications, 89
  elementary, 87
  transverse, 87
Acetabular labral tear, 96
  hip arthrography, 79
Acetabular labrum, normal, 96
Acetabulum, 69
Achilles tendon, 181–184
  computed tomography, 183
  inflammation, 182
  magnetic resonance imaging, 183
  routine radiograph, 183
  ultrasound, 183, 184
Achilles tendon tear, 182
  ultrasound, 17
Achilles tendonitis, 183, 184
Acromioclavicular dislocation, 248–249, 250
Acromioclavicular joint
  anatomy, 225
  arthrography, 238–239
Acromioclavicular joint injury
  child, 248, 249
  classification, 248, 249
Adduction, 175–176
Adductor muscle injury, 103
Adhesive capsulitis, arthrography, 236, 237
Alar ligament, 36, 37
Anger gamma camera, skeletal scintigraphy, 16
Angiography, 22–23, 24
  digital subtraction angiography, 23
  equipment, 23
  indications, 22–23
  technique, 23
Ankle
  ligament injury, 176–179
  ligamentous anatomy, 167–170
  osseous anatomy, 167–170
  soft tissue anatomy, 172–175
  soft tissue trauma, 176–190
  tendon injuries, 180–186
Ankle fracture, 190–201
  arthritis, 200
  child, 191–195
    classification, 191–195
    epiphyses, 191
    etiology, 191
    juvenile Tillaux, 191, 192
    triplane, 191, 192
  classifications, 196, 198
  clinical features, 196–198
  evaluation, 195
  malunion, 201
  mechanism of injury, 196
  nonunion, 201
  pronation-adduction injuries, 197, 198
  pronation-lateral rotation injuries, 197, 199
  reflex sympathetic dystrophy, 201
  routine radiography, 199–200
  supination-adduction injuries, 196–197
  supination-lateral rotation injuries, 197, 198
Ankle injury, 167–215. *See also* Specific type
  incidence, 167
Ankle sprain, differential diagnosis, 181
Anterior compression injury, pelvic fracture, 86–87
Anterior cruciate ligament, 109–110
Anterior cruciate ligament injury, 137–140
  clinical tests, 136–141
  magnetic resonance imaging, 137
  routine radiography, 137
Anterior drawer sign, 137
Anterior longitudinal ligament, 35, 36
Anterior talofibular ligament, 169
Anterior tendon injury, 185–186
Anterior (volar) lunate dislocation, 338, 339
Anteroinferior iliac spine
  avulsion fracture, 82, 83
  stress fracture, 85
Anterosuperior iliac spine, 67
  avulsion fracture, 82, 83
Anulus fibrosus, 35
Apical ligament, 36, 37
Arachnoid, 36
Arm
  articular anatomy, 224–225
  biomechanics, 225–226
  muscle tears, 258–259
  neurovascular anatomy, 225, 226
  neurovascular injuries, 259
  osteology, 221–224
  soft tissue trauma, 253–259
Arthritis
  ankle fracture, 200
  talar neck fracture, 203
Arthrography, 25–26
  acromioclavicular joint, 238–239
  adhesive capsulitis, 236, 237
  articular cartilage abnormality, 236, 238
  biceps tendon abnormality, 236, 238
  complications, 26

contrast medium, 25
elbow, 272–273, 274, 275
equipment, 25
glenoid labrum, 236–238, 242, 243
hand, 323–324, 325
hip, 76–80
arthritis, 78–79
indications, 78–80
knee, 117–119
labral abnormality, 236, 238
pelvis, 76–80
rotator cuff injury, 253–256
rotator cuff tear, 223–236
shoulder, 230–328
technique, 232–233, 234
shoulder capsule abnormality, 241–242
shoulder capsule injury, 253–256
wrist, 321–323
Arthroscopy, knee, 119, 146
Articular cartilage abnormality, arthrography, 236, 238
Atlantoaxial region, ligamentous anatomy, 36, 37
Atlantooccipital dislocation, 50
Atlas
fracture, 50–51. *See also* Specific type
posterior arch fracture, 50
rotary dislocation, 51
Atlas injury, 50–51. *See also* Specific type
Avascular necrosis
hand, 351
talar neck fracture, 202–203
wrist, 351
Avulsion fracture, 123. *See also* Specific type
anteroinferior iliac spine, 82, 83
anterosuperior iliac spine, 82, 83
cervical spine injury, 40–41
defined, 4, 5
hip, 81–83
humerus, 245
iliac crest apophysis, 82
ischium, 82
lesser trochanter, 82, 83
os acetabuli marginalis superior, 82–83
pelvis, 81–83
pubic symphysis, 82
Axial loading injury, cervical spine injury, 40, 41
Axis
hangman's fracture, 52–53
injury, 52. *See also* Specific type
pedicle fracture, 55

B

Barton's fracture, 327–328
Bennett's fracture, 341
Biceps injury, 256–257, 259
Biceps tendinitis, 256–257, 259
Biceps tendon abnormality, arthrography, 236, 238
Biceps tendon ruptures, 281
Blocker's diagnosis, 253, 254
Bone scintigraphy. *See* Skeletal scintigraphy
Bone vascularity, skeletal scintigraphy, 19
Bowing fracture, defined, 5, 6
Bursitis, 284–285
defined, 9
elbow, 284–285
hip, 93–94
knee, 148–149
pelvis, 93–94
shoulder, 258
Bursography, subacromial bursa, 238
Burst fracture, cervical spine injury, 56, 57

C

Calcaneal fracture, 206–209
computed tomography, 208, 209
routine radiography, 207, 208–209
stress fracture, 359
Calcaneofibular ligament, 169, 170
Calcaneus, 170–171
anatomy, 206, 207
classification, 206–208
Calf, 155–164
anatomy, 155–157
muscles, 172–173
neurovascular structures, 156
soft tissue injuries, 157–160
vascular injuries, 163
vascular syndromes, 163
Capitate fracture, 337
Capitellar fracture, 290–291
Carpal bone, 304–306
Carpal dislocation, 338–339
Carpal fracture, 331–338
Carpometacarpal dislocation, 339, 340
Carpus, 303, 304, 305
Cervical spine injury, 37–57
avulsion injury, 40–41
axial loading injury, 40, 41
burst fracture, 56, 57
compressive hyperflexion injury, 38–39
computed tomography, 48, 49
conventional tomography, 48, 49
disruptive hyperflexion injury, 37–38
flexion-rotation injury, 38
hyperextension injury, 39
hyperflexion injury, 37–39
imaging, 41–49
lower, 53
magnetic resonance injury, 48–49
major, 49–57
mechanisms, 37–41
minor, 40–41
routine radiography, 42–48
AP view, 44–45, 46
extension views, 46–48
flexion views, 46–48
lateral view, 42–44, 45
oblique views, 45–46
odontoid view, 45, 46
pillar views, 46
prevertebral fat stripe, 42–43
soft tissue injuries, 57
stinger injury, 40, 41
teardrop hyperflexion injury, 39
upper, 50–53
vertical compression injury, 40, 41
Cervical vertebra, 32
anatomy, 32–33
Chauffeur's fracture, 328
Check ligament, 36, 37
Child
acromioclavicular joint injury, 248, 249
ankle fracture, 191–195
classification, 191–195
epiphyses, 191
etiology, 191
juvenile Tillaux, 191, 192
triplane, 191, 192
phalangeal fracture, 346–347
physeal injuries, 346–347
proximal humeral fracture, 242, 244
radius injury, 329–330
ulna injury, 329–330
Chip fracture, vertebral body, 55
Chondromalacia patellae, 120–121
etiology, 121
magnetic resonance imaging, 126
symptoms, 120–121
Clavicle
anatomy, 221, 222
posttraumatic osteolysis, 252
Clavicle fracture, 250–252
Clenched fist position, routine radiography, 13
Closed fracture, defined, 4
Coccyx, 35, 68
Colles' fracture, 325–327
Comminuted fracture, defined, 4
Compartment syndrome, 164
leg, 162–163
thigh, 103
Complete fracture, defined, 4
Compound fracture, defined, 4
Compression fracture, vertebral body, 55–57

Compressive hyperflexion injury, cervical spine injury, 38–39
Computed thermography, 26
Computed tomography, 19–20. *See also* Tomography
  Achilles tendon, 183
  cervical spine injury, 48, 49
  equipment, 19
  femoral shaft fracture, 102
  hand, 316–317
  hip, 73–75
  humerus, 229–230, 231
  indications, 20
  knee, 114–115, 116
  medial tendon injury, 185
  myositis ossificans, 104
  patellar fracture, 126
  pelvic fracture, 91
  pelvis, 73–75
  principles, 19
  rotator cuff injury, 255
  routine radiography, 208, 209
  shoulder, 229–230, 231
  shoulder capsule injury, 255
  technique, 19
  thigh soft tissue injuries, 104–105
  thoracolumbar spine injury, 62–63
  ultrasound, 277
  wrist, 316–317
  x-ray dose, 20
Contact thermography, 26
Contusion, defined, 6, 8
Conus medullaris, 36
Coracoid fracture, 253
Coronary ligament, 109
Coronoid fracture, 294
Cruciate ligament, 109
Cuboid, 170, 171
Cuboid subluxation, 180
Cuneiform, 170, 171

D

De Quervain's tendinitis, 348
Deltoid ligament, 169
Dentate ligament, 36
Disc, 35
Disc herniation, traumatic, 41
Discoid meniscus, 145–146
Dislocation. *See also* Specific type
  defined, 4, 6, 7
Disruptive hyperflexion injury, cervical spine injury, 37–38
Distal femur, physeal fracture, 127, 128
Distal phalanx fracture, 346, 347
Distal radial epiphysis, 303
Distal radial fracture, 324–329
Distal radial metaphysis, 303
Distal radioulnar joint
  dorsal dislocation, 330–331
  volar dislocation, 331
Distal radius, 303–304
Distal radius dislocation, 330–331
Distal ulna, 304
Doppler ultrasound, 15. *See also* Ultrasound
Dorsal intercalated segment instability, 306
Dorsal ligament, 307
Dorsal perilunate dislocation, 338
Dorsiflexion, 175
Dura, 36

E

Elbow
  arthrography, 272–273, 274, 275
  fat pads, 270–271
  ligament injury, 278–280
  magnetic resonance imaging, 273–277
  muscle anatomy, 267, 268
  muscle injuries, 280–283
  nerve injury, 283
  neurovascular anatomy, 268
  osseous anatomy, 265–267
  routine radiography, 268–272
  soft tissue injury, 278–285
  tendinitis, 280–283
  tendon injuries, 280–283
  throwing injuries, 278
  ultrasound, 277
  vascular anatomy, 269
Elbow capsule, 265–266
Elbow dislocation, 279
Epicondyle fracture, 286–288, 289
  lateral, 286–287
  medial, 286–287
Eversion, 175
External rotation, 176

F

Facet joint, 36
Femoral head, 69
Femoral neck, stress fracture, 362–363
Femoral neck fracture, 91
Femoral shaft, stress fracture, 361, 362
Femoral shaft fracture, 100–101
  classified, 101
  computed tomography, 102
  magnetic resonance imaging, 102
  mechanism of injury, 100
  routine radiography
    AP view, 101
    lateral view, 101–102
  soft tissue injuries, 102–104
  tomography, 102
Femur
  anatomy, 99–100
  blood supply, 99
  growth plate fracture, 127
  muscle groups, 99, 100
  muscle–tendon injury, 102
  neurovascular structures, 99, 100
  soft tissue injuries, imaging, 104–105
  supracondylar fracture, 131–134
Fibula, 155–164, 168
  anatomy, 155–157
  blood supply, 157
  muscle attachments, 156
  muscle injuries, 157–160
  soft tissue injuries, 157–160
  spiral fracture, 159
  stress fracture, 361
  tendon injuries, 157–160
  vascular injuries, 163
  vascular syndromes, 163
Fibular fracture, 158
Fibular shaft fracture, 157
Fifth metatarsal base fracture, 212–213
Filum terminale, 36
Finger, routine radiography, 311–312
Flexion-rotation injury
  cervical spine injury, 38
  thoracolumbar spine injury, 58, 59
Flexor carpi radialis, 309
Flexor carpi ulnaris, 309
Flexor digitorum tendon tear, 185
Flexor hallucis longus tendon tear, 185
Foot
  accessory ossicles, 172, 173
  anatomy, 170–172
  arches, 171
  ligament injuries, 179–180
  normal variants, 171–172
  soft tissue anatomy, 172–175
  soft tissue trauma, 176–190
  stress fracture, 215, 358
Foot injury, 167–215. *See also* Specific type
  incidence, 167
Foramen transversarium, 32
Forearm
  magnetic resonance imaging, 273–277
  muscular anatomy, 267, 268
  neural anatomy, 269
  neurovascular anatomy, 268
  osseous anatomy, 265–267
  radius, anatomy, 265, 266, 277
  routine radiography, 268–272
  soft tissue injury, 278–285
  ultrasound, 277
  vascular anatomy, 269
Forearm fracture, 296–297, 298

Forefoot
hallux rigidus, 189
imaging, 190, 191
metatarsalgia, 188
metatarsophalangeal subluxation and synovitis, 188–189
neuroma, 189
osteochondritis, 188, 189
pain, 188–190
differential diagnosis, 188
sesamoiditis, 188, 189
Fracture. *See also* Specific type
defined, 4
Fracture-dislocation, defined, 6

G

Galeazzi's fracture, 328–329
Glenohumeral dislocation, 245–248
anterior, 245–246
complications, 248
posterior, 246–242
superior and inferior, 247–248
Glenohumeral joint, anatomy, 224–225
Glenoid, 224
osteochondritis, 253
Glenoid labrum, arthrography, 236–238, 242, 243
Greater tuberosity, 222, 223
Greenstick fracture, defined, 5
Growth plate fracture
defined, 5, 6
femur, 127
medial femoral, 128, 130
tibia, 127
Guyon's canal, 310

H

Hallux rigidus, forefoot, 189
Hamate fracture, 318, 335–337
Hamstring injury, 102–103
Hamstring tear, 92
Hand
arthrography, 323–324, 325
avascular necrosis, 351
computed tomography, 316–317
ligament injuries, 348–350, 351
ligamentous anatomy, 307–309
magnetic resonance imaging, 317, 321
muscular anatomy, 309–310
neurovascular anatomy, 310, 311
neurovascular injury, 351
osseous anatomy, 303–307
radionuclide imaging, 317, 318
routine radiography, 311
soft tissue injuries, 348–351
tendinitis, 348, 349
tomography, 316
Hangman's fracture, axis, 52–53
Hematoma, defined, 7, 8
Hemorrhage
defined, 7, 8
medial gastrocnemius, 160
Hill-Sachs deformity, 228
Hindfoot
anatomy, 170–171
lateral pain, 187
medial pain, 188
plantar pain, 187, 188
posterior pain, 187, 188
Hip
anatomy, 67–71
anterior dislocations, 90
apophyses, 68
arthrography, 76–80
arthritis, 78–79
indications, 78–80
articulations, 68–71
avulsion fracture, 81–83
bursitis, 93–94
computed tomography, 73–75
diagnostic injections, 76–80
dislocation, 89–90
fracture-dislocation, 89–90
ligaments, 68–71
magnetic resonance imaging, 75, 76
muscle attachments, 68, 71
musculature injury, 92
myositis ossificans, 92
osseous anatomy, 67–68
ossification centers, 68
overuse injury, 83
periarticular anatomy, 70
posterior dislocation, 89–90
routine radiography, 71–73
AP views, 71–73
lateral views, 71–73
oblique view, 73
skeletal scintigraphy, 75
soft tissue, 92–97
stress fracture, 83
tenography, 76–80
tomography, 73–75
Hip fracture, 80–91
major, 85–91
minor, 81–85
Hip pointer, 92
Humeral condyle fracture, 291–292, 293
Humeral head, 222
Humeral shaft fracture, 244
Humerus, 223
avulsion fracture, 245
computed tomography, 229–230, 231
routine radiography, 226–229, 230
ultrasound, 229
Hyperextension injury
cervical spine injury, 39
thoracolumbar spine injury, 59
Hyperflexion injury
cervical spine injury, 37–39
thoracolumbar spine injury, 58
Hypothenar muscle, 309, 310

I

Iliac crest, 67
Iliac crest apophysis, avulsion fracture, 82
Iliac wing fracture, 73
Iliofemoral ligament, 69–70
Iliopsoas bursa, hip arthrography, 79
Iliotibial band syndrome, 148
Ilium, 67
Incomplete fracture, defined, 4–5, 6
Infection, skeletal scintigraphy, 19
Injury site, epidemiology, 2
Innominate bone, 67
Interosseous ligament, 169
Interosseous muscle, 309
Interosseous talocalcaneal ligament, 171
Interphalangeal joint dislocation, 347–348
Intervertebral disc, 35
Intraarticular basilar fracture, 341
Inversion, 175
Ischium, 67–68
avulsion fracture, 82

J

Jefferson fracture, 50–51
Jones fracture, 213, 214

K

Kienbock's disease, 351
Knee. *See also* Patella
anatomy, 107–110
arthrography, 117–119
arthroscopy, 119
articular anatomy, 107–110
bone anatomy, 107–110
bursae, 109
bursitis, 148–149
capsule, 109
computed tomography, 114–115, 116
diagnostic injection, 117–119
fibrous capsule, 108
ligament injury, 135–141
ligament instability, 137
ligaments, 109
muscles, 110

neurovascular supply, 110
osteochondral fracture, 127–131, 132, 133
periarticular ligaments, 108
routine radiography, 110–114
AP views, 110–112, 113
lateral views, 110–112, 113
notch view, 112, 113
patellar views, 112–113, 114
synovial membrane, 107–108
tendinitis, 149
therapeutic injection, 117–119
tomography, 114–115, 116
ultrasound, 115
Knee injury. *See also* Specific type
arthroscopy, 146
common chronic, 146
plicae syndrome, 146–148

L

Labral abnormality, arthrography, 236, 238
Lachman test, 137
Laminar fracture, 53, 54
Laminography. *See* Tomography
Lateral compression injury, pelvic fracture, 85–86
Lateral meniscus, 109, 110, 141
Lateral plateau fracture, 116
Lateral talocalcaneal ligament, 171
Lateral wedge fracture, 57
Leg, compartment syndrome, 162–163
Lesser trochanter, avulsion fracture, 82, 83
Ligamentum flavum, 36
Ligamentum nuchae, 36
Linea aspera, 99
Lisfranc injury
mechanism of injury, 211–212
routine radiography, 212
Little League elbow, 281
Little League shoulder, 253, 254
Loose body, hip arthrography, 79
Lumbar vertebra, anatomy, 34, 35
Lumbrical muscle, 309
Lunate, 3045
Lunate fracture, 334–335, 336
Lunotriquetral ligament injury, 350

M

Magnetic resonance imaging, 20–22
Achilles tendon, 183
anterior cruciate ligament injury, 137
cervical spine injury, 48–49
chondromalacia patellae, 126
clinical applications, 22
clinical techniques, 21
coil selection, 22
elbow, 273–277
femoral shaft fracture, 102
forearm, 273–277
hand, 317, 321
hip, 75, 76
imaging parameters, 22
medial tendon injury, 185
meniscal cyst, 145
meniscal injury, 142–145
metallic implants, 21
neuroma, 190, 191
patellar fracture, 126
patient positioning, 22
patient selection, 21–22
pelvis, 75, 76
posterior cruciate ligament injury, 137
pulse sequences, 22
rotator cuff injury, 255–256, 257, 258
rotator cuff tear, 239–241
accuracy, 240–241
shoulder, 239–241
shoulder capsule abnormality, 241–242
shoulder capsule injury, 255–256, 257, 258
thigh soft tissue injuries, 104–105
thoracolumbar spine injury, 63
ultrasound, 115–117, 118
wrist, 317, 321
Magnification radiography, 14–15
equipment, 14
limitations, 15
principles, 14
radiation exposure, 14–15
Malunion
ankle fracture, 201
talar neck fracture, 203
Medial femoral condyle, shearing fracture, 131
Medial gastrocnemius, hemorrhage, 160
Medial malleolus, 167, 168
Medial meniscus, 109, 110, 141
Medial tendon injury, 184–185
computed tomography, 185
magnetic resonance imaging, 185
Medial tibial stress syndrome, 161–162
Median nerve, 284, 310
compression, 284
Meniscal cyst, magnetic resonance imaging, 145
Meniscal injury, 141–146. *See also* Specific type
magnetic resonance injury, 142–145
routine radiography, 142
Meniscal tear
bucket-handle, 144
clinical evaluation, 142
grading systems, 144
radial, 144
vertical, 144
Meniscus, 107, 108–109
Metacarpal, 306
Metacarpal fracture, 339–344
complications, 344
second through fifth, 342–344
Metacarpophalangeal joint dislocation, 344
Metacarpophalangeal ligament, 308
Metatarsal, 170, 171, 211
Metatarsal fracture, 212–214
Metatarsal ligament, 211
Metatarsal stress fracture, 358
Metatarsalgia, forefoot, 188
Metatarsophalangeal dislocation, 213
Metatarsophalangeal subluxation and synovitis, forefoot, 188–189
Microfracture, defined, 5
Midclavicle fracture, 252
Middle phalanx fracture, 345–346
Midfoot, anatomy, 170, 171, 209
Monteggia fracture, 296, 297
Motion artifact, routine radiography, 12
Myelography, 24–25
indications, 24–25
patient positioning, 24
technique, 24
Myositis ossificans
computed tomography, 104
defined, 9
hip, 92

N

Navicular, 170, 171
Navicular fracture, 210
Nerve injury, defined, 9
Neuroma
forefoot, 189
magnetic resonance imaging, 190, 191
Neurovascular injury
hand, 351
wrist, 351
Nonunion
ankle fracture, 201
talar neck fracture, 203
Nucleus pulposus, 35

O

Odontoid fracture, 48, 52, 53
type I, 52
type II, 52
type III, 52, 53
Open fracture, defined, 4
Os acetabuli marginalis superior, avulsion fracture, 82–83

Osgood-Schlatter disease, 123, 124
Osteochondral fracture
  Berndt and Harty classification, 131, 133
  knee, 127–131, 132, 133
Osteochondritis
  defined, 9
  forefoot, 188, 189
  glenoid, 253
Osteochondritis dissecans, 127–130
Osteoid osteoma, 75
Osteomyelitis, skeletal scintigraphy, 19
Overuse injury. *See also* Specific type
  defined, 9
  epidemiology, 2
  hip, 83
  pelvis, 83

P

Palmar ligament, 307
Patella, 107, 108. *See also* Knee
  anatomy, 119–120
  variations, 120
Patellar dislocation, 122
  lateral, 122
Patellar disorder, 119–126
  imaging, 124–126
Patellar fracture, 122–123, 124
  computed tomography, 126
  magnetic resonance imaging, 126
  routine radiography, 124–126
  stress fracture, 123
Patellar instability, 122
Patellar subluxation, 122
Patellar tendinitis, 123, 149
Patellofemoral pain syndrome, 120–122
  etiology, 121
  symptoms, 120–121
Pathologic fracture, defined, 6
Patient exposure, routine radiography, 12
Pectoralis muscle tear, 259
Pedicle fracture, 52, 53, 54
  axis, 55
  stress fracture, 364
Pelvic fracture, 80–91
  anterior compression injury, 86–87
  common patterns, 85
  complications, 89
  computed tomography, 91
  lateral compression injury, 85–86
  major, 85–91
  minor, 81–85
  routine radiography, 91
  vertical shear injury, 87
Pelvic hemorrhage, 89
Pelvis
  anatomy, 67–71
  apophyses, 68
  arthrography, 76–80
  articulations, 68–71
  avulsion fracture, 81–83
  bursitis, 93–94
  computed tomography, 73–75
  diagnostic injections, 76–80
  ligaments, 68–71
  magnetic resonance imaging, 75, 76
  muscle attachments, 68, 71
  musculature injury, 92
  osseous anatomy, 67–68
  ossification centers, 68
  overuse injury, 83
  routine radiography, 71
    AP angled views, 71, 72
    AP view, 71
  skeletal scintigraphy, 75
  soft tissue, 92–97
  stress fracture, 83, 363
  tenography, 76–80
  tomography, 73–75
Periosteal vessel, 157
Peripatellar pain, 123
Peroneal artery, 155
Peroneal nerve, 157
Peroneal tendon dislocation, 181
Peroneal tendon injury, 180–181
Peroneal tendon rupture, 181
Peroneus brevis, 174
Peroneus longus, 174
Phalangeal fracture, 212–214, 344–347
  child, 346–347
Phalanges, 307
Physeal fracture, 127
  defined, 5, 6
  distal femur, 127, 128
Pia mater, 36
Piriformis syndrome, 96–97
Pisiform fracture, 335, 336
Planography. *See* Tomography
Plantar flexion, 175
Plicae syndrome, knee injury, 146–148
Popliteal fossa, ultrasound, 16
Positioning, routine radiography, 12
Posterior arch fracture, atlas, 50
Posterior cruciate ligament, 109–110
Posterior cruciate ligament injury, 137–140
  clinical tests, 136–141
  magnetic resonance imaging, 137
  routine radiography, 137
Posterior longitudinal ligament, 36
Posterior sacroiliac ligament, 68
Posterior talofibular ligament, 169–170
Posterior tibial artery, 155
Posterior tibial tendon injury, 184–185
Posterosuperior iliac spine, 67
Pronation, 176
Pronator teres syndrome, 284
Proximal humeral epiphyseolysis, 253, 254
Proximal humeral fracture, 242–245
  characteristics, 243–244
  child, 242, 244
  classification, 244
  etiology, 242–243
Proximal phalanx fracture, 344–345
Proximal radial fracture, 292–293, 294
Proximal tibiofibular injection, 119
Proximal ulnar fractures, 294, 296
Pubic bone, 67
Pubic ramus, 67
Pubic ramus fracture, 74
Pubic symphysis, 67
  avulsion fracture, 82
  lesions, 93

Q

Q angle, 121
Quadriceps injury, 103, 104
Quadriceps tendinitis, 123, 149

R

Radial nerve, 283
  compression, 283
Radial styloid fracture, 328
Radiation protection, routine radiography, 12
Radiocarpal dislocation, 331
Radiography
  magnification, 14–15
  routine, 11–12, 13
Radionuclide imaging
  hand, 317, 318
  wrist, 317, 318
Radioulnar subluxation, 317
Radius injury, child, 329–330
Rhabdomyolysis, thigh, 103–104
Rotary valgus injury, 129
Rotator cuff, 224
  muscles, 224
Rotator cuff injury, 253–256. *See also* Specific type
  arthrography, 253–256
  computed tomography, 255
  magnetic resonance imaging, 255–256, 257, 258
Rotator cuff tear, 231
  arthrography, 223–236
  magnetic resonance imaging, 239–241
    accuracy, 240–241
Routine radiography, 11–12, 13
  Achilles tendon, 183
  ankle fracture, 199–200

anterior cruciate ligament injury, 137
calcaneal fracture, 207, 208–209
cervical spine injury, 42–48
AP view, 44–45, 46
extension views, 46–48
flexion views, 46–48
lateral view, 42–44, 45
oblique views, 45–46
odontoid view, 45, 46
pillar views, 46
prevertebral fat stripe, 42–43
clenched fist position, 13
equipment, 11
femoral shaft fracture
AP view, 101
lateral view, 101–102
finger, 311–312
fracture-dislocation, 209–211
hand, 311
hip, 71–73
AP views, 71–73
lateral views, 71–73
oblique view, 73
humerus, 226–229, 230
knee, 110–114
AP view, 110–112, 113
lateral view, 110–112, 113
notch view, 112, 113
patellar views, 113–114, 115
stress view, 113–114, 115
Lisfranc injury, 212
meniscal injury, 142
midfoot fracture, 209–211
motion artifact, 12
patellar fracture, 124–126
patient exposure, 12
pelvic fracture, 91
pelvis, 71
AP angled views, 71, 72
AP view, 71
positioning, 12
posterior cruciate ligament injury, 137
radiation protection, 12
shoulder, 226–229, 230
stress fracture, 357–358
tarsometatarsal fracture-dislocation, 212
thoracolumbar spine injury, 60–61
AP view, 60
lateral view, 60–61
thumb, 312–313
wrist, 313–316

S

Sacral fracture, 74
Sacroiliac joint subluxation, 74
Sacrum, 68
anatomy, 34–35
Scaphoid, 305
Scaphoid fracture, 331–334
Scapholunate angle, 305
Scapholunate ligament injury, 350
Scapula, anatomy, 221–222, 223
Scapular fracture, 231, 253
Sciatic nerve, 99, 100
Segond fracture, 130
Sesamoid fracture, 214
Sesamoiditis, forefoot, 188, 189
Shearing fracture, medial femoral condyle, 131
Shin splint, 160–161, 163
Shoulder
arthrography, 230–328
technique, 232–233, 234
articular anatomy, 224–225
biomechanics, 225–226
bursae, 224–225
bursitis, 258
computed tomography, 229–230, 231
magnetic resonance imaging, 239–241
muscle tears, 258–259
neurovascular anatomy, 225, 226
neurovascular injuries, 259
osteology, 221–224
routine radiography, 226–229, 230
secondary ossification centers, 222
soft tissue trauma, 253–259
tomography, 229
ultrasound, 229
Shoulder capsule abnormality
arthrography, 241–242
magnetic resonance imaging, 241–242
Shoulder capsule injury, 253–256
arthrography, 253–256
computed tomography, 255
magnetic resonance imaging, 255–256, 257, 258
Simple fracture, defined, 4
Sinus tarsi syndrome, 180
Skeletal scintigraphy, 16–19
^{67}Ga-labeled citrate, 16
^{111}In-labeled autologous white blood cells, 16
Anger gamma camera, 16
bone vascularity, 19
equipment, 16–17
hip, 75
indications, 17–19
infection, 19
osteomyelitis, 19
pelvis, 75
principles, 16
technetium-99m, 16
thoracolumbar spine injury, 63
trauma, 18
Smith's fracture, 327
Snapping iliopsoas tendon, 94
hip arthrography, 79
Snapping triceps tendon, 282
Soft tissue injury. *See also* Specific type
defined, 6
Soleus syndrome, 162
Spinal cord, 36
Spinal nerve, 36
Spine
anatomy, 31–36
ligamentous anatomy, 35–36
neuroanatomy, 36
osteology, 32–35
Spine injury
cervical, 31
etiology, 31
frequency, 31
location, 31
lumbar, 31
severity, 31
thoracic, 31
Spinous process, anatomy, 32, 33
Spiral fracture
fibula, 159
tibia, 159
Sports, 1
Sports injury
categories, 4–9
epidemiology, 1–4
high school athletics
injury severity, 2, 3
injury type, 2, 3
incidence, 1
incidence by gender, 1–2, 4
intercollegiate, 2–3
severity, 1
Sprain, defined, 8
Sternoclavicular dislocation, 250, 251
Sternoclavicular joint, 251
anatomy, 225
Stinger injury, cervical spine injury, 40, 41
Strain, defined, 7, 8
Stratigraphy. *See* Tomography
Stress fracture. *See also* Specific type
activities, 358
anteroinferior iliac spine, 85
classification, 358
defined, 5, 6, 357
femoral neck, 362–363
femoral shaft, 361, 362
fibula, 361
foot, 215, 358–360
hip, 83
incidence, 357

isotope studies, 358
location, 358, 363–364
patellar fracture, 123
pedicle, 364
pelvis, 83, 363
routine radiography, 357–358
tibia, 360–361, 362
Subacromial bursa, bursography, 238
Subclavian vein thrombosis, 259
Subluxation, defined, 6, 7
Subtalar dislocation, 206
Superior facet fracture, 53, 54
Supination, 176
Supracondylar fracture, 285–286, 287
femur, 131–134
mechanism of injury, 285
neurovascular injury, 285
Supraspinous ligament, 36
Symphysis injury, 93
Synovial chonchromatosis, 95
Synovial membrane, knee, 107–108

T

T condylar fracture, 289–290
Talar body fracture, 203–204
Talar dislocation, 206
Talar dome fracture, 204–206
Talar head fracture, 203–204
Talar neck fracture, 202–203
arthritis, 203
avascular necrosis, 202–203
complications, 202–203
incidence, 202
malunion, 203
nonunion, 203
radiographic diagnosis, 202
Talar neck fracture dislocation, incidence, 202
Talar process fracture, 203–204
Talus, 167, 168, 170–171
anatomy, 201–202
Tarsal stress fracture, 358
Tarsometatarsal fracture-dislocation, 211–212
mechanism of injury, 211–212
routine radiography, 212
Teardrop fracture, vertebral body, 55
Teardrop hyperflexion injury, cervical spine injury, 39
Telethermography, 26
Tendinitis, 161
hand, 348, 349
knee, 149
wrist, 348, 349
Tendinosis, 161
Tennis shoulder, 254–255
Tenography, 25–26
complications, 26
contrast medium, 25
equipment, 25
hand, 324–325
hip, 76–80
pelvis, 76–80
wrist, 324–325
Tenosynovitis, 161
defined, 9
Thenar eminence, 309–310
Therapeutic injection, knee, 117–119
Thermography, 26
indications, 26
Thigh
anatomy, 99–100
compartment syndrome, 103
fascial compartments, 100
femoral shaft fracture, imaging, 104–105
muscle-tendon injury, 102
muscular anatomy, 100
neurovascular anatomy, 100
rhabdomyolysis, 103–104
Thoracic outlet syndrome, 259
Thoracic spine, lateral view, 34
Thoracic vertebra, 32
anatomy, 33–34
Thoracolumbar spine injury, 57–63
computed tomography, 62–63
flexion-rotation injury, 58, 59
hyperextension injury, 59
hyperflexion injury, 58
magnetic resonance imaging, 63
mechanisms, 58–60
minor, 59–60
routine radiography, 60–61
AP view, 60
lateral view, 60–61
skeletal scintigraphy, 63
tomography, 62–63
vertical compression injury, 58–59
Thumb, routine radiography, 312–313
Thumb fracture, 339–342
Tibia, 155–164, 167, 168
anatomy, 155–157
blood supply, 157
growth plate fracture, 127
muscle attachments, 156
muscle injuries, 157–160
soft tissue injuries, 157–160
spiral fracture, 159
stress fracture, 360–361, 362
tendon injuries, 157–160
vascular injuries, 163
vascular syndromes, 163
Tibial plafond fracture, 198, 199
Tibial plateau fracture, 134, 135
Tibial shaft fracture, 157
Tibial spine fracture, 131, 132, 133
Tibial tuberosity fracture, 127, 128, 129
Tomography, 13–14. *See also* Computed tomography
blurring, 13
cervical spine injury, 48, 49
complex motion studies, 14
equipment, 13
femoral shaft fracture, 102
hand, 316
hip, 73–75
knee, 114–115, 116
pelvis, 73–75
section thickness, 13
shoulder, 229
simple motion studies, 14
thoracolumbar spine injury, 62–63
ultrasound, 277
wide-angle, 14
wrist, 316
Torus fracture, defined, 5
Transcondylar fracture, 285–286, 287
Transscaphoid perilunate dislocation, 338
Transverse process, 33
Trapezial dislocation, 339
Trapezium fracture, 337–338
Trapezoid dislocation, 339
Trapezoid fracture, 337
Trauma, skeletal scintigraphy, 18
Traumatic spondylolisthesis of C-2, 53
Triangular fibrocartilage complex, 307
Triangular fibrocartilage complex tear, 350, 351
Triangular fracture, vertebral body, 55
Triceps rupture, 281–282
Triceps tear, 259
Triquetrum fracture, 334, 335
Trochanteric fracture, 91

U

Ulna injury, child, 329–330
Ulnar artery, 310
Ulnar nerve, 283, 310
compression, 283
Ulnar styloid fracture, 329
Ulnar variance, 304, 305
Ulnolunate abutment syndrome, 350, 351
Ultrasound, 15–16
Achilles tendon, 183, 184
Achilles tendon tear, 17
computed tomography, 277
elbow, 277
equipment, 15
forearm, 277
humerus, 229

indications, 15–16
knee, 115
limitations, 15
magnetic resonance imaging, 115–117, 118
popliteal fossa, 16
principles, 15
shoulder, 229
tomography, 277
Uncinate fracture, 57

V

Valgus, 176
Varus, 176
Vertebral arch fracture, 53–54
Vertebral body
anatomy, 32
chip fracture, 55
compression fracture, 55–57
fracture, 54–57
teardrop fracture, 55
triangular fracture, 55
Vertebral foramen, 36
Vertical compression injury
cervical spine injury, 40, 41
thoracolumbar spine injury, 58–59
Vertical shear injury, pelvic fracture, 87
Volar intercalated segment instability, 306
Volar ligament, 307
Volar perilunate dislocation, 338–339

W

Wrist
arthrography, 321–323
avascular necrosis, 351
computed tomography, 316–317
ligament injuries, 348–350, 351
ligamentous anatomy, 307–309
magnetic resonance imaging, 317, 321
muscular anatomy, 309–310
neurovascular anatomy, 310, 311
neurovascular injury, 351
osseous anatomy, 303–307
radionuclide imaging, 317, 318
routine radiography, 313–316
soft tissue injuries, 348–351
tendinitis, 348, 349
tomography, 316

Y

Y condylar fracture, 289–290